AF567113

I. FAGARASANU, M.D., F.R.S.M. (London)

MEMBER OF THE ROMANIAN ACADEMY
ASSOCIATE MEMBER OF THE ACADEMY OF SURGERY, PARIS
HONORARY FELLOW OF THE ASSOCIATION OF SURGEONS
OF GREAT BRITAIN AND IRELAND

C. IONESCU-BUJOR, M.D., D. ALOMAN, M.D.
E. ALBU, M.D.

SURGERY OF THE LIVER AND INTRAHEPATIC BILE DUCTS

Revised and Americanized by HENRY J. HEIMLICH, M.D.

ASSOCIATE CLINICAL PROFESSOR OF SURGERY
DIRECTOR OF SURGERY
UNIVERSITY OF CINCINNATI COLLEGE OF MEDICINE

EDITURA ACADEMIEI
BUCUREȘTI

WARREN H. GREEN, INC.
ST. LOUIS

1972

Translated from the Romanian
by IOANA STURZA

This is the revised version of
"Chirurgia ficatului și a căilor biliare intrahepatice"
EDITURA ACADEMIEI REPUBLICII SOCIALISTE ROMÂNIA
str. Gutenberg 3 bis, București, 1967
Sole distributors in the English language
WARREN H. GREEN, INC.
10 So. Brentwood Blvd.
St. Louis, Missouri, U.S.A.

CONTENTS

FOREWORD TO THE ENGLISH EDITION

After publication of the 1st edition in Romania in 1967, and especially following the very favorable reviews published in various surgical periodicals in France, U.S.S.R., U.S.A., Italy, Belgium, etc., we received numerous suggestions from various surgeons to have the book reedited in a widely-spoken language. Among these were professors B. Petrov of Moscow, G. Arnulf of Lyon, H. Heimlich of Cincinatti and others.

Professor H. Heimlich was particularly kind and offered to supervise the translation of the book into English and to find an American publisher who would publish it together with the Publishing House of the Academy of the Socialist Republic of Romania.

We wish to acknowledge our warmest thanks to the translator, Mrs. Ioana Sturza, whose contribution to the American edition has been essential, and to our friend Professor H. Heimlich for the many hours spent in checking the translation and for his basic appreciation of the book in the recommendation sent to the American editors.

Thanks are likewise due to Warren H. Green Inc. and to the Publishing House of the Romanian Academy for their extensive editorial efforts in the co-editing of this book, a first step in the scientific cooperation between the United States and Romania in the field of surgery.

THE AUTHORS

INTRODUCTION

Surgery of the liver parenchyma and intrahepatic bile ducts, little known in the past, has rapidly progressed during the last years, owing to the studies carried out on the anatomy and normal and pathologic physiology of this organ, in different medical centers throughout the world.

Although segmentation of the liver is well known today, permitting prior ligation of the hepatic pedicles, although a number of severe operations are performed such as left and right controlled hepatectomy, broad hepatectomy, etc., in many surgical clinics all over the world, and in spite of the contribution of new methods of investigation (intraoperative cholangiography, splenal and portal angiography, liver scintigram, etc.), surgery of the liver is still far from being available to the general surgeon and remains a strict speciality, performed by a small number of surgeons specialized in this problem.

The purpose of the present volume is to render available to surgeons and investigators that wish to be informed on problems of hepatology, both the classical findings and especially the latest advance made in hepatic anatomy, normal and pathologic physiology, pathology and clinics, as well as on surgical indications and procedures that can be applied today in surgery of the liver.

The book including 11 chapters and 246 illustrations, many of which original, is an attempt to sum up our present knowledge on surgical hepatology, numerous data being wide spread throughout many publications but not gathered together in a single volume.

The work is based on a long personal experience and a vast clinical material, including more than 3000 hepatobiliary operations.

The progress made of late that has added to our knowledge of the anatomy of the portal, arterial and suprahepatic vascular trees and distribution of the bile ducts, permitting systematic grouping of the liver segments, has indicated the necessity of starting with a special chapter on anatomy. On the other hand, the normal and pathologic physiology of the liver is of the greatest interest to the surgeon who wishes to operate on this organ. We have attempted in chapter 2 to give a general outlook, so that the surgeons interested in this problem should not have to look up the data they want in the vast bibliography in which they are to be found. Fundamental processes are discussed: metabolic functions, neuroregulation of the liver functions, correlation of the anatomofunctional compartments; the liver and homeostasis, hepatic insufficiency and coma; response of the liver to surgery, preoperative preparation and anesthesia; shock and resuscitation in surgical hepatobiliary patients; healing of the operative wound; the pathologic physiology of hepatic regeneration, etc.

A separate chapter concerns injuries of the liver and their surgical treatment.

Particular attention has been paid to inflammatory processes and sclerosis of the liver, bearing in mind the gravity of cirrhosis and the necessity of carrying out experimental and clinical investigations in order to find a surgical solution in the treatment of this severe consequence of chronic hepatitis, that stands at the basis of cirrhosis, in front of which medical therapy is so disarmed.

Intrahepatic lithiasis, little known in the past, has proved far more frequent than expected. Chapter 5 deals with this severe complication on the basis of our experience and the many cases treated.

Hepatic alterations due to hernia and diaphragmatic relaxation have preoccupied us since as far back as 1957. A description is given of the causes of diaphragmatic relaxation, offering a new pathogenic explanation of the false cystic images which tempt the surgeon to operate when it is not necessary and he is not aware that they may exist. Methods of differential diagnosis are likewise dealt with in this chapter.

Hydatid cyst of the liver is one of the most severe diseases of the liver; its incidence is fairly high in Romania. The progress made of late in the surgical treatment of this condition has led us to reserve a special chapter, in which we have also reported on our own experience in many clinical cases.

Chapters 8 and 9 are concerned with benign and malignant tumors of the liver, discussing in detail the present surgical possibilities in this connection.

A separate chapter deals with resection of the liver, since this is the radical treatment of most diseases of the liver, such as benign tumors, malignant tumors of a single lobe, hydatid cyst, hepatic hemangioma, etc.

The techniques used today are described in detail for physiologic and non-physiologic hepatectomies. Particular attention has been paid to drainage hepatectomy, to which we have brought a contribution of our own.

The last chapter includes total hepatectomies and liver homotransplants. This question of such present interest is discussed for the first time in a volume on surgical hepatology.

We have attempted to report on the clinical and experimental results obtained during the last 3 or 4 years in this field. These results lead us to hope in the future possibility of successfully substituting the whole liver or at least grafting heterotopically the left liver in man, in cases in which it is completely destroyed by cirrhosis or another disease and the medical treatment can no longer be of any help.

This volume, richly illustrated, is a complete guide to diseases of the liver and their surgical treatment. It may be equally useful to the physician and surgeons who wish to study surgical hepatology in view of their doctor's thesis or diploma.

To the completion of this work, several other colleagues of our clinic have brought their contribution and we wish to gratefully acknowledge their assistance: Dr. Frida Constantinescu for problems of pathologic anatomy, Dr. Elisabeta Musta in questions of radiology and Anton Perussi for the figures.

Similarly, we should like to mention our indebtedness to Petre Velluda and Gabriela Dona for their extensive assistance with the illustrations and secretariat work.

THE AUTHORS

CHAPTER 1

ANATOMY OF THE LIVER AND INTRAHEPATIC BILE DUCTS

OUTER CONFORMATION

THE BILIOVASCULAR SYSTEM OF THE LIVER

- ✦ The portal pedicle
- ✦ The hepatic veins

INNER ARCHITECTURE OF THE LIVER

- ✦ Segmentation based upon the distribution of the portal pedicle
- ✦ Segmentation based upon the distribution of hepatic veins

HISTOLOGIC STUDY OF THE LIVER

The liver, an ancillary gland of the gastrointestinal tract, the heaviest and largest organ in the entire human body, is a central laboratory of biochemical analysis and synthesis for a large number of substances deriving from the general and portal circulation. The macroscopic and microscopic structure of the liver and its extremely massive vascularity are perfectly adapted to its functional role. Almost one third of the venous return in the right atrium comes from the hepatic veins (about 1500 ml/min under basal conditions). Intense nutritive changes take place through the walls of the arterioportal sinusoid pseudocapillaries, between this large amount of circulating blood and the liver cells, whose lamellar arrangement increases their active surface up to values comparable to those of the alveolar surfaces in the lungs. As an accessory gland of the gastrointestinal tract, the liver is closely related to the first portion of the small intestine from which it arises in the course of embryonic life.

OUTER CONFORMATION

In the adult, the average weight of the isolated liver is about 1200—1500 Gm; within the live body, the weight of the liver is much greater because it is full of circulating blood. It is the largest and heaviest of all the organs representing one-fiftieth of the adult weight and one-tenth of the weight of a newborn child. Almost 75% of the liver weight is represented by the portion situated to the right of the midline. Its outer aspect is oval and the lower left part appears to be resected obliquely, starting from the top left towards the bottom right. The long cross diameter measures 25—30 cm and the short, sagittal diameter 18—20 cm. The maximum thickness in the frontal plane is of 6—10 cm at the level of the right lobe.

The outer aspect of the liver is determined by the hepatic recess in which it lies. Due to its great plasticity, this organ bears not only the imprints of the solid surrounding anatomic structures, but also those of the neighboring viscera. The convex aspect *(facies diaphragmatica)* (Fig. 1), moulded upon the vault of the diaphragm, exhibits several lateral imprints of the costal grid. Most of it is covered by the visceral peritoneum, except for the posterior portion which, on the right half, adheres directly to the diaphragm *(pars affixa)*. In most cases, the convex aspect is directed cranioventrally, the liver exhibiting anteversion, that may be exaggerated in the ventropetal anatomical type of Didanski (Fig. 2). The dorsopetal liver presents lesser anteversion or even retroversion (Fig. 3). Surgical approach to the inferior aspect is more difficult in the ventropetal type and approach to the superior aspect is more difficult in the dorsopetal type. The part covered by the peritoneum *(pars libera)* is divided by the sagittal insertion of the falciform ligament into two unequal surfaces corresponding to the right and the left lobe, which is smaller. Through the intermediary of the diaphragm, the marginal zone of the *pars libera* comes into contact with the thoracoabdominal wall. To the right of the falciform ligament, the central zone is connected with the pleura and right lung and to the left with the pericardium and heart: at this level, the liver exhibits a cardiac imprint.

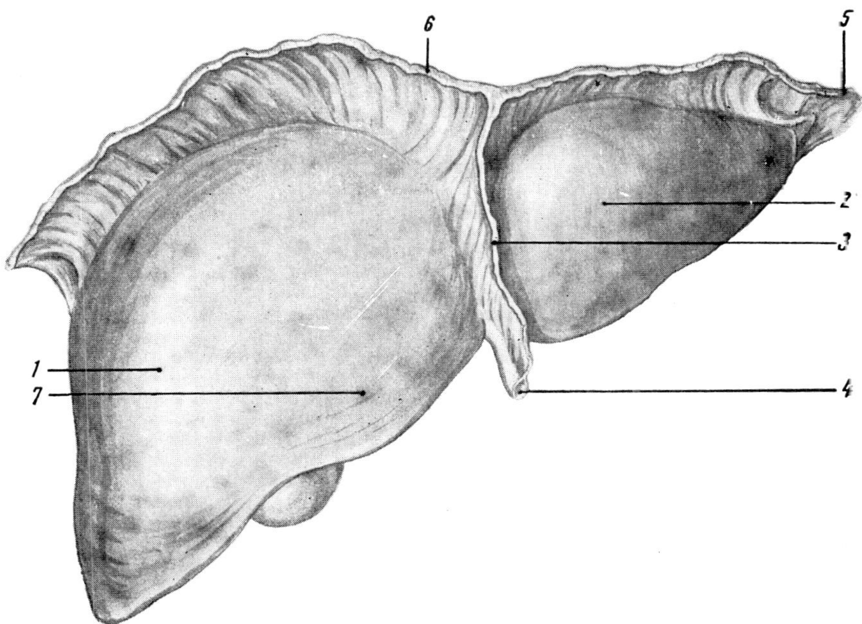

Fig. 1. — Diaphragmatic aspect of the liver, viewed ventrally.

1. Right hepatic area and quadrate lobe; *2.* left lobe; *3.* falciform ligament; *4.* round ligament; *5.* left triangular ligament; *6.* coronary ligament (with diaphragm); *7.* quadrate lobe.

The *pars affixa* corresponds to the level of vertebrae T10-T12: it is concave in shape as it moulds the spinal column. To the right of the midline there is a deep longitudinal depression called the *fossa of the inferior vena cava*, about 4 cm long, sometimes transformed into a canal, that is surrounded on all sides by hepatic tissue.

The *inferior aspect (facies visceralis)* (Fig. 4) is furrowed by two sagittal fissures and a transversal fissure which joins them together, forming an H. The right sagittal fissure *(fossa sagittalis dextrae)* is formed of the cystic fossa or hepatic bed of the gallbladder *(fossa vesicae felleae)* and *fossa venae cavae caudalis*, separated by the *processus caudatus*, a process of the caudate lobule.

The *left sagittal fissure (fossa sagitalis sinistra)* separates the inferior aspect of the right anatomic lobe from the left. The ventral portion is formed of the *fossa of the umbilical vein* in which the round ligament of the liver lies *(ligamentum teres hepatis)*, an obliterated rest of the umbilical vein which in the fetus joins the portal vein. The posterior portion *(fossa ductus venosi Arantii)* contains the remains of the venous canal of Arantius which in the fetus joins the portal vein to the lower vena cava.

The transverse fissure (porta hepatis) is the site of the hepatic hilus where the portal pediculum bifurcates. With reference to the anterior abdominal wall,

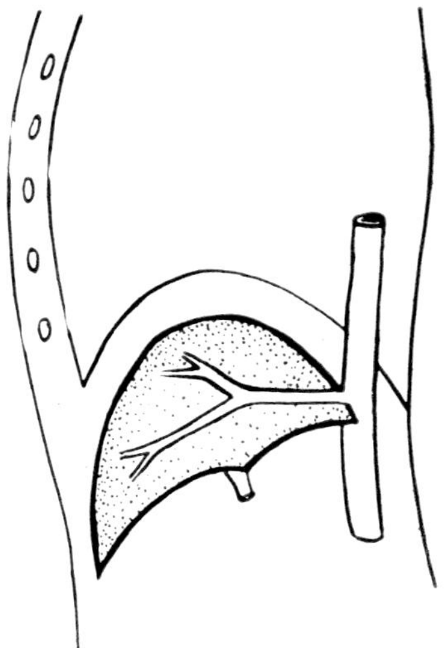

Fig. 2. — Schematic representation of the ventropetal liver (after Didanski).

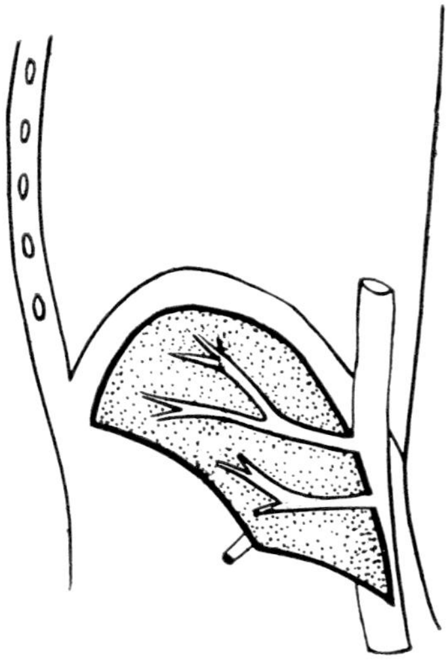

Fig. 3. — Schematic representation of the dorsopetal liver (after Didanski).

it is situated at a depth of about 15 cm, therefore closer to the posterior than to the anterior border.

These fissures divide the inferior aspect of the liver into the following anatomical regions:

The *right lateral zone* situated to the right of the sagittal groove includes three depressions of which the anterior one, *impressio colica*, is determined by the hepatic angle of the column. Dorsally is the *impressio suprarenalis* and between them the *impressio renalis*.

The *left lateral zone*, situated on the left side of the left sagittal fissure, covers part of the stomach and corresponds to the classical left lobe.

In the *central zone*, situated between the two sagittal fissures, are the quadrate lobe in front and posteriorly, the caudate lobe of Spiegel, separated from each other by the transverse fissure.

Spiegel's lobe, that protrudes into the *bursa omentalis* and whose main portion lies dorsally to the left of the inferior cava, belongs by its position to the posterior aspect of the liver. Part of it lies in a ventral oblique direction towards the right, describing an arch with the dorsal concavity, around the inferior cava with which

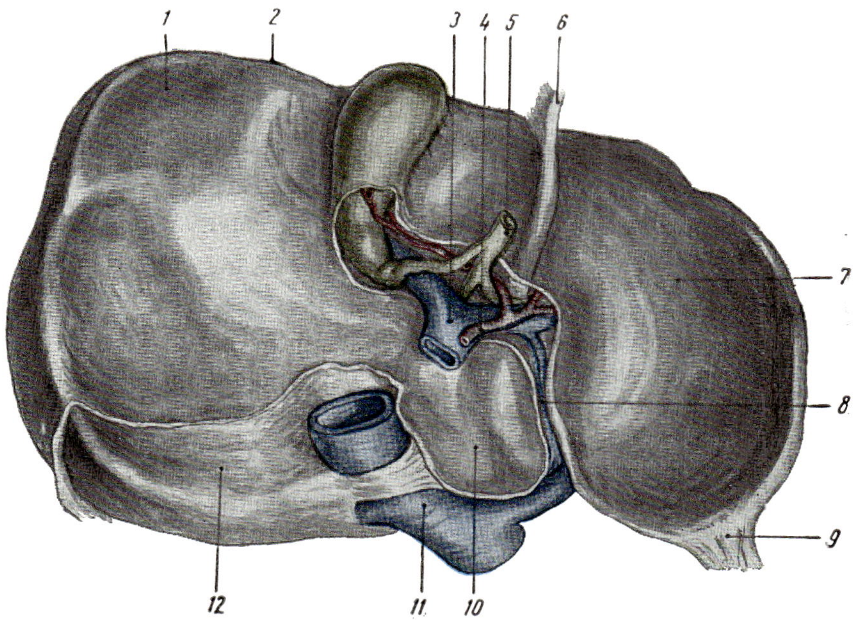

Fig. 4. — Visceral aspect of the liver.

1. Right lobe; *2.* anterior border; *3.* portal vein; *4.* hepatic artery; *5.* common bile cuct; *6.* round ligament; *7.* left lobe; *8.* left sagittal fissure; *9.* left triangular ligament; *10.* Spiegel's lobe; *11.* inferior vena cava; *12.* *pars affixa.*

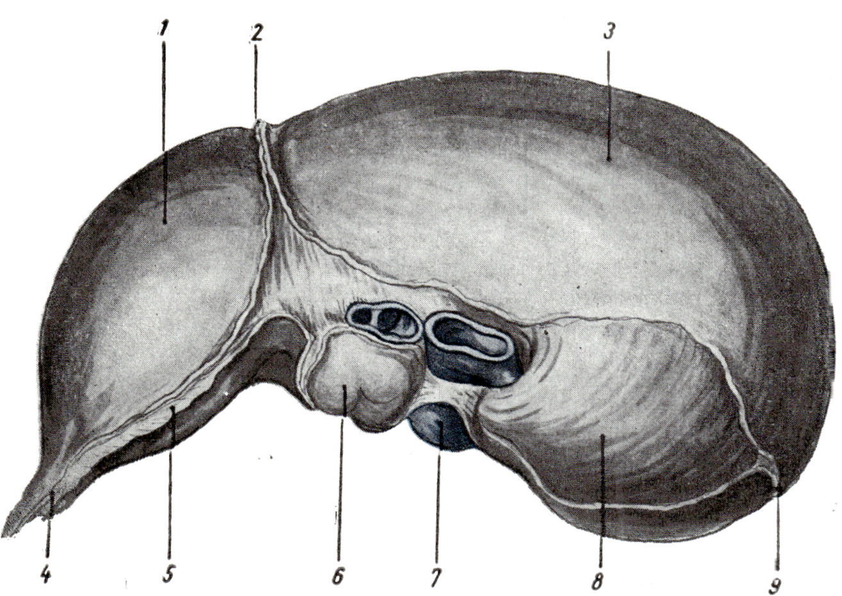

Fig. 5. — Posterior aspect (border) of the liver.

1. left lobe; *2.* falciform ligament; *3.* right lobe; *4.* triangular ligament; *5.* coronary ligament; *6.* Spiegel's lobe; *7.* inferior vena cava; *8.* *pars affixa*; *9.* right trangular ligament.

it comes into contact. The first portion of this process that forms the dorsal margin of the transverse fissure is called the *processus papillaris*. The second portion, the thin extremity of the caudate lobe, is called the *processus caudatus*, that separates the two segments of the right sagittal fissure.

The *quadrate lobe*, delimited by the gallbladder, transverse fissure and round ligament, covers part of the stomach, the pylorus and duodenum.

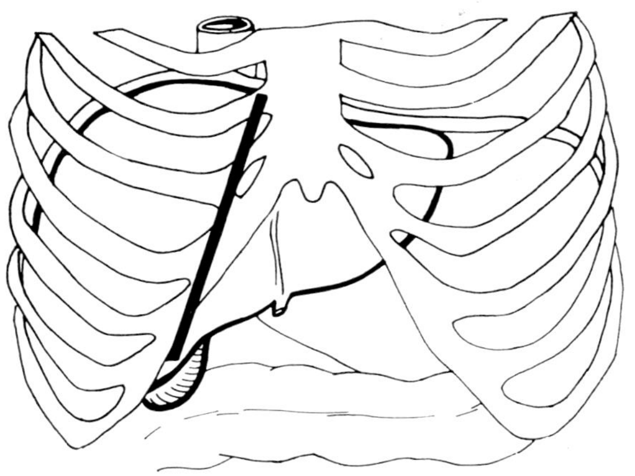

Fig. 6. — Projection of the liver on the ventral thoracoabdominal wall.

The two aspects of the liver are joined along an ovoid circumference that forms the ventral and dorsal borders of the liver. The sharp *ventral border* runs in an oblique, cranial direction towards the left, starting from the right extremity of the liver, along the costochondral border. It crosses the epigastrium 2—4 cm below the xyphoid process, the liver coming in direct contact with the abdominal wall in this region. The *ventral border* ends in the left extremity of the liver, 5—6 cm to the left of the midline. At the level of the right sagittal fissure is the *incisura cystica* and at the level of the left sagittal fissure the much deeper *umbilical incisura*.

The *dorsal border* is considered by many anatomists as a true dorsal aspect including the entire *pars affixa*, which we described as a part of the convex aspect (Fig. 5). According to this broader concept, the dorsal margin or aspect is about 4—5 cm thick at the level of the right lobe. It describes a dorsal concavity caused by the bulging of the spinal column, and comes in contact with the dorsal thoraco-abdominal wall, to which it adheres directly since it is not covered by the peritoneum. It is closely connected with the diaphragmatic crura, the lower cava vein, abdominal aorta and vagus nerves. To the left of the fossa of the cava vein there is a large incisure called *impressio oesophagea*. In the portion projected upon the inferior vena cava, the posterior aspect is crossed by the hepatic veins that emerge from the parenchyma.

In the anterior parietal projection (Fig. 6), the liver area corresponds cranially to a slightly oblique plane passing on the right side at the level of the fifth rib and on the left along the upper margin of the 6th rib. Caudally in the epigastrium the projection zone passes at half the distance between the xyphoid and the umbilicus but along the mammillary line it stops at the costochondral border or exceeds it by 1—2 cm. Along the mid-axillary line, the liver is projected between the 6th and 12th rib and along the posterior midline between T8 and T11 or T12 vertebrae. The limits of the projection area vary and are conditioned by respiration, the anatomic constitution and different physiologic or pathologic changes in the volume or position of the liver.

Fixation. The liver is maintained in its normal position by anatomic structures that fix it to the surrounding wall and organs, by the abdominal positive pressure and, to a much lesser extent, by the organs it comes in contact with along its visceral aspect. In an individual in a supine position, most of the liver rests upon the thoracoabdominal wall and the ligaments prevent it from gliding dorsoventrally or laterally below the diaphragmatic vault. In our opinion, the ligaments are not sufficient in a standing position to maintain the liver in its place. The strain would induce rupture of the portion of the parenchyma to which they adhere. The main factor that maintains the liver in its place, in a standing position, is the negative pressure in the potential space between the convex aspect and the diaphragm.

Actually, the hepatic ligaments represent peritoneal folds that join the visceral to the parietal serosa. The fibrous tissue of the ligaments is poorly represented either by processes of the subserous capsule of Glisson or by the vestiges of certain embryonic vessels. The *ligamentum falciforme hepatis* fixes the convex aspect of the liver to the diaphragm along a sagittal plane that joins the umbilical incisure to the inferior vena cava. Below the umbilical incisure, it exhibits a process inserted along the midline of the ventral abdominal wall and reaching up to the umbilicus.

The *ligamentum teres hepatis* or *chorda venae umbilicalis* (the round ligament) is situated in the umbilical process of the falciform ligament.

Ligamentum coronarium hepatis joins the dorsal aspect of the liver to the diaphragm and the dorsal abdominal wall where the visceral peritoneum of the convex aspect is reflected on the diaphragm, and the peritoneum on the visceral aspect is reflected on the dorsal abdominal wall. The coronary ligament runs in a cross direction tracing a large T along the convex aspect of the liver together with the falciform ligament. Between the two bands of the coronary ligament there is a large space that corresponds, on the surface of the liver, to the *pars affixa*.

Ligamenta triangularia dextrum et sinistrum are the lateral processes of the coronary ligament that are reflected over the vault of the diaphragm. The coronary ligament together with the triangular ligament separate the subdiaphragmatic peritoneal space from the subhepatic space.

The lesser omentum (omentum minus) is a peritoneal fold that joins the visceral aspect of the liver to the abdominal portion of the esophagus, the lesser curvature of the stomach and the duodenum. It is inserted on the liver, along the transverse fissure and the dorsal segment of the left sagittal fissure and is formed of three parts: *pars condensa* in the vicinity of the cardia; *pars flaccida*, the thin middle portion; *pars libera* or the *hepatoduodenal ligament* includes within its thickness the elements of the portal pedicle of the liver. Between the hepatic pedicle covered by the hepatoduodenal ligament and the inferior vena cava is *the foramen of Winslow*, a communication orifice between the *bursa omentalis* (lesser sac) and the large peritoneal cavity. Part of Spiegel's lobe protrudes into the *bursa omentalis* and can be seen on opening the lesser omentum.

THE BILIOVASCULAR SYSTEM OF THE LIVER

The vascular system of the liver consists in an *afferent* pedicle including the hepatic artery and portal vein and an *efferent* system formed of the hepatic veins. To these elements of the afferent vascular pedicle, are added the bile ducts, lymphatic vessels and hepatic nerves forming together the *portal pedicle*. The most important formations of the portal pedicle — the portal vein, hepatic artery and bile ducts — are called the portal triad of Glisson and are closely joined together along their ramified intrahepatic course. Glisson's fibrous capsule, after covering the whole surface of the liver with a very thin membrane, becomes thicker around the hepatic hilus where it is designated as *porta hepatis*, then turns inwards along all the branches of the portal triad which it covers in a fibrous sheath.

THE PORTAL PEDICLE

The hepatic artery *(arteria hepatica)* is the least consistent element of the portal triad, the one which exhibits the greatest variations, both along its afferent extrahepatic course and along its intrahepatic ramifications. About 20—25% of the afferent hepatic blood is supplied by the hepatic artery and about 75—80% by the portal vein. In most cases it arises from the celiac artery and is known as *arteria hepatica communis*. After passing along the cranial border of the pancreas, it branches off into a thick artery, *arteria gastroduodenalis*, then, after describing a loop, it runs in an upward direction towards the liver hilus under the name of the *arteria hepatica propria*, lying between the folds of the hepatoduodenal ligament, on the right side of the common bile duct and in front of the portal vein. One to two cm from the hilus, it divides into the right and left hepatic arteries that penetrate into the liver. From the *arteria hepatica propria* arises the *arteria gastrica dextra* (pyloric artery) and frequently from the right hepatic artery, the *arteria cystica*.

This anatomic distribution is very inconsistent since anatomical variants are encountered in 50—60 per cent of the cases.

1. *Arteria hepatica communis* may arise from the *arteria mesenterica cranialis*.
2. *Arteria hepatica communis* may branch off at any level into the right and left hepatic arteries.
3. *Arteria hepatica communis* may sometimes not exist, the right hepatic artery branching off directly from the cranial mesenteric artery, and the left hepatic artery from the *arteria coeliaca*.
4. Frequent branches of the hepatic artery arise from the superior mesenteric artery, but especially from the *arteria gastrica sinistra* (coronary artery of the stomach). Sometimes, the left gastric artery supplies blood to a large part of the left lobe of the liver.
5. *Arteria hepatica propria* or *arteria hepatica dextra* is situated ventrally to the juxtahilar portion of the hepatic duct in about 13 per cent of the cases.

The portal vein *(vena portae)* collects and transports to the liver the venous blood of the intraabdominal gastrointestinal tract, of the extrahepatic bile ducts, pancreas and spleen. The portal vein has the anatomical peculiarity of being situated between two vascular arborizations, one of the peripheral extremity of the digestive tract, the other at the central extremity of the hepatic parenchyma. Its initial tributaries are the *vena mesenterica cranialis*, *vena lienalis (splenica)*, and *vena mesenterica caudalis* to which is added the *vena coronaris ventriculi superior*, that joins the trunk of the portal vein or the *vena lienalis*. The confluence of these veins takes place retroduodenopancreatically at the level of the L2 vertebra.

The portal vein is about 5.5—8 cm long and has a diameter of 11 mm. After running upwards and slightly to the right, parallel and dorsal to the common bile duct and hepatic artery, it branches off into the *ramus dexter* and *ramus sinister venae portae* (right and left branches of the portal vein). The right branch receives blood from the *vena cystica*.

The *afferent* and *efferent collateral venous circulation* in the liver is particularly important in certain pathological states. In portal hypertension caused by intrahepatic obstruction (cirrhosis), or a Budd-Chiari syndrome (thrombosis of the hepatic vein), the venous blood from the portal area returns to the caval system through the natural portacaval anastomoses. As it can barely pass through the liver, the blood flows through the coronary vein, which anastomoses at the level of the cardia with the esophageal veins, through which it reaches the azygos and the superior vena cava. Similarly it passes through the inferior mesenteric and superior hemorrhoidal veins, then through the middle and lower hemorrhoidal vein, which are branches of the inferior cava system. The paraumbilical veins join the left branch of the portal vein to the superficial periumbilical branches of the epigastric vein. The vascular adhesions of the viscera in the portal area of the abdominal wall likewise behave as portacaval anastomoses.

In portal hypertension caused by extrahepatic obstruction but with maintained intrahepatic circulation, part of the portal blood may reach the liver through several groups of *accessory portal veins*: the gastrohepatic group, the cystic group and the veins proper of the portal triad. The veins of the falciform ligament and the umbilical vein, which may in principle transport blood either in an afferent or an efferent direction since they have no valves, cannot be considered as true accessory portal veins, since they do not bring visceral blood to the liver, but only systemic blood.

Among the elements of the portal pedicle, the portal vein presents the most constant type of intrahepatic ramification followed along general lines by the other formations, especially the ramifications of the bile ducts. Interior segmentation of the glandular hepatic mass is closely linked to the intrahepatic distribution of the main branches of the portal vein (Figs 7 and 8).

The *left branch* lying at first in the transverse fissure gives rise to several dorsal rami supplying the caudate lobe. After about 3—5 cm it reaches the umbilical fissure, then bends at a straight angle and under the name of *recessus umbilicalis* or *ramus ventroflexus* extends ventrocaudally and ends in a cul-de-sac 2 cm from the ventral border of the liver. It is continuous with the vein of the umbilical cord and several thin paraumbilical veins.

From the flexure described in the left branch of the portal vein, arises the *left lateral vein* supplying segment II; from the *recessus umbilicalis*, two or several lateral venous formations branch off to the right towards segment IV and to the left towards segment III.

The *right branch*, after extending 1—3 cm divides into two branches, the *right lateral vein* and the *right paramedian vein* that supply the lateral and paramedian segments of the right hepatic region. Each of these veins gives off a large ventral branch and a dorsal one. Although fewer in comparison to those of the hepatic artery, there are several variants of this pattern of the portal vein ramifications, especially in the intrahepatic distribution of the right branch (Fig. 9).

The names of the branches of the portal vein differ from one author to another. Rex, Melnikov, Krastin, Hjörtsjö, Elias and Petty, Netterblad, Gans, Rapp, Junès,

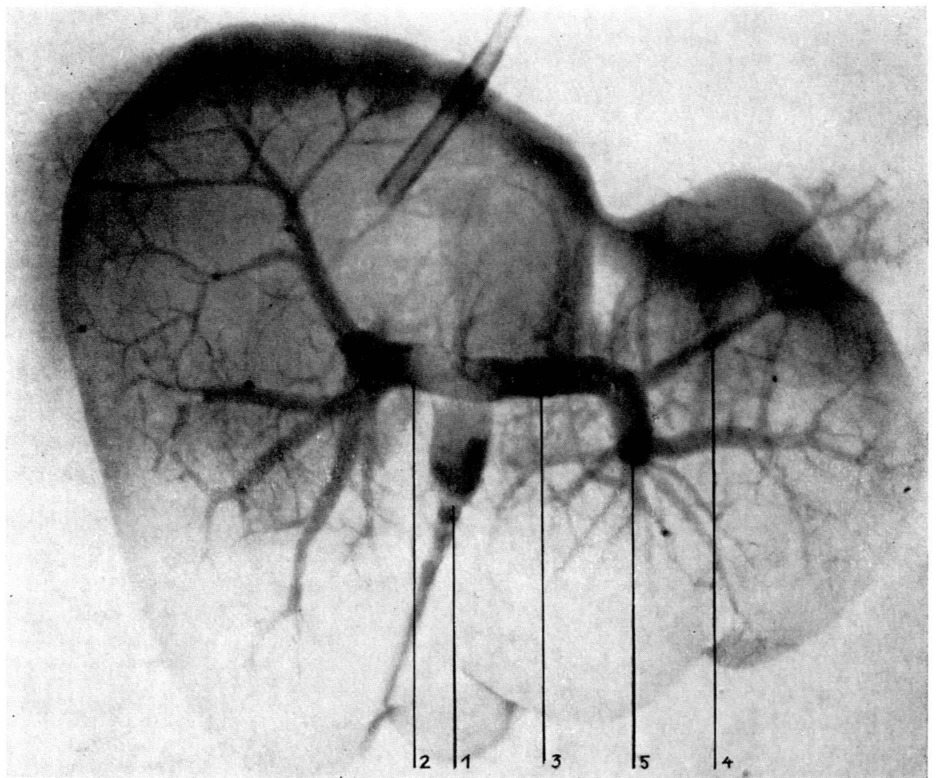

Fig. 7. — Radiographic aspect of the portal ramification (laboratory specimen). The contrast substance was introduced through a catheter into the portal vein. Another catheter was fixed to the vena cava to be subsequently used for hepatic venography.

1. Portal trunk; *2.* right branch of the portal vein; *3.* left branch of the portal vein; *4. recessus umbilicalis* ; *5.* left lateral vein.

Bourgeon and Couinaud use their own nomenclature. For the moment, we have adopted the nomenclature of Couinaud, with several additions from other authors.

Table 1 gives the nomenclature of the more important branches of the portal vein according to different authors.

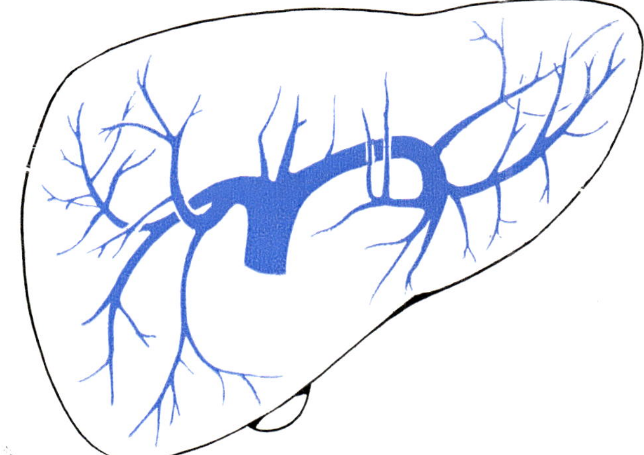

Fig. 8. — Intrahepatic ramification of the portal vein (after Healey and Schroy).

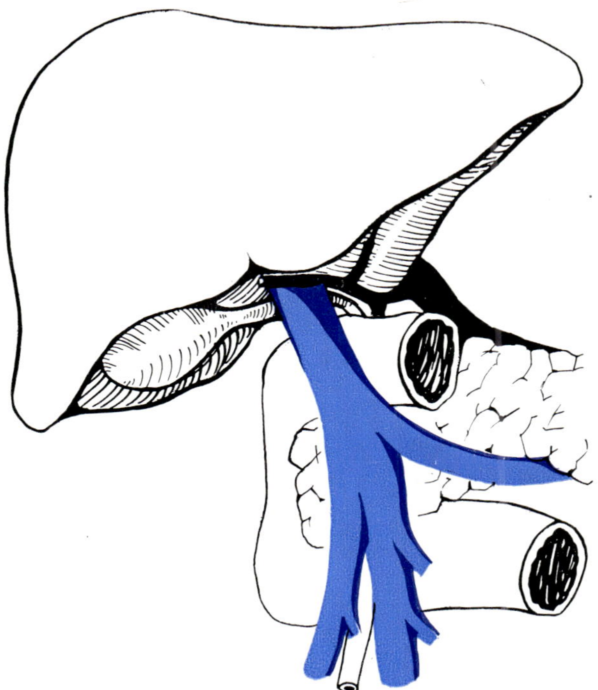

Fig. 9. — Rare variant of the portal vein trunk, lying on the ventral aspect of the duodenum.

Intrahepatic bile ducts. As a rule, the intrahepatic bile ducts run parallel to the ramifications of the portal vein, especially the large branches that stand at the origin of the right and left hepatic ducts. The right and left hepatic ducts *(ramus principalis dexter* and *ramus principalis sinister ducti hepatici)* join together at an angle of 60–105° (Hjörtsjö), forming the hepatic duct *(ductus hepaticus)* within the glandular parenchyma or immediately below the ventral aspect of the liver, in contrast to the hepatic artery and the portal vein that separate at a distance of 1–2 cm from the transverse fissure. In rare cases, the two hepatic ducts join more distally, at the site of convergence with the cystic duct, giving the aspect of a biliary trifurcation.

In general, the hepatic duct passes at first ventrally with regard to the right hepatic artery and right branch of the portal vein. After about 4 cm it is continued, after its confluence with the cystic duct, by the common duct. The hepaticocystic confluence takes place as a rule retroduodenally, or several millimeters higher up. Therefore, what is known as the supraduodenal portion of the common duct is the hepatic duct and choledocotomy is a hepaticotomy.

The anatomic pattern described is found in about 55% of the cases. In the remaining cases one of the numerous anatomical variants of the confluence of the hepatic ducts may be encountered (trifurcation, the right paramedian or right lateral duct join the left hepatic duct, etc.), to which are added the variants of the gallbladder and cystic duct.

Table 1

Hugo Rex (1888)	A. Melnikov (1924)	C. H. Hjörtsjö (1948)	C. Couinaud (1957)
Main right branch	*Ramus dexter venae portae*	*Vena portae, ramus horisontalis dexter*	Right portal vein
Ramus arcuatus	*Vena arcuata posterior dextra*	*Vena portae, rami segmenti dorsocaudalis*	Right lateral vein
Ramus ascendens	*Vena arcuata superior dextra*	*Vena portae, ramus principalis dexter*	Right paramedian vein
Main left branch	*Ramus sinister venae portae*	*Vena portae, ramus principalis sinister*	Left portal vein
Ramus angularis	*Vena arcuata posterior sinistra*	*Vena portae, ramus dorsolateralis*	Left lateral vein
Recessus umbilicalis	*Recessus umbilicalis*	Terminal arcuate position of the portal vein, *ramus principalis sinister*	Left paramedian vein

Cholangiography is a good means of anatomical and clinical investigation and supplies evidence of the intra- and extrahepatic distribution of the bile ducts and different variants (Figs 10 and 11). Fig. 12 gives an outline of some of these variants.

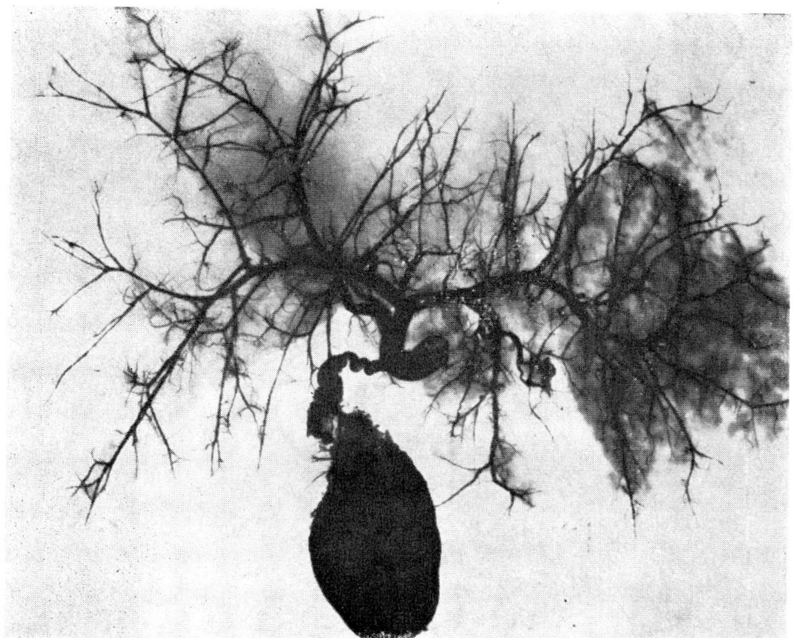

Fig. 10. — Intrahepatic ramification of the bile ducts (radiography of a laboratory specimen injected with contrast substance). This ramification corresponds to type *3*, Fig. 12.

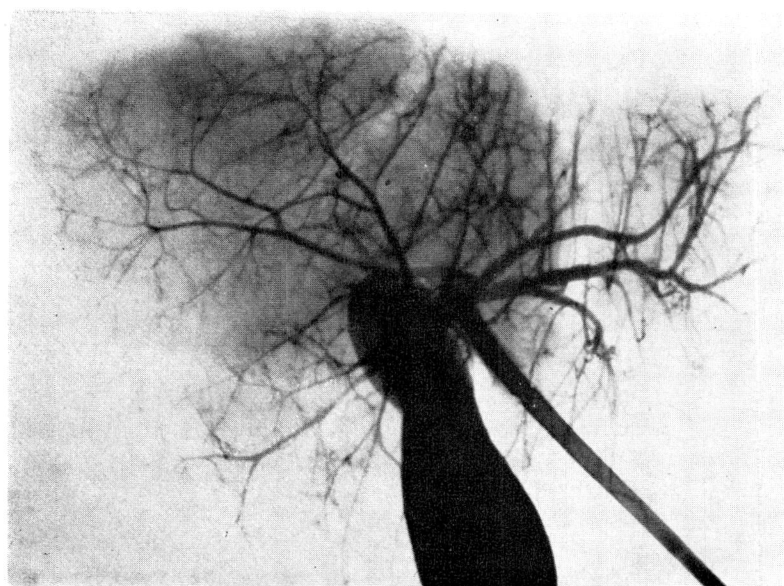

Fig. 11. — Another radiographic aspect of the intrahepatic bile ducts (laboratory specimen). Both the right and left hepatic ducts are double. By transposition one of the ducts on the right discharges into a left hepatic duct.

The aberrant bile ducts, described by Ferrein in 1753, by Toldt and Zuckerkandl in 1875, actually continue the intrahepatic duct which emerge at the periphery of the glandular mass, especially within the thickness of the left triangular ligament. These aberrant ducts were found by J. E. Healey in 5 per cent of the anatomic fragments studied. Since they have a large caliber, the surgeon should be well aquainted with them as they must be ligated after severing of the left triangular ligament, in the course of total gastrectomy, hiatal hernia, Heller or

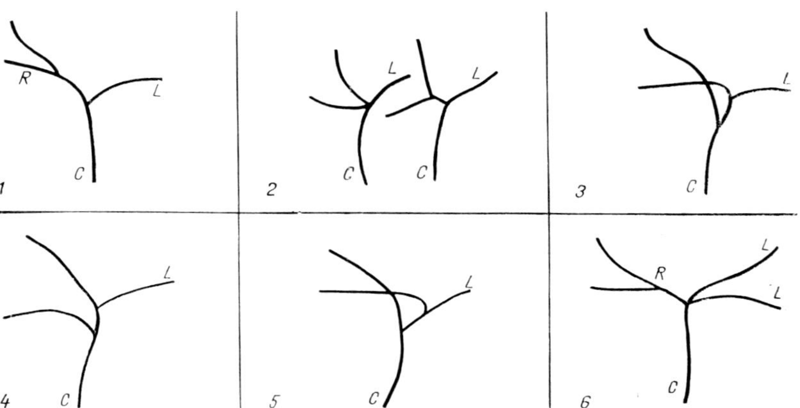

Fig. 12. — Principal modes of confluence of the bile ducts (after Cl. Olivier; the proportions after C. Couinaud).

1. The most frequent type (51%); *2.* short or double right hepatic duct (12%); *3.* (16%); *4.* (4%); *5.* (9%) — different forms of double right hepatic duct. By transposition one of the two branches may discharge into the left hepatic duct; *6.* double left hepatic duct (3%). *C* = common hepatic duct; *R* = right hepatic duct; *L* = left hepatic duct.

Dragstedt's operation. We likewise found a fairly voluminous aberrant bile duct in one of our anatomical specimens.

In almost 35 per cent of their cases, Healey and Schroy also found an aberrant bile duct above the gallbladder (not accompanied by arterioportal branches) lying in the hepatic recess of the gallbladder. This duct may be damaged in the course of cholecystectomy.

The lymphatic vessels and nerves of the liver. In the liver there is a dense network of lymphatic vessels that collect the lymph from Disse's perisinusoidal spaces. According to the hepatic areas which they drain, they may be divided into superficial and deep lymphatic vessels (Fig. 13).

Superficial lymphatic vessels. A group of superficial vessels pass through the falciform ligament, cross the diaphragm, join the internal mammary group and then flow into the thoracic duct. Another group crosses the coronary ligament and diaphragm and extends up to the supradiaphragmatic lymph nodes around the inferior vena cava. The lymphatic vessels on the visceral surface of the liver end in the lymph nodes lying along the hepatic pedicle.

The *deep lymphatic vessels* may be divided into an ascending group that closely follows the ramifications of the hepatic veins and then join together in a few trunks that accompany the cava in its trans- and supradiaphragmatic course, and a descending group that follows the ramifications of the portal triad up to the lymph nodes of the hepatic pedicle and then to the celiac lymph nodes.

The *liver nerves*, incompletely studied up to the present, have a multiple origin. The sympathetic innervation arises from the right splanchnic nerve and

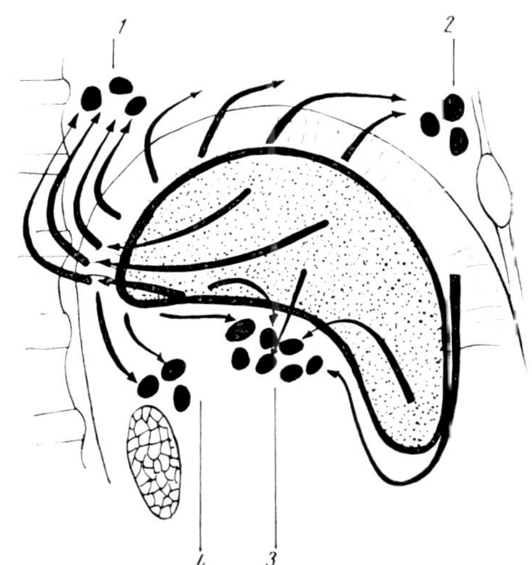

Fig. 13. — Regional lymph nodes of the liver (drawn after Testut).

1. Posterior mediastinal lymph nodes; *2.* anterior mediastinal lymph nodes; *3.* hilar lymph nodes; *4.* suprapancreatic lymph nodes.

the parasympathetic innervation from the left vagus nerve. These branches form an anterior and a posterior plexus around the hepatic artery, and also receive fibres from the right vagus nerve and the celiac ganglion. From this plexus, nervous fibers penetrate into the liver along the portal triad, up to the hepatic lobulus. Branches of the right phrenic nerve likewise penetrate into the liver along the ramifications of the hepatic veins.

THE HEPATIC VEINS

The mixed portal and arterial blood in the hepatic sinusoids is drained by the centrolobular veins, collected into the venules and increasingly larger veins that flow into the vena cava through the right and left hepatic veins (Figs 14, 15 and 16).

The left hepatic vein drains the classical left lobe. At a short distance before joining the left ventral aspect of the cava, it receives a voluminous affluent called the sagittal vein or, according to some authors, the middle hepatic vein, which sometimes flows directly into the inferior cava. The sagittal vein receives affluents from the middle part of the liver, from the right and left of the sagittal plane, that joins the cystic fissure with the inferior vena cava and is called the main fissure of the liver.

The original branches of the *sagittal vein* arise close to the ventral border of the liver, to the right and left of the main fissure. The sagittal vein lies almost on the visceral surface of the liver, sometimes in direct contact with the hilar fibrous plates, in the hepatic recess of the gallbladder. It then passes 1 cm above the hilus.

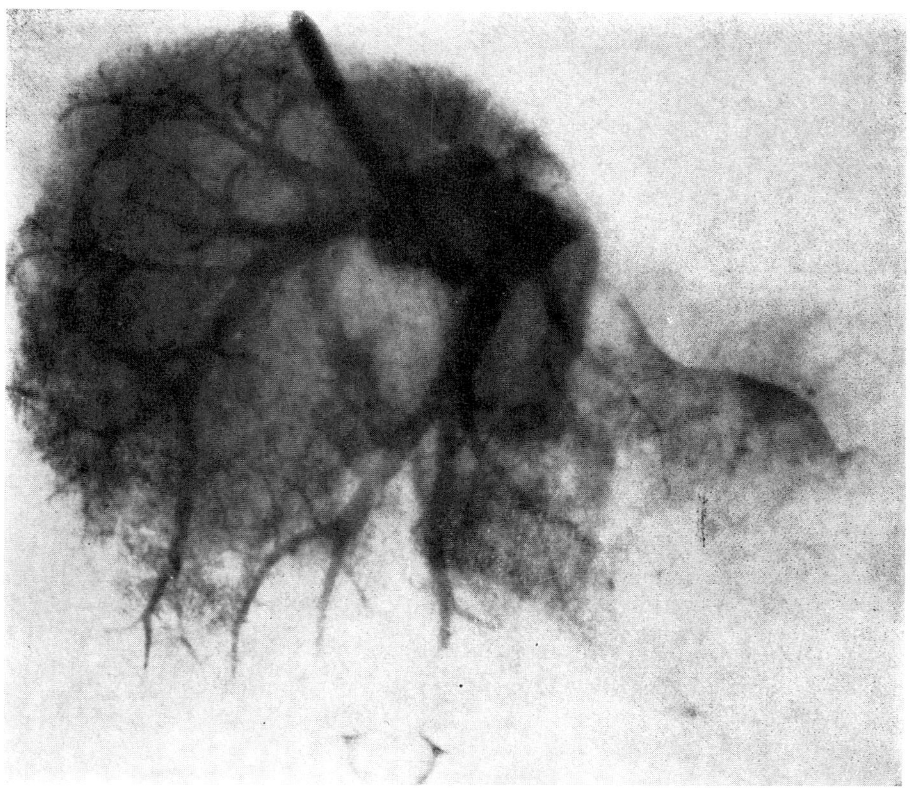

Fig. 14. — Radiologic aspect of the ramifications of the hepatic veins (laboratory specimen). Sagittal vein bifurcates after a shorter course than usual. The left hepatic vein is reduced or incompletely filled with contrast medium.

The same as the other voluminous hepatic veins, the sagittal vein has a pennate ramification, receiving numerous lateral affluents of reduced caliber, in contrast to the elements of the portal pedicle that have an arborescent ramification.

The right hepatic vein drains the venous blood from the dorso-lateral part of the classical right lobe. It corresponds to the right hepatic fissure in a relatively avascular oblique plane from the viewpoint of the afferent arterial-portal circulation. It receives affluents from the right and left of this fissure, then extends over the right ventrolateral aspect of the cava.

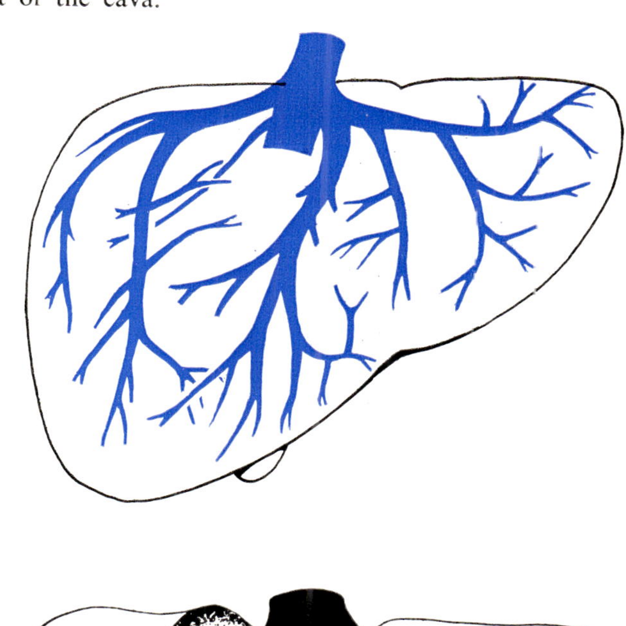

Fig. 15. — Ramifications of the hepatic veins (after Healey and Schroy).

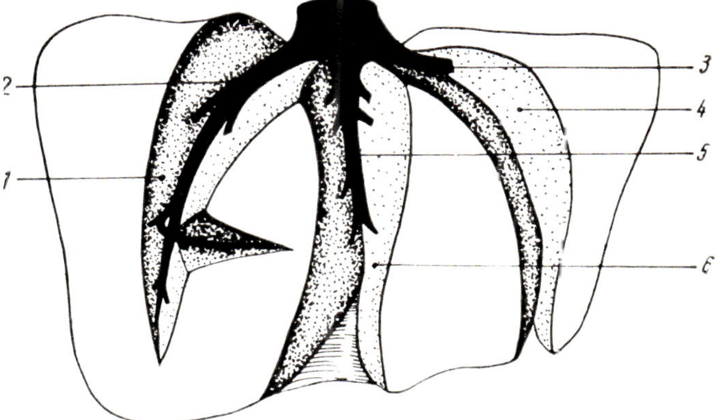

Fig. 16. — Ramifications of the hepatic veins (after Olivier). The hepatic tissue was incised along the fissures in order to reveal the deep veins.

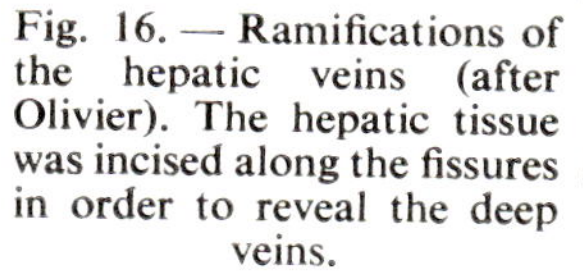
1. Right portal fissure; *2.* right hepatic vein; *3.* left hepatic vein; *4.* secondary fissure; *5.* sagittal vein; *6.* main fissure

Spiegel's lobe is drained by 15—20 *accessory hepatic veins*, of reduced caliber that flow into the vena cava.

There is no anastomosis between the branches of the hepatic vein or with the portal branches. The continuity of the afferent and efferent vascular system is ensured by the hepatic sinusoids. In rare cases in the normal liver, and more frequently in the cirrhotic liver, there are more or less voluminous anastomoses between the portal and hepatic branches that actually represent intraglandular portacaval shunts.

In humans, the existence of a sphincterial musculature where the hepatic veins join the cava, as described in the dog, has not been confirmed. It appears that in man the muscular fibres at this level are not sufficiently numerous to bring about an efficient contraction. Neither has the hypothesis of the two separate blood flows in the trunk of the portal vein been confirmed. According to this hypothesis, the blood draining from the region of the superior mesenteric vein circulates separately in the portal vein and does not mix with the blood from the splenic and inferior mesenteric vein. The two semicolumns of blood are then assumed to be distributed to the right and the left branch of the portal vein, each half of the liver being linked to the physiology and pathology of the respective area (carcinomatous metastases with a specific location in the right or left half of the liver according to the origin of the tumor). In most cases, radiologic arguments (splenoportography) invalidate this hypothesis.

Characteristic of the anatomic peculiarities of the hepatic circulation are the branches of the efferent venous system of the hepatic vessels which do not follow retrogradely the course of the afferent system of the portal vein and hepatic artery. The intrahepatic branches of the afferent system are distributed radially around a center situated in the hepatic hilum, whereas the hepatic veins are distributed fanwise with the tip towards the vena cava (Figs 17 and 18).

Therefore, the hepatic veins form a second vascular topographical system, differing from the distribution of the first topographic system (portal). The branches of the hepatic veins pass through the free zones between the branches of the portal pedicle crossing them in opposite directions, like the fingers of the hands when joined together (Fig. 19).

INNER ARCHITECTURE OF THE LIVER

Except for the hepatic artery, whose branches form an anastomotic network up to the surface of the liver, of no great importance from the functional and surgical points of view, the branches of the hepatic vessels and bile ducts do not anastomose. A more or less voluminous portal pedicle and one or several hepatic venous branches supply a given glandular area without important vascular connections with the neighboring areas. Ligation of the afferent or efferent pedicle may produce necrosis of the region drained by these branches since, although the pseudocapillary system of the sinusoid vessels exhibits a microanastomotic continuity throughout the hepatic mass it cannot ensure a sufficient afferent or return circulation.

Precise knowledge of the intrahepatic distribution of the first and second topographic vascular systems led to the conception of the existence of certain territorial units and subunits of the hepatic parenchyma, that do not correspond exactly with the classical anatomic divisions based upon the outer visible segmentation, especially on the visceral aspect of the liver. The liver may be divided into such units, both according to the intrahepatic distribution of the portal pedicle and

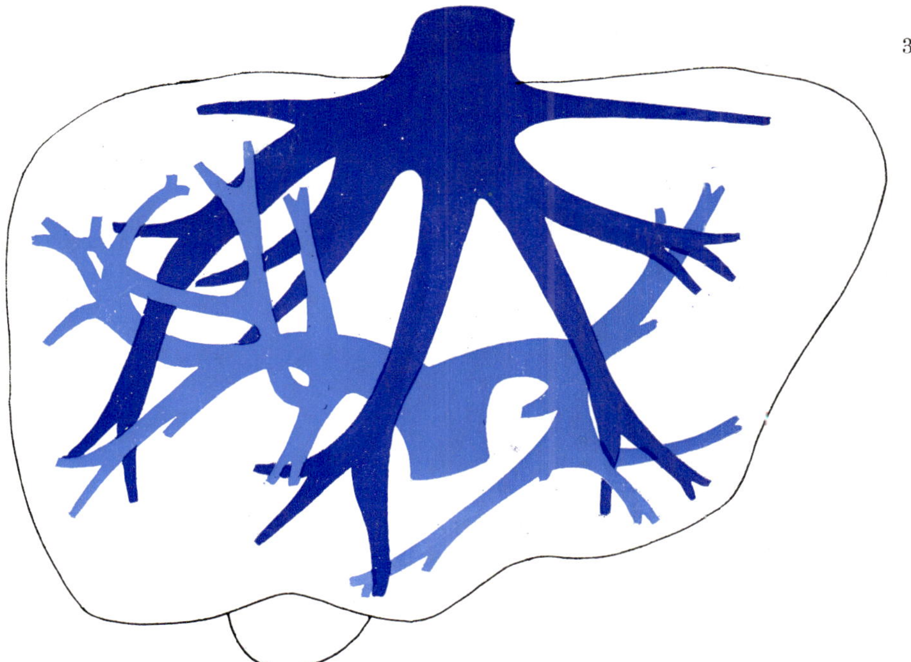

Fig. 17. — Schematic representation of the relationship between the portal ramifications (light blue) and hepatic veins (dark blue).

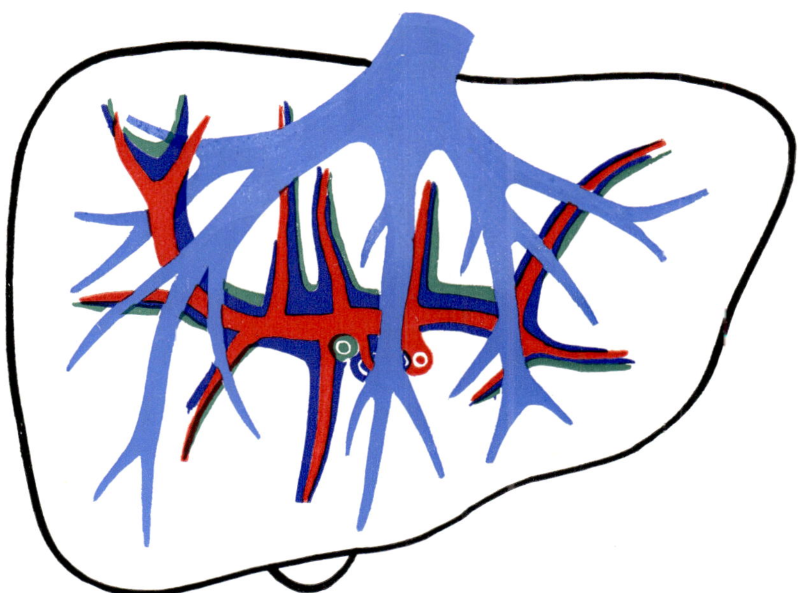

Fig. 18. — Schematic representation of the three elements of the portal pedicle and their relationship with the branches of the hepatic veins.

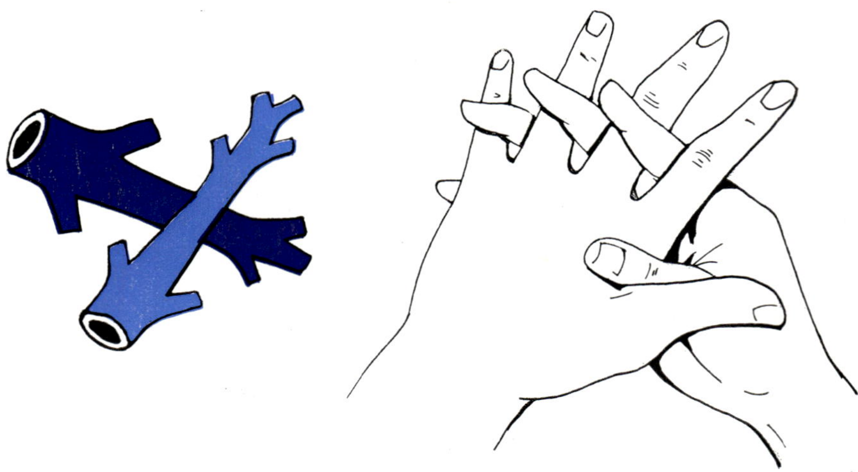

Fig. 19. — Anatomic relations between the branches of the afferent and efferent pedicle. Compare with the crossed fingers of the hands (after K. Stucke).

according to the distribution of the hepatic vein. Segmentation according to the portal distribution is not superposed exactly upon that of the hepatic vein ramifications. For instance segmentation based upon the ramification of the portal pedicle falls into two large areas: the right and left hepatic areas separated by the large fissure, whereas according to the second topographic system, the liver is divided into the right, middle and left lobes, the middle lobe belonging in equal part to the right and left liver.

The segmentary architecture of the liver was mentioned as far back as 1654 when F. Glisson published *Anatomia hepatis* which gives a surprisingly accurate description of the liver following a study of wax casts of the intrahepatic vessels. In 1888, Hugo Rex gave a detailed systematization of the liver, which was overlooked for a long time since the surgical possibilities of those times did not permit a practical application of these anatomical details. The anatomical study of the liver was taken up again by A. Melnikov who published several important works in this sphere in 1922 and 1924, which have become classical. Recent studies have been promoted by the similitude of the inner architecture of the liver to that of the lung, which is likewise segmented and presents a fourfold bronchovascular system, similar to the biliovascular system. In 1948 and 1951, C. H. Hjörtsjö published several works based upon hepatic segmentation, after studying numerous anatomic specimens, comparing the stereoscopic cholangiographies with the corrosion preparations of the bile ducts filled with plastic material. In 1953 P. E. Rapp and in 1955 H. Gans studied a segmentation based upon the ramifications of the hepatic veins. The anatomy of the intrahepatic biliovascular system has also been studied in Romania by Z. Iagnov and R. Georgescu, P. Andronescu, D. Făgărăşanu and N. Constantinescu and by S. Ciobanu (plates I—VI).

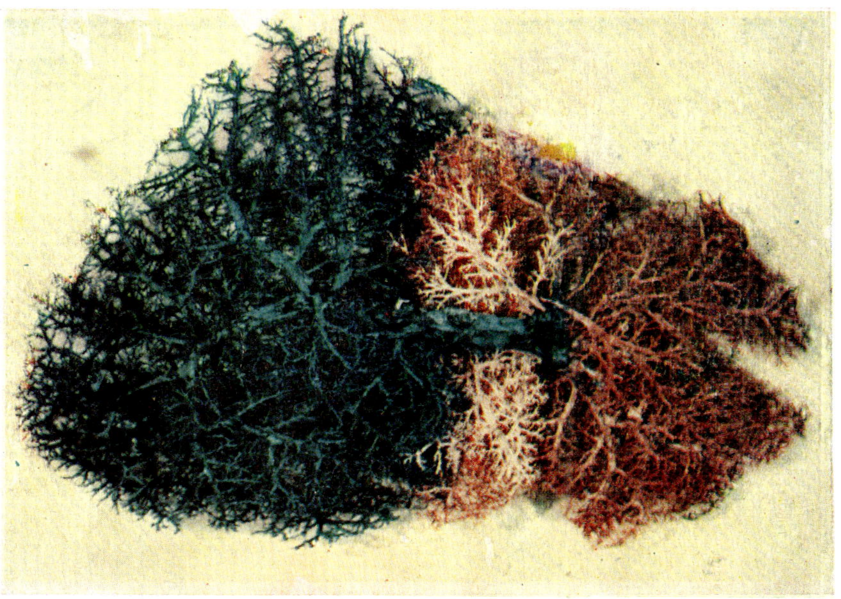

Plate I. — Liver of adult. Visceral aspect. Blue: right portal vein. Red: left portal vein, segment I and part of the quadrate lobe.

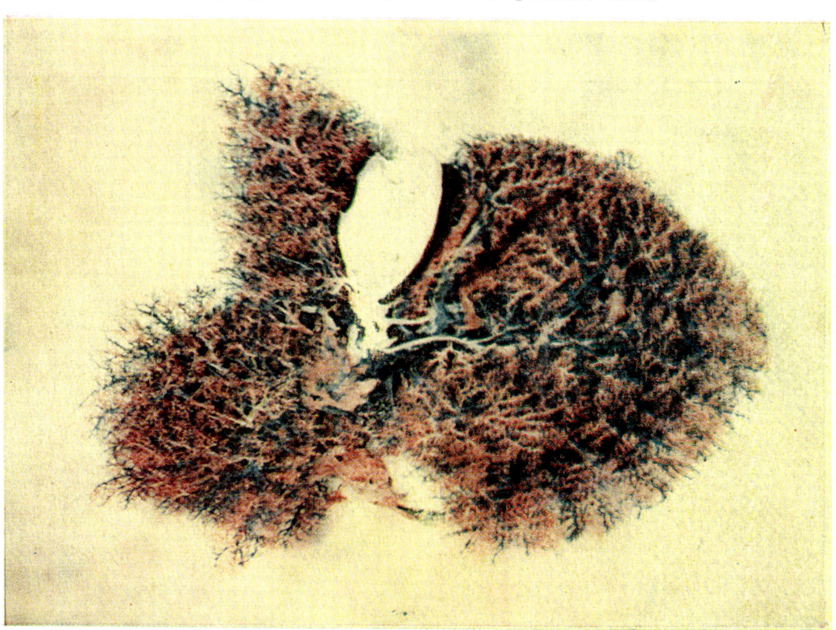

Plate II. — Liver of fetus. Visceral aspect. Blue: hepatic veins. Red: portal vein. White: bile ducts. Note the large volume of the left hepatic area.

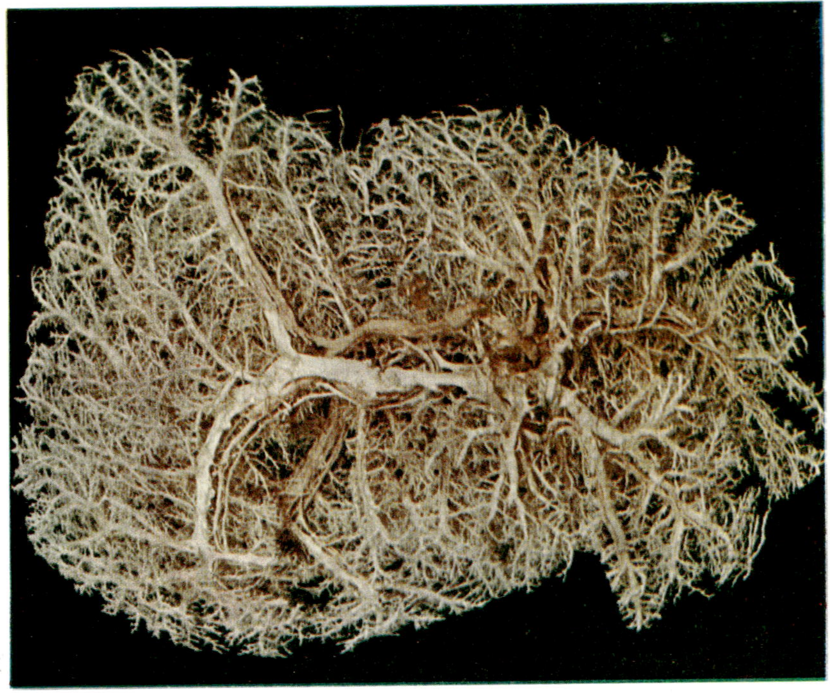

Plate III. — Liver of adult. Visceral aspect. White: portal vein. Yellow: bile ducts.

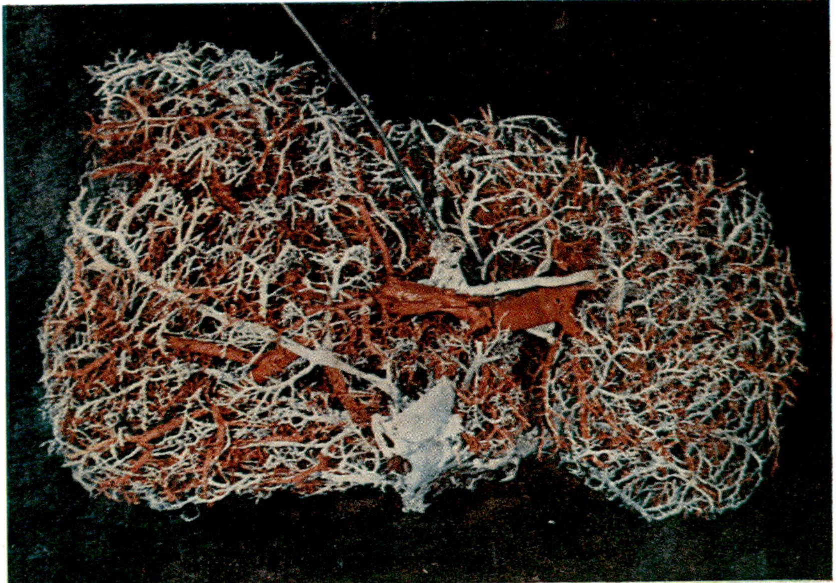

Plate IV. — Liver of adult. Visceral aspect. Red: portal vein. White (with indicator): bile ducts. Blue: hepatic veins.

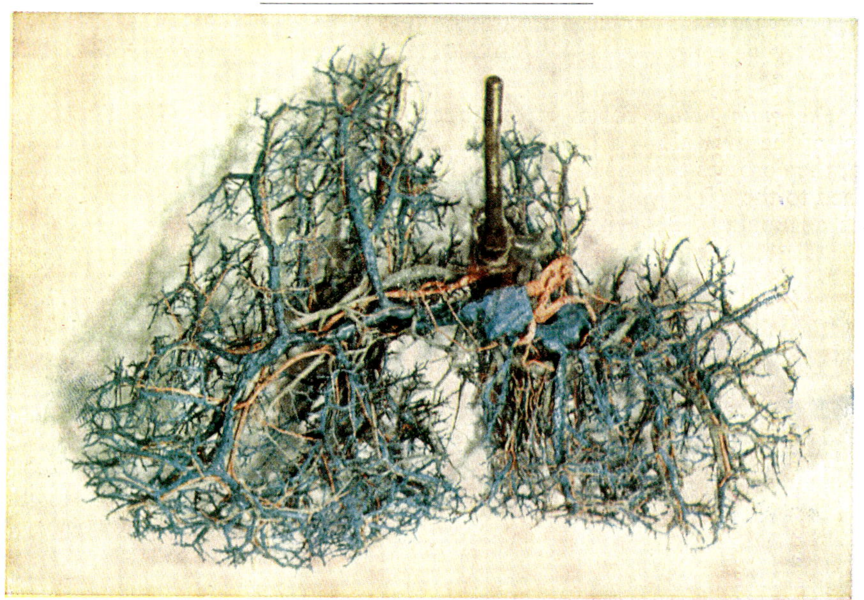

Plate V. — Liver of adult. Visceral aspect. Blue: portal vein. Red: hepatic artery. Green: bile ducts. The main fissure is marked by the relative absence of the branches of the portal pedicle.

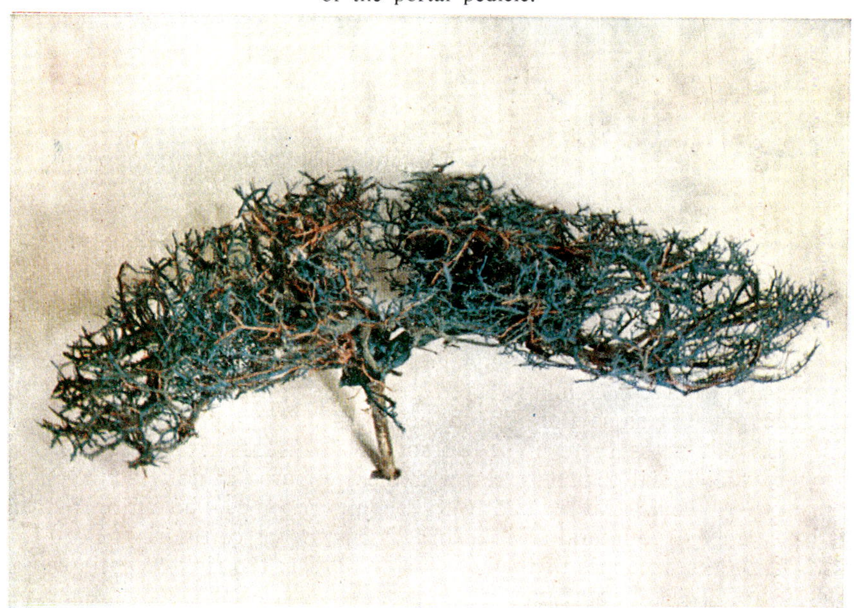

Plate VI. — The same specimen as in plate V, seen from the posterior border. The main fissure is fairly evident along a vertical line continuing the hilus.

SEGMENTATION BASED UPON THE DISTRIBUTION OF THE PORTAL PEDICLE

The main fissure forms an oblique plane (Fig. 20) that lies on the visceral aspect of the liver along a line that passes longitudinally to the fundus of the cystic fossa, then crosses the hepatic hilus and ends in the vena cava. This plane is slightly inclined to the left, forming with the transversal plane an angle of about 75°. It also forms an angle of 35° with the median sagittal plane, to the right of which this fissure is situated. On the diaphragmatic aspect of the liver, the main fissure is marked by a hardly visible groove at the level of which the liver is less consistent. In the liver the main fissure, the same as the other fissures, does not correspond to a fibrous plane. It is only a virtual plane characterized by the fact that it is not crossed by the larger branches of the portal pedicle. The fissure is avascular only from the portal point of view, since the sagittal vein runs along its entire length.

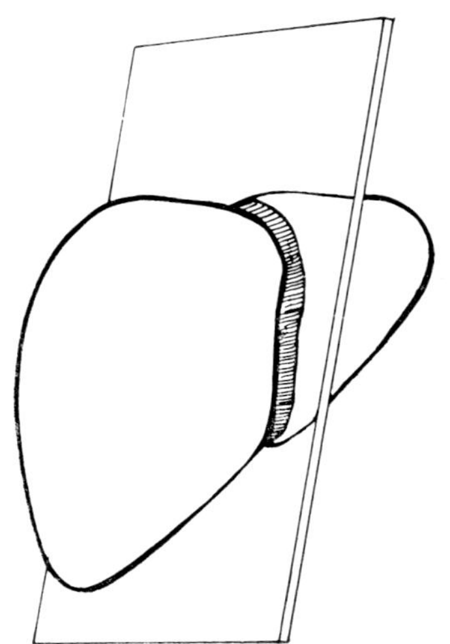

Fig. 20. — Hjörtsjö's plane separating the right hepatic area from the left, along the main fissure (after Child).

The secondary fissure runs almost parallel to the main fissure separating the classical lobe from the rest of the liver (Fig. 21).

The right portal fissure forms a curve with a ventromedial concavity projected upon the surface of the liver along a line that begins at half the distance between the cystic fissure and the right extremity of the liver and ends at the junction of the right hepatic vein with the cava.

The right hepatic area (Fig. 22) is situated to the right of the main fissure. We have used the term of Junès since the term of right and left liver would suggest a pair of organs separated from each other and the term of right and left half would imply an equal weight and volume of a symmetrical organ. The right part is divided by the right fissure into a right paramedian and a lateral part, the paramedian part being situated ventrocraniomedially and the lateral part being situated underneath, posteriorly, and to the right. Each of these parts are divided by the cross segmental fissure into a ventral and a dorsal segment, segments V and VIII in the paramedian part, segments VI and VII in the lateral part. Actually, these segmental fissures are not true grooves since they do not follow longitudinally the branches of the hepatic veins but cross them in a dorsoventral direction. Hence, the surgical approach to the dorsal segments through these fissures is not possible since the venous return of the ventral segment would be interrupted. The entire right hepatic area is irrigated by the lateral and paramedian branches of the right portal pedicle along which lie the branches of the right hepatic duct: the right hepatic vein drains the lateral area and adjacent part of the right paramedian area, and the original and right lateral branches of the sagittal vein drain part of the paramedian area next to the vein.

The *left hepatic region* (Fig. 24) is divided by the secondary fissures into a *left paramedian* and a *left lateral area*. The paramedian area is formed anteriorly by the classical quadrate lobe and the left half of the gallbladder fossa (segment IV)

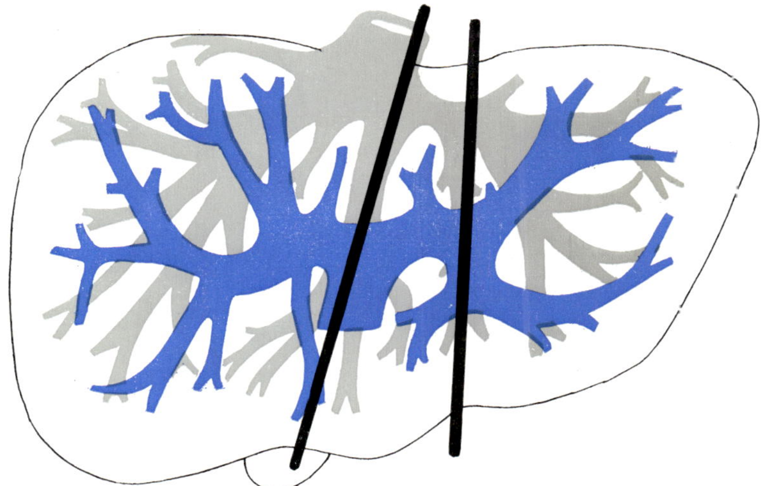

Fig. 21. — Main and secondary fissures (black lines) (after Stucke).

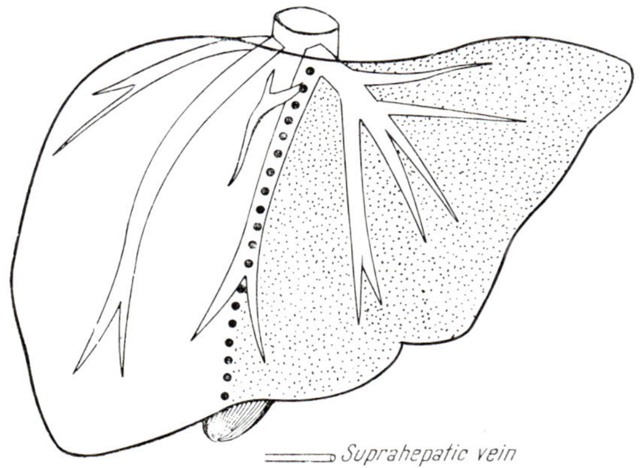

Fig. 22. — The borderline between the right and left hepatic areas on the diaphragmatic aspect (after Couinaud).

and posteriorly by the caudate lobe (segment I). The lateral area corresponds to the classical left lobe. It is divided by a transverse segmentary fissure into a dorsal segment (segment II) and a ventral segment (segment III). By its portal vascularization, the caudate lobe belongs to the right or to the left region, or to both.

Both the right and the left regions are irrigated by a single afferent pedicle and drained by a main efferent pedicle (left hepatic vein) and by numerous smaller pedicles, branches of the sagittal vein.

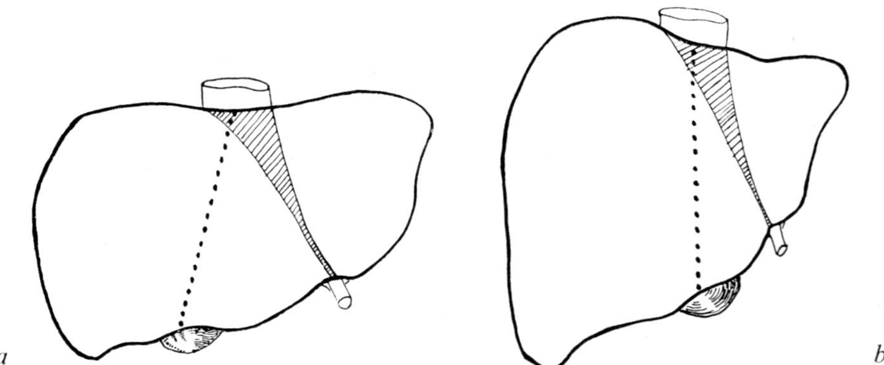

Fig. 23 a and b. — Compare liver with lengthened transverse diameter to that with shortened diameter. The main fissure, oblique in the first type, has an almost sagittal direction in the second.

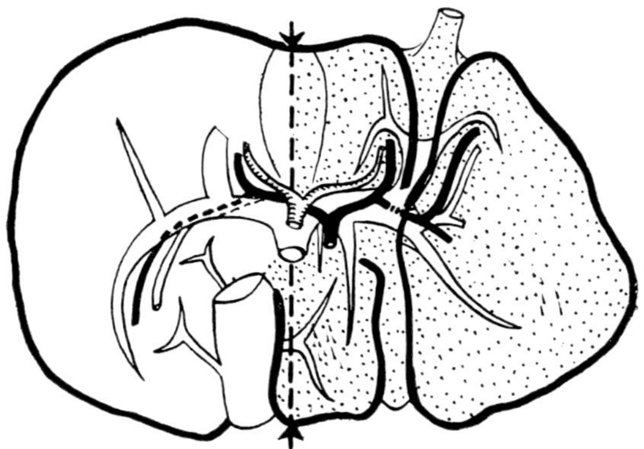

Fig. 24. — Borderline between right and left areas on the visceral aspect of the liver (after Couinaud).

The hepatic segments, designated by different authors according to their topographic location, were marked by Couinaud with figures, segment I conventionally denoting the caudate lobe. The other seven segments succeed one another along the contour of the liver counterclockwise (on the visceral aspect of the liver) (Fig. 25).

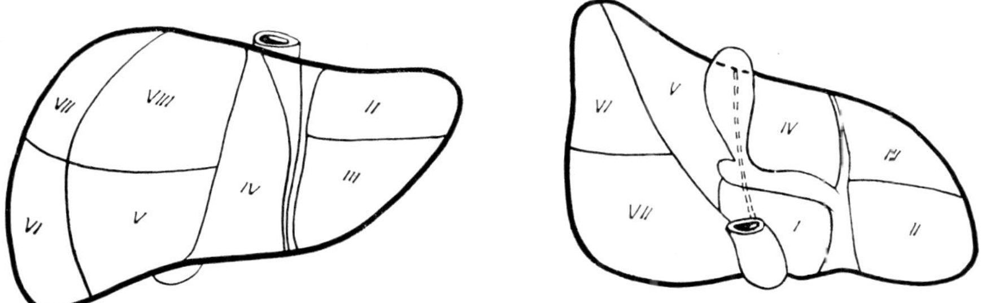

Fig. 25. — Hepatic segmentation. Projection of the intersegmentary limits on the diaphragmatic and visceral aspects (after Couinaud).

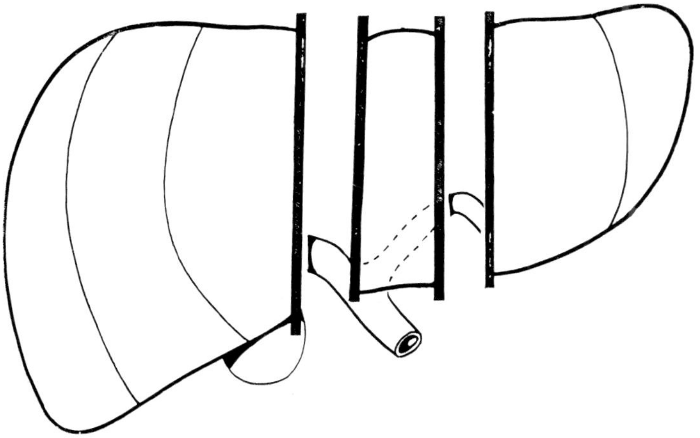

Fig. 26. — Segmentation of the liver according to Hjörtsjö (drawn after Stucke).

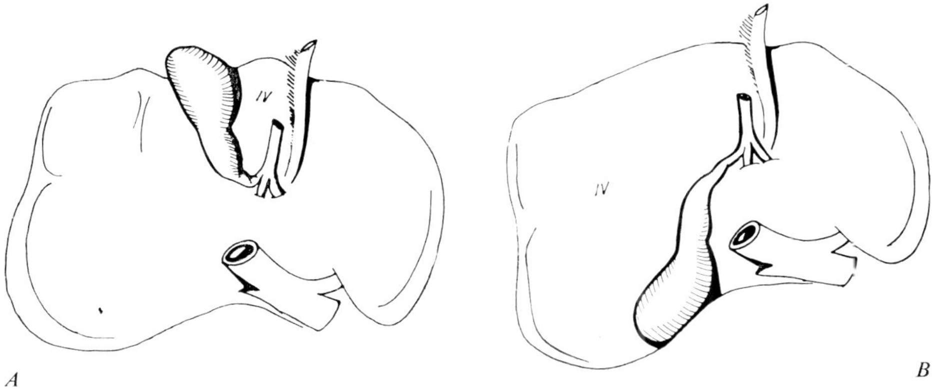

A

B

Fig. 27. — Rare variant of hepatic segmentation observed in one of our cases (*B*) in comparison to the normal aspect (*A*). The fundus of the gallbladder lies in the direction of the posterior border of the liver. Segment *IV* (quadrate lobe) is enormously developed due to complete absence of the right lobe.

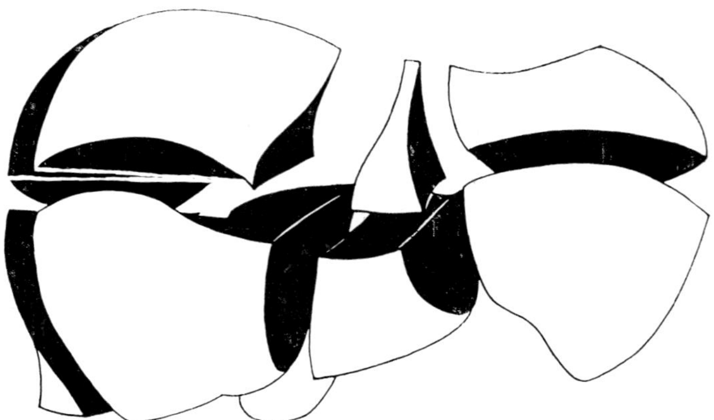

Fig 28. — Hepatic segmentation. Schematical representation according to Reifferscheid. Diaphragmatic aspect.

SEGMENTATION BASED UPON THE DISTRIBUTION OF HEPATIC VEINS

For practical reasons, the principal hepatic segmentation is that based upon the distribution of the first topographic system. This system is well known owing to the cholangiographies and portal phlebographies performed in the clinic, to the increased necessity of hepatic exeresis and approach of the bile ducts along their intrahepatic course. Although less important from the surgical point of view, segmentation based upon the hepatic veins must be known since it is an anatomic fact just as clearly defined as portal segmentation.

Phlebogram of the hepatic veins shows that between the ramifications of the three main trunks the existing avascular planes correspond to veritable fissures, one to the right and the other to the left, dividing the liver into the right, the median and the left lobe.

The right lobe includes the right portal lateral area and the right paramedian area, the remaining right paramedian area and the left paramedian area correspond to the medium lobe. The caudate lobe does not belong to any of these three lobes since it has a separate efferent circulation represented by 15—20 hepatic venules that flow directly into the cava.

As the left fissure corresponds to the secondary portal fissure, the left lobe of the hepatic segmentation is exactly superposed over the left portal lateral area, that is the classical left lobe. The left lobe has two afferent vascular pedicles (left lateral pedicle of segment IV and the pedicle of segment III) and a single efferent pedicle: the left hepatic vein.

HISTOLOGIC STUDY OF THE LIVER

After numerous microscopic studies, with contradictory results in many cases, it has been concluded that the basic elements of the liver structure, the liver cells, have a lamellar arrangement, lying in single layers that cross one another

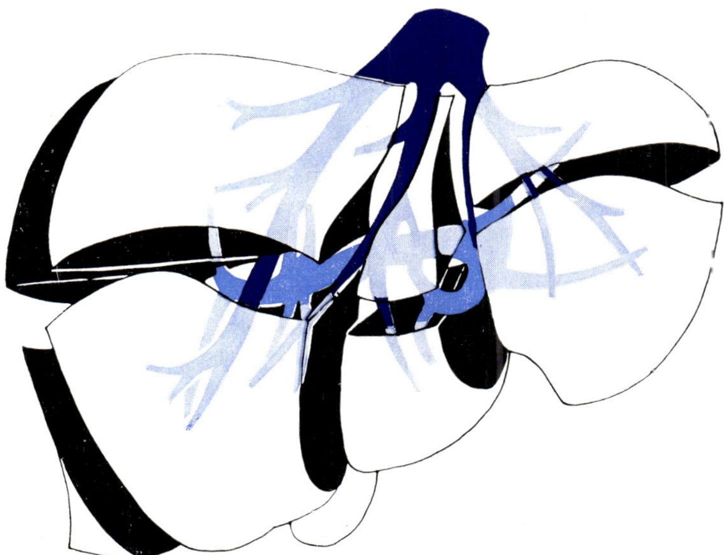

Fig. 29. — The same aspect as in Fig. 28 to which the portal branches and hepatic veins are added.

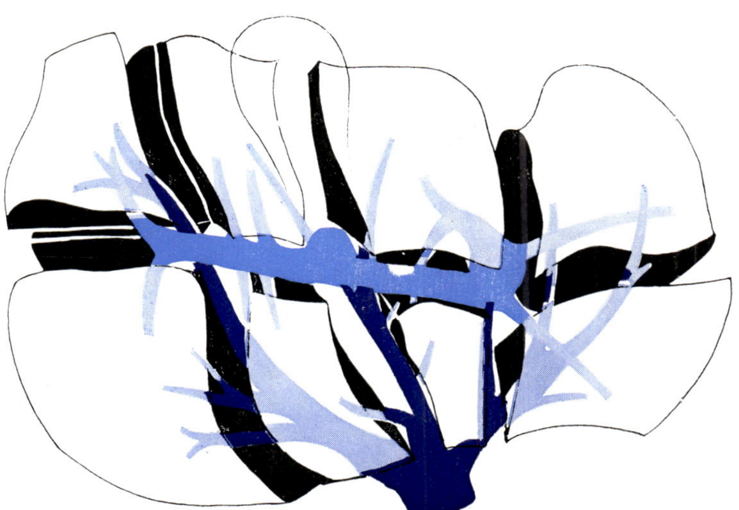

Fig. 30. — Segmentation of the liver (after Reifferscheid). Visceral aspect. Light blue: portal ramifications. Dark blue: hepatic veins, represented in the intraparenchymatous areas in a somewhat lighter tonality.

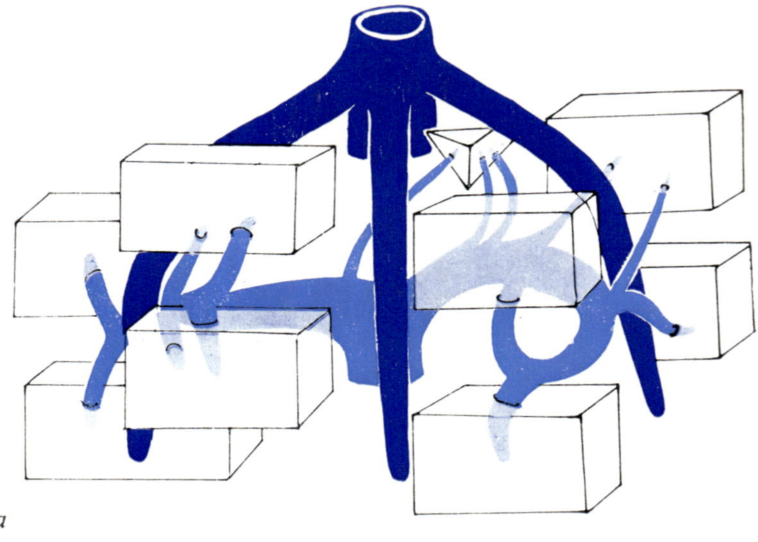

a

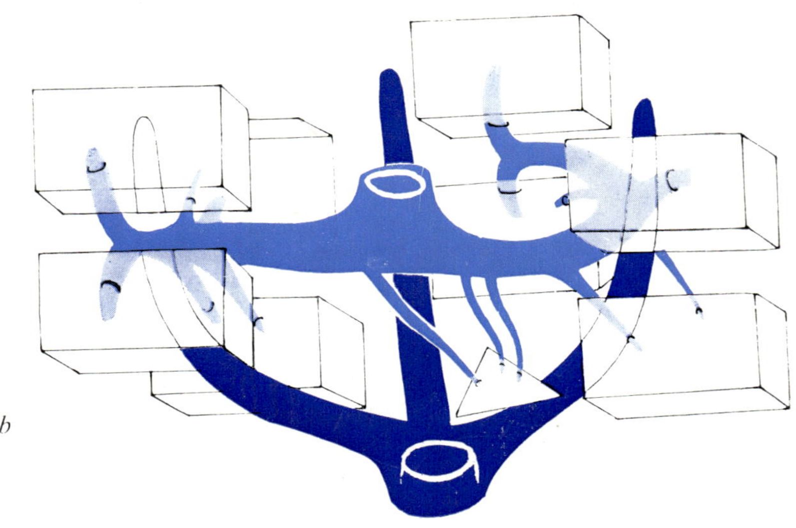

b

Fig. 31 a and b. — Other schematic representations of hepatic segmentation (after Reifferschied).

and between which large spaces occupied by vessels are included. The microscopic anatomofunctional unit of the liver is the *lobule* which is formed of portions of hepatic tissue supplied by the smallest branches of the afferent and efferent vascular system.

Elias (1952), who studied stereoscopically the hepatic lobule, compared it to a maze of rooms, representing the vascular terminations, separated by walls formed by the lamellae of the liver cells and which communicate with one another

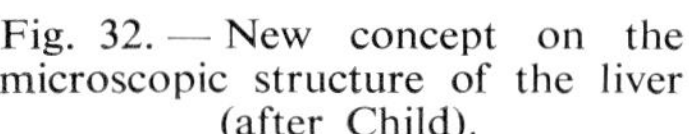

Fig. 32. — New concept on the microscopic structure of the liver (after Child).

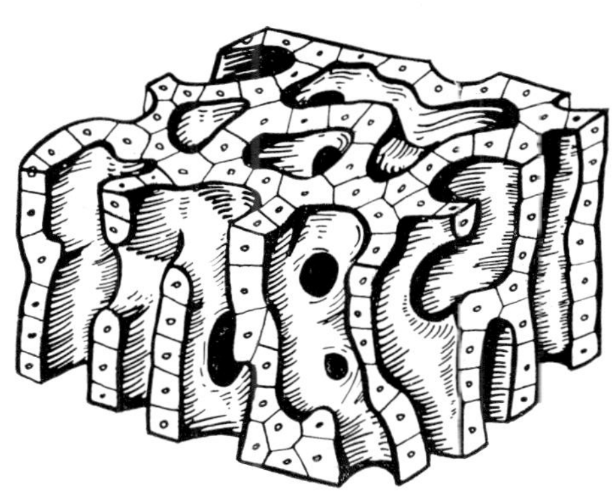

by numerous doors and windows by which the blood vessels enter and leave. The margin of the lobule is surrounded by a layer of liver cells, called the *placa limitans* which is likewise crisscrossed by afferent and efferent vessels. The *placa limitans* is continued with the neighboring lobules so that the continuity of the basic cellular element is ensured throughout the whole mass of the liver (Fig. 32). Since a true anatomic separation does not actually exist between the lobules, the hepatic lobule is a hypothetical unit, arising from the necessity of an anatomic scheme that can be readily understood.

The spaces contained between the lamellae of the liver cells are occupied by the following biliovascular structures (Fig. 33).

The portal venous system. The portal venule that irrigates a lobule represents a branch of 6—7th order of the portal vein. Before entering the lobule a sphincteral structure can be observed, which probably regulates the afferent portal output. In the lobe, the venule is divided into sinusoid pseudocapillaries which converge, perpendicularly towards the central vein, a branch of the efferent hepatic system.

The arterioles reach the liver lobe together with the portal venule through Kiernan's portal spaces. Some branch off into capillaries, supplying the anatomic structures in Kiernan's spaces, and others anastomose with the portal venules; most of them penetrate into the lobule, as shown by Chrzonszczewsky as far back as 1866.

In 1932, Knisely using the transillumination technique *in vivo* showed that each intralobular arteriole is anastomosed with a sinusoid. Therefore, the sinusoids represent the main portoarterial junction. Wakim and Mann in 1942 and Elias in 1952 confirmed these data and showed in addition that the arterioles possess

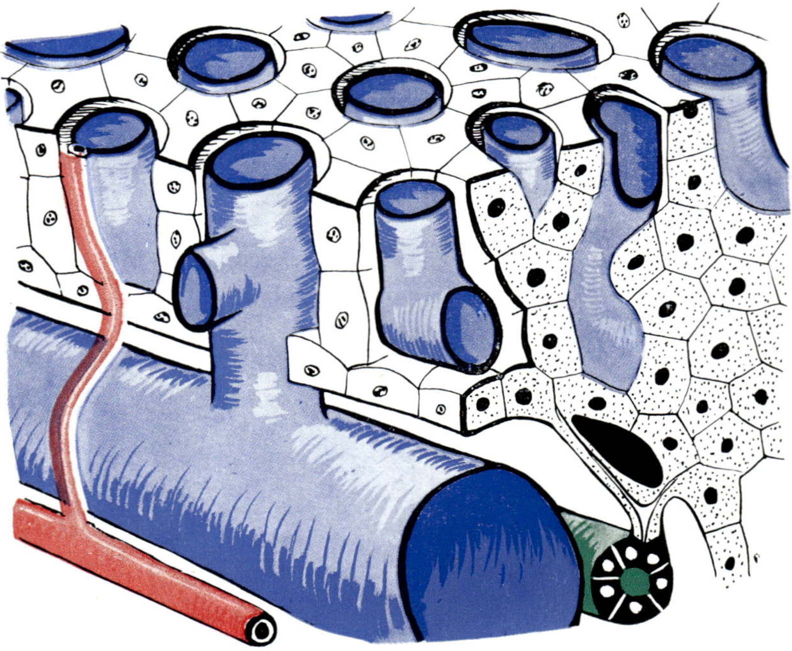

Fig. 33. — Schematic microscopic aspect of the intrahepatic biliovascular ramification (after Child, modified).

sphincteric structures which control the output. According to Wakim and Mann, at any moment 75% of the hepatic mass is inactive from the point of view of the circulation, but in each lobe the circulation varies from moment to moment, oscillating between a minimal and a maximum output, with an exclusive arterial or exclusive portal supply, or with an arteriovenous mixture in different proportions.

The sinusoids differ from the capillaries, with which they were confused for a long time, by their wider diameter and broad lateral openings through which they communicate with the neighboring sinusoids. According to C. G. Child, the sinusoid walls are not formed of two kinds of cells (endothelial and stellate), but only of Kupffer stellate cells which have a selective phagocytic capacity. According to Knisely, a particle that penetrates into the sinusoid is covered by a precipitate probably formed of a highly specialized protein. The coating, with long pennate processes is phagocytized by Kupffer's cells together with the foreign particle.

From the centrolobular vein, several efferent venules arise, with sphincteric structures that regulate the venous return and which probably confer upon the liver its role of blood reservoir for regulating the volume of the circulating blood. These data have not yet been fully confirmed in man.

The lymphatic vessels have only been followed up to the periphery of the lobules. A presinusoidal groove has been described — Dissé's space — which separates the sinusoids from the hepatic lamellae, and a periportal one — Mall's space — which appears to represent the first steps of the lymphatic drainage system in the lobule. No direct connection has been found up to the present between these spaces and the lymphatic vessels in Kiernan's portal spaces, the confluence of which gives rise to the large lymphatic trunks.

In the spaces between neighboring liver cells, anastomosed biliary canaliculi form a network that includes the whole lobe and, therefore, all the liver; from this network, an intralobular cholangiol arises which in turn continues with a small caliber bile duct, situated in the portal space.

REFERENCES

1. ANDRONESCU P. et al., Spitalul, 1957, *2*, 165.
2. BRAUS H., ELZE C., *Anatomie des Menschen*, Springer, Berlin, 1956.
3. CHILD G. C., *The hepatic circulation and portal hypertension*, W. B. Saunders, Philadelphia, 1954.
4. CIOBANU ST., Chirurgia, 1956, **5**, *4*, 495.
5. CIOBANU ST., Chirurgia, 1957, **6**, *3*, 434.
6. COUINAUD C., J. Chir., 1954, **70**, *12*, 933.
7. COUINAUD C., *Le foie. Etudes anatomiques et chirurgicales*, Masson, Paris, 1957.
8. ELIAS H., PETTY D., Amer. J. Anat., 1952, **90**, *1*, 59.
9. GOLDSMITH N. A., WOODBURNE R. T., Surg. Gynec. Obstet., 1957, **105**, *3*, 310.
10. HEALEY J. E., SCHROY P., SORENSEN R., J. int. Coll. Surg., 1953, **20**, *1*, 133
11. HJÖRTSJÖ C. H., Acta anat. (Basel), 1951, **11**, *4*, 599.
12. IAGNOV Z., REPCIUC E., RUSSU G., *Anatomia omului, Angeiologie, glande endocrine, sistem nervos*. Ed. Medicală, Bucharest, 1954; *Anatomia omului. Viscerele*, Ed. Medicală, Bucharest, 1958.
13. JUNÈS P., Rev. int. Hépat., 1956, **6**, *1*, 128.
14. NETTERBLAD S. C., Acta anat. (Basel), 1954, **21**, suppl. 20.
15. PATEL J., COUINAUD C., *Les bases anatomiques des hépatectomies réglées*, in *XVIe Congr. Soc. Internat. Chir.*, Copenhagen, 1955, p. 1015.
16. POPESCU C., Chirurgia, 1958, **7**, *3*, 381.
17. PAPILIAN V., PREDA V., *Embriologie*, H. Welther, Sibiu, 1946.
18. REIFFERSCHEID M., *Chirurgie der Leber*, G. Thieme, Stuttgart, 1957.
19. SEVKUNENKO V. N., MAXIMENKOV A. N., *Chirurgia operatorie și anatomia topografică*, Ed. Stat Lit. Științ., Bucharest, 1954.
20. STUCKE K., *Leberchirurgie*, Springer, Berlin, 1959.
21. TESTUT L., *Traité d'anatomie humaine*, 8th ed., Doin, Paris, 1931.
22. TESTUT L., JACOB O., *Traité d'anatomie topographique*, Doin, Paris, 1925.

CHAPTER 2

NORMAL AND PATHOLOGIC PHYSIOLOGY OF THE LIVER

FUNDAMENTAL ASPECTS IN NORMAL AND PATHOLOGIC PHYSIOLOGY

- ✦ Metabolic functions
- ✦ Neuroregulation of liver function
- ✦ Correlations of the anatomofunctional compartments
- ✦ The liver and homeostasis
- ✦ Hepatic insufficiency and hepatic coma

THE LIVER AND SURGERY

- ✦ Preoperative preparation and anesthesia
- ✦ Shock and resuscitation in surgical hepatobiliary patients
- ✦ Postoperative complications
- ✦ Wound healing in hepatobiliary diseases

THE PATHOLOGIC PHYSIOLOGY OF HEPATIC REGENERATION

- ✦ Importance of the experimental method for study of the normal and pathologic physiology of the liver
- ✦ Methods of study of hepatic regeneration

The documentary material referring to the normal and pathologic physiology of the liver has increased very much so that not even a list of the works published in this field during the last ten years could be included within a few pages.

This, however, is not our aim; we do not propose to discuss the physiology of the liver but only the aspects of importance to the surgeon, either because they are connected with the pathogeny of certain surgical conditions, or because they represent fundamental hepatic processes, without which existence is not possible.

FUNDAMENTAL ASPECTS IN NORMAL AND PATHOLOGIC PHYSIOLOGY

METABOLIC FUNCTIONS

a) **Carbohydrate metabolism.** Participation of the liver in carbohydrate metabolism was the first step in our knowledge of the physiology of the liver (Claude Bernard, 1853). From the intestine, polysaccharides reach the liver through the portal vein as monosaccharides; here they are retained and only a small part passes through the hepatic veins into the general circulation. It is considered that the liver may stock about 150—200 gm carbohydrates in polymerized glycogen form.

In the period of alimentary rest, the liver gradually releases, into the circulation, from its polysaccharide deposit, monose (glucose) which can be used by all the tissues of the normal organism. This can also be proved by the difference in glycemia levels in the portal and the hepatic veins (a difference that always exists but whose direction varies with the state of alimentary rest or digestive activity), which clearly shows the "efficiency" and importance of the liver, as an essential organ in glycoregulation. In addition, there are durable variations in peripheral glycemia in certain hepatic changes (moderate hyperglycemia in hepatitis of medium gravity, hypoglycemia in acute yellow atrophy), and severe, progressive hypoglycemia observed experimentally in total hepatectomy so that it is hard to understand how the role of the liver in glycoregulation has often been overlooked under the mirage of endocrine pancreatic glycoregulating activity.

Experimental studies have proved that glycemia levels can only be maintained in the hepatectomized animal by repeated glucose perfusions. The efficiency of fructose perfusions is limited within the first hours after hepatectomy but later the clinical aspect does not improve, and galactose perfusions are practically inefficient although the hypophysopancreatic system is intact. Moreover, in the hepatectomized animal, glucose perfusion gives a diabetic-like hyperglycemia curve, whereas in the pancreatectomized animal glucose loading gives a "normal" glycemia curve (Ekrem).

If it is borne in mind that maintenance of glycemia within normal limits is an essential condition of human life, then the particular role of the liver in carbohydrate metabolism will be readily understood.

Here, along general lines, is the metabolic chain of glucose, a hexose of first importance and its polymerized form — glycogen

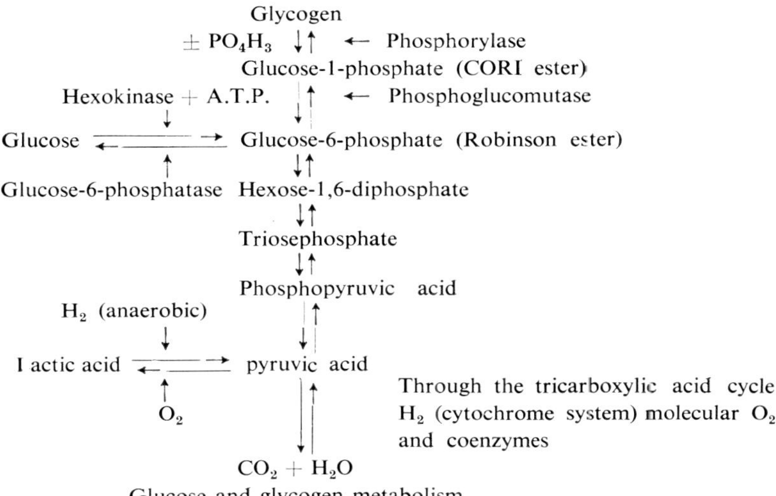

Glucose and glycogen metabolism
(according to Best and Taylor, completed)

Therefore, there is a main chain of reactions, from the polymerized form of carbohydrate (glycogen) to the ultimate forms of catabolism (O_2 and H_2O); similarly, there are two points of connection in the chain and two possible shunts:

— from glucose-6-phosphate (Robinson ester) to glucose (and conversely), and

— from pyruvic acid to lactic acid (and conversely).

This shows that, at any rate, in the glycogen-pyruvic acid segment of the chain, there are four final possibilities: glycogen, glucose, lactic acid and pyruvic acid, in terms of the internal medium and the momentary mode of action of the enzymes to certain proportion of the components.

These four substances normally occur in the human body and represent: an innocuous transport form *(glucose)*, a storage form *(glycogen)*, a transport form with a toxic effect above certain concentrations *(lactic acid)*, a connective form with the final stages of catabolic degradation *(pyruvic acid)* and other metabolisms.

On the other hand, a certain correlation exists between some of these elements: glycogen is present in many tissues, but especially in the liver and muscles; due to certain local enzymatic peculiarities, the metabolic chain of hepatic glycogen differs up to a certain point from that of muscular glycogen.

Hepatic glycogen (generated especially by hexoses but also by *lactic acid brought by the blood from the muscles* after muscular work) may be rapidly converted into hexose; on the other hand, muscular glycogen undergoes degradation in the anaerobic phase into pyruvic acid and then lactic acid (the proportions depending upon oxygen supply). However, in the muscles the converse process of glycogen synthesis from lactic acid cannot take place as it occurs only in the liver. Thus, between the two storage forms and the two transport forms there is a direct connection (as may be seen in the "Cori cycle").

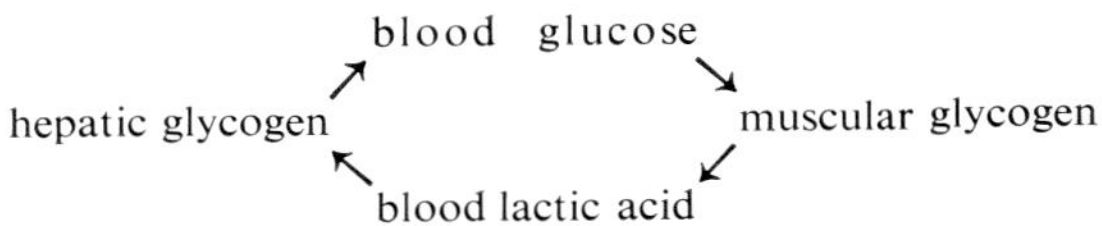

It is significant that, starting from glycogen, the energy released by degradation to lactic acid (gram molecule) is equal to about 29,000 calories, and oxidation of this amount of lactic acid into water and carbon dioxide releases about 320,000 calories. It results that *interruption of the chain of reactions with shunt to the lactic acid form* is extremely disadvantageous from the viewpoint of energy, apart from other drawbacks brought about by the increase in lactacidemia.

Other important aspects have also been revealed by biochemical investigations concerning carbohydrate metabolism in the liver.

From the scheme of biochemical reactions it results that glucose must be converted to glucose-6-phosphate under the action of *hexokinase* in order to take part in the chain of reactions, this being the first stage in glucose metabolism (glycogen is synthesized in the liver especially from hexoses). Conversely, glucose-6-phosphate (Robinson ester) may be broken down to circulating glucose under the action of hepatic glucose-6-phosphatase, this being the last stage in the release of glucose from glycogen. Thus, the two substances, free glucose and Robinson ester pass from one form into the other in terms of the predominant enzymatic action of the two enzymes, hexokinase and hexose-6-phosphatase, present in the liver. Hexokinase occurs in all the tissues, conditioning the utilization of glucose by the liver cells which possess in addition a glucokinase enzyme of their own (Lea, Walker); in the peripheral tissues, however, there is no glucose-6-phosphatase, which would explain why extrahepatic glycogen is not a source of blood sugars (Ekrem). Upon the balance between the activity of these two enzymes in the liver depends the importance of the hepatic glycogen storage and the role of the liver in glycoregulating mechanisms.

Insulin increases hexokinase activity, thus facilitating the peripheral use of glucose and the increase of hepatic glycogen storage.

On the other hand, glucagon (another pancreatic hormone) intensifies glucose-6-phosphatase (Ekrem, 1959) and phosphorylase activity (Sutherland and Cori, 1948), resulting in glycogenolysis and, consequently, in an increase in the amount of circulating glucose.

Glucagon (which might perhaps be released under the influence of the anterior pituitary) evidently acts upon glucose-6-phosphatase, whereas insulin appears to arrest the action of the *pituitary growth hormone* and *adrenocortical hormone*, which inhibits the normal activity of hexokinase; thus, insulin would *indirectly* release hypoglycemia-inducing glucokinase and hexokinase, protecting them against the influence of the adrenocorticohypophysis.

These aspects have not been studied from the viewpoint of experimental pathologic physiology, but in clinical laboratories, comparing the enzymatic activity of the human liver tissue obtained by biopsy puncture with its activity determined in the blood obtained by catheterization of the human hepatic veins

We have already seen some of the aspects of glucose metabolism and of its polymerized form — glycogen, as well as the role of the liver in this metabolism.

Bearing in mind the evident efficiency of glucose perfusions in the hepatectomized animal, the more reduced effect of fructose perfusions and the inefficiency of galactose in such animals, it has been deduced that the utilization of galactose in the organism is conditioned by its integral transformation into glucose in the *normal liver*.

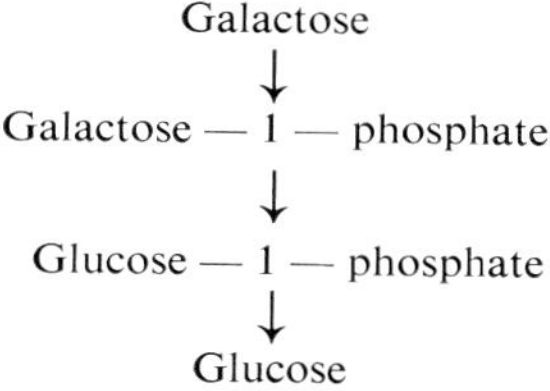

Galactose metabolism (Topper in I. Banu)

URIDINE — DIPHOSPHATE — GLUCOSE + GALACTOSE — 1 — PHOSPHATE ⇄
URIDINE — DIPHOSPHATE — GALACTOSE + GLUCOSE — 1 — PHOSPHATE

Galactose metabolism (Leloir in I. Banu)

This emphasizes the importance of the liver in carbohydrate metabolism and the possibility of using glucose tolerance tests for appraising the functional capacity of the liver. As stressed by Köhler, Lupu and Miasnikov, the administration of galactose in hepatocellular changes results in *marked, lasting* hyperglycemia.

Similarly, the necessity of partial transformation of fructose into glycogen and then into glucose, may likewise be deduced.

Finally, to conclude on carbohydrate metabolism, it should be mentioned that in the preoperative period, a maintenance ration of 2000—2500 calories is recommended, of which 75% carbohydrates (Pevzner); for the postoperative period it is rational to ensure the same amount of calories since the reparatory processes consume part of the energy supplied by food.

b) **Fat metabolism.** The chemical structure of fats or lipids is varied in the human body, which explains the numerous classifications proposed. A first separation into two categories may be accepted:

Simple lipids : fatty acid esters with different alcohols, for instance triglycerides or neutral fats;

Complex lipids : esters of fatty acids with different alcohols and other groups.

— Phospholipids (phosphatides) contain fatty acids, phosphoric acid and a base; in lecithin the base is choline, in cephalin it is amine-ethanol and in phosphatidylserine it is serine.

— Glycolipids (fatty acids + sphingosine + ose).

— Cholesterol esters, in which the base is cholesterol.

These complex lipids were grouped before under the heading lipoids, together with:

— Free cholesterol (which is an alcohol) and certain hydrocarbons (carotene), today studied separately in view of their chemical structure which determines different metabolic pathways.

Two categories of lipids may also be distinguished from another point of view: a) "constitution" lipids, in a fixed proportion in normal states, characteristic of each tissue and which take part in the formation of the cellular protoplasm (active role in certain metabolic chains), for instance *lecithins ;* and b) "storage"

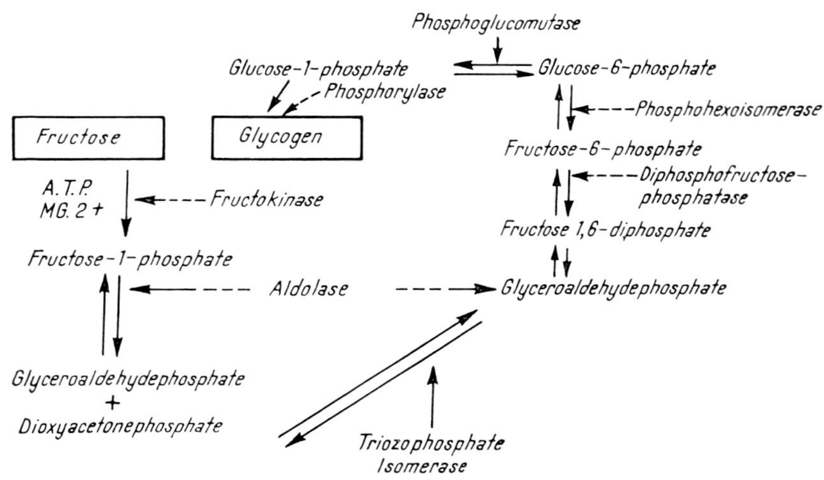

Fig. 34. — The metabolism of fructose (E. Soru).

lipids which appear in variable proportions and have a role in the metabolism of energy, being catabolized on necessity; these include triglycerides and many cholesterol esters, which are to be found in the form of fatty inclusions in the protoplasm.

A common factor is the presence of "fatty" acids in the structure of different products (except cholesterol and carotene). We shall deal firstly with the metabolism of triglycerides, particularly fatty acids.

The liver also participates in the digestion of triglycerides: bile facilitates the emulsion of fats, increasing the contact surface with the intestinal juices; bile likewise favors the activity of pancreatic lipase, which hydrolyses triglycerides into glycerine and fatty acids. The latter may be resorbed as such (Frazer) or as phosphatides (Verzar) and, finally, as cholesterol esters contained in the bile. Emulsioned triglycerides may also be resorbed since the esters of cholesterol and triglycerides may also be found on the other side of the intestinal epithelium (the enterohepatic cycle of Le Bréton).

The investigations of Chaikof (as well as those of Borgstrom) appear to prove that triglycerides containing fatty acids with a short chain (less than 12 carbon toms) penetrate into the capillaries and reach the liver together with the portal alood. On the other hand, triglycerides containing fatty acids with a longer chain bf 14 carbon atoms are taken up in the lymphatic stream of the chyliferous vessels and reach the general circulation through the thoracic duct without passing through the liver; only a small part will be stored and the rest will be catabolized in the lung (the lipodieretic function of the lung).

It has not yet been fully elucidated whether passage through the liver is absolutely necessary for fats to become apt to be stored in the subcutaneous adipose panniculum and at other sites, or whether they pass "directly into the deposits" (Kvyatkovskaya).

Experimental proof has accumulated showing that about 40% of the CO_2 deriving from the catabolism of fats is of extrahepatic origin (Chaikof and Geyer, in independent investigations). This was confirmed by the investigators who found lipolytic enzymes in different other organs: kidney, muscles, spleen, heart brain (Wolk and Cahn in independent investigations). Hence, the liver which is not the only consumer of fats is, notwithstanding, the most active *lipid oxidizer.*

The biochemical phases of fatty acid oxidation in the liver. Knoop's theory, according to which two carbon atoms successively split off from the fatty acid chain, is well known.

Normally, these two carbon units (in the form of "active acetate") are in the presence of sufficient oxalacetic acid (deriving from carbohydrate metabolism by the addition of CO_2 to pyruvic acid) to produce the condensation of acetic acid with oxalacetic acid and the oxidation of acetic acid *through* Krebs tricarboxylic cycle. A schematic representation of this cycle is given in Fig. 35 (according to Levy).

In pathologic states, the catabolism of fatty acids in the liver may result in the formation of ketone bodies, as will be seen further on.

The hepatic enzymatic system of fatty acid oxidation is located in the mitochondria. The activators of this phenomenon are: magnesium ion, ATP (adenosintriphosphate acid) and an oxidizable metabolite of the tricarboxylic cycle.

Coenzyme A interferes in the reaction by its SH groups; in the presence of ATP, the acetate chain is bound to *coenzyme A* by its substitution for H in the *SH group:* Co. A — S acetyl (or active acetate) results and will be oxidized in the Krebs cycle.

Phosphatides: investigations with ^{32}P labeled atoms or with ^{14}C-labeled choline shows that an intense and constant renewal of phosphatides takes place in the liver. These experimental and clinical findings point to the importance of choline as absolutely necessary for the normal metabolism of triglycerides.

Initially it was believed that lecithins are necessary for macromolecular complexes with triglycerides, for transport in the blood flow. However, it has been demonstrated experimentally that lecithin injected by intravenous route to the normal animal disappears within 6 hours, whereas in the hepatectomized animal in only about 100 hours. Hence, it may be assumed that different tissues may use blood lecithins (or eventually when combined with triglycerides) but that *the main consumer of lecithins is the liver.*

It has been clearly established that choline deficiency lowers the activity of the enzymatic system by oxidation of fatty acids. Moreover it was found that the addition *in vitro* of choline to the liver homogenate of an animal with deficient lipid metabolism does not stimulate the oxidation of fatty acids, although the administration *in vivo* to such deficient animals normalizes the catabolism of fatty acids. Therefore, neither choline nor phosphorylcholine are directly active, probably only lecithin; a proof is the depressor effect of lecithinase (from *Clostridium welchii*) which destroys the lecithins in the *normal liver homogenate* and consequently abolishes the fatty acid oxidation activity it initially possessed.

Hence, it may be concluded that lecithins probably *interfere as such, directly*, in the metabolism of fatty acids.

In the absence of choline, the catabolism of fatty acids does not take place at normal level. This has a double unfavorable effect: on the one hand, it withdraws from the circuit an important source of energy (1 gm lipid furnishes 9 calories,

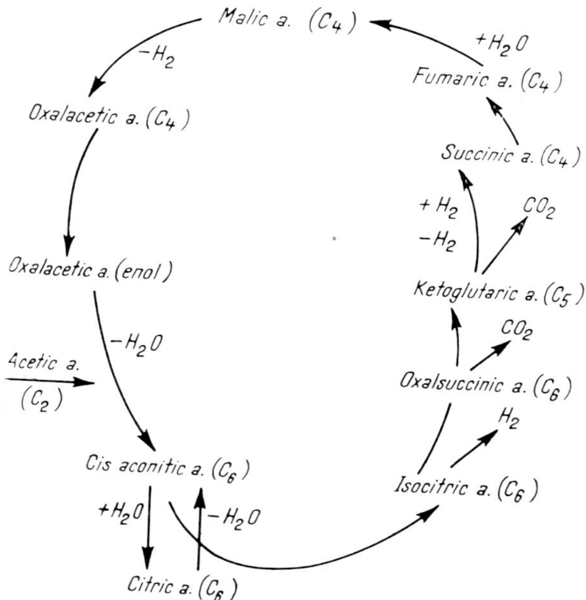

Fig. 35. — The Krebs tricarboxylic cycle.

1 gm fully used carbohydrate or protein gives only 4 calories), and on the other, triglycerides (but not sterids) accumulate in protoplasmic inclusions in the hepatic epithelial cell, giving rise to hepatic "steatosis" or "fatty liver". In terms of the amount of fatty accumulation, it may represent from the very beginning an index of metabolic deviation or may bear the stigma of severe metabolic alterations.

From the surgical point of view, the onset mechanism and existence of steatosis is *always characteristic* of a metabolic deviation which may at any moment be doubled by a consecutive deficient lipid metabolism, i.e. "ketosis", a severe clinical condition. Thus, the fatty liver may be the result of deficient nutrition, hormonal imbalance, the action of certain toxic agents.

Worthy of note among the deficient nutrition causes is the steatogenic effect of malnutrition, of a hypoprotein hyperlipid diet with excess carbohydrates, diets without essential fatty acids or with the addition of liver (containing cholesterol, with a steatogenic effect). Similarly, it should be emphasized that the unfavorable effect of a steatogenic diet is accentuated by the addition of vitamins B_1, B_2 and PP, as well as by vitamin B_6 or B_{12} deficiency. Among the amino acids, cystine added in a proportion of 12% to the normal diet confers upon it a steatogenic effect.

Among the causes of "hormonal imbalance with a steatogenic effect" are:

— insulin insufficiency and several postpancreatectomy states when insulin is not administered;

— excessive (or therapeutic) activity of the growth hormone type, ACTH or total retrohypophyseal extract.

It is naturally of interest to study the action of certain antisteatogenic factors, known under the name of lipotropic factors.

Choline is the most active lipotropic factor; its effect is clear-cut in most cases, excepting in fatty liver due to an antehypophyseal effect or to the toxic action of phosphorus. Choline may be replaced by methionine which plays the role of precursor, or by the pancreatic lipocaic hormone, which is actually efficient because of the large amount of choline it contains.

Choline lowers hepatic steatosis and reduces to normal ketogenesis, fatty acid enzymatic oxidation in the liver *(in vivo)* and hepatic glycogenesis.

Inositol, which may be found in phosphatides, can likewise be used as a lipotropic factor, efficient especially in biotin fatty liver (vitamin H), cholesterol fatty liver, fatty liver due to a hypoprotein, hyperlipid and hyperglucidic diet.

Cholesterol, listed among the lipids owing to certain physical properties, has the chemical property of a superior alcohol. In man, cholesterol biosynthesis has been unquestionably demonstrated; only part of the cholesterol derives from food, the rest being synthesized in the liver and adrenals from *acetyl* fragments, resulting from the catabolism of fatty acids. It is to be found in the blood in a proportion of 0.15 to 0.20 gm% and may increase very much in pathologic states, malnutrition and pregnancy. Increase in the amount of blood cholesterol may give the serum a lactescent aspect if there is not a corresponding increase in phosphatides.

In hepatobiliary pathology, cholesterol is of twofold importance:

— it is a component of the bile;

— it may supply information on the functional capacity of the liver; *in the blood*, cholesterol is partly free and partly esterified with superior fatty acids. *Esterified cholesterol* indices are normally 0.5—0.7, and may decrease pathologically to 0.4 or even 0.3, giving a warning of the patient's low resistance in the preoperative period or accounting for the unfavorable evolution of a postoperative complication.

In 1958, Garattini demonstrated experimentally that cholesterol biosynthesis is blocked by phenyl-ethyl acetic acid, which inhibits *coenzyme A* activity, pointing once again to the metabolic importance of this coenzyme.

Vitamin A (carbohydrate structure) is present in the organism in the form of an unsaturated alcohol — $C_{20}H_{30}O$ — and is derived from the plant pigment carotene. Under the favorable influence of lecithins and bile salts, carotene absorbed from the food in the intestines is converted 30 to 50% into vitamin A (perhaps in the intestinal mucosa), which is almost all (95%) stocked in the liver. Vitamin A appears to play the role of an oxidoreducing agent together with other, as yet, undetermined substances. Its indirect antiinfectious role (by a protective effect upon the epithelium) and its role in the function of the retina makes us pay particular attention to the cycle of vitamin A. The liver interferes in this cycle by facilitating provitamine resorption from the intestine; a functional hepatic deficit, even if it is mild, may be manifested by an insufficient extraction of carotene from the intestinal content resulting in hemeralopia and alteration of the integument, mucosa, etc. Since vitamin A absorption is not influenced by the bile and, therefore, a normal plasma concentration can be obtained in icteric patients by adding vitamin A to the diet, the quantitative determination of vitamin A cannot supply information on the functional state of the liver, as was expected at a given moment. Certain clinical aspects will be stressed further on; for the moment it should be recalled that the administration of active vitamin A may build up again vitamin A reserves in the Kupffer cells, even in the presence of a hepatobiliary deficit.

c) **Protein metabolism.** Proteins represent about nine tenths of the dry substance of the protoplasm and the actual indispensable substrate of the phenomena of cellular life.

Chemically, they are made up of amino acids in variable amounts *(simple proteins)* or of *simple proteins bound with chemical groups of another origin* (nucleoproteins, chromoproteins, etc.) and, finally, they may be *derivatives* due to splitting of the first two groups *(protein derivatives)*.

Life is conditioned by the constant change and renewal of the proteins which represent living matter, otherwise stated countless biochemical processes ceaselessly take place in each of the cells of an organism. Therefore, protein metabolism must be understood as a vast, complex phenomenon that occurs over an incalculable surface and throughout the whole depth of the substance which forms the living organism.

This is protein metabolism in its general aspect but it does not follow that the same phenomena take place in the same way in all the tissues: in the evolved organism, with differentiated tissues, all the phases of metabolic transformation *are not identical* in all the tissues. From the quantitative point of view (and even qualitative as regards certain biochemical phenomena) there are preferential or even exclusive sites of protein metabolism in certain metabolic stages.

Thus the liver, an organ with a complex metabolic activity, plays a particularly important role in protein metabolism, as may be seen from the following schematic description.

Amino acid metabolism : food proteins are broken down in the gastrointestinal tract to resorbable amino acid forms (negligible amounts may be resorbed as polypeptides, but play no important role in nutrition).

Biochemical study of amino acid concentrations in the portal blood and hepatic veins has shown that the liver retains most of the amino acids brought by the portal blood and that in the blood leaving the liver the amount of *urea* increases. Thus, a chain of biochemical transformations was established between the initial (amino acid) and the end form (urea) of amino acid metabolism.

In man, urea is the normal, end stage in the metabolism of the amino acid nitrate fraction, next to catabolism of the remaining "fatty acid" molecule to CO_2 and H_2O.

Ureogenesis represents, however, only one of the pathways taken by the amino acid molecule, its *complete disintegration with the supply of energy* and waste products. From the metabolic point of view, proteins are comparable to the other nutritive principles (carbohydrates and lipids), but they also play another role in the economy of the organism, that of building up morphologic structures. In order to be integrated in the protoplasm of the living organism, proteins must be brought into the circulation as amino acids or better said, *certain amino acids*, corresponding to those which undergo degradation by the wear and tear inherent to cellular life.

The human organism possesses a large capacity of amino acid conversion into one or other form, except *for 10 essential amino acids* which must be received as such in the gastrointestinal tract (threonine, valine, leucine, isoleucine, arginine, lysine, methionine, tryptophane, phenylalanine and perhaps histidine). The remaining 15 amino acids can be synthesized in the organism, transamination and transmethylation playing an important part in this synthesis. Points of contact exist between these two more important metabolic pathways (energy-producing and structural), as shall be seen.

The amino acid that reaches the liver may undergo *oxidative deamination* (a phenomenon which does not occur elsewhere in the human body); following the intervention of certain enzymes several biochemical phenomena take place (according to Best and Taylor):

$$\begin{array}{ccc} \text{R} & & \text{R} \\ | & & | \\ \text{CHNH}_2 & \rightarrow & \text{C} = \text{NH} + 2\text{H} \rightarrow \text{at the hydrogen acceptor} \\ | & & | \\ \text{COOH} & & \text{COOH} \\ \alpha\text{-amino acid} & & \alpha\text{-imino acid} \end{array}$$

Therefore, the α-amino acid (under the influence of α-aminoxidase, glycinoxidase, or L. glutamic acid dehydrogenase) loses 2 hydrogen atoms and is transformed into an α-imino acid.

Finally, the imino acid is hydrolysed into α-keto acid:

$$\begin{array}{ccc} \text{R} & & \text{R} \\ | & & | \\ \text{C} = \text{NH} + \text{H}_2\text{O} & \rightarrow & \text{C} = \text{O} + \text{NH}_3 \\ | & & | \\ \text{COOH} & & \text{COOH} \\ \alpha\text{-imino acid} & & \alpha\text{-keto acid} \end{array}$$

Deamination will finally give a *keto-acid* and *ammonia*. It is only at this point that ammonia enters the *ureogenesis* chain. Along general lines, the phenomenon of ureogenesis takes place according to Krebs in the following phases:

Ammonia is bound to CO_2 and ornithin (an amino acid), producing citrulline:

$$NH_3 + CO_2 + NH_2 - (CH_2)_3 - CHNH_2 - COOH \rightarrow O = \underset{\displaystyle NH - (CH_2)_3 - CHNH_2 - COOH}{\overset{\displaystyle NH_2}{\overset{|}{\underset{|}{C}}}}$$

Another ammonia molecule is bound to citrulline and produces arginine.

$$\underset{\text{citrulline}}{O = \underset{\displaystyle NH-(CH_2)_3-CHNH_2-COOH}{\overset{\displaystyle NH_2}{\overset{|}{\underset{|}{C}}}}} + NH_3 \rightarrow \underset{\text{arginine}}{HN = \underset{\displaystyle NH-(CH_2)_3-CHNH_2-COOH}{\overset{\displaystyle NH_2}{\overset{|}{\underset{|}{C}}}}} + \underset{\text{water}}{H_2O}$$

Finally arginine, under the influence of arginase (present in the liver of mammals) is hydrolyzed into urea and ornithine (the cycle can be taken up again with new ammonia molecules, formed in the course of deamination).

$$\underset{\text{arginine}}{HN = \underset{\displaystyle NH-(CH_2)_3-CHNH-COOH}{\overset{\displaystyle NH_2}{\overset{|}{\underset{|}{C}}}}} + \underset{\text{water}}{H_2O} \longrightarrow \underset{\text{urea}}{O = C\begin{matrix} \diagup NH_2 \\ \diagdown NH_2 \end{matrix}} + \underset{\text{ornithin}}{NH_2-(CH_2)_3-CHNH_2-COOH}$$

Discussions have arisen concerning the citrulline-arginine stage, reaction in which ammonia may not be necessary as such, but is produced by transamination, the nitrate donor being either glutamic acid (aerobic reaction in the presence of magnesium ions and adenosine triphosphate, according to Cohen and Hayana) or aspartic acid (anaerobic reaction also necessitating the presence of ATP and Mg ions, according to Ratner).

Transamination demonstrated by Kritzman and Braunstein, who incubated liver fragments with L. glutamic acid and pyruvic acid, consists in the transfer of the NH_2 group from the amino acid to the keto acid and results in another amino and another keto acid, as follows:

$$\begin{matrix} COOH \\ | \\ (CH_2)_2 \\ | \\ CH-NH_2 \\ | \\ COOH \end{matrix} + \begin{matrix} CH_3 \\ | \\ C = O \\ | \\ COOH \end{matrix} + \text{transaminase} \rightarrow \begin{matrix} COOH \\ | \\ (CH_2)_2 \\ | \\ C = O \\ | \\ COOH \end{matrix} + \begin{matrix} CH_3 \\ | \\ CHNH_2 \\ | \\ COOH \end{matrix}$$

L. glutamic acid + pyruvic acid ⟶ α-ketoglutaric acid + alanine

Transamination is of capital importance for the transformation of alimentary amino acids into the amino acids necessary for reconstruction of the living cell substance; similarly, transamination appears to play a part in the metabolic chain of ureogenesis and also takes place in tissues other than the liver.

On the other hand, deamination supplies the ammonia necessary for the first stage of ureogenesis and also supplies the *keto acids* which will subsequently take part in the transamination reactions; thus deamination is a key phenomenon both for directing the amino acid towards energy-releasing catabolism and for integration of the amino acid in the structural forms characteristic of the organism. Deamination occurs *in the liver* and it may, therefore be readily understood why amino acid perfusions in the hepatectomized animal cannot prolong existence even inasmuch as glucose perfusions.

The schematic representation of amino acid metabolism helps us to appraise the key-role played by the liver in the degradation and utilization of simple proteins (formed by peptide binding of a variable number of amino acids).

There also exists another category of proteins, the so-called *conjugated proteins*, among which the nucleoproteins deserve special attention. They are to be found in large amounts in the cell nuclei and two variants have been especially studied: deoxyribonucleic or thymonucleic acid and ribonucleic acid.

They are formed of simple basic proteins (histone or protamine) and a sequence of 4 nucleotides.

The nucleotide is formed of: phosphoric acid + pentose + a purine or pyrimidine base. To go into greater detail, thymonucleic acid contains a pentose: D.2-deoxyribose, two purine bases: adenine and guanine, and two pyrimidine bases: thymine and cytosine.

Deoxyribonucleic acid is concentrated in the chromosomes and, to a lesser extent, in the cytoplasm.

Ribonucleic acid has a pentose — D. ribose — and a pyrimidine base — uracyl instead of thymine; this acid is present especially in the protoplasm and nucleoli.

Modern studies have shown that in the phases of cellular multiplication significant variations appear in the concentration and distribution of these nucleic acids, both in the nucleus and protoplasm. These studies applied to the liver supplied histochemical indications concerning the regenerative or atrophic evolution of the hepatic epithelial tissue after certain toxic conditions and made it possible to appraise the intensity of the recovery phenomena after hepatic resection.

Nucleic acids are broken down by tissue nucleases into tetranucleotides, which the nucleotidases split into phosphoric acid and *nucleosides*; the latter, under the influence of specific cellular enzymes *(nucleosidases)* liberate pentose and the purine or pyrimidine base remains.

At present the catabolism of purines in man, whose end product is *uric acid*, is alone well known. The site of uric acid formation has not been well established, but it is known that its transition from the previous phase (xanthine) to uric acid is only possible under the influence of xanthine oxidase, which *is to be found in the liver alone*; this suggests that the liver plays a part in the uric acid cycle at least at a given moment. On the other hand, uric acid is destroyed to a great extent in the liver (resulting in unknown substances), which again shows the important role of the liver next to other tissues and the kidneys, as an essential organ in clearing the blood of uric acid and maintaining the uric acid balance.

From the above, it results that the liver also interferes in the metabolism of nucleoproteins, although less decisively than in that of simple proteins. These basic facts allow us to approach the question of the utilization of proteins.

The organism requires with its food supply the 9—10 indispensable amino acids and a certain amount of the other amino acids, which can be synthesized (especially in the liver) by transamination, using deamination products in the first place.

Therefore, the use of proteins with component amino acids differing very much from those of the body cell depends upon the capacity of the liver to synthesize the necessary amino acids to be found in only reduced amounts in the food. With the same food made of lower plant proteins (beans, maize), the ponderal curve will be more or less altered in terms of the capacity for functional effort of the liver.

On the other hand, when the necessary amino acids occur in the food but in reduced proportions, the organism will rapidly break down a large amount of proteins until it obtains the necessary amounts of these amino acids. Therefore, it will not be able to use the entire quantity of proteins ingested for repair of the tissues, because the organism needs these indispensable amino acids only in *a given proportion with respect to the other amino acids* and what remains in excess of the non-essential acids will be catabolyzed along energy-producing lines, with intense deamination, which is probably responsible for the specific, dynamic action of proteins. Under these conditions *heat and urea* are produced, and loss of body weight will occur if the food intake does not insure equal amounts of calories with a specific basal metabolism + dynamic action. Hence, in a patient whose liver has a limited or subnormal functional capacity, excess proteins in the food is not a good solution; it is preferable to administer reduced amounts of highly digestible proteins, rich in indispensable amino acids, together with hydrocarbons and lipids in adequate amounts for the necessary quantum of calories.

This question will again be mentioned when dealing with the relationship between fundamental metabolisms and preoperative preparation.

The three preceding paragraphs describe the more important stages in the metabolism of hydrocarbons, lipids and proteins; however, these three main metabolic lines have many common points or zones of interference.

Part of these common points or zones of interference are well known today; actually, the current observation that life can be maintained with very different diets suggests that the organism can synthesize (up to a given limit) certain nutritive principles from substances of another category.

In the following paragraphs we shall recall some of the main stages that take place in the liver.

Glycosynthesis in the organism. Under normal conditions, alimentation offers sufficient amounts of carbohydrates; carbohydrate metabolism expresses the transformation of ingested carbohydrates in the organism. When the food is predominantly protein, the organism can still maintain its normal function by deriving part of the amino acids into carbohydrate metabolism, i.e. the largest part of the fatty acid molecule remaining after amino acid deamination in the liver (Fig. 36). Not all amino acids are glycogenetic, only: glycine, alanine, aspartic acid, glutamic and hydroxyglutamic acids, serine, cystine (with a straight chain), proline and oxyproline (heterocyclic acids), and, to a lesser extent, arginine, valine and threonine.

For carnivores, the mechanism of glycosynthesis from proteins is fundamental; man, an omnivorous animal, uses this mechanism imperfectly and hence, an excessive meat diet is not to be recommended. Even the rabbit may change its dominant metabolism under certain particular conditions, as noted by Claude Bernard:

when starving, it will use up its own tissues for maintaining its life (it becomes carnivorous in its main metabolic functions).

In the organism, about half the proteins ingested can be converted into glucose, with certain variations that depend not only upon the individual but also upon some undetermined factors.

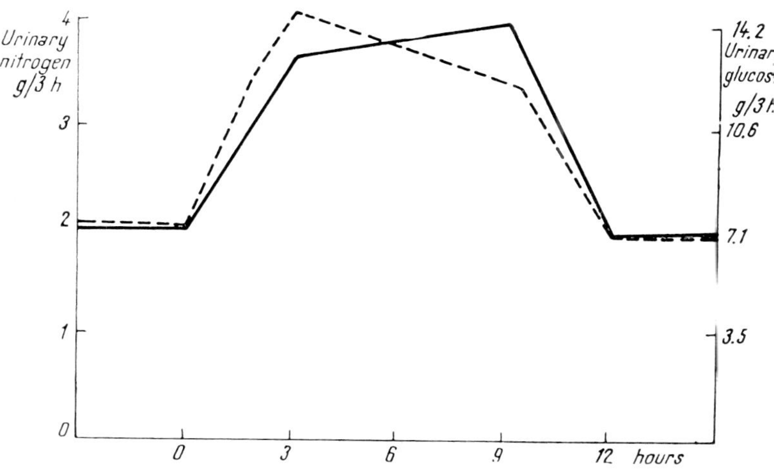

Fig. 36. — The formation of sugars from proteins (Lusk in Fulton). fluorhizinized dog fed on 500 g meat:
— — — urinary glucose;
——— urinary nitrogen.

It has been established by biochemical investigations and radioactive isotopes that the transition from fatty acids to carbohydrates occurs through an active acetate stage (acetyl-coenzyme A), after oxidation with splitting into segments of two carbon atoms of the fatty acid.

The acetyl-coenzyme A phase is fundamental in lipid metabolism and this shows how lipids can also contribute to the synthesis of glucose; however, at least in humans, the participation of lipids to carbohydrate synthesis is not very important as demonstrated by the studies carried out with radioactive isotopes.

Lipid synthesis. It is known that an increase in the adipose deposit can be obtained with a carbohydrate diet. It appears that the transition from carbohydrate to lipid metabolism likewise takes place through an *acetyl-coenzyme A* stage, after which the enzymes can catalyze the binding of carbon atom pairs fragments into long fatty acid structures. Fragments of the amino acid chain likewise pass through this stage. This stands true both for triglycerides and for cholesterol synthesis. Plasma cholesterol is chiefly synthesized in the liver and only a small part is supplied with the food.

Protein synthesis. As already mentioned, amino acid synthesis can be obtained in the organism by transamination starting from keto acids of the same chain length; the respective keto acids may sometimes derive from carbohydrate metabolism (for instance pyruvic acid from which alanine may derive).

Experimental incubation of liver fragments in certain nitrate and non-nitrate mixtures or perfusion of the liver rich in glycogen with an ammonium chloride

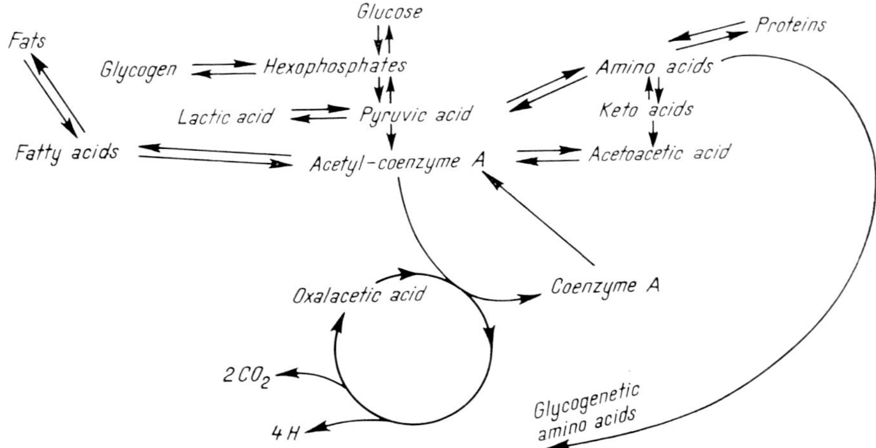

Fig. 37. — Metabolic interrelations (Fulton).

solution, demonstrates that amino acid synthesis, within the limitations of the human body, takes place mainly in the liver. Hence, to the extent in which the function of the liver is restricted, amino acid synthesis will be correspondingly deficient.

However, it should be recalled that the possibilities of the organism to synthesize amino acids are limited both qualitatively (there are 10—12 essential amino acids, indispensable to life, that cannot be synthesized) and quantitatively, hence the diet must obligatorily contain a minimal amount of proteins. Of the purines, arginine and histidine, which form part of the nucleoproteins, are indispensable for their synthesis.

From this brief outline, results the actual interference of the metabolic chains, as well as the importance of certain phenomena that occur predominantly or exclusively in the liver (such as deamination, fatty acid oxidation, acetylation of coenzyme A, etc. (Fig. 37). A practical consequence of this interference is the influence exerted by one category of foodstuffs upon the utilization of other nutritive principles (in the reserves of the organism). Worthy of note is the protein sparing action of carbohydrates and lipids since their presence relieves tissue protein of the necessity of furnishing energy.

In inanition, nitrate excretion is maximum and diminishes with administration of a diet richer in calories and more varied; in a protein-free diet with sufficient calories minimal nitrate excretion is obtained, expressing the inevitable disintegration of the body tissues (the wear and tear coefficient). There are two different aspects in this connection.

The calories supplied by carbohydrates or lipids avoid catabolism of the body's own proteins along energy lines (amino acid spoliation); in this instance, an inadequate fuel (tissue protein) is substituted by an adequate one (lipids or carbohydrates).

Carbohydrates also spare proteins since a strictly lipid diet does not lower the excessive utilization of the body's own proteins. Whereas a carbohydrate diet lowers nitrogen excretion very much (therefore protein catabolism).

Lipids, which do not protect body proteins, greatly enhance the protective action of carbohydrate when associated with them.

From these findings it must be concluded that in the diet of the normal subject, and all the more so in that of a subject with a limited hepatic functional capacity, proteins should be obligatorily included, but in restricted amounts in terms of the wear and tear coefficient.

Carbohydrates, the most adequate energy-producing material should be given in large amounts the more manifest is the alteration of the physiologic condition (bearing in mind the specifics of the case, for instance diabetes).

The introduction of lipids in the diet will be necessary the greater is the necessity of restricting nitrate extraction (with associated renal clearance deficit); when the patient's condition does not make it possible to associate lipids, carbohydrates must be used instead.

Reference has been made several times to *coenzyme A*; it is now pertinent to give a brief description of the known data referring to its nature and role.

Coenzyme A (acetylation coenzyme) was discovered at the same time by Nahmanson in the U.S.S.R. and Lippman in the U.S.A. (Şoimu). It has the following chemical structure (Best and Taylor):

```
            I
 ___________^___________
 H—S—CH2—CH2—NH
              |
              C = O      |       N—C—NH2              |
              |          |       |  |                 |
              CH2        |      HC  C—N               |
              |          |      ||  ||   \C           |
              CH2        |       N—C—N /              |
              |          |             |              |
              NH         | II          HC ——          | IV
              |          |             |     |        |
              C = O      |            HCOH   |        |
              |          |             |     |     OH |
              CHOH       |             HC —— | —O—P = O
              |          |             |     O     OH |
       CH3·C·CH3         | OH    OH    CH ———         |
              |            |     |     |              |
              CH2—O—P—O—P—O—CH2                        |
                      ||    ||
                      O     O
                     ___v___
                       III
```

Part I corresponds to thioethylamine, II to pantothenic acid, III to pyrophosphoric acid, IV to adenosine (with a phosphate radical at carbon 3 of ribose). Hence coenzyme A may be considered a nucleotide.

Coenzyme A takes part in the biochemical reactions by means of the HS group of thiolethylamine, which binds it to the labile acetyl group resulting in the macroergic thiolester-acetyl-coenzyme A bond (active acetate), which can be broken down by certain enzymes.

The following are the main biochemical phenomena conditioned by the intervention of coenzyme A:

In carbohydrate metabolism, the complete utilization of glucose can only take place in the presence of coenzyme A, which permits entrance of the pyruvic acid — lactic acid stages in Krebs cycle, integrally releasing CO_2 energy and water.

In the metabolism of fatty acids (resulting from lipids) the presence of coenzyme A is essential for oxidation. This normally takes place when there are sufficient amounts of oxalacetic acid (deriving from carbohydrate metabolism); an abnormal shift occurs towards the production of ketone bodies when the amount of oxalacetic acid is insufficient.

Thus, pyruvic acid appears to be a turn-table between the three main metabolisms, but it can only be taken up in Krebs cycle in the presence of coenzyme A.

The presence of coenzyme A is likewise essential in the synthesis of tripeptides, such as glutathione.

In the synthesis of glycoproteins *in the liver*, an acetic radical of acetyl coenzyme A is bound to glucosamine or galactose-amine, an initial stage in the synthesis of mucins and chondroitins.

In the synthesis of phospholipids: 3 stearin — coenzyme A + α glycerophosphate → 3 phospholipid + 3 coenzyme A.

In the synthesis of sterols: the sterol ring is synthesized from the acetyl coenzyme A groups in the liver, adrenals and testicles. In experimental application of this concept, Garattini and Paoletti blocked the synthesis of cholesterol with diphenyl-ethyl-acetic acid that inhibits coenzyme A, thus checking in practice the data supplied by physiology.

The synthesis of porphyrin (the first stage of hemoglobin synthesis) takes place in the presence of coenzyme A.

Hippuric acid synthesis can only occur in the presence of coenzyme A (the liver is the site of maximum synthesis).

The resynthesis of acetylcholine from choline is facilitated by the presence of acetyl-coenzyme A.

The acetylation of sulfonamides takes place in the liver under the action of coenzyme A.

Acetylation inactivating histamine likewise takes place in the liver under the action of acetyl-coenzyme A.

The biosynthesis of glucocorticoids with an antiphlogistic effect starts from cholesterol in the presence of codehydrase I and coenzyme A.

After having listed the main biochemical phenomena in which coenzyme A takes part, it should be emphasized that the *principal coenzyme A storage site is to be found in the liver*, which implicitly explains the importance of hepatic participation in the fundamental metabolic processes.

However, a specific of the enzymatic conditions in which the activity of coenzyme A takes place in the liver, is the existence of highly active deacylase which catalyses the following reaction:

acetoacetyl—S—CoA ⇄ acetyl acetic acid + HS—CoA (free coenzyme A), next to a less efficient enzyme which gives a converse effect:

acetyl acetic acid + succinyl—S—CoA⇄acetoacetyl—S—CoA + succinic acid.

In other words, in the liver, in carbohydrate deficit with an excessive supply of lipids, there exists a massive release of ketone body precursors, while in other organs (heart, kidney, muscles) there is another enzymatic dominance and hence a tendency to a rapid utilization of ketogenic substances brought by the circulation.

In carbohydrate deficit, ketone bodies can be used up to a certain extent by the extrahepatic tissues as a source of energy. However, their appearance in the inner medium soon brings about pH disturbances (they are relatively powerful acids), which can only be compensated for some time by mobilization of the bases, spoliation of the alkaline reserve, increased renal aminogenesis and rapid excretion through the urine, together with polypnea that removes the maximum amount of CO_2 from the blood. However, (neutralized) excretion of the ketone bodies represents a loss of energy, a further negative aspect added to acidosis, negative nitrate balance and dehydration, i.e. the nocuous effects of ketosis, state in which the liver plays an important part.

d) **Pigment metabolism and biligenesis in normal and pathologic states.**

The exocrine function of the liver is represented by bile secretion.

Normally, about 700—1000 ml bile are produced in 12 hours. Bile normally contains:

	%
Water	95.5 —97.5
Dry residue	2.5 — 3.5
Bile pigments	0.4 — 0.5
Bile acid salts	0.9 — 1.8
Cholesterine	0.06— 0.16
Mineral substances	0.07— 0.08

Once the bile has reached the gallbladder it is concentrated by the resorption of water, without any significant change in the proportion of the other components, although cholesterol may exhibit certain fluctuations which are independent of the other solid substances.

Today, the origin and physiologic significance of most of the bile components is well known.

Bile pigments. As far back as 1874, I. P. Tarkhanov proved experimentally that the bile pigments increase after hemolysis or hemoglobin injection, thus proving that bilirubin (the main bile pigment) derives from hemoglobin; he likewise showed that intravenous injection of bilirubin increases the elimination of this pigment from the bile, therefore proving that the liver takes up and eliminates this pigment even when supplied by other organs.

It has been demonstrated that from 1 gm hemoglobin, 40 mg bilirubin can be produced (Gordienko). Other negligible sources of bile pigment also exist, such as myoglobin and the respiratory enzyme cytochrome C, as shown by investigations with ^{15}N radioactive isotope, incorporated in the hemoglobin molecule (Sherlock).

The bile pigment is the only waste product:

hemoglobin ⇄ iron (stocked in the liver)	+	globin (passes among the proteins)	+	bilirubin (excreted in the bile)

These cardinal points, known for some time, are still valid but the same cannot be stated about the explanations given to the phases of biligenesis.

The various hypotheses, partly supported by biochemical findings gave rise to theories whose result is perhaps the great number of nomenclatures which maintain a fair amount of confusion in an already complicated problem.

For the moment, here is a list of certain chemical forms that are found in the products collected from man or living animals.

Bilirubin : the main bile pigment, with two forms that can be differentiated by the van den Bergh test in "direct and indirect" bilirubin.

Stercobilinogen : bilirubin modified under the influence of the intestinal microbial flora (more seldom the bacteria that penetrate into the bile ducts).

Stercobilin : an oxidized form of stercobilinogen.

Urobilinogen : identical in structure to stercobilinogen, is to be found in the fresh urine.

Urobilin : identical as structure to stercobilin, the oxidized form of urobilinogen, appears in the urine under the influence of atmospheric oxygen.

Therefore, in the blood there is bilirubin and one or the other derivative; conventionally, the bile pigments in the feces have been called stercobilinogen and stercobilin, and in the urine urobilinogen and urobilin, although their chemical identity has been established.

Let us now return to the phases of biligenesis.

Some time ago, Hymans van den Bergh found that in contact with Ehrlich's diazoreagent, serum bilirubin may give either a *delayed staining reaction* with the slow appearance of azopigment, or an *immediate reaction.*

Since the first type of reaction can be hastened by adding alcohol, it has also been called the indirect reaction and the second test, without the addition of alcohol, the direct reaction. This has led to the differentiation of two kinds of bilirubin:

— direct (producing the azopigment on direct contact with the diazoreagent);

— indirect (producing the azopigment with the diazoreagent when alcohol is added).

The finding that indirect bilirubin is to be found in large amounts in the serum of patients with hemolytic jaundice, without passing into the urine, and direct bilirubin is found in larger amounts in the serum and urine of patients with obstructive jaundice, points to the conclusion that actually two forms of pigment exist with different chemical properties and probably different genesis.

From the documented theories of Lemberg and Watson two erroneous conclusions, concerning the intermediary phases of biligenesis, resulted:

— From hemoglobin to indirect and then to direct bilirubin, a series of hydrolysis reactions take place with progressive simplification of the complex hemoglobin molecule.

— "Indirect" hemoglobin represents a pigment + globin complex, a large molecule whose magnitude prevents it from passing through the renal filter.

Both conclusions proved inconsistent.

Electrophoretic studies (Gray-Martin) have shown that both kinds of bilirubin migrate together with albumins, and in 1953 Cole-Lathe separated by chromatography two pigments, of which one elutes rapidly and gives the direct reaction and the other slowly, giving the indirect reaction; neither of these bile pigments contain proteins (Sherlock).

Finally, Schmid prepared azopigments A (corresponding to "indirect" bilirubin) and B (corresponding to "direct" bilirubin).

It should be emphasized that hydrolysis of azopigment B (from direct bilirubin) releases glycuronic acid, which is bound to the carboxyl group of propionic acid, so that today it is admitted that bile bilirubin, which appears in the urine in case of an obstacle in the bile ducts, is a *diglycuronoconjugated pigment* (Schiff), that passes through the renal filter, although it has a larger molecule, than indirect bilirubin just because the glycuronoconjugated form is more hydrosoluble (this also explains its rapid elution from the chromatographic column).

It is now easier to represent the pigment cycle. Hemoglobin is split into three components (iron-globin-pigmentary tetrapyrolic nucleus) by the cells in the reticuloendothelial systems throughout the organism and, as such, the hepatic Kupffer cells also take part in this phenomenon.

Iron is stocked in the liver, globin is encompassed in the protein fund of the organism and the pigment is "indirect" (or prehepatic) bilirubin.

The liver epithelial cells take up this pigment and conjugate it with glycuronic acid, excreting it into the bile ducts in the form of "direct" (or hepatic) bilirubin.

In the intestine, bilirubin is transformed by bacteria into stercobilinogen, part of which is eliminated through the feces (about 300 mg/day) and part is resorbed and returns to the liver with the portal blood. The normal liver retains stercobilinogen from the blood and excretes it as such, or in less studied forms (used perhaps for the resynthesis of hemoglobin or stimulating hematopoiesis-Gordienko), and a small part escapes from the liver into the general circulation and is excreted by the kidneys as urobilinogen (about 4 mg/24 hours).

When excessive amounts of prehepatic bilirubin reach the liver, they cannot be excreted at an unlimited rate, and hemolysis increases indirect bilirubin in the blood.

If the bile ducts are blocked, direct bilirubin is "regurgitated" (Rich) into the blood capillaries and then passes from the blood into the urine.

When the cells are altered the liver can no longer retain the indirect bilirubin supplied by the reticuloendothelial system (indirect bilirubin increases in the blood) and neither can it excrete all the direct glycuronoconjugated bilirubin produced, part of which returns to the blood: direct bilirubin likewise increases in the blood and will appear in the urine.

Urinary urobilinogen variations will depend upon:

— the appearance of stercobilinogen in the intestine, in the absence of which urobilinogen disappears from the urine (the interrupted cycle in obstructive jaundice);

— the capacity of the liver to retain stercobilinogen (urobilinogen) brought from the intestine by the portal vein; alterations of the liver cell lower the uptake of urobilinogen, which increases in the urine. As already mentioned, exaggerated hemolysis, even with a normal liver, exceeding its uptake capacity, increases urinary urobilinogen with increase of indirect blood bilirubin, which does *not* appear in the urine.

Bile acid salts. Steroids with a cholanic nucleus, differ by the number and position of their hydroxyl groups (Sherlock).

— Cholic (3,7,12-trihydroxycholanic) acid is the most important; and

— Chenodeoxycholic (3,7-dihydroxycholanic) acid, is less important.

In the bile they are conjugated with two aminated acids (glycine and taurine) in the form of taurocholic and glycocolic acid.

Sodium dehydrocholate (decholin) is not a normal component of the bile.

According to its chemical structure, it is considered to derive from cholesterol, but variations in the supply of alimentary cholesterol do not modify the production of bile acids (Gordienko). However, it is certain that they are produced, concentrated and destroyed only in the liver (Grey, cited by Nash), since experimental hepatic necrosis induced with phosphorus is always accompanied by a decrease of bile acids.

The salts of these acids have a very economical turnover in the liver: from the intestine they are resorbed almost integrally (90%) and on reaching the liver they are again secreted with the bile. About 10% is synthesized daily, therefore 10% must be approximately the daily loss. These experimental findings are confirmed by the clinical data which permit appraisal of the daily losses in man at 2 gm and the daily amount secreted by the liver at 10—20 gm.

Apart from the influence of the functional capacity of the liver (Grey — postoperatively the production of bile acids decreases, alteration which is more difficultly reversible the more the liver is damaged — Nash) it was found that a carbohydrate diet lowers the production of bile acid salts and a hyperprotein diet increases it. Actually, the most adequate stimulant is the introduction of bile salts into the intestine.

The main functions of bile acid salts are:

— cholagogue action;

— the emulsion of fats in the intestine;

— to stabilize cholesterol in the bile;

— to favor the absorption of vitamin K and D and carotene from the intestine (but not the absorption of vitamin A);

— to exercise a hydrotropic action on fatty acids and their calcium soaps;

— to activate pancreatic lipase, and, to a lesser extent, gastric lipase (without any influence on intestinal lipase).

As these effects depend directly upon the concentration in which the bile salts reach the intestine, and the bile collected from a bile fistula has a very low concentration, Crandall and Ivy insisted that instead of administering bile from the drained fistula, exogenous bile should be introduced (the best is gallbladder bile).

Bile lipids — phosphatides, lecithin (in man 0.02 or 0.05%).

— Free cholesterol (0.04 to 0.16%), is maintained in solution by the presence of bile salts at a ratio of 1:13 (normal 1/30).

— Fatty acids whose presence is also necessary for maintaining cholesterol in solution.

Cholesterol has an enterohepatic circuit similar to that of biliary acids and is their adjuvant in the emulsion of fats.

Increase in the concentration of biliary cholesterol does not appear to be significantly influenced by food, but rather by the effect upon the liver of the different alterations in the patient's general state of health. No parallelism exists between its concentration in the bile and in the blood; a proof is that its concentration in the bile increases very much in pregnancy, without any evident change in cholesterolemia. However, it should be mentioned that, conversely, in mechanical obstruction of the common bile duct, cholesterolemia progressively increases until the bile duct becomes patent and biliary stasis ceases.

Minerals. No special comments are necessary as minerals only intervene in the physiologic and pathologic processes in altogether abnormal states, such as total biliary fistula of long standing. In this instance it may be attributed to alteration of the patient's general condition, to nervous reactivity, to alterations in the circulation, function of the myocardium or electrolytes caused by the loss of ions (K and Na) in the bile.

However, in most cases, these disturbances with an insidious onset do not draw attention, especially as other phenomena monopolize by their gravity the entire therapeutic effort, such as the hemorrhagic syndrome due to vitamin K deficiency.

It is none the less true that attentive care of the patient with bile loss should also have in view the mineral salts in the bile.

e) **The defense and synthesis function of the liver.** In the literature there is a remarkable diversity in the understanding and mode of exploring of the defense function of the liver. In order to avoid confusion, it is necessary to approach the subject step by step.

The liver unquestionably plays an important role in the defense mechanisms of the organism; many of the bacteria that penetrate into the blood pass through the liver and are taken up by macrophages within a few minutes (Vîsocovici and Verigo), where they undergo marked changes and are finally digested. Most of the toxins produced by bacteria are likewise neutralized in the liver by as yet insufficiently elucidated mechanisms. On the other hand, the liver participates through its reticuloendothelial tissue in the elaboration of antibodies that neutralize antigenic toxins in the blood.

In the hepatectomized animal, toxic substances such as strichnine and nicotine are destroyed far more slowly, and simple substances such as amino acids, ammonia or lactic acid produce severe disturbances in contrast to the weak effect or lack of effect after their administration to the intact animal.

Part of the exogenous substances (toxic substances) are eliminated through the bile, in less harmful forms.

Another portion of the toxins, as a rule resorbed from the gastrointestinal tract, is modified in the liver by a sequence of phenomena with the consequent appearance of less toxic derivatives, which are more readily eliminated by the kidneys. In this connection, certain synthesis processes are of particular importance for the anti-toxic function of the liver, i.e. glycuronoconjugation and sulfoconjugation.

Benzoic acid, brought by the circulation to the liver, is conjugated with glycocol (glycine), forming hippuric acid, which is less toxic and rapidly excreted by the kidneys (at the first passage). However, the phenomenon is far more complex and may also occur in the kidneys; urinary elimination of hippuric acid also depends upon the integrity of the renal function. Hence, study of this phenomenon would not be a good method for investigating the hepatic function.

Therefore, the site of synthesis is in the liver and the kidneys, but for the synthesis to take place, glycine synthesized and stored only in the liver, is necessary. The glycine reserve and the speed of its formation depend directly upon the functional state of the liver, i.e. the damaged liver will have a reduced reserve and capacity of glycine synthesis; the benzoic acid test will reveal a lesser production of hippuric acid; however, the state of the kidneys should be established as the test may be falsified by renal alteration.

The existence of a U.D.P.G.A. factor has been discovered which, with the acceptor in the presence of the hepatic tissue, leads to the synthesis of the respective glycuronide. This factor (uridin-diphosphate-glycuronic acid) is not influenced by B-glycuronidase which is present in all the tissues, and the B inhibitors of glycuronidase (saccharolactone) do not modify the synthesis of glycuronides (Dutton, cited by Jayle).

Recently, the use of ^{14}C labeled glucose showed that it can be converted into glycuronide directly, whereas glycuronic acid is not a U.D.P.G.A. precursor.

In the liver, glycuronoconjugation is constant, because bilirubin (produced by the activity of the reticuloendothelial system upon the pigment in senescent red blood cells) undergoes glycuronoconjugation before becoming an actual bile pigment. As already mentioned, the existence of a glycuronoconjugated form explains the different behavior of the two forms of bilirubin both in renal excretion and in diazoreaction.

Among the steroids, estrogens exist in the glycuronoconjugated form.

Phenols follow another route of detoxification: in the liver, phenols undergo sulfoconjugation, and certain toxic products of intestinal putrefaction (indol, scatol) can be more readily eliminated through the kidneys in these more filtrable, more hydrosoluble and less toxic forms.

In independent investigations Hilz, Robbins and Bandurski showed that phenols with an "active sulfate" take part in the reaction, i.e. 3-phosphoadenosin-5-phosphosulfate (P.A.P.S. — Jayle) deriving from ATP + Mg ions and SO_4 in the presence of certain catalysers. The last reaction is P.A.P.S. + ROH + sulfokinase $\rightleftarrows$ ROS (ester sulfate) + P.A.P. (3 phosphoadenylic acid).

Sulfoconjugation not only interferes in the cycle of certain toxic products but also in the very important cycle of certain adrenocorticohormones: corticosterone exists in sulfoconjugated form (Jayle), as aldosterone also seems to appear in the urine.

It is now possible to interpret the antitoxic and defense function of the liver. Different harmful chemical substances, toxins or even microbes encounter, in their passage through the liver, all the complex phenomena that characterize the normal function of the liver and may be taken up by one or other of the chains of these phenomena, substituting one of the normal stages.

Bacteria are phagocytized by cells that usually phagocytize red blood cells, some substances undergo glycuronoconjugation (a normal stage in the metabolism of pigment) and others sulfoconjugation, which as we have seen confers solubility to certain hormones.

Bromsulphalein (BSP) is conjugated in the liver cell with glutathione, an accelerated form of transfer from the cell into bile. A protein-free diet lowers both hepatic glutathione and the enzyme that catalyses BSP conjugation with glutathione (Combes, 1965).

In other words, at least for part of the phenomena listed, the antitoxin and defense function of the liver results from the incidental interference of certain aggressive agents with some of the phenomena characterizing the normal synthesis activity of the liver (Levy, cited by Jayle). In this sense, evaluation of the antitoxin function of the liver is a good means for measuring its functional capacity.

From the above it is concluded that the defense function of the liver is actually integrated within the complex metabolism of the liver and represents only a casual, particular instance of these permanent fundamental metabolic phenomena.

On the other hand, it should be borne in mind that excessive stress of certain normal metabolic changes by the antitoxin function will diminish the efficiency of the respective chain. Practically this may occur in patients with a functional hepatic deficiency subjected to a highly complicated therapy (Chester).

NEUROREGULATION OF LIVER FUNCTION

It is of interest to know that although Claude Bernard discovered, more or less at the same time, the role of the liver in the carbohydrate cycle and the existence of the neuroregulation of glycemia, the attention of research workers was almost exclusively concentrated on the biochemical phenomena of glycogenolysis and glycogenosynthesis. The same occurred with the study of other fundamental metabolic chains so that after a hundred years of scientific study of the liver much knowledge has been accumulated concerning the stages and the details of the biochemical phenomena but little is known about their neuroregulation.

Notwithstanding, an organ in which so many biochemical reactions occur, part of which are independent but very many interdependent, an organ that so readily adapts its multiple activities to the very requirements of the body as a whole, cannot function without a particular system of regulation. It is true that certain phenomena are governed along general lines by biochemical determinants, as proved *in vitro* by the repetition of certain of the metabolic stages on liver sections. Thus, glycogenolysis, deamination, transamination, etc. have been observed; a liver perfused with solutions rich in glucose retains glucose and, under certain conditions, may retain amino acids, etc.

Can these disparate aspects, under working conditions so far removed from the normal, lead to the conclusion that the "enzymatic systems, acceptors, donors, substrates and nutritive principles, enter and leave the reaction as an ideal robot?" In other words the question arises of the role of the nervous system in regulation of the liver functions. We shall not insist upon the well-known role of hormones but will deal especially with certain factors that must be emphasized in connection with neuroregulation.

The innervation of the liver is very rich; vital staining and argentic impregnation have shown that the terminal arborizations of the nervous fibers end not only in the vessels and bile ducts, but also in each epithelial cell (Fig. 38), pointing to the material support of the functional connexions between the neurax and the liver.

Adrenaline, as already stated, mobilizes the carbohydrate reserves of the liver (glycogenolysis), a phenomenon that has also been observed after stimulation of the sympathetic nervous system, cerebral cortex or subcortical neuroendocrine nuclei.

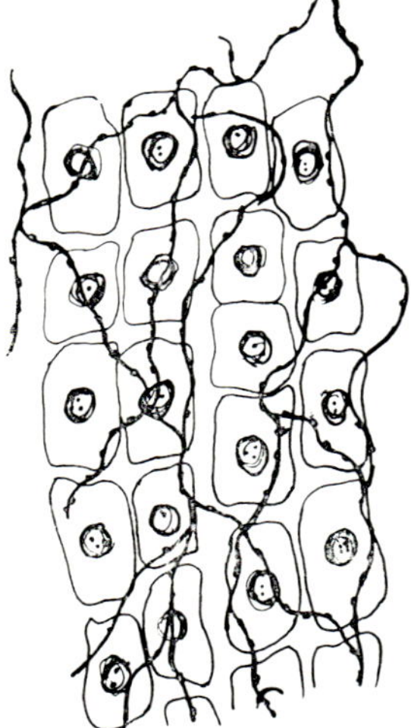

Fig. 38. — Intrinsic hepatic innervation (after Brătianu).

Pavlov's school demonstrated experimentally the existence of a regulation system governing the formation and degradation of glycogen in the liver, a system made up by the interoceptive connections of the internal organs (Kvyatkovskaya).

Breitzburg and Sedina obtained by alimentary conditioned reflexes hyperglycemia in which the liver plays a primordial part (Tucherstein), and E.B. Zakrjevskii, applying the produre of perturbation of the coordinating activity of the cortex (by "conflicts" between contrary conditioned reflexes) observed an increase in galactosuria following the administration of galactose; concomitant changes occur in the dynamics and amount of hippuric acid in the Quick-Pîtel test, which shows that at least one of the synthesis functions of the liver is disturbed.

Hence, it is no longer surprising that certain vagotropic substances (parasympathicolytic atropin and parasympathicomimetic carbocholine) influence the results of the galactose test (Tucherstein); actually, in Botkin's disease, atropine improves the results of the galactose test and carbocholine alters it still more.

Thus, without diminishing the importance of the insulinohypophyseal system in maintaining glycemia, it should be regarded in its due place as a link in the regulating chain controlled by the cortex (influenced by interoceptor variations) and mediated by the subcortical nuclei and pituitary, the liver being the true fundamental organ for the retention or release of circulating glucose; the pancreas is one of the intermediary factors that modify the activity of the liver.

Neuroregulation of lipid metabolism has been studied to a lesser extent; however, a steatogenic diet, administered to an animal kept in *the cold* avoids fatty loading of the liver (Levy). Since thermoregulation and the metabolic alterations of adaptation to the cold are based upon the adaptation function of the nervous system, it results in the last instance that the latter influences the metabolism of fats in the liver.

With reference to protein metabolism, mention has already been made of changes in the synthesis of hippuric acid brought about by nervous disturbances, in other similar experiments glycocol metabolism and the transamination of certain elective amino acids in the liver were arrested, whereas in the rest of the organism they took place almost normally (Kvyatkovskaya).

Bykov and Usievich proved that bile secretion is subjected to the most delicate influences on the part of the nervous system, and Ivanova showed that bile formation and reaction can be influenced by conditioned reflexes (Tucherstein, Saragea and Foni).

Hence, it is not surprising that parasympathicomimetics and parasympathicolytics modify bilirubinemia in the course of hepatitis (Tucherstein).

We believe it pertinent to mention here the clinical attempts and experimental studies which demonstrated that reflexotherapy and acupuncture influence the amount of bile discharged.

We have listed the facts known today concerning the neuroregulation of some of the fundamental metabolic functions of the liver; they leave no doubt as to the reality and importance of neuroregulation but they also point to the necessity of further studies for elucidating all the details of this regulation. The problem is further complicated by the fact that the liver also influences the activity of the cortex (and subcortical nuclei) by multiple pathways, both by hepatic interoceptor impulses and by the release of substances, that are necessary or harmful to the central nervous system. Owing to this interdependence, the controlled organ (liver) is fairly well known, the control organ (central nervous system) is sufficiently well known, and as regards their interaction many of the elements involved have been established, the principal ones having already been listed; several others will be mentioned at the respective sections (homeostasis, hepatic coma, the liver and surgery).

CORRELATIONS OF THE ANATOMOFUNCTIONAL COMPARTMENTS

The normal liver is mainly an epithelial organ but the importance of the reticuloendothelial tissue distributed between its vascular network should not be underestimated; the epithelial gland discharges its bile into the network of bile ducts, with a differentiated structure.

On the other hand, the intratrabecular capillary bed is fed by two sources of inflow blood and disposes of efferent blood (hepatic veins) and lymphatic vessels.

Therefore, in the liver there are a series of intricate anatomofunctional compartments. Though in nature they intermingle and the disturbance of any one of them influences the functions of all the others, for a better understanding we shall describe the following pairs:

a) epithelial tissue and reticuloendothelial system (RES);

b) gland and excretion pathways;

c) inflow (vena porta — hepatic artery) and outflow circulation (hepatic and lymphatic veins).

a) **Interrelation between the epithelial tissue and the hepatic reticuloendothelial system.** In protein synthesis it is well known that the diseases involving the hepatic parenchyma are associated with a decrease in plasma albumin; moreover, morphologically, the liver becomes richer in connective tissue (at least in the chronic forms) while globulins increase in the plasma. This would suggest that the epithelial element supplies albumin while the connective tissue (i.e. the RES) supplies globulin; however, experimental data have shown that the Kupffer cells are particularly involved "in the elaboration of albumin" (Best-Taylor), which would prove that the two categories of tissues intimately cooperate in the synthesis of albumin; there is less available information concerning the globulin.

In pigment metabolism, it is known that the senescent red cells are taken up by the RES (therefore by Kupffer cells, too) which produces from hemoglobin the bile pigment called "prehepatic bilirubin"; this pigment is converted into glycuronoconjugated pigment, i.e. "hepatic bilirubin", only in the liver (i.e. the epithelial cell). This is perhaps the clearest example which proves that the different compartments of the liver do not stand side by side but complete one another in their activities (the Kupffer — hepatic relationship — I. Pavel).

At other times, the same substance, according to the phase in which it is to be found, may be retained by one or other of the two compartments; for instance, the exogenous alimentary cholesterol reaches the liver in the form of kilomicrons and is fixed by the Kupffer cells, while the endogenous (plasma) cholesterol bound to β-globulin is bound to the parenchymatous cells (Byers, mentioned by Mincu).

However, there are also some aspects of independent activity: study of hepatic clearance soon showed that the activity of the glandular tissue and that of the RES should be explored separately; hence, there are certain methods for determining parenchymatous clearance and others for the Kupffer clearance (Mincu).

b) **Interrelation between the gland and the excretory pathways.** As an exocrine gland, the liver produces its secretions by a complex physiologic process in which the mechanical factors also play a certain part. "Bile is continuously secreted . . . at reduced rates and low pressure" (Nash).

By experimental studies, Prokopenko (1949) reached the conclusion that "biliary secretion and bile elimination cannot be considered as independent processes; these processes are closely interconnected". In extreme situations which occur only in pathologic conditions, an obstacle that completely obstructs the extrahepatic bile ducts may lead to the complete arrest of bile production. If this situation lasts longer, the liver undergoes structural changes and at the same time a strange phenomenon of pigment resorption occurs, even of bile cholesterin, within the dilated bile ducts (white bile; liver in a state of hydrohepatosis — Bockus).

Therefore, here again we find the same close interdependence between the compartments, the activity of one compartment being closely dependent upon that of the other.

c) **Interrelation between the in-and outflow circulation.** The liver receives blood from two well-known sources: the hepatic artery and the vena porta, and delivers it through:

— the hepatic veins with a well-known function,

— the lymphatic vessels, whose distribution and functions are but poorly known.

Interposed between the two circulations is a wide network of sinusoids with entrance and exit sphincters (Knisely), situated at the junction of the portal venule with the vena porta and at the junction of the sinusoids with the central vein.

Although the connection between the intralobular lymphatic spaces and the actual lymphatic vessels in the portal space is not yet clear, the existence of these connections has been proved:

— Nix observed in normal dogs (by draining the lymphatics with a cannula), that the hepatic lymph produced in 24 hours is equal to 47% of the plasma volume and contains 35% of the total circulating proteins; in experimental cirrhosis the hepatic lymph output reaches 258% (Child).

— Bollman shows that ligation of the common bile duct is soon followed by the appearance of bile in the hepatic lymph; it is moreover well known that previous ligation of the thoracic duct prevents the occurrence of experimental obstructive jaundice (ligation of the common bile duct).

The liver is not a passive recipient whose venous outflow is mechanically subordinated to the sum of the two inflow pathways, but on the contrary, plays an active regulating role (by the damming mechanisms of the two kinds of intrahepatic vascular sphincters).

Therefore, filling of the capillary-sinusoidal bed does not substantially change when the hepatic artery or the vena porta alone is ligated, as proved by maintenance of the hepatic volume under these conditions. Opening and closing of the intrahepatic vascular sphincters, regulated by very fine corticovisceral connections, may considerably change the quantity of blood received by the liver within a time unit. In man, the normal hepatic circulation is of about 1500 ml blood/minute with wide functional variations.

Other sphincters have also been described (Dale) in the hepatic veins, at their junction with the inferior cava. Contraction of these sphincters may considerably reduce the transhepatic blood flow. These suprahepatic sphincters are contracted by histamine and β-methylcholine and released by epinephrine. The activity of these chemical mediators only reveals one side of the complex effects of the neuroflex control of intrahepatic circulation.

The study of intrahepatic circulation is particularly important, among others, because the level of metabolic activity of the liver depends to a large extent upon the circulatory conditions.

The problem of anatomofunctional compartments in the liver has been described by A.M. Rappaport in a series of papers. In a synopsis of his own data, corroborated with the results obtained independently by other workers, he developed in 1963 a unitary concept on the hepatic morphofunctional unity, rejecting the classical concept of the hexagonal hepatic lobule.

Starting from the finding that for the hepatic parenchyma the arterioportal blood received is the starting point of specific metabolic activity, and the hepatic veins are the terminal points, Rappaport demonstrated, anatomically, that around the preterminal arterioportal branches there are small masses of parenchyma (simple acini) whose periphery ends on both sides near the initial branches of the hepatic veins (the classical "centrolobular vein"). The simple acini have zone I of maximum nutrition and metabolic activity (the oxidative processes of Krebs cycle, the appearance of glycogen, the site of entry of proteins into the cells); then, an intermediary zone II in which the activity of the oxidative processes in Krebs-cycle is less intense (Zamfirescu), and finally a peripheral zone III where reserve [glycogen is stored and where the TPN diaphorases, lipase and the glicolytic]

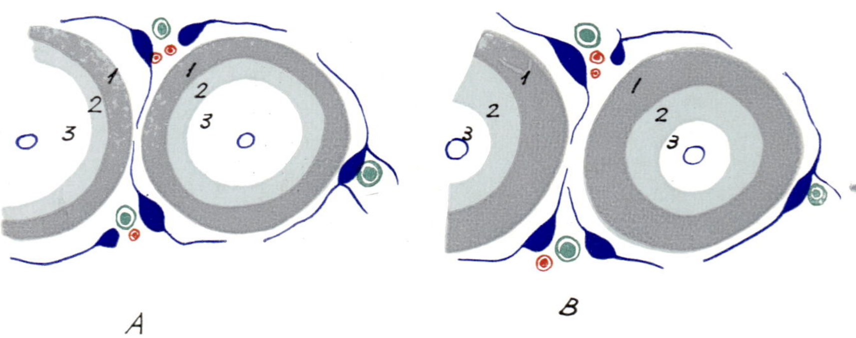

Fig. 39. — Functional zones in the hepatic parenchyma in terms of the blood inflow and outflow.

1 — Zone of maximum hepatocellular function; *2* — zone of medium hepatocellular function; *3* — zone of minimal hepatocellular function; *A* — at rest; *B* — postprandial functional stress (or hepatic arterial postneurectomy).

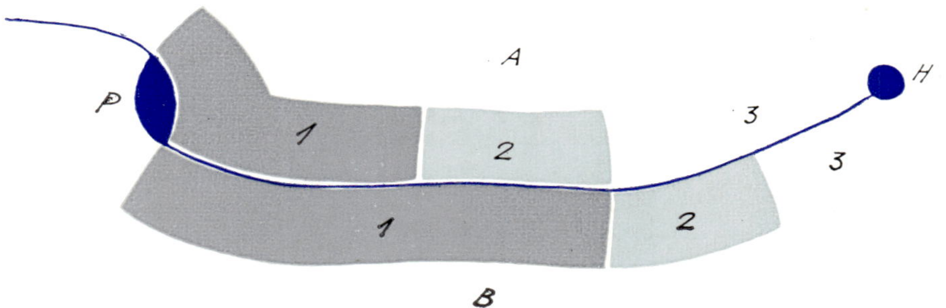

Fig. 40. — Displacement of the functional zones along the hepatic sinusoidal capillary.

1 — Zone of maximum hepatocellular function; *2* — zone of medium hepatocellular function; *3* — zone of minimal hepatocellular function; *A* — at rest; *B* — postprandial functional stress; *P* — portal presinusoidal vessel; *H* — centrolobular vein (hepatic postsinusoidal vein).

enzymes are also to be found (Zamfirescu); here, too, fats are stored (the site where fatty loading appears) (Figs 39 and 40). If zone I were considered cytogenetic (intense DNA metabolism) the cells would gradually migrate towards zone III (near the "centrolobular" vein), which is also cytoclastic (Scheppers, 1961). Normally zones III are in anatomic contact and sinusoidal continuity but in pathologic states they are the first to be destroyed. Thus, the inverted lobule, centered around the arterioportal branches and separated from the centrolobular vein, reveals in fact the true hepatic structure by destruction of zone III (the simple acini remain isolated). Normally, the simple acini are joined together in complex acini and acini clusters. Therefore, the old hexagonal lobule made of several simple acini halves is but an image arbitrarily selected from the hepatic morphologic mosaic, without any reason to be considered a morphofunctional unit. The new morphofunctional concept helps us to understand hepatic regeneration.

THE LIVER AND HOMEOSTASIS

a) **The liver and water metabolism**: control of volemia. Already in 1882 Stolnikov observed that animals with Eck's fistula readily developed circulation insufficiency and died soon after hepatectomy.

In 1921, Lamson and Roca were able to establish (experimentally in dogs) that, in the liver, retention of large amounts of fluid from the circulation takes place after injections with saline sera. The fluid is temporarily retained in the liver, then partly, slowly delivered to the circulation through the lymphatics and thoracic duct and partly eliminated through the bile.

In fact, the liver exercises its role of regulating the volume of circulating blood less actively upon the fluid incidentally penetrating into the vessels (perfusion) than on that normally penetrating with the food into the portal system. Discussions still exist concerning the intimate mechanisms of this regulation (Knisely valve mechanism, rejected by Seneviratne-Child). Experimental studies (in dogs) confirm that even on a fasting diet the liver retains water (4.3—7 per cent), as results from the difference in composition of the portal and suprahepatic blood, both as regards the hematocrit and salts (Bujor, Velican, Beroniade, Florea, Constantinescu, communication at the Institute of Therapeutics, 1958).

Thus, the liver may modify volemia by the retention of fluid (water or plasma), concomitant to an increase in hematocrit.

But the liver can also change the composition of blood by an elective action on the blood cells; Merkulova (1943) observed reflex changes in arterial blood pressure after applying stimulators directly upon the liver surface.

Moiseeva (1954) noticed that the stimulation of hepatic chemoreceptors causes leukopenia by a redistribution mechanism with elective retention of leukocytes in the liver (phenomenon which no longer occurs after anesthesia of the chemoreceptors) and then leukocytosis. The liver may actually retain electively "certain white cells", for instance eosinophils (Bujor et al.).

The liver exercises a far more complex action on the number of red cells; in the normal adult man, the liver does not produce red cells.

Denervation of liver entails progressive anemia without morphologic changes, reticulocytosis or myelogram alterations (experimentally in cats — Moiseeva).

The products of pigment metabolism seem to be physiologic activators of erythropoiesis in which blood bilirubin plays an important part (Moiseeva).

The role of the antipernicious factor and the interrelation with vitamin B_{12} are well known.

The synthesis of *hemoglobin* (consisting of porphyrin with iron and a protein-globin) appears to take place in the nuclei of the bone marrow cells (Best) but globin may be synthesized to a certain extent in the liver too.

The iron resorbed particularly from the duodenum and to a lesser extent from the jejunoileum is mostly stored in the liver but iron resorption depends on the general condition of the iron reserves in the organism, and in this regard the liver holds an important place.

The liver, which as we have already seen may change the composition of the blood by an elective action exercised upon its various elements, may also modify the volume of the circulation; thus, it is acknowledged that the normal adult liver may supply, if necessary, a volume of 1—2 liters of blood and in pathologic conditions it may store up a volume of blood representing 60 per cent of its weight (circulation insufficiency); under the influence of adrenaline, the liver delivers a blood volume equal to about 59 per cent of its weight.

Most of the mechanisms by which the liver participates in the control of the blood volume or that of its main figured elements and water, are governed neuroreflexly and seldom mechanically (such as cardiac liver in right ventricular insufficiency).

b) **Glycemia** in the normal man is of about 0.1% (varying between 0.080 and 0.120 gm%) and this level is maintained with slight variations although carbohydrate metabolism is complex and carried out with the participation of numerous organs and physiologic mechanism. This constancy implies a continuous adaptation of glucose release to the extent in which it is withdrawn from the circulation by the vital requirements of the various tissues (particularly the liver) during the periods in which intestinal resorption introduces carbohydrates into the body. In the chapter on metabolism, mention was made of the complexity of intrahepatic processes and, in the paragraph on neuroregulation, stress was laid on the importance of the nervous system in glycoregulation.

The rate of glycogen breakdown is accelerated by adrenaline and the rate of gluconeogenesis is influenced by the internal secretion of the anterior pituitary, adrenal cortex, thyroid and pancreas (Best-Taylor).

Clinical practice confirms the experimental data, emphasizing the importance of the liver in this complex mechanism of glycoregulation in diseases involving the hepatic parenchyma. The more perturbed the activity of the epithelial cells, the further from normal the responses to the induced hyperglycemia test.

This is of importance since it proves that carbohydrates considered to play a therapeutic role in the diet, should be administered sparingly to patients with a severe hepatic functional deficit.

c) **Lipemia.** Its normal values of about 0.50 gm% are fairly constant (measured at least 12 hrs after meals).

Neutral fats represent about one third. As already mentioned, the liver is the site of intense oxidation of the superior fatty acids and at the same time the site of fatty acid synthesis. However, the role of the lung in reducing postprandial hyperlipemia (lipodieretic function) should not be underestimated.

Phospholipids represent a little more than one third and it is generally admitted that they are entirely supplied by the liver.

Cholesterol represents one third of the total amount of lipids and the liver plays an important part in the regulation of blood cholesterol by its synthesis, retention (in the RES and epithelial cells) and esterification. Of these mechanisms, esterification alone is entirely subordinated to the liver and reflects fairly accurately one aspect of the functional state of the liver.

d) **Proteinemia** and the metabolic activity of the liver.

In the normal adult the plasma contains 6.03—6.72 gm proteins/100 ml plasma; 3.32—4.04 gm% albumins; 2.23—2.39 gm globulins%; 0.34—0.43 gm fibrinogen %.

Albumins are certainly synthesized in the liver and this explains their decrease in all the major alterations of the liver.

Fibrinogen is synthesized by the liver and this accounts for its increase in the diseases with slight involvement of the liver (with an irritating effect) and its persistent or definite decrease in accentuated hepatic alterations.

Globulins appear to be produced by the liver (experiments on isolated organ) but in all hepatic diseases, associated with a decrease of the other two protein fractions, an increase of plasma globulin levels is noticed; no valid explanation has been found so far for these facts of clinical observation.

Therefore, it results that the liver has a direct influence upon the level of the various blood protein fractions and upon proteinemia itself, which proves the importance of blood protein determinations in order to appraise the functional state of the liver, as well as the importance of maintaining a normal functional state of the liver in order to keep the values of these fractions within normal limits. Total blood protein determinations are less conclusive than determination of each separate fraction, since the same hepatic alteration which lowers albumin level, brings about an increase in globulins, so that the total figure may not significantly change. If we add the fact that the biologic value (maintenance of osmotic pressure) is incomparably higher for 1 gm albumin than for 1 gm globulin, it appears absolutely necessary to determine the different plasma protein fractions separately.

e) **Liver and blood clotting.** As stressed by Quick (1938), four substances are necessary in blood coagulation (Nash): prothrombin, thromboplastin, calcium ions and fibrinogen.

Actually, at present, a series of "factors" are known to participate in coagulation — either accelerating or preventing it; the list is far from complete since not all these factors are generally accepted and the same factor may be known under 2—3 names.

It is not our intention to describe the whole series of complicated (and at times unsubstantiated) biological reactions which take place in the course of coagulation, but only to mention the main stages and to emphasize the way in which the liver may influence the respective factors or stages.

— *Thrombin* is found as inactive prothrombin in the plasma and is a glucoprotein complex (Seegers) synthesized by the liver in the presence of vitamin K (a mechanism not yet fully elucidated). Normally, in the blood there are 25 mg of prothrombin/100 ml, and from the blood it is continuously taken up by the lung. Therefore, normal blood prothrombin levels are maintained by continuous production of the respective amounts by the liver. Morphofunctional changes, resections, as well as surgical shock lower the rate of this synthesis in the liver. Similarly, vitamin K deficit causes an immediate decrease of prothrombin synthesis. This may occur in: a vitamin K-free diet (seldom), arrest of vitamin K biosynthesis in the colon (more often — due to antibiotics), lack of vitamin K resorption in the intestine (biliary fistula, jaundice) and hepatic morphofunctional changes (the most common cause).

The normal level of blood prothrombin (considered to be 100% or over 85%) exceeds by far absolute requirements; only when prothrombinemia falls 80% below *normal levels*, which represents 20% of the normal level, there occur changes in the coagulation time, which may, however, soon become very important. When blood prothrombin is below 10%, severe hemorrhage is imminent. If account is also kept of individual variations, all patients with a prothrombinemia below 50% should be considered in a *danger zone* (Nash) because the surgical trauma may cause its decrease below the safety limit (Anderson) between the 4th and 7th day after operation.

— Plasma *thromboplastin* is found only in traces or inactivated and it seems to be produced by all the body cells (in the lung as lecithin and in the brain as phospholipid). The liver does not interfere directly in its production.

— *Calcium* ion levels are regulated by the parathyroids and by bone marrow metabolism, and are, therefore, always to be found in sufficient amounts in the blood *(in vivo)*.

— *Fibrinogen*, a protein with a large molecule, is produced by the liver.

The essential diagram (leaving out stimulating factors and interactions) is:

Prothrombin + thromboplastin + calcium $^{++}$ ——→ thrombin.

Thrombin + fibrinogen ——→ fibrin.

Thrombin in small quantities lyses the platelets triggering thromboplastinogenase which activates the inactive plasma thromboplastinogen, converting it into active thromboplastin. The latter can now act on the prothrombin produced by another, less active, precursor (prothrombinogen) in contact with a rough surface. The action of thromboplastin on prothrombin occurs in the presence of calcium ions and of a certain stimulating globulin (factor V = labile factor). This is a somewhat more complete modern concept on coagulation. As the liver does not modify the activity of these factors, they will not be discussed here.

Heparin occurs in the liver, more than in any other organ, and, therefore, the liver may be justly considered as "an essential organ in the regulation of proteins and of blood coagulation".

HEPATIC INSUFFICIENCY AND HEPATIC COMA

There are two categories of hepatic functional insufficiency:

— with a blatant clinical symptomatology; as a rule hepatic plurifunctional disturbances;

— with attenuated or clinically latent symptoms (detected by careful functional exploration).

However, one should not underestimate the importance of latent hepatic insufficiency or that with a less important symptomatology of *unknown origin*, since certain chronic diseases of other organs may be detected.

As regards the material substrate in the milder forms (latent or oligosymptomatic), we sometimes fail to detect the pathohistologic changes, but in the severe forms important structural changes are generally found.

Severe hepatic insufficiency may end in "hepatic coma".

If "hepatic coma" represented total insufficiency of the liver, a vital organ, medical treatment would have but little effect.

At present, it is generally accepted that against the background of hepatic insufficiency, hepatic coma occurs as a severe and dreaded complication but not necessarily fatal.

This can be illustrated by a clinical case having the value of an experiment: TL portocaval anastomosis was performed in a patient after pancreatoduodenectomy with resection of the portal trunk. The patient had repeated hepatic comas, every time preceded by an increase in ammoniemia (Chester).

Gastrointestinal hemorrhage in patients with portal hypertension is particularly dangerous since the increase of colic putrefaction leads to resorption of ammonia and toxic products which are incompletely neutralized by the deficient liver. The evolution may readily be complicated by hepatic coma.

No matter whether the increase in ammoniemia is only an indication of hepatic insufficiency and exaggerated resorption of toxic products from the colon (Sherlock), or whether the resorbed ammonia itself is neurotoxic (Dessman), blocking a ketoglutamate which breaks up Krebs cycle, altering the general metabolism of the brain (Galea), it should be remembered that the increase of blood ammonia (heralding coma) can be attenuated by the use of antibiotics. Hence, the modern curative treatment in hepatic coma is meant:

— to ensure an energy and tissue recovery relationship with the final products of metabolism (glucose, amino acids), water and salts (K^+);

— to control intestinal ammoniogenesis with antibiotics;

— to diminish the effect of increased ammoniemia (with glutamic acid);

— to improve hepatic cellular metabolism (choline associated with methionine, vitamin C, vitamin B_{12});

— to favor glycopexis, reduce capillary permeability and increase serum albumins by corticotherapy.

Hepatic coma, considered as a complication of hepatic insufficiency, must be treated, and success may be obtained. If the patient has an old irreversible hepatic insufficiency, success is transient but if this complication occurs subsequent to portocaval anastomosis in patients with portal hypertension and moderate hepatic insufficiency, the success may become permanent if the treatment is associated to an adequate diet and if exaggerated intestinal putrefaction is controlled.

THE LIVER AND SURGERY

Each of the points listed up to the present represent subjects that cannot be dealt with in detail and completely along general lines, but which must be directly connected with the precise conditions in which a *given* patient, with a *given* disease and hepatic functional state will have to undergo a *certain* operation.

Hence, some of the subjects will be taken up again in the chapters on pathology and therapy.

However, there are certain aspects of major importance that form a common pathophysiologic background against which the characteristics of each case and each intervention stand out.

PREOPERATIVE PREPARATION AND ANESTHESIA

a) **Preoperative preparation** of hepatobiliary patients should improve the functional level of the liver. Depletion of the glycogen and protein reserves (with fatty deposition) in the liver cells, insufficient prothrombin synthesis and limitation of the glycuronoconjugation capacity should be considered as the main causes of function deficiency. An insufficient supply of calories and especially a protein-low diet accentuate these disorders.

In order to build up again glycogen reserves, a high caloric input is necessary, i.e. a mixed, predominantly carbohydrate diet.

A standard ration of 2000—2500 calories per day, in which about 20% are proteins, 75% carbohydrates and 5% fats, is recommended in the preoperative period for patients in general. The lithiasic patient with jaundice (obstructive or hepatocellular) and the patient with biliary fistula should not be given lipids and his diet will only consist of carbohydrates and proteins. However, the hazard of hypokalemia secondary to the exaggerated administration of parenteral glucose, should be borne in mind. Potassium balance will be maintained by the administration *per os* of fruit and vegetable extracts, or by intravenous administration of potassium chloride when necessary.

A particular aspect is that of the patient with obstructive jaundice, cholangitis and oligoanuria due to toxic renal involvement. In such case azotemia increases, revealing the intensity of the catabolism of the body's own proteins while the anorexic patient refuses any kind of food. Potassium must not be given, only i.v. glucose (200—400 gm/24 hours) to arrest the increase in azotemia and spare as many of the body's own proteins as possible. Perfusions with aminated acids may also reduce the wear and tear of one's own tissues without, however, preventing it altogether (inevitable "renewal").

To give an example, here is a brief description of the evolution and treatment of such a complex case.

Patient (M) aged 65, was admitted to a medical clinic with a diagnosis of obstructive jaundice, cholangitis, auricular fibrillation, myocardosclerosis.

Subfebrile course, 15,000 leukocytes, in the urine — rare granular casts and very rare red blood cells. Dysproteinemia tests — negative; blood bilirubin: 22.19 mg% (I = 8.25 mg% and D = 3.94%).

Blood urea, high from the beginning (0.162 gm%) gradually increased and signs of azotemia developed with alteration of the general condition (agitation, hiccoughing, vomiting).

The carbohydrate dose was increased (200 gm glucose) and a low protein supply with controlled fluid balance was allowed. As soon as diuresis exceeded 500 ml, vegetable soup was given. Within 5 days, urea fell to 0.030 gm% and 0.028 gm%. Cholangitis which was the cause of the renal toxic alteration only improved after 10 days treatment with antibiotics when the leukocyte count fell to 6,400. The patient was then referred to the surgical clinic. After 3 weeks the patient had recovered sufficiently to undergo the operation successfully (choledochoduodenostomy after removing numerous calculi from the common duct). The patient fully recovered and was discharged after ten days.

The amounts of lipids and carbohydrates are readily established, but it is very difficult to establish the necessary amount of proteins. Clinical and experimental studies clearly prove that a low protein diet is harmful; but a double amount of proteins in the diet (in comparison to average values) will reduce the glycogen reserve in the liver (experimental investigations). Thus, the drawbacks of an excessive or deficient protein supply are very clear.

A mixed diet of about 3200 calories contains:

101 gm	proteins
73 gm	fats
520 gm	carbohydrates

with the addition of fresh cheese (200—400 gm) and briar tea according to the doctor's prescription (L. B. Berlin in Pevzner).

The long-standing experience of clinicians, who used a purified insulin product, proved that the treatment with glucose + insulin is not advantageous as it sometimes diminishes the glycogen reserves in the liver.

In order to increase tolerance to carbohydrates, vitamin C is added to the diet in large amounts (200—400 mg/24 h).

As already shown in the section on coagulation, vitamin K should be administered parenterally to all the patients with hypoprothrombinemia, with jaundice (and decolored stools) and to those to whom wide spectrum-antibiotics are administered. Vitamins in large amounts should also be given to patients with biliary fistulas.

b) **Anesthesia.** Although chloroform is no longer used, anesthesia in hepatobiliary patients still remains an open question. Oxygenation will be dealt with in the chapter on shock-resuscitation and here, only a brief description of the current methods of anesthesia will be given.

The basic anesthetic is morphine and its derivatives, and, although it is conjugated in the liver (and to a lesser extent in the kidneys), this does not take place with the participation of glycuronides, but with other as yet unknown substances.

On the other hand *Dolantin* (Pethidine) is destroyed by the normal liver (deesterification, demethylation) and should be used with the utmost care because hepatic insufficiency may explain the exaggerated effects of normal doses.

Atropine may be prevalently used in patients with hepatocellular alterations.

Anesthesia can be *potentiated by:*

Largactyl. Jaundice occurs only after prolonged administration of Largactyl so that the use of a single dose for potentiation need not be taken into account. However some authors consider hepatic insufficiency as a possible contraindication (Moyer, 1954 — cited by Goodman).

Phenergan has a powerful antihistaminic action and may obviate the suprahepatic barrier (See "Shock").

Dolantin has already been mentioned.

Of all these substances, Phenergan appears to be the best drug for potentiating anesthesia in hepatobiliary patients.

Anesthesia, shall be examined from the point of view of tolerance of the liver to general, local and spinal anesthesia.

General anesthesia may be obtained either by inhalation of a gaseous mixture rich in oxygen, or by i.v. injection of certain barbiturates.

Injectable barbiturates (Evipan-Thiopental) do not offer a sufficiently deep anesthesia, of long duration, as necessary for most of the major operations on the liver and bile ducts. As regards their use for other categories of operation in patients with a hepatic functional deficit, the duration and intensity of their effect depends upon the functional state of the liver since they are inactivated especially by the latter. In other words, in patients with hepatic insufficiency, however mild, one cannot foresee whether the usual dose will induce anesthesia of short duration or whether it will be followed by a prolonged hypnotic effect. For this reason it is recommended to avoid barbiturates for operative anesthesia, reserving them especially for the induction of anesthesia. Gaseous anesthetics: although liposoluble, ether when correctly administered with oxygen does not appear to cause important functional or morphological changes; in some patients with preoperative alterations, the deficits became more accentuated postoperatively but this appears to be the consequence of surgical aggression and not of the anesthetic.

Nitrous oxide can only produce surgical anesthesia in anoxemia-inducing concentrations, therefore dangerous for the liver. It may be used for induction or associated with curare.

Cyclopropane, an efficient anesthetic may give discrete hepatic deficiency especially when alterations existed prior to the operation.

Fluothane is perhaps the most innocuous volatile anesthetic and can be used even in marked hepatic alterations.

It is worthy of note that both ether and cyclopropane mobilise hepatic glycogen by *adrenosecretion ;* it is likewise known that depletion of the glycogen reserve in the liver has an unfavorable influence on its functional capacity.

Curarisers do not modify the metabolic aspects mentioned.

Therefore, general anesthesia performed by means of up-to-date techniques presents a series of drawbacks:

— Barbiturates should be as a rule avoided (except for induction);

— Efficient gaseous anesthetics (ether-cyclopropane) do not avoid the mobilisation of glycogen due to adrenosecretion;

— *Local anesthesia* has for many years been considered "innocuous". The substance generally used is novocaine (procaine) which is hydrolyzed by procainesterase in different tissues and especially in the liver, resulting in paraaminohippuric acid and diaminoethanol.

Paraaminohippuric acid is partly conjugated and partly eliminated in the urine.

Many patients with a functional hepatic deficit may exhibit a low tolerance to novocaine and some authors have even proposed a hepatic functional test with novocaine (Richaud-Hazard). In large hepatobiliary operations, to be efficient local anesthesia must include large areas of the abdominal wall and numerous intraabdominal reflexogenic zones; consequently infiltration of the tissues must be done with large amounts of novocaine which may sometimes give rise to manifest intolerance (hypotension, agitation, etc.).

Therefore, local anesthesia when efficient is no longer "innocuous".

Spinal anesthesia. It is recomended to use a mixture of 1—1.5 ml 8% novocaine and 1 ml 0.5—0.6% percaine. The patient lies in the Trendelenburg position and the site of the puncture must be at least as high as D. 6, blocking the somatic and visceral areas and the roots at D 6 — D 12 from which the *rami comunicantes* emerge with the preganglionic fibres of the larger and lesser splanchnic nerves. Blocking of the splanchnic nerves prevents nervous induction of adrenosecretion and consequently avoids hyperglycemia with the mobilization of hepatic glycogen. Therefore, spinal anesthesia is advantageous for the patient when followed by correct fluid (glucose perfusion) and respiratory resuscitation (permanent oxygenation. This anesthesia gives perfect muscular relaxation, offering optimal conditions to the surgeon and shortening the duration of the major operations very much. Spinal anesthesia with 5% xylin (2 ml) offers the same advantages.

On comparing the different methods, it may be concluded that spinal anesthesia offers the best conditions for uncomplicated hepatobiliary operations performed by the abdominal approach. The same good conditions can be obtained with general, closed-circuit anesthesia (Fluothane-Oxygen), potentiated and with the addition of curare in relaxing doses, therefore a far more complicated procedure, indicated in operations of long duration.

For the operations which necessitate opening of the thoracic cavity it is necessary to resort to closed-circuit orotracheal anesthesia that insures optimal conditions for the respiratory function in the open thorax.

SHOCK AND RESUSCITATION IN SURGICAL HEPATOBILIARY PATIENTS

Up-to-date studies in the field of shock have revealed the decisive role of he central nervous system (especially the cortex) in the onset and evolution of raumatic, hemorrhagic or mixed shock. According to Asratian, a neuroendocrino-humoral disturbance first takes place and is followed by anoxia of the tissue, stasis, hypercapnia and finally metabolism in anaerobiosis. In the past, a central role in the pathogeny of shock was attributed to functional deficit of the liver, at a time when each pathologic process was assumed to be localised within a single organ; thus the fact that the cat, rabbit or dog die quickly after ligation of the portal vein was considered to prove that removal of the liver from its physiologic circuit is incompatible with life (Schiff, 1877).

Eck showed by means of a portacaval fistula that the liver can be removed from the physiologic circuit and death does not occur when return of the portal blood to the general circulation is ensured; hence, ligation of the portal vein kills the normal animal by the retention of a large volume of blood in the splanchnic circulation.

Dale (1910) coined the term histaminic shock showing that this substance disturbs the circulation in the liver, with the retention of an important volume of blood in the portal system.

Studying hemorrhagic shock, Pilcher (1914) showed that gradual repeated bleeding results in an irreversible stage when the therapeutic measures which were formerly efficient have no longer any effect. The irreversibility of shock was attributed to depressor substances produced by the anoxic liver (Fine). The argument raised was that in the animal with acute anemia, shock does not become irreversible when oxygenation of the liver is maintained by cross circulation.

Friedman showed that in severe shock vasoconstriction occurs in the intrahepatic network of the hepatic artery and the portal vein.

Frank proved experimentally that Eck's fistula may avoid rapid death after ligation of the portal vein but does not avoid irreversibility of repeated hemorrhagic shock against which only constant oxygenation of the blood supplied to the liver is efficient.

Wiggers (1946) observed that in hemorrhagic shock the blood supply to the liver diminishes more than expected if account is kept of the decrease in arterial blood pressure. Knisely and Seneviratne established, separately, that alteration of the circulation in the liver sinusoids in shock is due to the activity of the vascular sphincter on entering and leaving the sinusoid network.

Therefore, it has generaly been accepted that in shock unfavorable circulatory changes occur in the liver, resulting in disturbances of the metabolic functional state of this organ (Child).

Changes in intrahepatic circulation are known to be under the control of a neurohumoral complex. On the other hand, it is also known that the liver possesses a large number of interoceptors (Merkulova, Moiseeva, I. T. Niculescu) and that injury of the liver may produce a series of distant alterations.

The functions of the liver are disturbed by operative aggression; injury of the liver lowers its capacity to synthesize prothrombin and when the insult exceeds a certain intensity, the administration of vitamin K is no longer efficient in correcting hypoprothrombinemia (Bollman, cited by Nash).

From the above data and recent clinical and experimental investigations it may be concluded that the liver plays an important role, either as an organ from which nociceptive impulses start, disturbing the activity of the cortex and of the liver itself, or in the stage of anoxic tissue disturbances when it is particularly involved and may jeopardize reversal of shock.

If we bear in mind the sensitivity of the liver to anoxia and the fact that numerous neuroreflex mechanisms aggravate anoxia in the liver, we can readily understand the gravity of mixed shock (traumatic + hemorrhagic) in hepatobiliary patients in which the irreversible phase is very soon reached.

Therefore, in the resuscitation of these patients particular attention should be paid since insufficient (or delayed) and excess resuscitation are just as dangerous.

Oxygenation should be constant and intravenous perfusion with 5% glucose should be started at a low rate of perfusion.

Isogroup blood will be administered in equal volumes and all plasma substitutes, such as dextran or soldextrin, should be avoided because they are gradually retained by the reticuloendothelial system (therefore also by the Kupffer cells) which they temporarily block. Hence glucose serum, plasma or isogroup blood will be administered according to requirements.

Today, adrenaline is no longer used since it depletes liver glycogen, but endogenous hyperadrenalinemia caused by emotion, pre-anesthesia, pain, hypercapnia, hypoventilation, etc. must be avoided. Among the other stimulating substances, ephedrine should only be used *in extremis* because it has many of the side effects of adrenaline (even if more attenuated).

Actually, attentive fluid and respiratory resuscitation with correct anesthesia help the hepatobiliary patient to withstand complex operations without shock (hepatectomy, gastrocholecystostomy with patent distal common duct, etc.).

Among the methods of prevention of shock is the stabilizing of blood pressure. This can be obtained in hypotension or by efficient potentiation, or finally by maintaining the blood pressure at almost normal values.

Controlled hypotension appeared to some investigators (Bertrandt, 1955) as less certain against anoxia than hypothermia (as regards resistance to anoxia).

Efficient potentiation, by moderately lowering metabolism and especially by autonomic stability, avoids the appearance of unfavorable intrahepatic phenomena which are the causes of shock. However, efficient pharmacodynamic potentiation is difficult to obtain in practice in these patients, who tolerate no kind of "cocktail".

Clinical experience and the data in literature attribute an important place in the prophylaxis of anoxic hepatic disturbances to high spinal anesthesia that diminishes (or inhibits) the discharge of adrenaline and lowers basal metabolism.

The experimental investigations carried out during the last five years and certain clinical applications showed that circulatory, metabolic and vegetative stability can be obtained by combining antihistaminics (Phenergan) with ganglioplegics (of the hexamethonium type) and an antiadrenalytic, with a vasopressor and hypometabolizing effect (Ergotoxin). Present investigations will establish the value of this association, together with anesthesia, in comparison to the simpler, and probably just as efficient, association of spinal anesthesia with ergotoxin (as premedication).

POSTOPERATIVE COMPLICATIONS

Apart from the usual complications, certain characteristic ones may develop in hepatobiliary patients due to the specific of their pathophysiology:

a) Severe hepatic insufficiency that may sometimes occur without preliminary signs in a patient whose evolution is normal during the first 3—4 days. This may be probably due to the absence of food (caloric deficit) within the first days after the operation and to overloading of the liver with autolysis products resorbed from the operative wound.

b) Hemorrhagic syndrome due to the accentuation of hypoprothrombinemia caused by surgical trauma.

These two complications appear to be combined in gastrointestinal hemorrhage, followed by hepatic coma. As already mentioned, the treatment will consist in tetracycline (which lowers colic putrefaction and ammoniogenesis), associated with vitamin K (to increase prothrombine synthesis) and vitamin C.

c) Evisceration (rare).

d) Bed sores, a consequence of hypoproteinemia.

WOUND HEALING IN HEPATOBILIARY DISEASES

The liver plays an important metabolic role in supplying the body with the necessary elements for the healing of wounds. In biliary patients with an efficient functional liver, no peculiarities appear in the speed and aspect of the reparatory processes; on the other hand, in hepatic insufficiency, alterations of the reparatory processes develop with the accentuation of hypoproteinemia. At a given level of deficiency, the patients show a tendency to dehiscence; in the more advanced forms evisceration may also be observed. Today, even in the departments with a hepato-biliary profile, evisceration is very rare due especially to correct pre- and post-operative care.

The capacity of the organism to heal a wound is enunciated by the state of the blood. Anemia with hypohemoglobinemia shows that the body has a reduced capacity to build up cells and tissues. In such cases surgery should be put off (i possible) until the circulating volume is improved by repeated transfusions (isogroup) Although apparently paradoxical, it is known that plasma transfusions are not very efficient because foreign proteins must be transformed before being used, whereas whole blood furnishes not only proteins but also the red blood cells which immediately improve the oxygen supply to the liver.

If marked hemorrhage occurs in a patient with moderately, limited hepatic function, the hepatic deficit will be worsened and recovery, after the hemorrhage has ceased, will be very slow; in such cases the liver cannot ensure the normal rhythm of healing of the operative wound. Here is an example:

The patient (M), aged 75, was admitted to a medical clinic after a massive gastrointestinal hemorrhage; he suffered from mild diabetes mellitus (controlled by diet) and for some time also from auricular fibrillation.

On admission, the hematocrit was 19.3% (as compared to the normal 45%) and 2,000,000 red blood cells. The response to the medical treatment and transfusions was very slow. After one month, the hematocrit value was 32.6% and red blood cells 3,370,000. Hemoglobin increased to 62% from 48% on admission. The roentgenogram revealed the cause of the hemorrhage: a neoplastic process on the lesser curvature of the stomach.

The clinical examination revealed an irregular surface over the liver suggesting hepatic metastases, which eliminated the idea of a radical operation.

Explorative laparotomy for biopsy confirmed the existence of a gastric tumor and hepatic metastases. The pathohistologic examination pointed to a diagnosis of adenocarcinoma.

The evolution was not complicated by diabetes (although ketonuria appeared immediately after the operation) but by delayed healing of the operative wound; on the 4th day evisceration occurred and the wound was again sutured.

Great difficulties were encountered during the reoperation as the tissues had become friable and were cut by the sutures. Notwithstanding, the abdominal wall was closed. One end of the suture line opened on the 6th day, but after a very slow 21-day course, the wound was healed.

In this case, the liver altered by diabetes and auricular fibrillation was further affected by the tumor metastases so that it was no longer able to help recovery or a normal evolution of the operative wound after the hemorrhage.

A difficult problem is that of patients with biliary fistulas in which digestion is disturbed. A diet rich in calories and the administration of bile is necessary (bile from bovine gallbladder, because the fistula bile is poor in bile salts).

The capacity of the liver to compensate certain deficits is remarkable, since severe disorders in healing seldom occur, although functional deficits are fairly frequent. However, even moderate functional deficits may influence the quality of the wound ("weak" scar), and this should be kept account of before surgery, when the patient's condition must be improved as much as possible.

THE PATHOLOGIC PHYSIOLOGY OF HEPATIC REGENERATION

IMPORTANCE OF THE EXPERIMENTAL METHOD FOR STUDY OF THE NORMAL AND PATHOLOGIC PHYSIOLOGY OF THE LIVER

Reference has frequently been made to experimental investigations and not only to clinical findings. Experimental studies have always been instrumental for a closer understanding of the functions of the normal or pathologic liver. It should be recalled that experimental research work stands at the basis of Claude Bernard's knowledge of the liver functions; without the cardinal experiments of Eck, Pavlov, Mann and Magath, many of the complex aspects of the liver functions would not have been understood.

The *acute experiment* is less used today *in vivo ;* however, *in vitro*, liver tissue cultures and especially liver slices and triturate permit study of the most delicate problems of biochemistry, the key to different metabolic stages (glycogenosynthesis, glycuronoconjugation, etc.).

The *chronic experiment* has led to basic research work on certain functions or groups of functions.

Biliary fistulas have made it possible to follow up the dynamics of hepatic participation in different metabolisms.

— Eck's fistula pointed to the role of barrier played by the liver against certain digestion products resorbed from the intestine.

I. P. Pavlov, who modified Eck's operation, anastomosed the cava to the porta (not the porta to the cava) and then sutured the cava above the anastomosis; with time, a large number of collaterals developed, shunting the blood from the portal network into the superior cava network and bypassing the liver. At this moment, total hepatectomy can be performed without risking immediate disorders of the general circulation, and the evolution can be followed up (8—10 hours without treatment or 1—2 days with glucose perfusions) until coma and death with severe nervous disturbances and hypoglycemia occur.

Rostovtsev, by his devisceration method, supplied unquestionable evidence that total hepatectomy, with an intact gastrointestinal tract, brings about two interrelated groups of phenomena: on the one hand, hepatic insufficiency; on the other, the appearance in the circulation of some nocuous products resorbed from the intestine. Even with devisceration, it is not possible to avoid complications following the appearance of nocuous tissue metabolites, with decrease in the blood pH, so that neither in this instance is i.v. glucose efficient and the animal dies in convulsions.

Both clinical and experimental findings have revealed not only the complexity of the liver functions but also the "remarkable functional reserves" of this organ (Mann). Similarly, it has been demonstrated that the liver possesses a certain functional plasticity and the capacity to reestablish some functions after aggressions which do not exceed a given limit.

Some experimental results, which showed that part of the liver can be resected and may almost reach its initial volume with time, as well as the functional plasticity, already mentioned, have served as arguments for the "hepatic regeneration" theory. In this connection, some authors (Palmer) asserted that the "liver can even regenerate lobes''. However, not all investigators have found evident aspects of regeneration (Mallet-Guy, 1954). The divergence of opinions appears to reside in the various methods used and in the different meanings given to the same terms.

METHODS OF STUDY OF HEPATIC REGENERATION

In order to study hepatic regeneration, a number of very different methods have been used, which only supplied answers to some of the questions raised:

— does "hepatic regeneration" exist;
— the fundamental mechanism of regeneration of the damaged liver;
— the factors that influence the intrahepatic reparatory processes;
— the role of hormones;
— the role of the circulatory output;
— the role of the nature of the blood supplying the liver;
— the role of functional stress;
— the role of the nervous system in reparatory processes;
— the role of the condition of the liver at the moment of the injury.

We shall first show the possibilities offered by the most frequently used methods, and then give the answers to these questions as far as our present knowledge makes it possible.

a) **The method of liver destruction** in multiple foci.

The administration of small, repeated doses of carbon tetrachloride (and other toxic substances) results in epithelial cellular alterations (vacuolar and fatty degeneration), nuclear damage, vasodilatation and interlobular infiltration with small or long cells (with a vesicular nucleus). Although some alteration foci may be very small, they are disseminated throughout almost all the lobules and give rise to important functional alterations (galactose test, etc., increase in non-protein nitrogen). Subsequently, the interlobular infiltrates are resorbed to a certain extent, but mostly become fibrous. The zones of epithelial alteration may be replaced by connective tissue or cellular cords. The most readily followed up aspect, i.e. alteration of the epithelial cell after prolonged fasting, was studied in the electron microscope, in the rat. It was observed that the liver cell may lose part of its mass, which it then recovers. This true regeneration (Fawcett-Don, 1956) only occurs *in the less modified cells*. On the other hand, the partly destroyed cellular cords can replace the losses also with epithelial liver cells. In this case, a partly damaged *lobule is regenerated.*

b) **The method of partial hepatic destructions.** In lower animals important portions of the liver lobes can be resected or cauterized, and after some time, the liver will regain its prior volume, by increase of the other lobes and of the parts that have remained intact in the damaged lobes (Ponfick and Meister in 1894, cited by Child). Determination of the blood constants (especially urea) revealed no signs of functional limitation even after resection of 80% of the liver in the dog (Mann).

Detailed examination of the local phenomena after these non-anatomic resections showed that the remaining portions of the lobes subsequently undergo necrosis due to interception of their vessels. This led to study of the technique of anatomic resections. Sometimes, especially after cauterization, the eschar itself is resorbed and it was deduced that a relationship may exist between the size of the eschar and the stimulation effect of cellular multiplication in the neighboring areas (Repciuc et al.). Due to the very complexity of the factors that combine unpredictably, non-anatomic resections cannot give a categorical answer, not even to the question of whether "the neoformation of lobes exists", but they demonstrate that the regeneration of lobules does exist, since the newly formed portions of the resected lobes have the same structure as the normal ones.

Study of the composition of the peripheral blood does not seem adequate.

c) **The method of anatomic limited resections** of a known volume, is the latest method used and has supplied many data.

With this method, the surface of the lesion is reduced to a minimum; in the animals with a lobate liver and deep fissures, there is hardly any lesional surface, apart from ligation of the lobar pedicles.

Similarly, the question of subsequent alteration of the remaining territories no longer arises, because the pedicles of the remaining lobes are spared with this technique.

This method is used alone or combined with other operations and makes it possible to approach numerous aspects of the regeneration process in the liver.

Some authors have studied the rate of regeneration of the liver after resection, in terms of the portal supply; a decrease in the latter reduces the rate of regeneration of the remaining liver (Sénèque).

Further studies concerning the dependence of hepatic regeneration on portal supply by shunting the portal blood (especially Eck's fistula before resection) showed that liver diminishes after the fistula is carried out and no longer recovers its volume after resection (Child, 1953). When, in the animal with Eck's fistula a relative constriction is applied to the inferior vena cava above the liver (increasing pressure in the portal vein), hepatic resection will again be followed by a rapid increase in the volume of the remaining liver.

The conclusion was drawn that a given output and pressure of the portal circulation are necessary to sustain active recovery of the volume of the remaining liver.

Integral substitution of the portal blood flow by the inferior cava blood (Fig. 41) resulted, after hepatic resection, in a far more rapid increase in regeneration than in the animals with Eck's fistula, attaining about 50% of the recovery in hepatectomized animals with a normal portal supply.

Comparing these results with those obtained in the animals with Eck's fistula, it was concluded that venous supply is indispensable for hepatic regeneration after hepatectomy (Child), and the role of functional metabolic stress in this process is much less important.

However, there is certain proof lending support to the importance of the functional factor.

G. H. Whipple showed that a carbohydrate diet favors regeneration whereas a fatty diet slows it down.

Rogers found that the unfavorable effect of fats may be attenuated by adding proteins.

Finally, Davis and Whipple established that proteins stimulate reparatory processes to a lesser extent than carbohydrates.

Some endocrine glands influence the reparatory processes of the liver: hypophysectomy or adrenalectomy slows down these processes, while thyroidectomy does not influence them.

In the normal mouse, the administration of deoxycorticosterone enhances the reparatory processes after hepatectomy (Child).

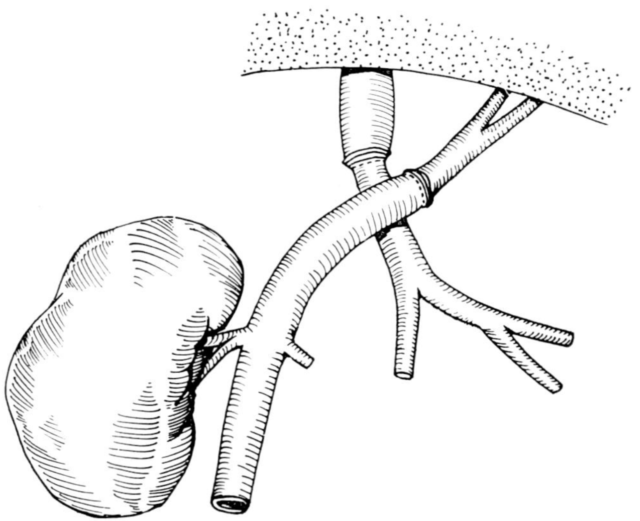

Fig. 41. — Portacaval transposition.

Prior alteration of the liver (post carbon tetrachloride cirrhosis) almost completely arrests the appearance of reparatory processes after hepatectomy (Mann).

This appears to show that between the functional element and recovery of the volume of the liver after hepatectomy there exists a certain correlation and interdependence.

We took up again the experimental study of recovery phenomena after anatomic hepatectomy in dogs. *

After establishing the normal morphology of the liver in the dog, intrahepatic arrangement of the vasculobiliary elements and the ponderal relationship between the lobes and the whole liver or the body weight, anatomic hepatectomy (43% of the total liver weight) was performed.

Postoperatively (the animals were followed up 4 days to 8 months), the animal and the remaining liver were weighed, the structure of the remaining liver and its

* C. Ionescu Bujor, I. Velican, V. Beroniade, C. Florea and C. Constantinescu: *Morpho-functional Alterations after Anatomic Hepatectomy*, communication read at the Institute of Therapeutics of the Academy, 2 February 1959, Bucharest.

function were examined, testing the blood collected from the portal vein and inferior vena cava, where they join the hepatic veins.

Results. The animal's body weight showed a phasic variation, the deficit being of 20% in the first days, 28% after 2 months and returning to initial or even higher values after 3 months. Therefore, on referring the weight of the remaining liver (variable evolutive value) to the weight of the animal after hepatectomy (another variable value), confusions may arise. If we apply the curve of the phasic

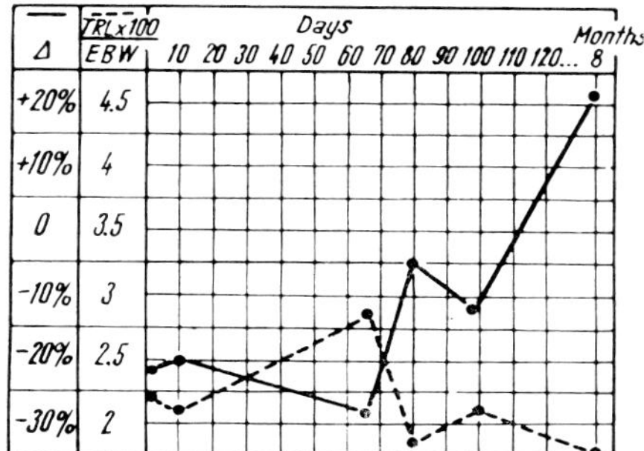

Fig. 42. — Evolution of the ponderal curve (——) and residual liver at the moment of resection/body weight ratio (. . . .), variable in time.

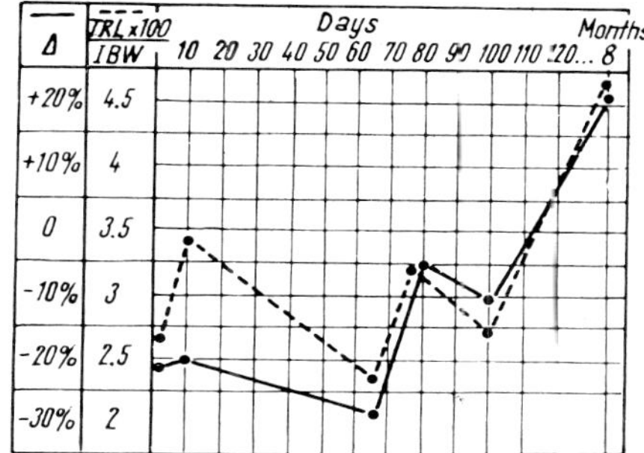

Fig. 43. — Evolution of the ponderal curve (——) and residual liver at sacrifice/initial body weight ratio (. . . .). Note parallelism between recovery of the liver and body weight.

evolution of the body weight of an animal to that of a "10-kg ideal dog", the remaining liver, after resection of the two left lateral lobes (43% of the total liver weighing 315 gm, i.e. 3.15% of the body weight), will weigh after the operation 174.5 gm. If it were admitted that the weight of the liver is invariable and we refer it to the evolutively variable weight of the body, then two mirror image curves (Fig. 42) are obtained. The actual curves never correspond to these theoretical curves of evolution of the $\frac{\text{remaining liver} \times 10}{\text{body weight}}$ ratio, hence the liver also modifies its weight, according to its own laws.

In order to avoid this fallacy (inherent when two variables are involved), the weight of the remaining liver will be referred to a fix value, that of the initial body weight. Thus, there is a ratio of two values that can be measured directly, of which only one is variable (the weight of the remaining liver); the ratio will express the comparative evolution of the weight of the remaining liver in different animals. Fig. 43 shows the evolution of this ratio, i.e. the evolution of the weight of the remaining liver (dotted line) and the evolution of the body weight (solid line). The close relationship between the evolution of the two processes is evident and it may be concluded that recovery of the liver is indispensable for recovery of the body. A certain difference is noted in the first period when the deficient weight of the liver is less accentuated than that of the body; the significance of this period will be discussed later on. It is now possible to interpret the apparently capricious evolution (dotted line, Fig. 44) of the weight of the remaining liver *(RL)* in terms of the actual body weight of the animal *(BW)*. Both values are measurable and variable. The ratio of the comparatively small weight deficiency of the *RL* to the greater deficiency of the *BW* will give values above the normal for the liver; in the middle period when the weight deficiency of the *RL* and of the body become more accentuated the curve also shows low values for the $\frac{RL \times 100}{BW}$ ratio, and runs comparatively close to the *BW* curve.

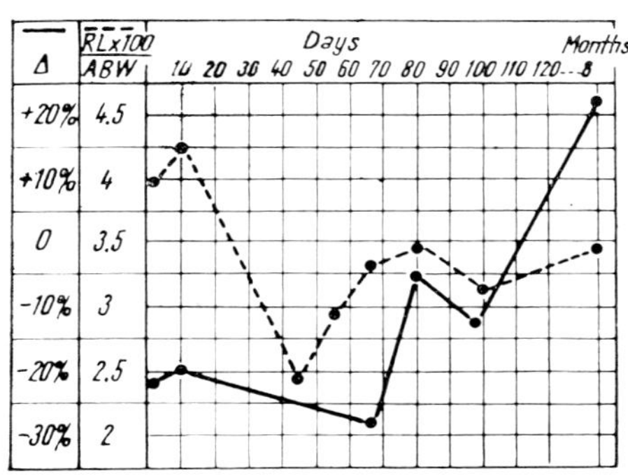

Fig. 44. — Evolution of the ponderal curve (——) and residual liver at sacrifice/present body weight ratio (. . . .). Graphical analysis of the recovery of the liver in the dog.

This graph clearly shows the accuracy of our method of analyzing the results, therefore the practical value of referring the weight of the remaining liver to the initial weight of the animal.

Critical analysis of our material unquestionably confirms "recovery of the liver weight" after anatomic resections. Which is the substrate of this process?

Morphologically, the resected liver is not built up again (in the dog), that is the liver which had 7 lobes, of which 2 were resected, remains with 5 lobes at whatever interval after the resection it is controlled. It is the remaining 5 lobes that increase in weight, and not the 2 resected lobes that form again, thus invalidating the older belief that the liver can build up its lobes again. The fact that the organ as a whole regained its weight led to the erroneous conclusion that the resected lobes had formed again.

Histologically, no aspects of tumultuous proliferation were noted (either by Mallet-Guy or by us), only in the middle and late stage there were some aspects which suggested more intense proliferations. With the techniques used we could not assess the existence of moderate proliferations and can only deny that of intense proliferations.

Radiologic studies have elucidated certain points in this connection. In the normal liver (Fig. 45), the front view shows the branches of the portal tree separated into two fields (right and left liver), with two important branches on the right side and a smaller trunk with two long branches for the left lateral lobes, on the left side; in addition there is a smaller branch in the left posterior paramedian area. The near side-view of the cholecystocholangiography (Fig. 46) reveals the location of the gallbladder projected on the liver.

After 45 days, the portogram (Fig. 47) shows the outspread ramifications of the right territory; the vascular stump of the resected lobes is short; the diameter of the portal branch of the paramedian area is almost equal to that of the ligated vascular stump.

In the cholecystocholangiography (Fig. 48) performed after the same interval, the gallbladder appears to be raised, corresponding to a new spatial distribution of the remaining lobes that occupy almost all the hepatic recess; the two small, remaining paramedian lobes of the left liver are displaced and push the gallbladder up and leftwards.

An almost similar situation was found in a patient with agenesis of the right liver: the left liver occupied all the right subphrenic space and the gallbladder was displaced backward and to the right, paravertebrally (I. Făgărăşanu).

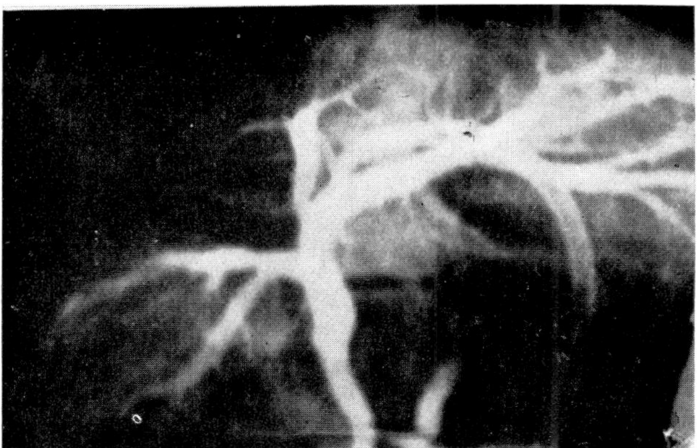

Fig. 45. — Portal venography of the normal liver (dog).

At 90 days the portogram (Fig. 49) in the dog showed: wider spread portal branches in the right area, overlying paramedian lobes, deviated to the left.

After 8 months, the portogram (Fig. 50) image *simulated the aspect of a normal liver*, but with a less widespread portal tree.

As regards the importance of the volume or quality of the blood supply, it is worthy of note that after anatomic resection of two of the four left liver lobes, the two small paramedian lobes represent only 20% of the total remaining liver, and this proportion remains the same throughout the postresectional evolution (followed up for 8 months). Therefore, although the two lobes receive more blood and one even has a portal branch of its own, they do not grow more than the rest of the remaining liver. This is, we believe, an argument against the decisive importance of the *volume* of the blood supply. As regards the quality of this supply, all the remaining lobes receive the same kind of portal blood; this proves that the same quality of blood and the same way, irrespective of the volume supplied, ensure the same liver restoration.

From the functional point of view, the portal and suprahepatic blood determinations pointed to the existence of

— a first period of metabolic disturbances (4—10 days);

— a second period in which some metabolisms are reestablished (carbohydrate, water, etc.) but others still remain deficient (ureogenesis);

— finally, in the late period all the hepatic functions were reestablished (appraised in "digestive rest", without "overloading").

Comparison of the functional aspects and the evolution of the weight of the remaining liver and of the body weight, might lead to the following interpretation:

In the first period, the functional hepatic deficit is greater than the loss of parenchyma, probably due to the brutal stimulation of the interoceptors, in spite of all the measures taken (potentiated general anesthesia in hypotension). The loss

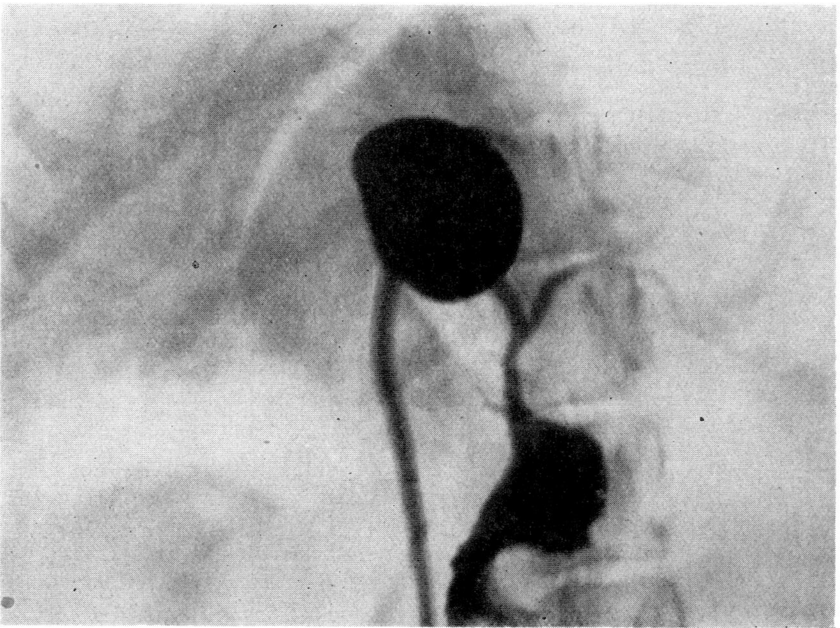

Fig. 46. — Cholecystocholangiography (normal dog).

of body weight is very great owing to the hepatic deficit. The weight of liver is falsely increased (probably congestion). To this congestion of the remaining liver transient hyperbilirubinemia after right hepatectomy in man has been attributed by some authors (Abdol-Islami). The recently traumatized remaining liver, inhibited to a certain extent, may be considered to retain insufficiently the bilirubin produced by the reticuloendothelial system; this may also be considered a contributing factor. At any rate, we attribute the functional deficit to a probable inhibition plus congestion, and masking of the ponderal hepatic deficit likewise to congestion.

In the second phase, the functional deficit reflects fairly exactly the absence of hepatic parenchyma, which accentuates the loss of body weight. As only 43% of the liver is resected, some of the functions are reestablished at an early date (in digestive rest), after attenuation of the initial inhibition; this explains why the

Fig. 47. — Portal venography 45 days after anatomic resection of the liver (absence of the left liver); the residual liver only occupies the right half of the subphrenic space (dog).

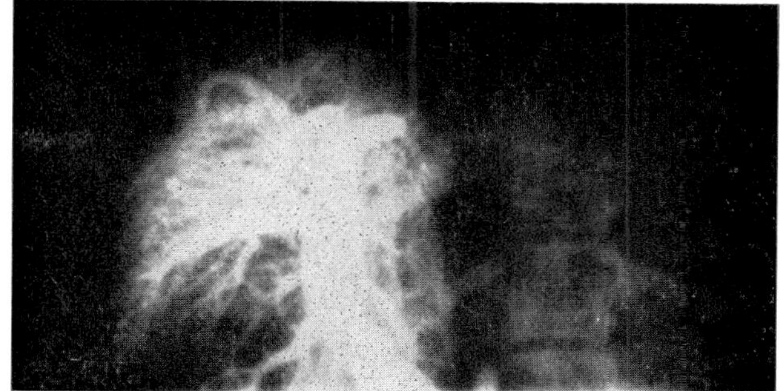

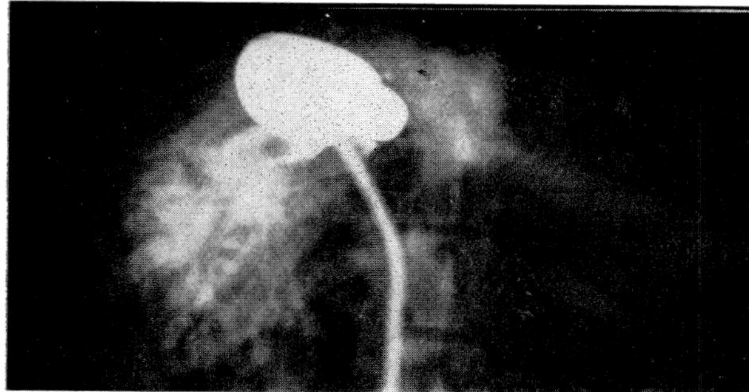

Fig. 48. — Cholecystocholangiography 45 days after anatomic resection of the liver: raised gallbladder (compare with Fig. 46).

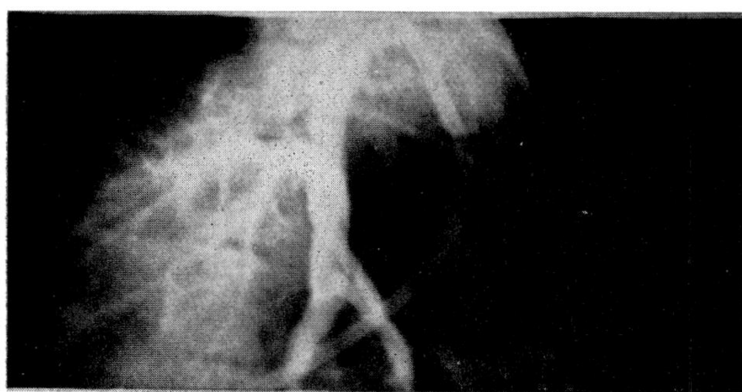

Fig. 49. — Portal venography 90 days after hepatectomy (dog); outspread of the residual lobes.

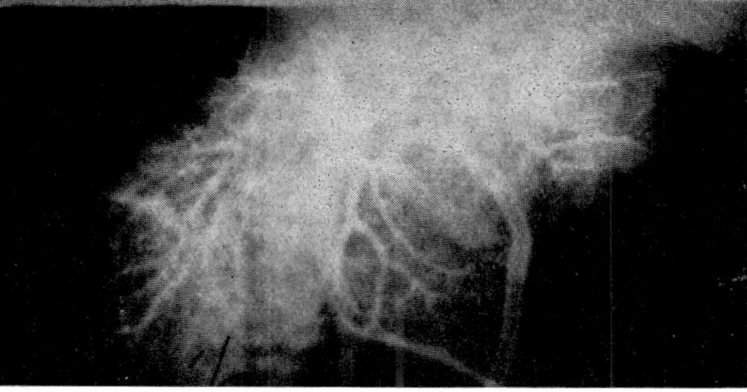

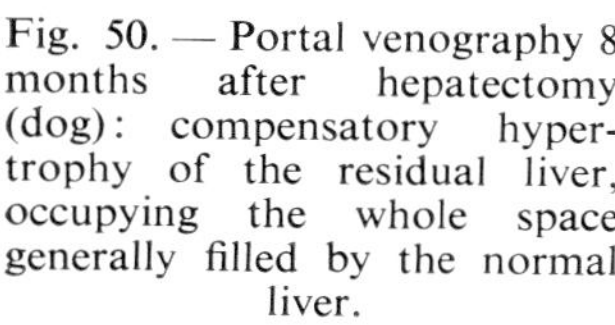

Fig. 50. — Portal venography 8 months after hepatectomy (dog): compensatory hypertrophy of the residual liver, occupying the whole space generally filled by the normal liver.

relative functional improvement is not accompanied by an improvement in the deficient body weight.

Finally, when the liver recovers its volume, all the functions recover, permitting integral recovery of the body weight. Similarly, we believe that the results obtained after resections in the normal dog or the dog with an Eck fistula (or with portocaval transposition) should also be interpreted from the viewpoint of the importance of the functional factor; the fact that the blood flow from the cava only gives a recovery of 50% of that brought about by the portal blood, shows that apart from the volume the quality of the blood supplied is also of importance since the portal blood is the normal functional stimulator of the liver cells.

The material supplied by different investigations and especially by anatomic hepatectomies, allows us to answer the questions put at the beginning of the chapter:

— Hepatic (organ) regeneration does not exist, the liver definitely bearing the imprint of the resection performed.

— After resection, the liver recovers its volume and weight by compensatory hyperplasia of the remaining lobes in case of anatomic hepatectomy, or of the remaining viable parts of the injured lobes in case of non-anatomic hepatectomy.

— Morphologic and functional recovery after resection depends upon:

a) certain hormones (adrenals, pituitary);

b) the input of the blood supply (the lower it is, the more slowly the liver recovers its volume);

c) the composition of the blood supplied to the liver or the functional stress: the portal blood is the necessary activator of morphofunctional recovery. A carbohydrate diet protects the proteins, permitting a more efficient reconstruction of the liver cells;

d) the neurogenic factor has been studied to a lesser extent. From our investigations it appears to be obviously important, at least in the first period (functional postoperative inhibition);

e) the state of the liver; a pathologic (cirrhotic) liver recovers its weight far more slowly.

✦

The importance of the liver, a deeply located organ, that plays a part in all the vital functions of the organism, need not be further emphasized.

The studies of the last 30 years have furnished vast material which could not even be outlined in the available space. However, it is of surgical importance to recall that the participation of the liver in some of the stages of basal metabolism, in maintaining the blood constants and in certain intra- and extrahepatic surgical diseases is of major importance.

In the chapters on pathology (cirrhosis, hepatectomy, etc.) the respective normal and pathophysiologic aspects will be dealt with in detail.

The surgeon's knowledge of normal and pathophysiology will be verified by the supreme test: the hepatic operation, especially resection. The data briefly summed up in the preceding pages will then become of particular importance and upon their putting into practice will depend the very life or the rapid recovery of the patient.

We have also attempted to touch upon some of the most important gaps in our knowledge, which will probably represent for many investigators the scope of future research work.

REFERENCES

1. ALEKPEROV M. A., Probl. Endokrin. Gormonoter., 1955, *4*, 33.
2. ALEKPEROV M. A., Probl. Endokrin. Gormonoter., 1955, *6*, 34.
3. ALPERN D. E., *Fiziopatologie*, Ed. medicală, Bucharest, 1956.
4. BEST C. H., TAYLOR N. R., *The physiological bases of medical practice*, Williams Wilkins, Baltimore, 1955.
5. BRATU I., STOICESCU C., PREDESCU V., Viaţa med., 1959, **6**, *6*, 357.
6. BULIGESCU L., Viaţa med., 1958, **5**, *12*, 1079.
7. CHESTER M. J., Proceedings of the staff meetings of the Mayo clinic, 1952, **27**, *26*, 553.
8. CHILD G. CH., *The hepatic circulation and portal hypertension*, W. B. Saunders, Philadelphia, 1954.
9. CHIOSA L., NEUMAN M., *Vitamine şi antivitamine*, Ed. Medicală, Bucharest, 1955.
10. COMBES B., J. clin. Invest., 1965, **44**, *7*, 1214.
11. EKREM SERIF ESELI, Med. int., 1959, **11**, *3*, 373.
12. GALEA GH., RĂDULESCU M., Viaţa med., 1957, **4**, *3*, 19.
13. GARATINI S., PAOLETTI R., Minerva med., 1958, **59**, *36*, 1731.
14. GAVRILESCU ŞT., MUNTEANU M., Viaţa med., 1959, **6**, *3*, 257.
15. GOODMAN L. S., GILLMAN A., *Bazele farmacologice ale terapeuticii*, Ed. medicală, Bucharest, 1960.
16. GORDIENKO A. N., *Rukovodstvo po patologhiceskoy fiziologhii*, Gosmedizdat, Kiev, 1955.
17. HEGGLIN R., *Diagnosticul diferenţial al bolilor interne*, Ed. Medicală, Bucharest, 1964, p. 695.
18. ICHINHOROIKO V., Khirurghiya, 1958, **12**, 34.
19. JAYLE M. F., Therapia, 1958, **13**, *2*, 37.
20. KVYATOVSKAYA A. N., Pediatria (Mosc.), 1959, *3*, 3—9.
21. LAVEDAN P., *Mythologie et antiquités grecques et romanes*, Hachette, Paris, 1931.
22. LEVY M., BONVALLET M., DELOST P., DONTCHEFF L., HUGGETT G., MINZ B., *Récents progrès en physiologie*, Presses Universitaires de France, Paris, 1956.
23. LUPESCU C., VOICILOIU T., TIGARAN C., Viaţa med., 1959, **6**, *11*, 1029.
24. LUPU N. GH., RUNCAN V., Viaţa med., 1959, **6**, 303.
25. MARINESCU VOINEA, IONESCU-BUJOR C., Anal. rom. sov., 1957, *3*, 5.
26. MINCU I., GEORGESCU R., ICNESCU N., Viaţa med., 1959, **6**, *12*, 1131.
27. MOISEEVA O. I., Byul. eksp. Biol. Med., 1954, *6*, 33; Byul. eksp. Biol. Med., 1954, *8*, 29; Byul. eksp. Biol. Med., 1954, *10*, 19.
28. MOMMSEN TH., MARQUARDT J., *Manuel des antiquités romaines*, vol. XII/1, Thorin, Paris.
29. NASH JOSEPH, *Surgical physiology*, Ch. C. Thomas, Springfield, Illinois, 1953.
30. PAVEL I., *Icterele*, Ed. Medicală, Bucharest, 1957.
31. PEVZNER M. I., *Bazele alimentaţiei dietetice*, Ed. Stat Lit. Ştiinţ., Bucharest, 1953.
32. POPPER H., FENTON SCHAFFNER, *Liver — structure and function*, Hill Book, New York, 1957.
33. PROKOPENKO G. B., *Reguliatsii pischevaritelnovo aparata*, Izd. Akademii Nauk SSSR, Moscow, 1949.
34. RAPPAPORT A. M., POTVIN P., Rev. int. Hépatol., 1963, **13**, *5*, 291.
35. ROGER G. H., BINET L., *Traité de physiologie normale et pathologique*, vol. III, Masson, Paris, 1939.
36. RUNCAN V., *Probleme de hepatologie*, Ed. Medicală, Bucharest, 1964.

37. Saragea M., Foni I., *Cercetări de fiziologie şi fiziopatologie hepato-biliară*, Ed. Acad., Bucharest, 1955.
38. Schiff Leon, *Bolile ficatului*, Ed. medicală, Bucharest, 1966.
39. Sherlock Sheila, *Diseases of the liver and biliary system*, Blackwell, Oxford, 1955.
40. Şoimu I., Viaţa med., 1957, **4**, *4*, 13.
41. Startsev I. V., Klin. Med., 1954, *1*, 91.
42. Toparskaya N. V., Klin. Med., 1952, *12*, 46.
43. Tucherstein O. R., Terap. Arkhiv., 1951, *6*, 43.

CHAPTER 3

INJURIES OF THE LIVER

The outstanding development of industry and transportation in the course of this century has considerably increased the hazard of labour and especially of street accidents. Injuries of the liver occupy an important place among the traumas produced by these accidents, owing both to their frequency and to their gravity demonstrated by the high mortality rate, particularly following closed injury, notwithstanding the obvious therapeutical progress of the last two decades.

HISTORY

Up to the end of the last century, surgeons were almost completely disarmed when faced by injuries of the liver. In wartime, detached fragments of liver parenchyma, protruding through an abdominal wound, were found. As far back as the Romans, Cornelius Celsus recommended the extirpation of such liver fragments. Giovanni Berta, and probably other surgeons, proceeded in this way in 1716.

In the latter half of the 19th century the first operations on the liver began to be performed, corresponding to a certain extent with the modern concept of the treatment of injuries of the liver. Bruns, in 1870, is considered to be the first to have cleaned a bullet wound of the liver surgically. In 1886, Burckhardt was able to control bleeding from a stab wound in the liver. However, injury of the liver was not as a rule treated surgically. In 1887, L. Edler found 543 cases of liver trauma reported in literature not treated surgically, with a mortality rate of 66.8%.

After the first attempts, considered as very daring for those times, a new stage developed in the surgery of injuries of the liver, that of suture and hemostatic tamponade. Later on, tamponade was gradually replaced because of the poor results obtained, and suture of the liver wound was increasingly improved upon.

After the two world wars, during which a vast experience in hepatic traumatology accumulated, new medicosurgical techniques were developed, representing a starting point for steady improvement of the results to be expected following the treatment of these injuries: the discovery of antibiotics, the progress of anesthesia and resuscitation, and perfecting of hepatectomy techniques.

ETIOPATHOGENY

The liver is the intraabdominal organ most exposed to injury because of its volume and the large contact surface with the thoracoabdominal wall. Another decisive factor in connection with the high incidence of injuries of the liver is the fragility of this organ and its relatively limited elasticity. The capsule that envelops it does not offer sufficient protection and it is thin and not distensible. Although situated intraabdominally, most of the liver is protected by the wall of the chest. It is certain that injuries of the liver would be more frequent and severe without the protection of the chondrocostal grid. However, whether the thoracic wall is pierced or is injured, with or without fracture of the ribs, or is traumatized without evident parietal lesions, the liver is always exposed to injury.

In children, injuries of the liver occur more seldom, but are more severe. The chest wall is less resistant, the liver more friable and, proportionally, more voluminous than that of the adult with a relatively larger surface exposed to harm.

The older classification, comprising *closed and open trauma* of the liver, is still generally accepted, because it is the most practical. In closed trauma, the injury is indirect, without a disruption of continuity of the thoracoabdominal wall. An open injury of the liver is produced directly by the injuring agent which has penetrated through the thickness of the thoracoabdominal wall.

The most frequent closed traumas are caused by *street and labour accidents*, especially in countries with a highly mechanized industry and transport system. The motorcycle is one of the most dangerous means of transport owing to its speed, and lack of stability and protective covering. The causes mentioned in classical treatises occur far more seldom today: the kick of a horse, the prod of an animal's horn, of a cart shaft, a blow while boxing, etc. The impact surface being reduced, these traumas almost exclusively involve the part hit directly. Today injuries are as a rule severe, due both to their violence and to the broader application surface; in most cases, the patients with injury of the liver are generally cases of polytrauma, with one or several associated lesions of the organs close to or further from the liver.

According to the circumstances in which the accident occurs and the way in which the traumatic agent acts, closed liver injuries may be divided into the following groups:

1. *Direct blow* in the region of the liver by a hard object in motion or by propelling of the body against a hard object. This category includes most street accidents, those produced by deceleration included, i.e. by sudden putting on of the brakes, when the body may be thrown against the steering wheel. This category also includes blows, kicks, thrusts, etc.

2. *Crushing* is due to a direct blow, when the injured organ is caught between two hard planes of which one at any rate is mobile. In crushing, the force of the missile depends especially upon its mass, whereas in direct blows the force depends especially upon the velocity of the impact. Some of the most common examples of crushing are the accidents in which somebody is caught under the wheels of a car in motion, or between the buffers of a railway car, or under a falling wall.

3. A *fall* from on high is a fairly frequent occurrence on building sites, in faulty landings with the parachute, etc.

4. An *underwater explosion*, with its shock wave, may produce more or less severe lesions to swimmers in the neighborhood, from simple visceral contusion up to disrupting of the abdominal cavity or parenchymatous organs, such as the liver.

5. *Obstetrical ruptures* of the liver in newborn infants may occur during a difficult birth or when artificial breathing is practiced with too much strength. Rupture of the liver is a rare occurrence in the mother during labor; the mechanism of this rupture is a crushing of the liver between the pregnant uterus and the strongly contracted diaphragm.

Open injuries of the liver in peacetime are caused both by firearm wounds and by stabbing with a knife or sharp object. Even objects with a blunt tip may penetrate into the liver if thrust with enough strength. In modern warfare, injuries of the liver are almost exclusively caused by firearms, bullet or gunshot wounds. There is no essential difference between the injuries of war- and peacetime, but the reduced possibility of transport from and treatment on the battlefield render the former far more severe. The injuries caused by gunshot are more severe than bullet wounds.

In order to assess the gravity of a wound, it is well to know from the beginning the nature of the missile: the kind of side-arm or projectile, the distance from which it was fired, the caliber, etc. But in severe cases, anamnestic data must be considered of second interest so that no time should be lost.

In World War II, injury of the liver produced by shells in the armed forces was almost double that caused by bullets. Bipolar wounds, especially those produced by shell splinters, were only observed in 27% of the cases, the remaining 73% being blind wounds. The comparatively small number of bipolar wounds is explicable by their gravity: most of those wounded die on the battlefield and never reach hospital.

IATROGENIC INJURIES OF THE LIVER

The modern means of exploration of the liver and peritoneal cavity, as well as certain means of resuscitation or treatment recently introduced into practice, were followed in some cases by more or less severe or even fatal complications. The injuries produced by rough handling during exploration or by pulling of the retractors with the fumbling hands of an assistant during a laparotomy are well known, but these injuries are generally recognized during the intervention and the remedy immediately found. But medical exploration of the liver may also cause injuries and complications. Simple puncture, biopsy puncture, simple laparoscopy or that accompanied by biopsy puncture, or laparoscopic cholangiography, transhepatic percutaneous cholangiography, etc. are sometimes followed by serious complications: hematoma, hemoperitoneum, choleperitoneum, hemothorax, hepatic or subphrenic abscess, biliary peritonitis, etc. In some cases, simple biopsy puncture of the liver was followed by arteriovenous fistulas or intrahepatic aneurysms.

These complications have already been reported in biopsy exploration of the spleen and especially of the kidney, but iatrogenic injuries of the liver are almost unknown.

It is absolutely necessary to be acquainted with these injuries in order to be able to interpret the, at times dormant, symptomatology that follows upon these explorations in some cases.

Although hemorrhage is generally mild, a transfusion being sufficient for the patient to recover, it must not be forgotten that fatal cases have also been reported. For biopsy puncture, R. Terry reported a mortality rate of 0.12% and an incidence of 0.32% major complications.

Rupture of the liver has also been reported following artificial respiration and especially after external massage of the heart during resuscitation, injuries which must likewise be included in the chapter of iatrogenic injuries, described by us for the first time.

PATHOLOGIC ANATOMY

CLOSED TRAUMA

Several kinds of injuries of the liver are known, determined to a great extent by the nature of the trauma.

Ruptures are produced especially by direct blows over a large portion of the upper abdominal and/or lower thoracic region. Simple ruptures may also be caused by crushing, when the impact is not too violent. In lateral trauma, the rupture is usually

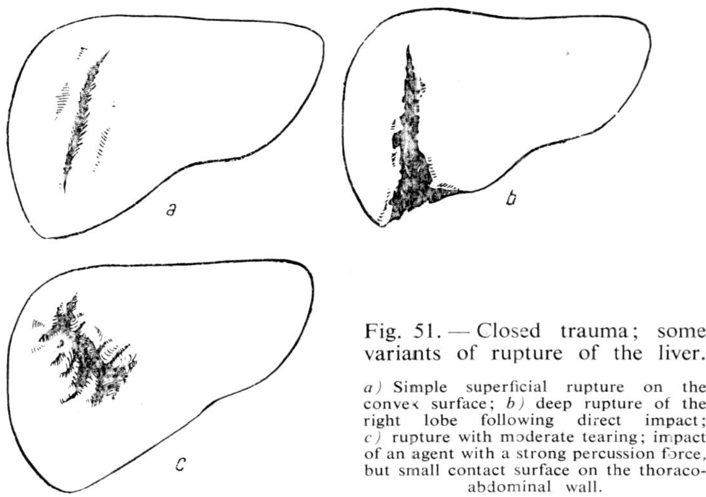

Fig. 51. — Closed trauma; some variants of rupture of the liver.

a) Simple superficial rupture on the convex surface; *b)* deep rupture of the right lobe following direct impact; *c)* rupture with moderate tearing; impact of an agent with a strong percussion force, but small contact surface on the thoraco-abdominal wall.

sagittal, on the convex surface of the liver. Transverse ruptures are produced by ventral trauma, particularly when the patient bends sharply forward at the moment of the accident (Fig. 51).

Crushing is characterized by a number of irregular, more or less deep fissures in the liver parenchyma, breaking up the tissue into fragments and jeopardizing the circulation of the blood.

Complete or incomplete **avulsion** of a tissue fragment is produced by falls from on high. The detached fragment is held by one of the ligaments that fix the liver to the abdominal wall.

Disruption is a rupture with numerous stellate fissures. The blow is generally sharp and powerful over a small area, on the lower part of the chest, for instance a strong blow with a walking stick. Disruption is caused by the shock wave transmitted through the thoracoabdominal wall to the liver, without literally deforming the wall by compression at the moment of the blow. The capsule is not always ruptured, but subcapsular or central ruptures and hematomas may appear in the parenchyma.

OPEN TRAUMA

Side-arm or firearm wounds may be divided into simple or *blind* wounds, *transfixing* or bipolar and *tangential* wounds. In side-arm injuries the wound is simple, with clear-cut margins, whereas the wounds produced by projectiles are

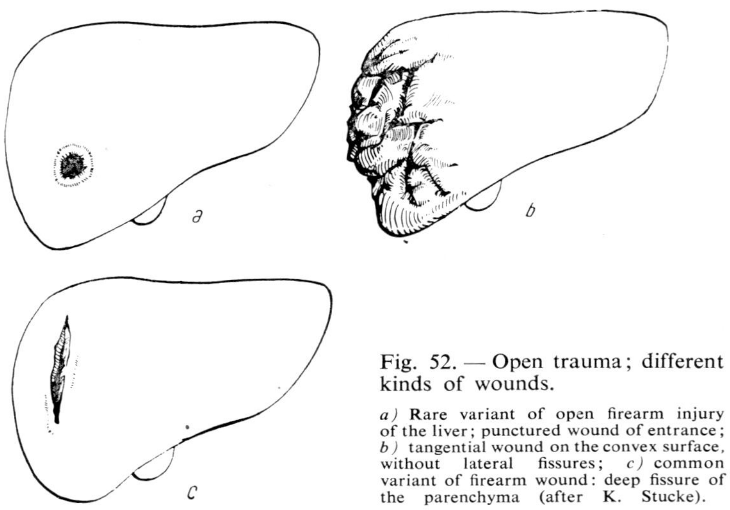

Fig. 52. — Open trauma; different kinds of wounds.

a) Rare variant of open firearm injury of the liver; punctured wound of entrance; *b)* tangential wound on the convex surface, without lateral fissures; *c)* common variant of firearm wound: deep fissure of the parenchyma (after K. Stucke).

far more complex. The wound of entrance in the liver is seldom punctiform; it is as a rule stellate because of the radial fissures on the surface of the organ, that continue downwards along the pathway of the missile. When it is voluminous and the kinetic force very strong, a large number of deep, broad fissures are produced, literally appearing as an explosion of the organ. Still more severe are the supplementary fissures, developing perpendicular to the radial ones. Soon after the accident, the fissures are transformed into cavities full of blood and bile. In bipolar wounds, the exit wound is as a rule very large.

In tangential wounds, that leave a groove on the liver surface, prolonged fan-like fissures develop within the mass of the liver. When the missile comes with great force, fissures are produced even when the bullet passes only through the thoracoabdominal wall without hitting the liver directly.

In firearm wounds, fracture of the ribs is an aggravating factor, as bone fragments may penetrate into the liver together with the missile, considerably broadening the wound and increasing tissue destruction. Another factor that conditions the gravity of the lesions is the extent to which the liver is filled with blood at the moment of the accident. In periods of maximum digestive activity, when the flow of blood to the liver is very high, trauma produces severe lesions.

ASSOCIATED WOUNDS

Injuries of the liver are considerably aggravated by concomitant damage to other organs. In open trauma the organs in the vicinity of the liver are as a rule involved, and in closed trauma distal lesions of the skull or limbs may be encountered. According to K. Stucke, associated lesions of the other organs occur in 80% of the closed traumas produced by street accidents.

R. W. Crosthwait showed, in a study of 640 cases, that only 32.8% of the cases had injuries exclusively of the liver; and 86% of the latter were stab wounds. In order of their frequency, the authors found associated injuries in the thorax, stomach, small intestine, colon, kidneys, pancreas, skeleton, spleen, extrahepatic bile ducts, central nervous system, urinary bladder. The diaphragm is also involved in a number of cases, in both open and closed trauma.

In a series of 829 accidents, G. F. Madding found associated visceral wounds in 60% of the cases. The extrahepatic bile ducts, and especially the gallbladder, were injured in 1—2% of the cases.

The common bile duct is seldom involved, although it is so close to the liver, but the bile duct is generally torn together with the large vessels cf the hepatic pedicle and the patient dies before being admitted to the hospital.

PATHOLOGIC PHYSIOLOGY

The immediate consequence of a rupture of the liver or a penetrating wound is hemorrhage; the more massive the injury, the larger the ruptured vessels. Spontaneous hemostasis only occurs when the injury is not too extensive and when large vessels are not involved. Hemorrhage leads to shock and death if surgical hemostasis is not accomplished.

The intrahepatic bile ducts are ruptured together with the vessels. At first, a small amount of bile is discharged through the damaged ducts, probably due to reflex inhibition of bile secretion. However, secretion soon increases and bile accumulates in the peritoneal cavity or, in open trauma, runs out through the abdominal or thoracic wound. Biliary peritonitis or pleurisy, at first aseptic, develops.

Rupture of the bile ducts results in infection of the damaged liver tissue, which is then propagated to the peritoneal or pleural cavities. In closed trauma, infection of the bile in the intrahepatic ducts is due to latent bacteria, whose virulence is awakened in contact with the damaged tissues. In open trauma, other factors contributing to infection are associated: projectile in the liver, pieces of material or dirt, necrosis of the tissues, etc.

To this destructive tissue action, induced from the beginning by the missile, may be added necrosis of the liver parenchyma fragments, devitalization due to involvement of the large vessels that supply arterial blood or drain the venous blood. Necrosis is accompanied by resorption of a large amount of toxic substances, with a general effect upon the organism. When necrosis is restricted to small fragments of liver tissue and the patient survives, there follows a phase of spontaneous elimination of the necrosed portions, resorption and then regeneration of the liver, that occurs rapidly in comparison to that of other tissues.

Devitalization is caused not only by interruption of the afferent or efferent circulation of a liver fragment, but also because of the powerful tissue motion, for instance along the pathway of a missile penetrating at high speed. Strong vibrations modify the delicate tissue architecture of the liver, resulting in inhibition of the metabolic exchanges within the liver cells. Some cells survive, but remain impaired to a certain extent. Lindner and Abendroth recently described late diffuse hepatic dystrophy after closed trauma without rupture. The authors explain this dystrophy by intrahepatic vasomotor disturbances due to rapid motion.

SYMPTOMATOLOGY

Patients with closed or open injuries of the liver are generally brought to the hospital in a state of shock, with circulatory respiratory and nervous disturbances characteristic of this syndrome. Since shock is caused first of all by hemorrhage, the laboratory tests will show a decrease in the number of red blood cells, hemoglobin and hematocrit. As in any internal hemorrhage, a leukocytosis of 15,000 to 20,000 cells/mm^3 will be found. In injuries of the liver, the state of shock is hardly ever of the purely hemorrhagic type since traumatic elements are added, which by the tendency to hemoconcentration mask acute anemia to a certain extent. An exception are stab wounds, with section of the large vessels, in which the hemorrhagic aspect is very evident and tissue trauma of much lesser importance.

In closed trauma, the local examination reveals abrasions, ecchymoses, parietal deformities produced by blood or serous collections, depression of the lower part of the chest wall due to rib fractures, with or without a mobile chest wall. In open trauma, the wound of entrance and of exit can be seen. From the wound, blood or blood mixed with bile may run out. The omentum or fragments of liver parenchyma may protrude through large open wounds. The outer wound does not always correspond with the zone of projection of the liver upon the thoraco-abdominal wall. The missile or side-arm may sometimes penetrate into the liver through a wound of entrance high up on the thorax or low down in the abdomen. The oblique route of the injury may be approximately established by the route of the injuring agent and the position of the patient at the moment of the injury. Apart from the exterior signs, the abdominal symptomatology is determined by the presence of blood in the peritoneal cavity, by peritoneal irritation due to the biliohematic exudate, by associated lesions of the neighboring organs and, finally, by different complications.

The pain is not characteristic; more accentuated at the level of the injury, it becomes diffuse and includes the whole abdomen, but seldom radiates towards the right shoulder (less than 10% of the cases).

The presence of blood in the peritoneal cavity may be detected by palpation or percussion, rectal or vaginal examination and peritoneal tap. Percussion reveals dullness in the flanks, especially on the right side, but it changes with a change in the patient's position. Rectal or vaginal palpation may reveal increasing filling of the pouch of Douglas. Peritoneal tap, recommended by E. Wright in 1947, is used by American surgeons in the diagnosis of intraperitoneal hemorrhage. In Europe it is seldom practiced.

The most frequent signs of peritoneal irritation are rigidity of the abdominal wall, Blumberg's sign and paralytic ileus. In the first days after the accident it is difficult to say whether the signs reflect mere peritoneal irritation or an actual peritonitis. Rigidity of the abdominal wall, especially in the right upper quadrant, is helpful but not decisive for the diagnosis, since it may be caused by simple contusion of the thoracoabdominal wall without visceral involvement, or may be absent even when injuries of the underlying organs exist. When present, rigidity involves not only the parietal muscles but also the diaphragm whose mobility is reduced or abolished; the resulting superficial respiration aggravates respiratory insufficiency in shocked patients.

The frequency and diversity of the injuries associated with open or closed trauma are very great. In severe trauma it is not possible to draw up an exact evaluation of all the injuries, but the central nervous system must be examined as rapidly and completely as possible (wounds, compression of the vault, signs of fracture of the base of the skull, coma, paraplegia due to fracture of the spine, etc.); similarly, it is necessary to detect any damage to the chest wall and the lungs (subcutaneous emphysema, signs of pneumo- or hemothorax). Massive hematuria reveals rupture of the kidney, generally on the right side. Associated injuries of the abdominal viscera can be examined directly by the surgeon by clinical, radiologic or surgical control.

The following clinical case, observed by us in a provincial hospital, shows how varied and misleading the associated injuries and their mechanisms of production are. A farmhand jumped from the top of a cart full of hay, about 8 feet high, directly onto the handle of a hayfork which penetrated into the pelvis through the anus. The fork handle was pulled out and he was admitted to the hospital a few hours later in a severe state of shock and with abdominal rigidity. Several small abrasions around the anus were noted. Nobody could say how deep the handle had penetrated. Pre- and peroperative antishock treatment was given. Laparotomy revealed rupture of the anterior rectal wall, which was sutured; there was no other intestinal lesion; rupture of the liver on the posterior aspect of the right lobe, with moderate intraperitoneal bleeding. The liver wound was cleaned and sutured. Shock worsened postoperatively and the patient died three hours later. At the postmortem examination, the route of the injury was determined. The handle had penetrated through the liver and the diaphragm and into the right lung, rupturing the lower and middle lobes. Incomplete surgery was due to masking of the thoracic symptomatology by the other symptoms, among which rigidity and shock were foremost; the history data were incomplete, hemoptysis absent and the accident itself unusual.

DIAGNOSIS

Injuries of the liver caused by open trauma are more readily diagnosed than in closed trauma. In most cases in which the wound of entrance and eventually of exit correspond to the area of projection of the liver upon the thoracoabdominal wall, the diagnosis does not give rise to any difficulty. As the missile may follow an oblique pathway, the surgeon must think of possible injuries of the liver not only in the presence of thoracoabdominal wounds in the area of the liver, but also when they are situated higher up on the chest or lower down on the abdomen. Discharge of bile through the wound is a pathognomonic sign, but is not obligatory for establishing a diagnosis of open trauma of the liver. Apart from the site and path of the wound, general and local signs of internal hemorrhage and peritoneal irritation should be looked for. A detailed diagnosis is not necessary, since wounds in this region demand surgical exploration in all cases, as a more accurate evaluation of the injuries can be established.

In closed trauma, the diagnosis is likewise based upon the history, signs of shock and local signs of internal hemorrhage and peritoneal irritation. In some cases, in spite of the apparent gravity of the trauma, these signs appear fairly late or are not sufficient to be able to reach a conclusion. The surgeon is faced with a dilemma hard to solve: is it a contusion or is there also an injury of the liver ? The only efficient method in such cases is to keep the patient under constant observation, to repeat the clinical examinations and laboratory tests at short intervals, every quarter of an hour, in order to appraise the evolution of the general and local signs. As shown by Kirschner (1938), the patient may be followed up for 3 or 4 hours before signs of internal hemorrhage develop.

In contusion, gradual improvement of the general and local condition is to be expected; in case of internal hemorrhage, aggravation occurs. It is obvious that a delay until convincing signs are obtained should be avoided, since a constant hazard of irreversible shock exists.

In multiple injuries with shock, in which rupture of the liver with internal hemorrhage is suspected, the clinical examination and especially the local signs are far more important than the laboratory tests, at least in the first phase when the tendency to hemoconcentration in traumatic shock is compensated by hemodilution produced by bleeding. Notwithstanding, the laboratory tests may come in very useful in uncertain cases when the laboratory data (hemogram, hemoglobin and hematocrit), followed up every quarter of an hour, point to the progressive hemodilution of internal hemorrhage.

In some cases of multiple injury, the abdominal symptomatology is masked by craniocerebral or thoracic wounds. In all craniocerebral trauma accompanied by shock the origin of the latter, whether abdominal, thoracic or of another kind, must be determined; in injury of the brain, without associated injuries, shock is exceptional. In thoracic trauma without or with minimal hemothorax, the hemorrhagic shock syndrome can probably be accounted for by an intraperitoneal hemorrhage. Injuries of the liver are more likely, the lower the thoracic trauma. In case of massive hemothorax, a concomitant injury of the liver is difficult to diagnose. In such cases peritoneal tap may be useful. When the diaphragm is ruptured, thoracentesis may aid in the diagnosis when small amounts of bile are mixed with the blood withdrawn from the pleural cavity.

X-ray examination is only indicated in severe injury of the liver when it does not delay resuscitation or imply transport maneuvers. Several views can be taken in the resuscitation division or on the operation table. These may reveal a "ruptured contour" of the diaphragm corresponding to the injury. Certain air-fluid levels may also be discovered in the region of the liver when internal hemorrhage occurs concomitantly with rupture of a cavity organ.

Laparoscopy in abdominal injuries. Although explorative abdominal puncture is used by American surgeons in the cases in which the symptomatology is not very clear, it has of late been replaced by laparoscopy (Larny and Sarles, Boquien, Debray et al.). It is recommended before laparoscopy to perform an abdominal radiography: the presence of gases in the peritoneal cavity indicates the probable presence of the rupture of a cavitary organ and contraindicates laparoscopy.

Laparoscopy will supply information of two kinds: in most cases it will evidence a more or less accentuated hemoperitoneum. The presence of blood evidently implies an emergency laparotomy. In some cases laparoscopy also reveals the source of the hemorrhage (liver, spleen), thus indicating the direction of the incision, and in other cases a digestive exudate may be found in the peritoneal cavity or an injury to one of the abdominal organs appears. There are cases in which no visceral injury is found and laparotomy would have been useless. In patients with multiple injuries who are very difficult to examine and whose symptoms are difficult to interpret, laparoscopy is widely applicable because of the state of shock of these patients, who would undergo with great difficulty an explorative laparotomy.

COMPLICATIONS

HEMORRHAGIC COMPLICATIONS

After surgically treated or untreated injuries of the liver, the following comparatively rare but exceptionally severe hemorrhagic complications may occur:

1. **Secondary hemorrhage due to rupture of a subcapsular hematoma.** Subcapsular rupture of the liver is seldom diagnosed in unoperated patients. When the hematoma is voluminous and occupies a position accessible to abdominal palpation, rupture may be suspected. Improved general condition permits the X-ray examination and a bulging of the diaphragm may be observed. The patient's condition may continue to be satisfactory, with at most low grade fever and slight jaundice. During coughing or a change in position, the distended liver capsule may rupture and the content of the hematoma is discharged into the peritoneal cavity. Accentuated pain, signs of internal hemorrhage, then a state of hemorrhagic shock rapidly develop. Up to the moment when the capsule is ruptured, the hemorrhage is spontaneously tamponed by increase in the intracavitary pressure. Rupture produces renewed bleeding from the damaged intrahepatic vessels.

In such cases, the diagnosis is based upon the following: the spontaneous onset of an internal hemorrhagic syndrome with shock in a person who has recently suffered from thoracoabdominal trauma. The prognosis of these patients, incompletely recovered from the initial trauma, is not favorable.

2. **Traumatic hemobilia.** This complication was concomitantly described in 1948 by H. K. Owen and Ph. Sandblom, who coined the name of traumatic hemobilia. Up to 1962, 28 cases were published in the literature, as found by Ph. Détrie.

Traumatic hemobilia develops after closed trauma in patients with central rupture of the liver. Autolysis in the lesional focus may erode one of the large vessels and the neighboring bile duct, resulting in a vasculobiliary communication. In most cases, the right branch of the hepatic artery and right hepatic duct are involved. The arteriobiliary communication seldom occurs in the branches of the left side. In some cases, a triple arterial-portal biliary communication may develop. The vasculobiliary communication takes place either through the cavity produced by the rupture, or directly through an arteriobiliary or arterioportobiliary fistula.

From the initial injury and up to the appearance of hemobilia there is a free interval of 2—4 weeks, but at times shorter or longer, 16 hours to several weeks. Hepatic trauma and the free interval are important history data for the diagnosis. Some patients, operated immediately after the initial accident, apparently exhibited only superficial ruptures of the liver, that were sutured.

Clinically, hemobilia is characterized by a symptomatic triad: pain, jaundice and intestinal hemorrhage. Pain, of the gallbladder colic type, is caused by filling and distension of the bile ducts. Jaundice, which is not accentuated, is caused by obstruction of the bile ducts with blood clots. Intestinal hemorrhage — hematemesis and melena — is massive and repeated. With hemorrhage pain disappears, then jaundice, as the blood is no longer retained in the bile ducts.

The history and clinical examination are sufficient to establish a diagnosis of traumatic hemobilia, without being able to determine the site of the lesion. The location of the vasculobiliary communication is difficult to determine, even intraoperatively, except for the rare cases in which the surface alterations correspond to the deep lesional focus. In such cases, the hepatic cavity is opened and packed with gauze. Cholecystostomy is performed in all the patients to decompress the bile ducts. Peroperative T-tube cholangiography sometimes reveals diffusion of the contrast medium in the traumatic cavity, or stenosis of the injured bile duct. As a rule, cholangiography is not satisfactory and, in order to locate the injury, hepatic arteriography has been attempted. Ph. Détrie was able to find the lesional focus by injecting the contrast substance through a catheter introduced into the hepatic artery through the sectioned pyloric artery. An area of diffusion revealed the site of damage to the artery.

In only 8 of the 28 cases published was it possible to determine the site of the injury peroperatively. Tamponing was done in 2 cases, ligation of the common hepatic artery and pyloric artery in 1 case, ligation of the right hepatic artery in 4 cases. In the 8th case, G. Thomeret performed right controlled hepatectomy, with transfusions (32 liters in all) before the operation, to compensate for repeated hemorrhage. All these 8 patients recovered following surgery.

The other 20 patients were considered to have been insufficiently treated, since even if some of them were operated, only a simple cholecystostomy or choledochotomy with T-tube drainage was performed to decompress the bile ducts, without discovering the bleeding site. Ten patients died from loss of blood and ten recovered spontaneously.

COMPLICATIONS DUE TO NECROSIS OF THE LIVER TISSUE

Fragments of the liver tissue of various size may be torn adrift from the liver or remain attached by a narrow strip of tissue. Insufficiently nourished, or lacking any blood supply, these fragments undergo necrosis, forming sequestra which generally lie in the middle of a pool of blood. Autolysis produced by proteolytic enzymes does not permit the formation of liver sequestra when the fragments are small, but when they are large the necrosis process exceeds the autolytic capacity of the fragment. Hepatic sequestration is generally accompanied by local infection and intrahepatic or subphrenic abscess. The treatment consists in removal of the sequestrum and drainage of the purulent collection.

SEPTIC COMPLICATIONS

Intra- and extrahepatic blood collections, mixed with bile, fragments of devitalized liver tissue and sometimes foreign bodies, generally become infected. In some cases the septic process involves the right pleural cavity or the peritoneal cavity, with all the severe consequences of empyema or generalized acute peritonitis. As a rule, suppuration is localized in the form of an abscess, intrahepatic, subphrenic or situated in other regions of the peritoneal cavity, distal to the liver.

1. **Hepatic abscess.** This complication appears after central or subcapsular ruptures, when the capsule is more resistant or less strained by the intracavitary pressure exercised by the blood collection. Fever, chills, local pain or pain irradiating towards the right shoulder, are not characteristic and insufficient for the diagnosis. Of greater importance is the association of this symptomatology with a free interval, after a recent injury of the liver. Sometimes, the importance of the free interval escapes the clinician's attention, especially when the injury occurred 2 or 3 months previously. In the X-ray, a certain immobility or limitation of the diaphragm movements, segmentary bulging of the cupola or fluid level may be observed. Explorative puncture is definitely contraindicated, except when the surgeon is prepared to operate as soon as the pus is discovered. Surgery consists in evacuation of the purulent collection and drainage of the remaining cavity.

2. **Subphrenic abscess.** The blood collections that appear around the liver after closed or open trauma, not treated surgically, may resorb spontaneously when they are not too large or infected with highly virulent bacteria; otherwise, suppuration of the hematoma takes place. The symptomatology, diagnosis and treatment of the latter do not differ from that of any other subphrenic abscess.

COMPLICATIONS DUE TO OVERFLOW OF THE BILE

Apart from its septic potential, the bile strongly irritates the tissues with which it comes in contact when the bile ducts are ruptured. The irritating and septic action mutually potentiate each other, increasing the hazard of overflow of the bile into the tissues or the serous cavities. The complications caused by the deleterious action of the bile depend upon the amount of bile discharged from the damaged ducts, the capacity of the organism to limit the pathologic process and the extent of the initial traumatic lesions.

Biliary peritonitis is the most feared complication.

Biliary pleurisy occurs in the cases in which rupture of the liver and intrahepatic bile ducts is accompanied by rupture of the diaphragm and of the peritoneal and pleural serous membranes. It is a frequent complication in open trauma, especially in firearm wounds.

External biliary fistulas occur after open injuries or closed operated trauma. The amount of bile lost depends upon the caliber of the ruptured bile duct, the fistula opening, or eventual obstacles located towards the terminal portion of the bile ducts (dyskinesia, stenosing odditis, etc.).

Biliobronchial fistula is likewise an external biliary fistula in which the bile is discharged through the respiratory pathways. These fistulas generally develop after open thoracoabdominal wounds, with concomitant hepatobiliary, diaphragmatic and pleuropulmonary injury. Biliobronchial fistulas seldom develop after closed trauma, but they may appear as a primary or secondary complication after a free interval. In secondary complications, the bronchial trunk is at first intact, the communication being gradually produced by erosion.

Residual, pseudocystic intrahepatic cavities filled with a biliary fluid may appear late, after resorption of the hematic content from a bile-blood pool subsequent to central or subcapsular rupture. These cavities are maintained by a fistulized intrahepatic bile duct or extravasation of the canalicular bile from the collapsed walls of the residual cavity. Such a cavity is well tolerated as long as there is no infection. Its presence, however, may bring about the late development of a hepatic abscess.

OTHER COMPLICATIONS

1. **Hepatobiliary complications.** The following hepatobiliary complications, more seldom encountered, have been reported:

Cholangitis. Infection of the bile ducts may be caused by stasis produced by compression or by a fistulous communication between the intrahepatic bile ducts and a septic cavity.

Stenosis of the intrahepatic bile ducts. This is a late complication caused by faulty healing of the injured bile ducts. The stasis that develops in the afferent bile branches of the stenosed duct predisposes to infection.

Diffuse hepatic dystrophy is likewise a late complication caused by strong turbulence of the liver tissue in closed trauma. It has been described by Lindner and Abendroth. M. Gerger and F. Byloff recently published data on the late results of isolated ruptures of the liver produced by closed abdominal trauma; in 7 patients they found different disturbances not observed before the accident: anorexia, pain, gaseous distention, intolerance of fats, headaches, serum protein alterations. All the 7 patients were operated after the accident and no pathologic hepatic alterations, apart from the traumatic injury, were found.

2. **The complications of associated lesions** exhibit a great anatomopathologic and clinical diversity. They are difficult to systematize or to foresee in the posttraumatic evolution.

3. **Pulmonary embolism.** In injuries of the liver, more or less numerous isolated liver cells or groups of cells are liberated and may penetrate into the damaged hepatic veins, then are transported by the blood stream through the lower cava vein to the right heart and from there to the branches of the pulmonary artery. Because of the state of shock, it is not possible to determine to what extent these microembolisms aggravate the patient's general condition.

4. **Hepatorenal syndrome** is a very severe complication that develops in cases with extensive injury of the liver. The syndrome was differentiated clinically by C. H. Heyd (1931), and was then studied from the viewpoint of pathologic physiology by F. C. Helwig (1931) and T.G. Orr (1932). They assumed that the disturbances were caused by the toxins produced by autolysis of the liver cells in the lesional focus. Other possible causes envisaged were bacterial toxins, endocrine alterations caused by shock, functional exclusion of the renal cortex in shock, transfusion accidents, etc. The clinical picture of the hepatorenal syndrome is dominated by a symptomatic triad: fever, jaundice and anuria, and a comatose state. Some patients pass small amounts of weakly concentrated urine, containing albumin and red blood cells. Petechial bleeding of the skin has likewise been noted.

EVOLUTION AND PROGNOSIS

Many open and closed traumas are incompatible with life because of extensive injury of the liver and other associated injuries. The severely wounded die on the battlefield or on the street in an accident, and only some of them are brought to hospital. The following data give us an idea of the mortality rate among hospitalized casualties: towards the end of the last century, Edler in a statistics of 543 injuries of the liver of various degrees of gravity, not treated surgically, because of the lack of possibility in those times, gives a mortality rate of 66.8% (1887).

In World War I, most wounds of the liver were operated. According to G.W. Beebe and M. DeBakey, the mortality continued to be very high: 66.2%. The statistics published between the two world wars showed only a slight decrease — to about 60%.

In World War II, however, there was a net decrease, down to 27%, according to the statistics of G.F. Madding on 829 cases.

After the war, due to improved treatment of the severe cases, the mortality rate steadily fell to 10% according to Sparkman, 13.5% according to Madding and 16.4% according to Fogelman. Associated injuries represent the most important factor, determining the evolution and prognosis of injuries of the liver. The injuries involving the liver alone give a fairly low mortality rate: 4.8% in the statistics of R.W. Crosthwait et al. (1962) in comparison to the general mean proportion of 17.3%, calculated on 640 various hepatic traumas. At present, most authors analyze the mortality rate per group of patients, in terms of the number of organs involved. Thus, Crosthwait found a mortality rate of 11% when the liver plus one organ was involved; 23.6% when the liver plus 2 organs was involved; 28.4% the liver plus 3 organs, and 38.1% and 84.6%, respectively, when the liver plus 4 or 5 organs was involved.

In an extremely interesting study, Crosthwait, in his clinic in Houston, found that stab wounds gave the lowest mortality: 3.4% as compared to bullet wounds, 25.6%, and closed trauma, 44.8%. In most of the cases, death was caused by hemorrhage from the liver and especially the neighboring organs, injured concomitantly.

TREATMENT

In principle, any injury of the liver, open or closed, necessitates surgery when the diagnosis is certain or even doubtful. Surgery must have two important objects in view: 1) to arrest bleeding, and 2) to prevent complications.

SURGICAL INDICATIONS

Many discussions have arisen of late concerning surgery in severe injury of the liver: should the operation be performed immediately or after prior treatment of shock? L. Wright, A. Prigot and L. Hill (1946) propose the following indications:

1. In case of massive bleeding, threatening the patient's life directly, and with signs of severe shock in spite of intensive treatment, the operation should be carried out immediately under the protection of massive blood transfusions during surgery.
2. In casualties with moderate bleeding, with a state of shock that gradually deteriorates, but which responds favorably to the antishock treatment, the operation is performed after the treatment.
3. In repeated hemorrhage, with successive improvement and aggravation of the general condition, the patient is operated at a moment in which his condition has improved, therefore, as a rule after previous treatment of shock.
4. In slight hemorrhage, with the probability of spontaneous recovery, it is recommended to follow the patient attentively, the surgical team being ready at any moment for transfusion and operation.

According to D.F. Madding (1955), in severe states of shock the patient is operated only after receiving 1 to 2 litres of blood. When the state of shock is less severe, the treatment of shock and the operation are performed concomitantly.

M. Reifferscheid (1958) sustains the priority of antishock treatment over surgery. The patient is put on the operating table as soon as he is admitted to hospital. Transport of the patient from the admission room to the ward and from there to the operating theatre may aggravate the hemorrhage and the state of shock. The antishock treatment with oxygen, blood, plasma, plasma substitutes, started on the operating table, is continued until the patient's condition improves. A valuable indicator of the efficiency of the treatment is the resumption of diuresis: urine begins to pass through the indwelling catheter. If the shock treatment does not succeed within 2 hours, the operation should be no longer delayed. E.F. Nicolayev and Saegesser proceed in the same way.

I.A. Sichkaruk (1962) is an adept of immediate surgery, with concomitant massive transfusion.

R.W. Crosthwait et al. (1962) proceed as follows: in the admission service, the patients with abdominal or thoracic, closed or open trauma, are examined rapidly for signs of internal hemorrhage. At the same time, an intravenous route of administration is established, for instance the saphenous vein. Until the blood group is determined, colloidal solutions are administered in shock. Penetrating wounds of the chest are rapidly closed by suture or occlusive dressing. Emergency pleurotomy is applied in case of marked pneumothorax or hemothorax. X-ray examination is performed when possible and when the patient's state permits it. Transfusion is continued in the operating theatre. Surgery should not be put off in an attempt to raise the blood pressure or to establish the diagnosis in detail.

On analyzing the procedure of other authors, it may be concluded that the main preoccupation of the surgeon is to establish the sequence or concomitance of the antishock treatment and the operation. The most rational attitude appears to be:

Antishock treatment, applied at the moment of admission of casualties in a state of shock. In this connection, the promptness of Crosthwait and associates is remarkable, but it is questionable whether the admission service is the most suitable place for its application.

Surgery, performed as soon as the diagnosis is established or when the likelihood of an internal hemorrhage exists. The operation may be delayed only in uncertain cases, therefore with small or moderate bleeding. In accentuated bleeding, with an acute hemorrhage syndrome, in casualties with thoracoabdominal trauma, without a hemothorax abundant enough to justify the hemorrhagic shock, the clinical and eventually the laboratory data will be sufficient to establish a diagnosis of injury of the liver and the necessity of immediate surgery.

Delay when the diagnosis is certain or very probable, in view of prior antishock treatment, is an aggravating factor in ruptures of the liver when the patient continues to lose blood. The interval between admission and the operation can be used for the administration of oxygen and the necessary amounts of fluid and blood, at a rate imposed by the circumstances. This interval should likewise be used for establishing the diagnosis, preparation of the surgeon and anesthetist, etc. In severe thoracic trauma associated with injury of the liver, intravenous administration of fluids should be done with the greatest care; a rapid rate of administration might induce acute failure of the right heart.

In milder injuries of the liver, such as stab wounds or closed trauma with minimal rupture and hemorrhage, the operation should not be put off because of the patient's general condition, but only when there is a chance of spontaneous recovery. Instead of an "armed expectation", tiring for the surgeon and dangerous for the patient, it appears more reasonable to resort to surgery from the beginning when injury of the liver is certain or very probable. Theoretically, an armed expectation has in view the timely detection of signs of aggravation of the hemorrhage or the onset of severe complications such as biliary peritonitis. Actually, this detection does not take place in due time.

PREOPERATIVE PREPARATIONS

Apart from the treatment of shock, other preoperative therapeutic measures must be taken. Synthetic analgesics are administered for assuaging the pain, avoiding opiates. Morphine induces spasm of Oddi's sphincter, biliary stasis and discharge of bile from the injured ducts. An indwelling vesical catheter will reveal the gravity of the shock and efficiency of the treatment. Of late, a permanent pre-, intra- and postoperative gastric tube has been recommended for emptying the atonic stomach, relieving respiration and the return circulation. The toxic products of gastrointestinal stasis, difficult to bear for the injured liver, are thus eliminated. *Tetanus antiserum* can be started before the operation in open trauma, using the dilutions recommended for persons with a low tolerance. The following, more concentrated doses, will be administered in the course of narcosis, when the serum is well tolerated. Broad spectrum *antibiotics*, plus penicillin are administered by intravenous route, together with the first infusion. Fractures of the limbs are temporarily fixed, as well as a mobile chest wall. Tracheostomy is performed in case of accentuated respiratory insufficiency, especially in case of severe associated thoracic trauma.

ANESTHESIA

The best indicated type of anesthesia in injury of the liver is tracheal intubation with muscle relaxants and assisted or controlled respiration. Fluothane is considered to be well tolerated by the liver; barbiturates are contraindicated.

INCISION

In open trauma, the site and size of the parietal injury will indicate the incision. In closed trauma, the incision will be chosen by the surgeon in order to have a wide route of access to the liver. The incision, whether transverse, longitudinal or oblique, can be broadened if necessary when the lesions found on exploration of the liver require a larger approach. The incision may branch off on the abdomen or on the chest wall, along an intercostal space, usually the 8th, giving both thoracic and abdominal access to the liver. The thoracic incision has been used more frequently of late. In spite of the progress of anesthesia and resuscitation, it has not been fully accepted when the patients are in a state of deep shock. In the statistics of Crosthwait (1962), comprising 611 operated cases, the abdominal incision was practiced in 96% of the cases, and the thoracoabdominal incision in only 4% of the cases.

EXPLORATION OF THE INJURIES

Initially, exploration of the peritoneal cavity will show what is the main source of bleeding. Damaged vessels may be found that bleed more than the liver. Hemostasis is, therefore, carried out in the order imposed by the abundance of the bleeding.

If no active hepatic hemorrhage is found, therefore if bleeding has been temporarily and spontaneously arrested, as occurs in most casualties with shock, the organs in the peritoneal cavity are explored and any perforation is rapidly sutured. In case of active hemorrhage, priority is given to hemostasis.

In order to be able to examine the liver, the blood and clots are removed from around the liver. The aspirator is not of much use, as it is socn obstructed with clots. These are removed by hand and the blood is absorbed with gauze.

Autotransfusion with blood from the peritoneal cavity was successfully used for the first time in a case of rupture of the liver by E. Kreuter (1917). C.S. White (1923) and G. Rosarie (1932) demonstrated experimentally that retransfusion of the blood is not dangerous if performed within the first 6 hours after rupture of the liver. For retransfusion, the blood should be filtered ten times. Most authors are against autotransfusion; I. Scott (1951), M. Saegesser (1955), G.F. Madding (1955) and M. Reifferscheid only recommend autotransfusion on the following conditions:

— when without transfusion there is imminence of death;

— when there is no possibility of transfusion with other blood;

— when not more than 6 hours have elapsed after the accident, since within this interval little bile has had time to mix with the blood and there are not yet large amounts of hepatic autolysis products. Autotransfusion is definitely contraindicated when the blood is infected with the content of perforated organs.

OPERATIVE TECHNIQUE

The operative technique must correspond with the therapeutic principles listed previously: hemostasis and prevention of complications. The measures to be taken in order to prevent complications are the following: closure of the biliary fistulas and resection of the devitalized liver fragments or of the fragments threatened by devitalization. To this may be added evacuation of the blood from the peritoneal cavity, the removal of foreign bodies, drainage, etc.

When injuries occur in the hilar region, accompanied by massive bleeding, it is of paramount importance to clamp the hepatic pedicle. When the aorta is not concomitantly clamped (Fig. 53) above the emergence of the celiac trunk, or at any rate the superior mesenteric artery, shock develops soon after clamping of the hepatic pedicle, or the existing state of shock worsens because large amounts of blood accumulate within the portal system, equivalent to an abundant internal hemorrhage. Within the brief moment when the hepatic pedicle can be clamped, the injured branches of the hepatic artery or portal vein can be sutured or ligated in the hilus. In the literature a single case of suture of the vena porta trunk, by P. Hallopeau in 1911, is cited.

Choice of the surgical treatment depends upon the kind of injury of the liver, its location, the abundance of the hemorrhage and skill of the surgeon. There are four principal methods of treatment: suture of the liver wound, tamponade, simple drainage and resection of the liver. These can be applied separately or combined. Irrespective of the method applied, any bleeding vessel or ruptured bile duct should be ligated. Similarly, any detached liver fragment, or fragments attached only by reduced bridges, should be removed. Temporary hemostasis is accomplished by manual compression or with long elastic clamps that do not crush the liver tissue.

Suture of the liver wound is indicated especially in clean, linear incisions, superficial or of moderate depth. Suture can also be applied in infractuous wounds, after cleaning the sides of the wounds and ligating the vessels and bile ducts. In order to arrest bleeding, the sutures should be tightened as much as the resistance of the liver tissue permits. Thicker sutures can be tightened more than thin sutures, which tear the tissue. The thickest catgut is used in approximating sutures or U-shaped sutures at 2 to 3 cm distance from the edge of the wound. In order to avoid the formation of a residual cavity, the suture must be placed deep in the tissue (Fig. 54 *a*, *b*).

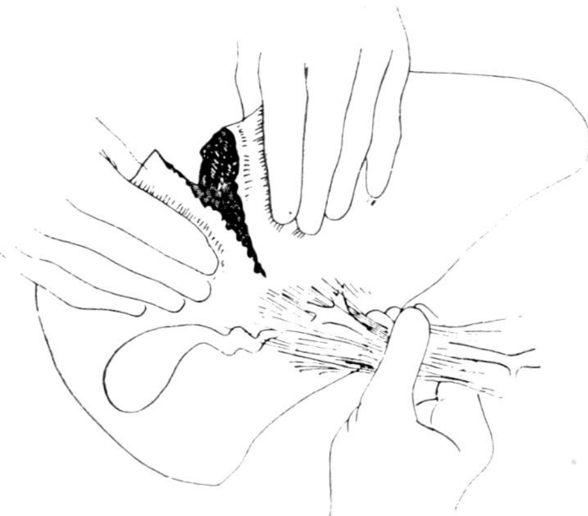

Fig. 53. — Temporary hemostasis in severe injuries, with abundant bleeding: digital compression of the hepatic pedicle and of the ruptured liver (after K. Stucke).

Tamponade. *Tamponade with gauze* was the traditional method used before World War II. Today it is considered as the least indicated method. It is only used as a heroic hemostatic means in deep, bleeding wounds, difficult of access, with a great loss of substance, when the vessels cannot be ligated directly and the wound cannot be sutured. This method is also indicated in subcapsular hematoma that presents hazard of secondary hemorrhage if it is not removed; the liver capsule is incised, the hematoma evacuated, the deep, bleeding vessels are ligated and the cavity is packed with gauze and drained with a rubber tube.

Tamponade with gauze has gradually been given up not only because its efficiency as a hemostatic is minimal, but also because it predisposes to complications, the most severe of which is secondary hemorrhage on removing the gauze. Moreover, the gauze saturated with blood and bile favors infection.

Tamponade with resorbable hemostatic material. In deep infractuous wounds of the liver, with lack of substance and active hemorrhage, simple suture is either impossible or inefficient. Tamponade with gauze treated with thrombin solution or powder is likewise uncertain, since it is never sufficiently compressive to control an abundant hepatic hemorrhage.

After World War II, a marked progress was made in the treatment of liver wounds by tamponade. Today, resorbable hemostatic material can be sutured in the wound, e.g. oxycel, sorbocel, gelfoam, etc., that increase the hemostatic action of the tampon (Fig. 55). This method of treatment is indicated in deep wounds or in wounds with a great loss of tissue, in which simple suture cannot ensure a satisfactory hemostasis. The technique for the application of resorbable hemo-

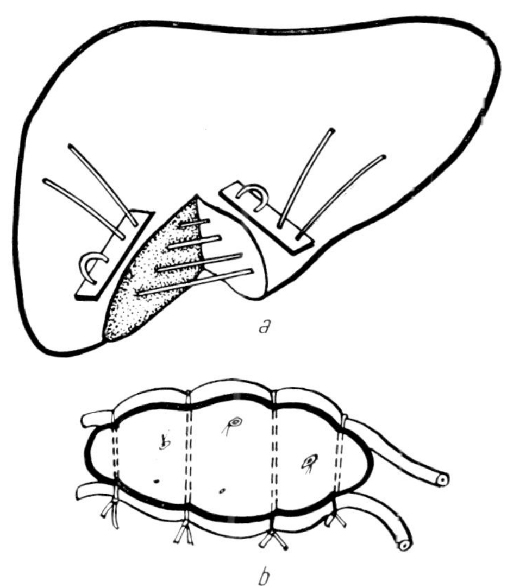

Fig. 54. — Special hemostatic suture techniques.

a) compressive sutures with magnesium strips; *b)* compressive suture of a bleeding portion, over rubber tubes.

static material is simple: thick catgut sutures are passed through the two sides of the wound as for simple sutures, without drawing them together. The cavity between the two sides of the wound is filled with resorbable sponges or gauze, and then the catgut sutures are drawn tight. The resorbable material being caught within the two sides of the wound, the sutures hold much better.

This method is not ideal, but is superior to tamponade with gauze (Fig. 56). In the wounds for which it is recommended there probably is no ideal method, i.e. wounds in which suture is insufficient and resection implies too great an intervention. Various complications have been reported after the use of resorbable material: infection, biliary fistulas, residual cavity, foreign body reactions, etc.

Tamponade with pedicle flaps from the diaphragm or omentum is likewise combined, the same as the preceding method: tamponade + suture (Fig. 57). Viable material being included within the suture, the method appears in principle superior if the following conditions are complied with: the sutures must be drawn sufficiently close to ensure hemostasis of the two parts and sufficiently lax for the flap sutured in the wound not to become necrosed. It is difficult to meet such conditions concomitantly.

Drainage. Drainage of the residual cavity is done in the following circumstances:

— *Associated with other methods of treatment*, especially with tamponade. The rubber or polyethylene tube, with multiple perforations, is introduced among or under the gauze within the cavity produced by the rupture.

— *Simple drainage*, only with a drainage tube, is recommended by Madding in deep hepatic wounds, produced by stabbing and without abundant bleeding.

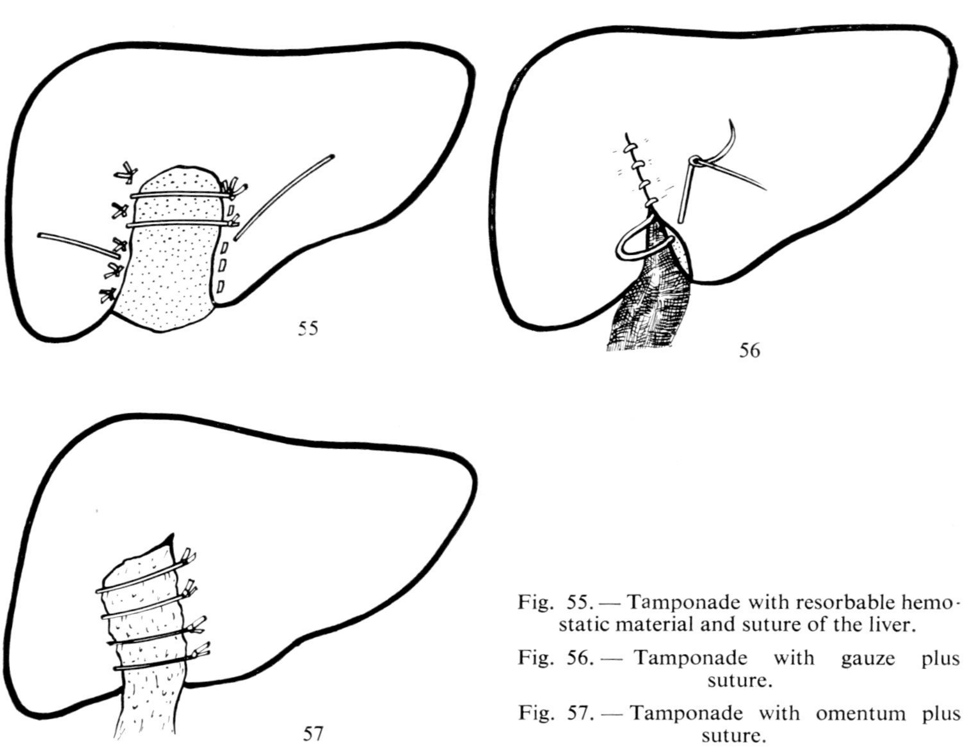

Fig. 55. — Tamponade with resorbable hemostatic material and suture of the liver.

Fig. 56. — Tamponade with gauze plus suture.

Fig. 57. — Tamponade with omentum plus suture.

When the wound of entrance on the liver surface is larger than the tube, it is sutured around the tube.

— *Drainage of the peritoneal cavity* is recommended by most authors, although it is not always used. Drainage was applied in only 138 of a series of 611 operated cases published by Crosthwait; apart from other complications, biliary peritonitis developed in 2 cases and one patient died. The author considers that it is wise to drain bullet wounds or ruptures of the liver, as the amount of bile discharged by even a small bile duct cannot be predicted. Other workers, such as Madding with his vast experience, Sparkman and Fogelman, etc. consider drainage as an essential method for preventing the complications produced by retention of the pathologic products in the peritoneal cavity.

There are few surgeons who do not use either hepatic or peritoneal drainage (G.W. Papen, L.V. Scott, etc.). Their arguments are rather of a theoretical order: drainage predisposes to bleeding due to erosion of the liver, to secondary infections, biliary fistulas, eventration, etc. We believe that systematic drainage after cholecystectomy is certainly exaggerated, but after most injuries of the liver it is a necessity.

— *Peritoneal drainage as single method of treatment.* When the approach to the wound is difficult and there is no bleeding at the moment of the operation, some surgeons do not stress the necessity of suture or tamponade, but drain the peritoneal cavity with a rubber tube. In a statistics of 300 cases published by G. Hellström (1961), this method was applied in 91 cases, obtaining better results than by the other methods of treatment, except tamponade with resorbable material.

Resection of the liver. In injuries of the liver, resection is indicated in deep broad wounds, with more or less voluminous detached liver fragments. When these fragments are sutured to the remaining liver, the patient is exposed to the most severe complications: necrosis of the devitalized fragments of the liver, hemorrhage and bilirrhage from the other part, infection, etc.

Theoretically, resection is also indicated in the rare cases of traumatic hemobilia, when hemorrhage is abundant, when the hemorrhagic focus has been located and when bleeding cannot be arrested by other hemostatic methods. Up to date, we have found a single case of traumatic hemobilia treated by hepatectomy cited in the literature (that of Thomeret).

The amplitude of the resection, determined by the extent of the macroscopic lesions, may attain right or left hepatectomy. In appraising the viability of a partly detached liver fragment, it is not so much the color of the injured portion that counts, as the whole liver changes its aspect due to hypoxia, but the quality of the parenchyma bridge that attaches it to the remaining liver and which may or not contain the vessels necessary for a sufficient afferent irrigation and venous drainage. When the fragment is considered non viable, it is sectioned below the ligature of the parenchyma bridge joining it to the remaining liver; hemostasis is then accomplished by direct or transfixing ligatures.

At times it is not a single fissure that partly detaches a fragment of the liver, but multiple, crossed fissures with numerous bleeding fragments. Such wounds often impose an atypical or controlled hepatic resection, in terms of their gravity and location. It is no longer a question of sectioning a bridge of liver tissue joining a fragment to the remaining organ, but an actual hepatectomy, within the liver parenchyma, according to the rules of typical or controlled resections.

Hepatectomy is seldom practiced in injuries of the liver. It is avoided by most surgeons, since the hazards are considered too great in severe trauma accompanied by shock. As a rule, resection is restricted to removal of the visibly non-viable fragment, that is almost completely detached, and does not raise any particular problems of surgical technique or imply shock inducing operative maneuvers.

POSTOPERATIVE TREATMENT

The antishock treatment must be continued until hemodynamic equilibrium is obtained and blood pressure is stable. Antibiotics are administered until all danger of septic complications has disappeared. Particular attention should be paid to eventual secondary hemorrhage, evidenced through the drainage tube. Similarly attentive observations of respiration, excretion and blood coagulability are of the greatest importance.

REFERENCES

1. Atanasiu I., Mareş E., *Chirurgia de campanie*, Bucharest, 1956.
2. Brittain R. S., Surg. Clin. N. Amer., 1963, **43**, *2*, 433.
3. Carlson P., Averbook B. D., Pearson S., Amer. Surg., 1962, **28**, *2*, 74.
4. Coban N. et al, *Hemobilia traumatică*, Communicated at the Surgery Society, Bucharest, April 1964.
5. Crosthwait R. W., Allen J. E., Murga F., Beall A. C., DeBakey M. E., Surg. Gynec., Obstet., 1962, **114**, **6**, 650.
6. Debray Ch., Leymarios J., Martin E., Hernandez Cl., Carayon J., Coste F., Presse Méd., 1968, **76**, *16*, 737.
7. Debray C., Pironeau A., Paolaggi J. A., Papi E., Herzaft R., Arch. Mal. Appar. digest., 1968, **57**, *12*, 971.
8. Delom P., Mém. Acad. Chir., 1953, **79**, *19—20*, 501.
9. Denischi A., Ionescu I., Neagu V., Papahagi E., *Traumatologie practică*, Ed. Medicală, Bucharest, 1963.
10. Détrie Ph., J. Chir. (Paris), 1962, **83**, *2*, 185.
11. Făgărăşanu I., *Les traumatismes iatrogènes du foie*, in *Congrès français de Chirurgie*, Paris, Sept. 1969.
12. Hellström G., Acta chir. scand , 1961, **122**, *6*, 410.
13. Hervé P., Lyon chir., 1955, **50**, *6*, 730.
14. Madding G. F., Arch. Surg., 1955, **70**, *5*, 748.
15. Melnikov A. V., Anal. rom. sov. (Chir.), 1956, **10**, *3*, *(11)*,78.
16. Pessereau G., *Traumatismes du foie*, in *Encyclopédie médico-chirurgicale*, ch. 7014—S. 10.
17. Reifferscheid M., Dtsch. Z. Chir., 1958, **288**, *4*, 361.
18. Sandblom Ph., Surgery, 1948, **24**, *4*, 571.
19. Sichkaruk J. A., Vestn. Khir., 1962, **88**, *5*, 40.
20. Sparkman R. S., Fogelman M., Ann. Surg., 1954, **139**, *6*, 690.
21. Stucke K., Langenbecks Arch. Klin. Chir., 1956, **284**, 629; 1957, **287**, 791.
22. Stucke K., *Leberchirurgie*, Springer, Berlin, 1959.
23. Terry R., Brit. Med. J., 1952, **1**, 1102.
24. Williams L. F., Byrne J. J., Amer. J. Surg., 1966, **112**, *3*, 368.
25. Zamcheck N., Klausenstock O., New Engl. J. Med., 1953, **249**, 1062.

CHAPTER 4

HEPATIC INFLAMMATORY PROCESSES AND SCLEROSIS

A. HEPATIC ABSCESS

HEPATIC ABSCESS DUE TO PYOGENIC BACTERIA

AMEBIC ABSCESS

B. HEPATIC CIRRHOSIS AND ITS SURGICAL TREATMENT

ASCITES SYNDROME

PORTAL HYPERTENSION SYNDROME

A. HEPATIC ABCESS

The liver abscess is a circumscribed suppuration of the hepatic parenchyma, in which part of the tissue, necrosed following the action of certain pathogenic agents, undergoes purulent lysis under the influence of histolytic enzymes liberated by the invading organism and by leukocytes.

The clinical picture, course, prognosis and therapeutic indications differ from case to case and are influenced to a great extent by the nature of the pathogenic agent (microbial or parasitic) and by the portal of entry into the liver. If we attempt to describe as many etiologic entities as there are pathogenic agents and portals of entry, we will come up against many repetitions and not against opposed homologous elements. An extreme attempt (Eolian) at describing in a single chapter all the forms of hepatic abscesses led to an obligatory differentiation into two categories: abscesses due to pyogenic bacteria and those due to ameba. This shows that at present it is necessary and also useful to separate hepatic abscesses into two categories, in agreement with many authors (Bockus, Brzhozovskiy, Sherlock, etc.). We shall adopt this classification of the material in the present chapter, the more characteristic aspects being illustrated by demonstrative clinical cases selected from our statistics.

HEPATIC ABSCESS DUE TO PYOGENIC BACTERIA

Definition. The hepatic abscess is a purulent collection either single or multiple, due to penetration and multiplication in the liver of the common bacteria of suppuration. The hepatic lesion is chiefly a complication of an infection that has developed in another part of the body. Irrespective of the importance of the first localization, hepatic involvement brings a particularly severe element in the evolution of the infection, which often threatens the patient's life. Due to the gravity of hepatic involvement the surgeon must be well acquainted with the clinical and therapeutic aspects of these abscesses.

Bacteriology. In principle any bacterium may bring about hepatic suppuration, but some bacteria have only exceptionally been encountered in the liver (gonococcus) and others with constant frequency by all authors, in the course of time.

In the order of their statistical importance, we may list *Escherichia coli* 30%, streptococcus 26%, staphylococcus 20%, association of these bacteria 13%, and then varied bacteria (*Bacteroides funduliformis*, etc.). Of late, a particular importance has been taken on by *Bacillus Friedländer*, which was seldom isolated in the past from hepatic abscesses, but which today is frequently associated with a ifatal evolution (in 10 of 14 deaths from hepatic abscess according to Baehr, or in 23% of the abscesses according to Bockus).

Etiology and pathology. The incidence of hepatic abscess differs according to the community investigated. There is no exact evidence because not all cases are examined postmortem, especially in case of regional (gangrenous appendicitis) or general (septicemia) infection whose gravity accounts for the disease. According to necropsy protocols, the incidence was of 0.45—1.47% up to 1938 (when chemotherapy began to be applied), 0.56% în 1948 (Kinney—Ferebee in Debakey—Schiff). In hospital statistics, the incidence of hepatic abscess ranged between 0.04 and 0.007%.

According to different statistics, the frequency of hepatic abscesses is steadily decreasing due to the increase in therapeutic efficiency, the progress of medicine in general and that of chemotherapy and surgery in particular.

This is particularly evident in the statistics of the U.S.S.R., explicable by the complex systematic preventive and treatment measures taken by the medico-sanitary staff.

A similar situation occurs in other socialist countries; in Romania, hepatic abscess is seldom encountered in surgical practice (in our statistics 6:12,000, i.e. 0.05%).

Both sexes are equally affected, males somewhat more frequently.

The age at which a hepatic abscess may occur is very varied; however, the maximum frequency appears to be around the age of 30.

Mechanism of production. The following are the portals of entry of the bacteria:

Arterial blood route. The bacteria penetrate along this route in septicemic states or confirmed septicemia, when numerous abscesses are produced in the liver. They are sometimes so numerous that they appear like punctiform, flickering, pale yellow dots against the darker background of the liver. Part of them become confluent forming larger disseminated cavities between which numerous small, isolated abscesses, that have formed later, may be seen.

These phenomena generally appear after important, primary localizations of the pyogenic infection in other organs (osteomyelitis, septic endocarditis), but may also appear after more common localizations (anthracoid furuncle). However, although the liver receives a significant volume of blood through the hepatic artery, it has two specific characteristics: a) it represents less than half of the total blood supply; b) it represents a volume of blood that has already been filtered through the pulmonary capillaries with an intense phagocytic activity (except for the bacteria mobilized by the valvular vegetations in endocarditis of the left heart). This probably also explains the rare occurrence of metastatic hepatic abscesses produced by way of the arterial blood supply. For these abscesses to develop, the density of the bacteria per ml of blood must be very high, or else the decrease in humoral defense mechanisms must be very low; in both instances, this means an important stage in aggravation of the general disease, frequently verified in practice.

Portal blood vessels are the portal of entry into the liver in 10 to 30% of cases (Ochsner — in DeBakey-Schiff). Inflammatory diseases of the gastrointestinal tract and its adnexae are a source of infection; the blood collected by the branches of the portal vein from the abdominopelvic viscera brings bacteria into the liver, either isolated or more often as a septic embolus. Many of the bacteria are retained and destroyed, but in terms of their number, virulence and other factors, part of them are fixed in the sinusoids, multiply and give rise to a small focus of inflammatory necrosis that represents the beginning of a hepatic abscess.

The preceding disease may be acute appendicitis, that was not operated in time (more seldom now than in the past), ulcerative colitis, etc. Exceptionally, in children, the bacteria may reach the liver through the umbilical veins.

It is worthy of note that from the primary visceral focus to the liver, the bacteria are usually carried through the portal flow in a septic embolus from the lesser thrombophlebitic areas of the original branches of the portal vein. This intermediary phase has been called by some "portal pyemia"; as will be seen further on the septic process can be intercepted in this phase of thrombophlebitis of the original portal branches (case 2).

The thrombophlebitis phase may sometimes be particularly severe (affecting the portal trunk), since obstruction of the porta threatens the patient's life directly and very swiftly. The bacteria coming by portal route are either bacillus coli, or a streptostaphyloenterococcal association, or different anaerobic bacteria.

Bile route. The bacteria that occasionally cross the hepatic filter to the bile ducts are discharged together with the bile without a characteristic symptomatology or cause cholangitis episodes, temporary in most cases. It is sufficient for a given cause to produce a relative (or accentuated) biliary stasis for these bacteria to multiply and produce cholangitis with alarming clinical signs; masked by the latter the slight inflammatory cholangitis reaction may develop into smaller and then larger hepatic abscesses with a starting point in the pericanalicular inflammatory infiltrate. The biliary tree being ramified throughout the liver and the density of the bacteria being approximately the same in all the lobular ramifications, it can be readily understood that adequate conditions exist for the simultaneous appearance of numerous, initially small, abscesses against a background of cholangitis (case 3). Today, when cases of septic infections (generating septicopyemia) and neglect of important diseases of the abdominopelvic viscera are very rare, the incidence of hematogenic, arterial and portal hepatic abscesses are likewise very rare. The frequency of conditions inducing biliary stasis (lithiasis, tumors of the pancreas, etc.) has not decreased to the same extent, cholangitic hepatic abscesses are proportionally more frequent today than in the past (the increase is relative, not absolute), i.e. about 22% (Kinney) and even 37% according to some authors.

There are also other portals of entry into the liver, likewise through the bile ducts: certain parasites — ascarides — that penetrate into the bile ducts or their ramifications, where they die and necrose. They bring with them intestinal bacteria that multiply within the biliary territory blocked by the body of the parasite in putrefaction (Djabadian). The difference consists in the number of abscesses that are far less numerous in hepatic ascariasis, since a limited number of parasites invade the liver, than in cholangitic abscesses; moreover the preceding general disease (intestinal ascariasis) is better supported than a neglected lithiasic cholangitis, so that surgery is often efficient (case 4).

Injuries to the liver may induce hepatic abscesses. In a penetrating abdominal wound the traumatic agent almost always introduces bacteria into the body. A hepatic abscess may be caused by a varied flora, including skin bacteria (staphylococcus, streptococcus) and telluric bacteria (anaerobic), especially in shell wounds during wartime. In open abdominal injuries, there may be a deep dissociation of the liver tissues, where blood and bile accumulate. Bacteria from the general circulation, or from the bile ducts will find in these hemobiliary collections favorable developmental and multiplication conditions; the hemobiliary collection is then transformed into voluminous hepatic abscess at times.

Up to 10% of the total number of hepatic abscesses are attributed to a traumatic factor, with the mechanisms outlined higher up.

A particular form of this traumatic factor is the liver biopsy puncture during a cholangitic episode which favors the appearance of an abscess at the site of the puncture (case 5).

These are the main routes of penetration of bacteria into the liver, but the question of how hepatic abscesses are produced is not complete. In some cases the possibility of a retrograde infection (superior cava — inferior cava — hepatic veins — hepatic abscess) has been incriminated in order to explain hepatic abscesses after inflammatory conditions of the cephalic extremity. These form the so-called "idiopathic" or "cryptogenic" category of abscesses (which are not numerically negligible), that cannot be listed in the above categories.

Cryptogenic abscesses represent 17 up to 60% of the cases of hepatic abscesses according to certain statistics (Alain-Mouchet). The clinical course starts with a poorly outlined primary infection and hepatic involvement that only becomes clearly delineated with time. This gradual succession, with an attenuated symptomatology renders the sequence of the phenomena and, therefore, their interpretation very difficult.

From the practical standpoint, the progressive evolution of these abscesses makes it possible to establish the diagnosis and start an active therapy, with greater chances of success.

In view of the number of diseases that may give rise, by various routes of access, to hepatic abscesses, the question arises of why this localization is relatively rare? Many authors emphasize the resistance of the liver to infection (Eolian: the role of the liver as generator of antimicrobial substances; Beaver: massive hepatic irrigation, the localization of infection due to the action of the sinusoidal reticuloendothelial cells).

Eolian supplied experimental proof that infection results in the appearance of hepatic abscesses only when prior sensitization of the liver occurs following a long-standing action of the pathogenic agent.

Pathology. Macroscopically, the abscess may be single (especially in the right lobe) or multiple (approximately uniformly disseminated), small or voluminous. The center of the abscess if fluid, viscous or nonhomogeneous (purulent exudate); around it the wall is formed of hepatic tissue, with accentuated peripheral inflammation and necrosis towards the inner aspect where the color and consistency gradually approaches that of the abscess content. In abscesses with a longer evolution the wall takes on a peculiar aspect, that of a granulation tissue, formerly called pyogenic membrane (an improper designation according to Crăciun). Microscopic examination shows a structureless substance in the central part, within which drops of fat, nuclear ghosts of polymorphonuclear leukocytes, cellular remains and stainable bacteria or bacteria with a modified tinctorial affinity (in the course of destruction), can be discerned. Within the wall of the abscess, towards the cavity, there is a predominant polymorphonuclear infiltrate that masks and dissociates the hepatic tissue; towards the outer aspect hepatic trabeculae, partly dissociated by edema or bands of leukocytic infiltrates can be discerned. The liver cells exhibit various stages of structural alteration, from fatty loading or steatosis to granular, vacuolar degeneration and tinctorial structural changes in the nucleus, and finally karyolysis and karyorrhexis.

Between the leukocytic ring and the still viable parenchyma there is a fibrogenetic tendency that represents a mode of morphologic limitation of the inflammatory-destructive process. In recent abscesses, the connective fibers hardly outline the contour of the abscess and some penetrate between the hepatic trabeculae; older abscesses sometimes present a dense, sclerous connective tissue that surrounds the cavity, lining the inner aspect with granulation tissue.

Inflammatory lesions in the form of leukocytic infiltrates and a historeticulocytic reaction can also be noted around the venules and small branches of the bile ducts; they are of importance since they mark the portal of entry of the infection into the liver;

— post-thrombophlebitic abscess: a small abscess limited to a portal space in the center of which one can still discern the thrombosed portal ramification with the partly lysed clot in the course of purulent transformation (Letulle);

— cholangitic abscess (Crăciun): the bile ducts monotonously contain bile mixed with altered polynuclears, pus globules and here and there amorphous material and bile thrombi. Along the bile ducts there is a mixture of bile and disintegrated leukocytes (pus), limited by the neutrophil infiltrate and histocytic reaction of the sustaining tissue. Around the acute inflammation, thromboses of the smaller vessels can be discerned (Crăciun; Letulle). The existence of small, multiple abscesses without marked lesions of the bile ducts or portal rami, but with the presence of diffuse, turbid intumescence, is evocative of a severe general disease, as for instance septicemia or septicopyoemia. The hepatic abscess, either initially or after a subsequent evolution comes in direct contact with Glisson's capsule. The visceral serosa is invaded by lymphatic route; it loses its shiny aspect and fibrin is deposited, forming symphyses with the diaphragm and neighboring viscera, i.e. perihepatitis. It is of importance for the surgeon to remember that the maximum intensity of the perihepatitis process occurs at the level where the abscess is closer to the capsule.

Clinical and laboratory study. It may be asserted that hepatic abscesses have no pathognomonic sign or symptom.

Moreover, in the initial phase, the more important signs of the preceding disease are superposed; only when the abscess has fully developed do the general signs of infection become dramatically accentuated and the patient will himself point to the site of maximum pain at the level of the liver. However, there are also cases with an insiduous onset and subclinical evolution; these cases generally correspond to deeply situated abscesses.

In the following pages mention will be made of the most important signs and symptoms, and inasmuch as possible, in the order of frequency with which they appear in the clinical picture.

Symptoms. Fever (present in 95.8% of cases) is often the first symptom, but takes on different aspects from case to case (recurrent, intermittent). In many cases, during the first period chills occur almost daily (especially in multiple abscesses) and are followed by profuse perspiration that exhausts the patient; these chills occur at very different hours and are encountered in 33—66% of the cases. With time, the fever shows a tendency to fall especially in patients whose resistance permits a chronic evolution (particularly in single abscesses). The pulse is as a rule in keeping with the fever in the phase of high fever, but is more accelerated than warranted by the fever in the hours of remission (indicating the gravity of the toxic involvement of the myocardium). However, the pulse curve is no longer clinically significant in the patients with a certain degree of jaundice.

Spontaneous pain (present in 92—96% of the cases) often appears late (especially in single abscesses) and has a wide range of variations: in many cases it starts with a deep, indefinite pain situated along the right thoracoabdominal borderline; as the hepatic lesion develops, the pain becomes more definite and is at times hardly tolerable; it is accentuated by the extreme phases of breathing and certain postures when the ribs press upon the liver.

The pain is classically described as radiating to the right shoulder, but in many cases it radiates to the right subscapular or right lumbar region.

The patient's general condition is altered. When the preceding disease is fairly severe, the patient will have already lost part of his working ability and appetite and as soon as the liver is involved by the infectious process, these symptoms become more accentuated. The facies marks a suffering that far exceeds the pain and fever, the skin is pale-yellow and asthenia and lack of dynamism reveal even to the uninitiated the severity of the disease.

Vomiting and nausea are functional symptoms, rarely encountered in hepatic abscess (10—20%); hepatic abscess is one of the rare digestive diseases that evolve as a rule without vomiting.

Physical signs. The tenderness (induced pain) of the liver to mild abdominal pressure in the right hypochondrium or powerful percussion at the base of the right posteroinferior hemithorax is almost constant (92—100% of the cases).

To this tenderness is related muscular hypertonia observed in the upper right quadrant of the abdomen; a weak defense sets in at this level, covering the entire upper half of the anterior abdominal wall (60%). This indicates as a rule the onset of perihepatitis, an inflammatory process followed by the formation of adhesions between the liver and other viscera or (especially) the parietal peritoneum. As already mentioned, perihepatitis is more intense at the level of the abscess close to Glisson's capsule, therefore the defense reaction and the site of maximum pain may supply information concerning the location and direction of evolution of the hepatic abscess. This is particularly pertinent in the single abscess.

Hepatomegaly is frequently encountered at the beginning (61%) and almost constantly in the advanced stages of the disease (91%). Although hepatomegaly accompanies all chronic hepatic inflammations and is not a pathognomonic sign, in hepatic abscess the enlargement takes place along vertical lines both up and downwards, an aspect seldom met with in other diseases. The amplitude of this enlargement is variable, because in the incipient periods it may be little accentuated (in some small, deep abscesses), or difficult to interpret when the abscesses develop following cholangitis with prolonged biliary stasis, in which case hepatomegaly appears before the onset of the abscesses.

It is worthy of note that the enlarged liver follows the traction of its taut ligaments which act together with several forces that gradually rotate the organ around its transverse axis. With time, a large part of the convex aspect of the liver comes in contact with the anterior abdominal wall and can be palpated directly. This change in position is a temporary mechanical effect brought about by artificial enlargement of the liver; hence, after evacuation of the collection, the liver tends to return to its normal position and volume. This accounts for certain cases in which there is a lack of agreement between the parietal incision and hepatotomy, aspect that will be dealt with in the paragraphs on treatment.

In the cases with a long-standing evolution, the liver occupies a large part of the abdomen; the deformity of the abdomen becomes more evident with emaciation.

Thoracopulmonary changes. From the beginning, respiratory mobility is reduced in the lower half of the right hemithorax. Then, in about two thirds of the cases the base of the hemithorax becomes broader with the development of hepatomegaly.

Immobility of the right pulmonary base is determined by percussion and auscultation (in 40% of the cases) and is accompanied in 60% of the cases by dullness and often by subcrepitant rales or pleural friction (68%).

Notwithstanding, pleural exudate and especially pleural empyema are seldom observed, probably due to the early development of pleural symphyses. Other physical signs are seldom encountered, or only in special situations: jaundice, met with in 8—36% of the cases (Bockus), has an altogether different significance from the moment in which it appears.

In hepatic cholangitis abscesses, jaundice accentuates the subclinical icterus always present in such cases; it does not, therefore, supply information concerning the gravity of the case.

In abscesses of other origin, jaundice appears late and is always of prognostic value; it announces complication of the abscess with diffuse, toxic cellular alteration or compression of the main bile ducts. In such cases jaundice impairs the prognosis.

Ascites is rare and may occur in thrombophlebitic abscesses in which portal hypertension has developed consequent to narrowing of the portal lumen due to pyelophlebitis. When ascites is present, the disease is in its final stage and the patient can no longer be saved.

Splenomegaly is very rare and considered to appear only very late in abscesses with a prolonged evolution (Eolian). However it should be emphasized that it may precede the appearance of the hepatic abscess or thrombophlebitis of the portal branches, especially in septic states (case 2). In these cases it indicates the existence of thrombophlebitis of the splenic vein or pyelophlebitis which will involve the liver if adequate treatment is not immediately started.

Laboratory tests. Leukocytosis is usually accentuated and may reach subleukemic values (30,000—40,000), with 89% neutrophils. It is closely linked to the evolution since chronic abscesses have been described in which leukocytosis tended to return to almost normal values (but with persistance of polynucleosis around 80%).

The results of urine tests do not agree; sometimes slight albuminuria alone is found, as in any septic state. In other cases, bile pigments may be found, with the same significance. The presence of urobilirubinuria is more constant; some authors even uphold that the absence of urobilin in the urine excludes a diagnosis of hepatic abscess (Hirschowitz — in DeBakey-Schiff).

Alkaline phosphatase increases in the blood, especially when the hepatic abscess follows cholangitis.

Positive hemoculture only indicates the existence of a septicemic state but does not point to the moment at which the hepatic localization appears; it indicates the gravity of the case but does not fully elucidate the diagnosis. A negative hemoculture has no significance whatsoever.

Explorative hepatic puncture may be considered as the only pathognomonic examination but is contraindicated when the existence of a hepatic abscess is suspected for the following reasons:

— Transpleural puncture exposes the pleura to septic seeding with severe consequences for the patient (empyema).

— A puncture through the abdominal wall exposes the patient to perforation of a loop which eventually adheres to the liver, or to seeding of the large peritoneal cavity. The resulting peritonitis is particularly dangerous for the patient whose general condition is already very poor (even under the protection of antibiotics).

Finally, a negative puncture does not exclude the presence of a hepatic abscess. In order to illustrate the negative aspects of hepatic puncture in patients with cholangitis, a description will be given of case 5 (biopsy puncture, followed by hepatic abscess).

The radiologic examination supplies valuable information concerning the size, position and relationships of the liver in 82% of cases. However, this implies a complex examination: fluoroscopic and simple or contrast radiography (barium meal) in the standard position and oblique or side views.

The radiologic examination will show:

— Elevation and immobility of a hemidiaphragm (especially the right one).

— Intrahepatic air-fluid level in case of infection with gas-producing bacteria (not necessarily anaerobic), an aspect seldom encountered (Eolian).

The lesser gastric curvature is displaced or elongated in case of left hepatic abscess (Miles, 1936).

By means of the radiologic examination it is possible to differentiate a hepatic abscess with subphrenic abscess from an isolated subphrenic abscess (Granger-Ochsner).

	Isolated subphrenic abscess	Hepatic abscess with subphrenic abscess
In anteroposterior position	Narrowing of the costophrenic sinus	Narrowing of the cardiophrenic angle
In lateral position	Narrowing of the posterior costophrenic sinus.	Narrowing of the anterior costophrenic angle.

Splenoportography for visualization of the liver makes it possible to identify the size, site and number of the abscesses whose opacity is less accentuated than that of the normally vascular parenchyma. This will be again dealt with under the heading "Diagnosis".

Direct visualization of the abscess by evacuatory puncture, followed by injection of the contrast substance exposes the patients to the injustified hazard of all punctures. This is only indicated when a fistula already exists. Fistulography will reveal the site and magnitude of the intrahepatic cavity, directing the operative approach along the optimal route of access. Ultrasonic examination determines the site, size and homogenicity of the content (Warg, 1964).

Evolution, complications. In most cases hepatic abscess is a severe, progressive disease, ending in death of the patient. The evolution is manifest, fever intense and loss of body weight runs parallel to rapid alterations of the patient's general condition (softening of the soft parts). This is the case of multiple abscesses occurring after severe diseases (septicemic state, thrombophlebitis of the original portal branches, pylephlebitis, cholangitis). In a limited number of cases the evolution may be severe but very slow, taking on the aspect of a chronic disease; these are the chronic abscesses (as a rule cryptogenetic).

Certain complications may develop in the course of this severe condition, hastening the fatal end.

A rupture of the abscess into the free peritoneal cavity (7.2%) with fatal peritonitis, is a rare accident prevented by the early onset of perihepatitis.

Still rarer is the subphrenic abscess (3.9%) produced by seeding of the hepatophrenic space. When both the hepatic and the subphrenic abscess are large, it is difficult to determine which is the cause and which the effect.

Perforation of the abscess into a cavitary viscus initially permits partial evacuation of the abscess, with transitory improvement, but is soon followed by aggravation due to suprainfection of the abscess with other bacteria.

Pleural empyema (mostly on the right side) is an extremely rare complication because pleural symphysis precedes necrosis of the diaphragm.

Hepatobronchial fistula, accompanied by secondary pulmonary abscesses is a more frequent complication (15%).

Diagnosis. In spite of the many clinical symptoms and signs and the contribution of auxilliary tests, a hepatic abscess is frequently not diagnosed during the patient's life, but only at necropsy. This stands true especially in multiple abscesses following upon a severe disease with manifest symptoms.

However, in single abscesses an early diagnosis is likewise difficult; even after seven days in the hospital a diagnosis of hepatic abscess was established preoperatively in only 7 of 24 patients (Rottenberg).

Bearing in mind the gravity of the disease, we must endeavour to establish an early diagnosis and improve the efficiency of the treatment. An early diagnosis permits in some cases a preventive-abortive therapy (case 2). Therefore, the surgeon must have a thorough knowledge of such cases. If we refer to the present level of our knowledge, the clinical diagnosis would be possible in about 80—90% of the cases.

History is important for the diagnosis; it will point to the existence in the past history of the case of:

— Furuncles, osteomyelitis, infected wounds, after which multiple metastatic abscesses will develop (more seldom thrombophlebitis of the portal vein or its branches).

— Intestinal or pelvic septic condition (appendicitis, ulcerohemorrhagic rectocolitis, septic abortion) may lead to a suspicion of postpylephlebitic abscesses.

— Cholecystitis, obstructive jaundice, gallbladder colic, ascariases point to the cholangitic phase that precedes cholangitic hepatic abscesses.

— Penetrating wounds or abdominal contusion, often at a long interval before a solitary voluminous abscess develops.

There are several stages in establishing a diagnosis: diagnosis of the disease; diagnosis of the variety (multiple or single), of the location, simple or complicated; the etiopathogenic diagnosis.

Diagnosis of the disease : the signs of the hepatic localization (painful hepatomegaly) make it possible to differentiate hepatic abscess from general diseases with recurrent (septicemia) or intermittent fever and chills (malaria).

— It is more difficult to differentiate a hepatic abscess from other hepatobiliary inflammations:

— in cholangiocystitis palpation induces maximum pain over the distended gallbladder or the liver; the diaphragm is not immobile.

— Portal thrombophlebitis is accompanied by sharp alteration of the patient's general state of health and rapidly increasing ascites. The liver is not enlarged until seeding takes place.

— Thrombophlebitis of the original branches of the portal vein: the general state of health, fever and antecedents are the same as in hepatic abscess but there is no painful hepatomegaly. Pain is felt at a distance over the site of inflammation (appendix, splenic vein, etc.). However, it should not be overlooked that septic seeding of the liver frequently takes place in this period.

— Single subphrenic abscess sometimes develops following a characteristic disease (frequently after perforated gastroduodenal ulcer). This has already been mentioned in the paragraphs concerning differential radiologic diagnosis with hepatic abscess accompanied by subphrenic abscess.

— Solitary hepatic cyst or tumor: this diagnosis should be taken into consideration in solitary abscesses with a chronic evolution. An efficient diagnostic means is splenal and portal venography which reveals zones of lesser visualization with a hazy contour, sometimes surrounded by a denser band in case of hepatic abscess and zones of lesser opacification with a clearly outlined contour in case of hepatic cysts or full tumors. The clinical data and complementary tests (the presence of marked neutrophilia even in the abscence of leukocytosis in hepatic abscess) will help to establish the diagnosis.

— Perforated duodenal ulcer is as a rule preceded by a well characterized clinical period and always has a severe onset (perforation) and immediate, subsequent contraction (board-like abdomen), which totally differs from the muscular hypertonia that gradually develops in case of hepatic abscess. Notwithstanding, this confusion has often occurred. Radiologic examination on an empty stomach elucidates the question since pneumoperitoneum appears in case of perforated ulcer and a deformed, enlarged liver in case of abscess.

— Mention should also be made of acute abdomen with which a hepatic abscess is sometimes confused (Bockus; see case 2).

In acute abdomen due to perforation, the clinical aspect is the same as in perforated ulcer, mentioned above.

In acute abdomen due to progressive septic seeding from a visceral inflammatory process, incipient peritonitis has certain common signs with hepatic abscess (immobilisation of the diaphragm, fever, leucocytosis) but at least at the beginning there is *contraction* and not *muscular defense*, and the liver is clinically and radiologically within normal limits. Vomiting, ileus become obligatory, whereas in hepatic abscess they are extremely rare.

Diagnosis of the variety. The history of a case helps to determine the possible existence of a hepatic abscess and it has been possible to differentiate if from other conditions with the same characteristics; it now remains to determine the localization, probable number of abscesses and whether complicated or not.

Localization: the most frequent localization is in the right lobe and is accompanied by right pleuropulmonary alterations: in the left lobe gastroduodenal radiologic changes are noted;

— A right posterosuperior abscess has a thoracoabdominal clinical expression, whereas an abscess with an anterior evolution produces maximum abdominal modifications in the right hypochondrium and flank.

The location of medium and large abscesses can be determined by hepatic scintigram with radioactive gold.

Number: multiple abscesses are accompanied from the beginning by a severe general condition, manifest evolution and appear soon after one of the diseases that causes them. Solitary abscesses develop more torpidly, chronically, with less fever and leucocytosis and in many cases it is not possible to determine the primary site of the infectious focus (cryptogenetic abscesses).

The existence of complications will be suspected whenever sudden aggravation of the evolution of the abscess takes place or when the pleuropulmonary or peritoneal symptoms become more evident.

Etiopathogenic diagnosis: there are two important questions:

— to establish the nature of the disease that preceded the hepatic abscess. In general, conclusions may be drawn concerning the number of the abscesses or gravity of the condition according to the mode of penetration of the bacteria into the liver, and the latter may be correlated to the nature and site of the primary inflammatory focus. The anamnesis and general examination of the patient will be of the greatest value.

— to determine the pathogenic agent — to a certain extent this problem is automatically solved once the site and nature of the preceding condition is determined (staphylococcus after osteomyelitis, bacillus coli after cholangiocystitis, etc.). In other cases it will be necessary to await operation in order to collect pus from the abscess for bacteriologic determinations and antibiograms. Until the results are obtained, the choice of the antibiotic should be based upon statistical data, using the most efficient antibiotics against bacillus coli, streptococci and staphylococci (for the diagnosis of amebic hepatic abscess see the following chapter).

Treatment. The preventive treatment is of particular importance in this severe condition. It consists in correct, intensive treatment of all inflammatory diseases that can be followed by hepatic abscess, especially: acute gangrenous appendicitis; acute cholecystitis; ulcerohemorrhagic rectocolitis; peritonitis (and pelviperitonitis).

In these diseases, surgery should be applied together with antibiotics administered at an early date and over a long period, especially to patients whose biologic resistance is visibly deficient (posthepatitis states, etc.).

Particular attention should be paid to the early detection of thrombophlebitis of the original branches of the portal vein. In such cases a combined treatment (antibiotics and anticoagulants) may have an abortive effect upon thrombophlebitis and prevent hepatic septic seedings (see clinical cases).

Curative treatment: from the beginning it should be stated that the only treatment which may lead to recovery is surgery, but not all cases can be operated.

Indications. Solitary abscess: optimal indication for surgical drainage (case 5). Hepatic resection may be necessary in exceptional cases (older chronic abscess, with a sclerous wall) but particular attention should be paid to assess correctly the resistance of the patient to such a major operation (Mackensie-Gray).

— Rare medium sized abscesses (ascariasis): drainage may give good results (case 4).

— Multiple postcholangitic abscesses: the treatment with antibiotics (according to the antibiogram) gives doubtful results and may sometimes be improved by drainage of the bile ducts (DeBakey), but in most cases the hepatic organofunctional alteration is already irreversible (case 3).

— Multiple hematogenic abscesses: surgery does not give results and intensive antibiotic therapy should be applied although its efficiency remains questionable (case 1).

— Formerly a general consensus existed concerning surgical drainage in hepatic abscesses in two stages: 1) exposure of the liver and identification of the abscesses, inducing adhesions; 2) drainage after 5—7 days. Other means of extraserous access were attempted. At present there are still authors who recommend this procedure (Eolian, Alain Mouchet) but the method in two stages or one stage (Meshalkin) is also used with the protection of hepatoparietal sutures. Antibiotics are also considered to protect the peritoneum. (DeBakey).

At present there is no basic argument sustaining that hepatic collections with pyogenic bacteria should obey rules other than those applied to any visceral focus (pyosalpynx, pyocholecyst, gangrenous appendicitis, etc.). On the other hand, the condition is so severe that it is irrational to expose the patient to a double operative and anesthetic trauma when the operation can be performed properly in a single stage under protection of a barrier of isolating gauze strips moistened in an antibiotic solution (streptomycin + penicillin). In the first place the operation consists in exploration of the liver in order to determine the site and number of the abscesses; this implies a broad approach and good anesthesia (without hepatotoxic effect). It is recommended to fix the liver to the parietal serosa in case of a single voluminous abscess, or to leave a ring of gauze strips arround the hepatotomy sites when several abscesses are opened. These measures and the use of antibiotics protect the peritoneal serosa from subsequent contamination.

Anesthesia should be preferably endotracheal (protoxide oxygen — curare) or local, potentiated, and when possible a neuroleptic + analgesia. In other words the anesthesia should be efficient and without any hepatotoxic effect.

When resuscitation is applied under correct conditions spinal anesthesia may be used with good results.

Operative techniques. The surgical approach will be chosen according to the probable location, after a detailed radioclinical study.

Two large categories may be distinguished: abscesses with a posterosuperior development and abscesses with anterior development.

— Abscesses with a posterosuperior development are situated in the right lobe and can be reached by transpleurodiaphragmatic approach (Knowsley-Thorton). Position of the patient: left lateral decubitus in Trendelenburg position (Huard-Meyer-May). The incision, parallel to the ribs exposes the costal arch 8—9, or 10; 10—15 cm of the arch is resected from 1 or 2 ribs. Pleuropleural suture is started in the sinus, then continued if necessary to the upper part of the costophrenic sinus with double suturing of the diaphragm to the thoracic wall (Lacase artifice), so as to be able to perform phrenotomy without opening the pleura.

The liver is thus accessible over its entire posterosuperior surface. The abscess is identified and treated without fixing the liver to the abdominal wall, isolating it, however, all around with gauze strips in order to avoid contamination of the peritoneal cavity. The gauze strips are gradually withdrawn after 5—7 days, leaving behind a barrier of adhesions.

For abscesses of the right liver, with a strictly posterior evolution the subpleural, transdiaphragmatic route of approach may be considered advantageous (Boeckel-Elsberg-Pacheco-Mendes). An 8-cm incision is carried out along one of the last four ribs and the abdomen, sectioning the oblique and dorsal muscles, and resecting the exposed rib and its cartilage; laparotomy is performed in the anterior part of the incision (small oblique and transverse muscles), opening the peritoneum in order to explore the liver. When necessary, the soft parts of the chest are incised, cutting through the costal periosteal bed (two valves resulting) and phrenotomy may be performed directly if we are below the pleural cul-de-sac. If the symphysed pleural cul-de-sac is within the operative field, then a double phrenoparietal suture is performed (approximating the diaphragm to the wall with the hand introduced into the peritoneal cavity) and the operation is continued by transpleurodiaphragmatic approach.

In the abscesses with an anterior evolution or those whose exact location is not known, the anterior route of approach is used for exploration, performing a xyphoumbilical or right subcostal incision, parallel to the costal margin (Constantini).

The exposed liver is carefully examined and palpated even after an abscess had been identified, in view of the high incidence of multiple abscesses.

In general, the following attitudes may be adopted in the treatment of hepatic abscesses:

— isolation of the peritoneal cavity with large surgical drapes and hepatotomy performed in one stage;

— isolation of the peritoneal cavity by hepatoparietal suture around the area involved, and hepatotomy in one stage;

— isolation of the peritoneal cavity by gauze strips left 5—6 days, to form a barrier of adhesions, then hepatotomy in two stages;

— for cholangitic abscesses: external drainage of the bile ducts through a T-tube introduced in the common bile duct, or in cases of poor condition: cholecystostomy (the current technique).

For hepatic resections (exceptionally indicated in the treatment of hepatic abscesses), see the chapter on "Hepatic Resections".

There is no general consensus concerning the treatment of complications; however, the following therapeutic patterns appear most rational:

— pleural empyema: is treated by thoracotomy, evacuation, repair of the phrenic gap (when evident) and aspiration-drainage of the pleura. The hepatic abscess is drained by another incision, dictated by the site of the abscess (DeBakey);

— Hepatobronchial fistula: direct treatment of the hepatic abscess (drainage) usually drains the pulmonary pus and results in recovery (with the aid of selective antibiotherapy). When this is not the case, pulmonary resection should be resorted to.

— Subphrenic abscess: the route of approach must be chosen so as to be able to drain both collections simultaneously (by extra - or subpleural route);

— Hemorrhage that may occur postoperatively, has two mechanisms of production with a different significance:

— the detachment of an eschar; is treated by tamponade and coagulants;

— hepatic insufficiency, in which case it may be very severe (case 3).

Prognosis and Results: untreated progression of a hepatic abscess results in death.

The prognosis in a treated abscess depends upon the surgical possibilities, and, therefore, upon certain factors made evident in several of our clinical cases.

The prognosis will be discussed in terms of the following factors: the number of abscesses; the existence of thrombophlebitis; cholangitic origin; lithiasis origin; ascariasis; injury as a contributing factor.

Number of abscesses: multiple septicemic abscesses are not operable and even under antibiotic treatment the mortality rate is still about 95%.

Case 1. Patient *I.M.*, aged 19, was admitted to the Surgical Department of the Brîncovenesc Hospital from April 17 to April 22, 1951 being referred to the Medical Clinic from the same hospital for recurrent fever (39.5° — 40°C/103 . 1° — 140°F), markedly deteriorated general condition, painful hepatomegaly, subclinical icterus.

The onset dated back 14 days with chills, fever and rapid deterioration of the general state of health.

After about 12 days she was admitted to the Medical Clinic where accentuated leukocytosis was found (12,000) with 82% neutrophils, tender hepatomegaly (the liver descended below the costal margin by about three finger-breadths), slight splenomegaly (the inferior splenic pole could be palpated below the costal margin and was slightly tender). In view of the recurrent character of the fever, the presence of subclinical icterus and tender hepatomegaly (in a patient without hepatic antecedents) and deterioration of the patient's general condition, a preoperative diagnosis of hepatic abscess was made and the patient was referred to the surgical department. At operation the liver was enlarged, pale yellow, and dotted with countless miliary or lenticular greyish-yellow spots over its entire surface. Each spot was round, slightly raised and surrounded by a fine congestive area, i.e. metastatic hepatic abscesses in the course of a cryptogenic septicemia. The exudate from an abscess was collected for bacteriologic examination and antibiogram. The case being evidently beyond the resources of surgery, the abdomen was closed.

The patient's state worsened postoperatively, penicillin therapy yielded no improvement and the patient died of toxicoseptic shock after 3 days.

The existence of clinically evident *thrombophlebitis* of the portal vein and its branches greatly worsens the prognosis. Pyelophlebitis in itself is a very severe condition. However, diagnosed in time, thrombophlebitis of the original branches of the portal vein may benefit by proper treatment.

Case 2. Patient *I.I.*, aged 26, was admitted to the Surgical Clinic of the Davila Hospital on December 24, 1959 (up to January 14, 1960); he was referred to the hospital with a diagnosis of: left subphrenic abscess? left diaphragmatic pleurisy?

Presenting signs: fever (around 39°C/102.2°F), pain in the left hypochondrium and left flank, dry cough, diarrheal stools.

Antecedents: appendectomy 8 years previously.

History of the case: for several weeks the patient suffered from a heel sore on the left foot, that developed slowly in spite of antibiotic therapy. He gradually became febrile and began to complain of pain in the left flank and hypochondrium (12 days before admission). The stools were soft and the patient complained of asthenia and abundant perspiration after the evening increase in temperature, which convinced him to go to the polyclinic, from where he was sent to the hospital.

Presenting signs: pale facies; mobile, palpable inguinofemoral lymph nodes on both sides. Dullness and reduced respiratory movements at the base of the left hemithorax. Tachycardia (115), regular pulse. Blood pressure 100/75 mm Hg. Auscultation: unmodified sounds.

Gastrointestinal tract: saburral tongue. Painful abdomen, spontaneously and tender on pressure in the left hypochondrium, where the inferior pole of the spleen could be palpated about 4 finger-breadths below the costal margin, of elastic consistency, tender on palpation. On inspiration, the lower pole of the spleen descended slightly. The liver was within normal limits and non-tender. Intestinal transit was normal but the stools soft. The renal recesses were free and micturition physiologic.

Radiologic examination: the barium meal showed nothing worthy of note in the stomach, duodenum, small intestine; at 24 hours, left aerocoly, lienal and descending angle displaced towards the midline.

Pulmonary radioscopy: ascension and hypomobility of the left hemidiaphragm. Slight haziness at the left base, especially in the left cardiophrenic angle. E.S.R. 124 mm/h. Dysproteinemia tests: Takata-Ara slightly positive; Greenstedt slightly positive; formaldehyde gelification positive at 24 hours; thymol turbidity test 6 U.M.L.

Hemogram (on day 3 and 5 after admission): red blood cells 3,890,000; leukocytes 19,800 with 88—80% neutrophils. Thick drop test for hematozoa — negative. Examination for Obermayer spirochaeta negative.

Treatment with 1.50 gm/day Chlorocide *, given for 4 days gave no results. This treatment associated with heparin 25,000 I.U., in 6 injections, led to disappearance of the fever within 24 hours (Fig. 58). This treatment was given for another 4 days. The patient was kept under observation for 6 days, during which there was an isolated peak of fever.

Pulmonary radiologic control on January 14, 1960 showed no pleuropulmonary lesions. The general condition was good. The patient was referred to the medical clinic for confirmation of the result obtained and long-term clinical follow up.

Multiple cholangitic abscesses are particularly severe. According to Brzhozovskiy, "surgical biliary drainage may be attempted to save the patient's life", but the mortality rate in these cases is of 95%.

---

* Chloramphenicolum.

Case 3. Patient *M.T.*, aged 42, was referred to the Surgical Clinic of the Davila Hospital from May 7, 1959 to June 23 1959, by the medical clinic, with a history of fever, chills, intense pain in the right hypochondrium, jaundice (and dark urine).

The hepatobiliary history of the patient was positive.

Jaundice (assumed to be due to hepatitis) was partially influenced by medical treatment applied 8 years previously.

In 1952, he was operated for recurrence of the jaundice and cholecystogastrostomy was performed for a presumed cancer of the head of the pancreas. Jaundice persisted after the operation.

The episodes of fever and jaundice were repeated after 1, 3 and 4 years.

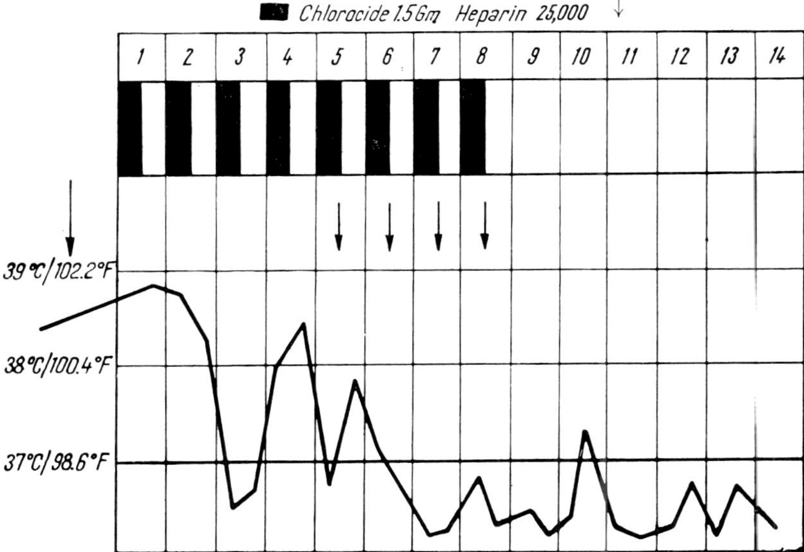

Fig. 58. — Febrile curve in thrombophlebitis of the splenic vein. Effect of the anticlotting treatment.

Five years after the cholecystogastrostomy, cholecystography showed a deformed gall-bladder, not communicating with the stomach but with normal evacuation. There were no calculi shadows in the gallbladder.

In 1959, 7 years after cholecystogastrostomy, the patient had a new febrile episode and jaundice gradually developed; he complained of vague pain in the right hypochondrium. In the medical clinic, duodenal intubation was performed and was followed by sharp pain and high fever (39°C/102. 2°F). Treatment with antibiotics was inadequate and he was referred to the surgical clinic.

The general condition was that of a toxic, icteric state.

At the site of maximum spontaneous pain the liver was enlarged (about 2 finger breadths below the costal margin) and below it an area of tender induration was found.

Laboratory tests showed moderate leukocytosis (6700) with 77% neutrophils; E.S R. 60 mm/h; bile pigments and granular casts in the urine.

Emergency operation, under spinal anesthesia. The gallbladder, which no longer communicated with the stomach, was released with difficulty from a compact subhepatic adhesion. In the gallbladder, bile mixed with pus was found. On the surface of the liver, which had the greenish-yellow aspect of biliary stasis, numerous lenticular yellow spots, surrounded by a congestive ring, represented cholangitic abscesses in the course of formation. Peroperative cholecystocholangiography showed that the gallbladder communicated with the common bile duct, in which no characteristic images of calculi were observed. In view of the desperate condition of the patient and as no calculi

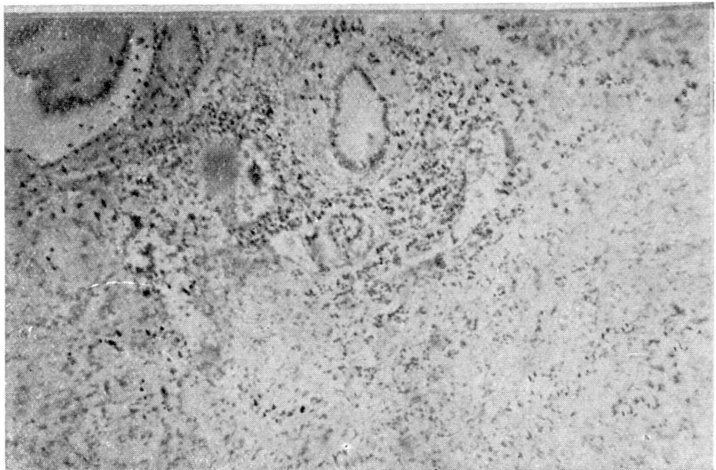

Fig. 59. — Cholangitic abscess in the liver (with low tinctorial affinity) with diffuse lesions of granular dystrophy and steatosis. Massive polymorphonuclear infiltrate around the dilated bile canaliculi in which purulent and pigmentary thrombi can be seen.

could be palpated in the dense hepatic pedicle, cholecystostomy with external biliary drainage was performed.

Clinical improvement followed, the temperature fell, and bilirubinemia decreased from 27 to 23 mg% in 17 days. The leukocytic count fell to 5000/mm^3, but 76% neutrophils persisted. Cholecystocholangiography through the drainage tube showed free passage into the duodenum, without outlining the intrahepatic branches. External drainage was discontinued after previous progressive clamping. The patient, without fever and a good general condition, but still subicteric, appeared to have recovered for the moment.

Twenty days after cholecystostomy and 3 days after removing the drain, the patient complained of subhepatic pain radiating in the right lumbar and subscapular regions, with the character of gallbladder colic; the temperature rose sharply and chills signalled reactivation of the cholangitis.

Reintervention under local potentiated anesthesia: peroperative cholangiography showed a vague, nonhomogeneous appearance of the common hepatic duct, without clearly outlined calculi; palpation through the infiltrated hepatic pedicle did not identify calculi. However, choledochotomy revealed numerous small pigmentary calculi (2—3 mm), encompassed in dense bile mixed with pus (suppurative cholangitis). After extracting about 200 calculi from the extra- and intrahepatic bile ducts, choledochoduodenostomy was performed and the subhepatic drainage closed.

The patient's condition did not improve postoperatively, although the temperature did not rise above 38°C/100 . 4°F. On day 2 after the operation, he lost about 750 ml bilious fluid through the subhepatic drainage site and on day 3 severe hemorrhage developed (hematemesis, bleeding of the operative wound) and he died within 90 minutes in spite of the rapid resuscitation (June 23 1959).

Necropsy: in the liver, rare residual calculi could be identified in the smaller bile ducts and blood and clots in the intra- and extrahepatic bile ducts. Microscopic examination: biliary stasis and cholangitis, interstitial hepatitis, marked fatty dystrophy (Fig. 59). Therefore, biliary stasis due to chronic pancreatitis; intra- and extrahepatic lithiasis complicated with suppurative cholangitis, and cholangitic abscesses in the process of formation.

The medicosurgical treatment did not prevent severe hepatic insufficiency (pericanalicular cellulohepatic alteration in the liver modified by chronic bile stasis). The terminal hemorrhage was due to severe hepatic insufficiency.

The less numerous cholangitic abscesses of hepatic ascariasis can be treated surgically with good results when diagnosed in time, in spite of their gravity, recognized by several authors (Startsev-Djabadian).

Case 4. The patient *G.S.*, 4 years old, was admitted in March (2—16) in the hospital.

He was referred from the Children's Hospital with fever, painful hepatomegaly, subclinical icterus.

The onset of the disease was insidious a few weeks previously; the pediatrician found hepatomegaly and fever, which were not modified by the treatment with broad spectrum antibiotics. Leukocytosis (9,000) with neutrophils (78%) raised the problem of a localized infection with pyogenic bacteria, eventually intrahepatic. Explorative laparotomy revealed an enlarged liver, with yellowish-grey spots, measuring 8—12 mm in diameter, less prominent on the convex aspect. On opening an abscess for bacteriologic examination and antibiotic susceptibility, a small necrosed ascarid was found. All the abscesses were opened and an ascarid extracted from each one. The abdomen was partly closed and drained with gauze strips and a tube. Following intense antibiotic therapy, the temperature fell, bile drainage through the wound diminished, then ceased and the child was afebrile, when discharged, with urine free of pigment, but a still enlarged liver.

Traumatic abscess usually has a good course and moreover, being solitary, forms part of the category with over 50% recovery. This is illustrated by case 5.

Case 5. Patient *M.S.*, aged 56, admitted to a medical department with a diagnosis of "hepatic tumor". Explorative puncture with a thick needle did not yield any exudate or a sufficient fragment for histologic examination. The patient, with low grade fever up to the moment of the puncture, became febrile and complained of increasing pain in the liver. She was referred to a surgical clinic with a diagnosis of suspected infected hepatic hydatid cyst (August 16 — September 10, 1962).

At operation, a lithiasic pyocholecyst was found included in a single adherential block and, at the site of the puncture, 3—4 cm from the vesicular fossa, a hepatic abscess measuring 3—4 cm in diameter. Drainage of the hepatic abscess and cholecystectomy were performed. Within 20 days, bile drainage ceased and drainage was discontinued. The patient recovered and was discharged.

Hepatic puncture represented in this instance the injury which allowed the bacteria from the bile ducts (cholangiocystitis) to invade the parenchyma, producing the abscess.

From the foregoing pages it is concluded that a hepatic abscess with pyogenic bacteria is always a severe disease, prevention is of the utmost importance since the curative treatment (surgery) is only applicable in certain types and localizations.

AMEBIC ABSCESS

Definition. The amebic hepatic abscess is caused by the necrosing histolytic action of *Entamoeba dysentaeriae* carried from the colon by the portal blood. After detailed description of the pyogenic abscess, mention shall now be made only of the distinctive particularities of hepatic amebiasis (rarely encountered in Romania).

The pathogenic agent is the parasite *Entamoeba dysenteriae*, still called today histolytic in its most aggressive form. It was described by Councilman and Lafleur in 1895. Three forms are known: the cyst, a resistant form (characterized by 4 nuclei and siderophil bodies); the minute form, a low pathogenic, regressive form, and the histolytic form, actually that which causes dysentery and the hepatic abscess.

Etiopathogeny. Classically, amebiasis is considered a tropical-subtropical disease. In tropical countries it causes up to 80% of the hepatic abscesses and cases of dysentery. But this disease is also of interest to the doctors in temperate countries, because:

— former patients from tropical countries returning home often remain carriers of the minute or cystic forms and anything that lowers the resistance of the body may produce a hepatic or colic localization;

— latent amebiasis due to incidental inoculation also exists in temperate countries; among these patients a small number may develop the characteristic disease (the 1933 Chicago epidemic-Sheila Sherlock).

The entameba that reaches the liver causes necrosis of a limited area (perhaps by gradual infarction) and then the specific histolytic action of the protozoan becomes manifest. The amebae are to be found at the margin of the live tissue, therefore in the abscess wall and only exceptionally in the abscess itself. With time, the abscess may became autosterilized (the chocolate-like content takes on the aspect of mastic) or suprainfection with pyogenic bacteria may occur (the content is greenish-yellow and has a strong odor when it contains *bacillus coli*).

Clinical studies. The onset (amebic hepatitis), characterized by fever and chills, painful hepatomegaly and leukocytosis, is suggestive when it occurs soon after a period of quiescence; it may, however, be completely masked by dysentery symptoms in the phase of activity. About 50% of the patients develop amebic hepatitis at a long interval after the dysenteric episode (up to 30 years).

In the acute stage, fever varies and tends to disappear in some cases (without suprainfection). Hepatomegaly becomes progressively more accentuated along the vertical line and is increasingly painful. The patient's general condition is better than in abscesses with pyogenic bacteria.

Leukocytosis is more moderate than in the latter condition and eosinophilia is present. The functional tests are not characteristic.

The radiologic examination reveals aspects analogous to those of the pyogenic abscess. Pleural reaction appears to be more frequent (at the puncture, red blood cells can frequently be found simulating neoplastic pleurisy).

Repeated coprologic examinations may help to discover the histolytic form or cyst.

Proctoscopy is valuable since it supplies evidence of superficial ulcerations, and biopsy makes it possible to identify the parasite in the submucosa.

Evolution and complications. The amebic abscess shows a tendency to become chronic, with progressive emaciation of the patient, but the course is often modified by complications that shorten the duration of the disease, hastening the end. Bronchial fistula is well tolerated until incidental suprainfection of the abscess occurs when the course is very severe.

Perforation into the pleura or peritoneum is fatal.

Suprainfection of the abscess is always followed by death within a short interval.

The diagnosis is easily established in endemic regions in the patients with a recent history of amebiasis or in patients who have come back from tropical zones.

The diagnosis is very difficult in temperate countries and frequently established retrospectively, postmortem. Needle biopsy is prohibited before the operation. Apart from the aspects discussed in the chapter on pyogenic abscess, mention should also be made of the differentiation between amebic and non-amebic abscess. In amebic abscess one may expect moderate fever, rare or no chills, a good general state of health as compared to accentuated hepatomegaly. Of major importance is a past history of dysentery. Suprainfected amebic abscess cannot be at first differentiated from pyogenic abscess.

The prognosis in amebic hepatitis is excellent (recovery under amebicide treatment).

In correctly treated, solitary non-infected amebic abscess the mortality is about 25%.

In multiple non-infected amebic abscess almost all cases end in death.

In suprainfected amebic abscess the prognosis is extremely severe.

Treatment. Medical treatment is adequate in the case of amebic hepatitis. Emetin in doses of 3×12 cg/day up to 0.80 Gm in 7—8 days, can be advantageously replaced by chloroquine (10 Gm in 21 days). Tetracycline, an amebicide for the intestine, has little effect on hepatic abscess but may be resorted to for suprainfections, as a surgical adjuvant. The non-infected amebic abscess should be treated with drugs for 7—8 days (as in amebic hepatitis) and then operated.

In case of a large solitary, well localized abscess surgery may be performed *a minima* with exposure of the liver and partial closure, with gauze strips around the site of the abscess, and daily needle aspirations done postoperatively; after 7—8 days the gauze strips are removed and aspiration is no longer necessary. This avoids suprainfection from outside. Multiple abscesses require a broad route of approach with precautions for isolating the serosa from contamination (see pyogenic abscess).

The suprainfected amebic abscess is opened under the protection of tetracycline. The route of approach and the attitude adopted in suprainfected abscess are the same as in pyogenic abscesses. The gravity of this form may be illustrated by the following clinical case.

The patient *H.C.* aged 45, from Vietnam, was referred to the surgical department (March 10 — March 16, 1960) with fever, alteration of the general state of health, pain in the right abdomen and right lumbar region, hepatomegaly, subclinical icterus; dysentery in the past history. The patient had been suffering for 20 days (fever, chills, right thoracic pain). Treatment with antibiotics was ineffective. Leukocytosis 15,500 mm; 88% polynucleosis; oliguria with granular casts in the urine. Abnormal hepatic tests indicated hepatic insufficiency. Emergency operation: postero-superiorly on the convex aspect of the liver, a large abscess, the size of a fist, containing 250 ml of thick, greenish-gray, fetid pus was found. Drainage of the abscess and subhepatic drainage was performed. In spite of the restorative treatment and antibiotics the general state worsened and the patient died on the fourth day after the operation.

Necropsy: multiple abscesses in the liver, many with a chocolate-like content but some with a hemopurulent content. Therefore, autosterilized amebic hepatic abscesses, suprainfected; the fatal course in spite of the medicosurgical treatment applied confirms the gravity of the prognosis in suprainfected amebic abscess.

REFERENCES

1. Bockus L. H., *Gastroenterology*, vol. III, W. S. Saunders, Philadelphia, 1953.
2. Brzhozovskiy A. G., *Chastnaia khirurghiya*, Medghiz, Moscow, 1958.
3. Crăciun E., *Introducere în morfologia patologică*, Ed. Medicală, Bucharest, 1958.
4. Fey B., Mocquot P., Oberlin S., Quénu, J., Truffert P, *Traité de technique chirurgicale*, vol. V, Masson, Paris, 1942—1944.
5. Hegglin R., *Diagnosticul diferențial al bolilor interne*, Ed. Medicală, Bucharest, 1964.
6. Letulle M., *Anatomie pathologique*, vol. III, Masson, Paris, 1931.
7. Mouchet A., *Nouveau précis de pathologie chirurgicale*, vol. V, Mason, Paris, 1957.
8. Sambron J., Gastard J., Arch. Mal. Appar. digest., 1965, **54**. *10*, 1071.
9. Schiff L., *Diseases of the liver*, Lippincott, Philadelphia, 1956.
10. Sherlock Sheila, *Diseases of the liver and biliary system*, Blackwell, Oxford, 1955.
11. * * *, *Klinicheskie ocherki operativnoy khirurghii*, Medghiz, Moscow, 1954.
12. * * *, *Mnogotomnoe rukovodstvo po khirurghii*, vol. VIII, Medghiz, Moscow, 1962.
13. Wang H. F., Wang C. E., Chang C. P., Kao J. Y., Yu L. M., Chiang Y. N., Chin. med. J., 1964, **83**, *3*.

B. HEPATIC CIRRHOSIS AND ITS SURGICAL TREATMENT

"Hepatic cirrhosis represents the final stage of certain hepatic degenerative and inflammatory processes, that lead to diffuse alterations in the parenchyma and stroma of the organ, intrahepatic ducts and vascular network of the liver" (V. V. Vinogradov).

The varied causes that may lead to this final stage certainly acted also in the remote past of mankind. Even if we attribute a prevalent role to alcoholism, as Savy does, we must admit the existence of this disease since ancient times. For many years cirrhosis was not recognized as such, but certain of its complications which drew attention were included in the ill defined group of hydrops (ascites) or blood vomiting, from which so many independent morbid entities have since been differentiated.

The real history of cirrhosis only began in 1819 when Laënnec described in a text of 15 lines the necropsy of soldier Jean Eidme, 42 years, who died from hemorrhagic pleurisy and ascites. Laënnec chose the term of cirrhosis, referring to the yellowish-orange color which in Greek is called *kirrhos*. Others perhaps, besides Laënnec foresaw the connection between hepatopathy and alcoholism or ascites (John Browne in Bockus) or described cirrhotic nodules (Morgagni "tubercles"), but the clear description of Laënnec precisely outlined the entity in which typical cases can be readily included. Systematic studies, at first morphologic and then functional, gradually completed our knowledge of this disease whose complexity and varied manifestations still raise, today after 154 years, problems that have not been settled. The most important stages are represented by:

— the studies of Rokitanski (1842) who established cirrhosis as a final episode in certain inflammatory processes.

— The contribution of R. Bright (1827) who stressed the etiologic role of alcoholism still accepted today by many clinicians as an adjuvant cause in cirrhosis.

— The morphologic studies of Kiernan (1833), who showed the importance of connective hypertrophy next to cellulose-dystrophic processes.

— Individualization of hypertrophic cirrhosis (Hanot, 1875), next to Laënnec's atrophic form

Gradually, the coexistence of cirrhosis with certain forms of intestinal hemorrhage were recognized, although at first, cases of death from rupture of esophageal varices were described anatomically, completely omitting the aspect of the liver (Power, 1840); soon, however, the relationship was established between morphologic changes of the liver and increased portal pressure (Gilber-Weil, Villaret, Pichancourt, 1913). Now, following the advance in physiology, much material has accumulated revealing the varied functional and circulatory disturbances in cirrhosis and establishing their correlation with morphologic changes. The numerous clinical descriptions, with individualization of various forms and types, with a nomenclature linked to classifications based upon widely different criteria make it impossible to maintain most of the clinical types described in the past as individual entities.

Therefore, eminent clinicians today conceive and speak about cirrhosis in the singular and not in the plural. This disease is considered as being caused by multiple factors and consequently manifested by different modes of evolution and different clinical aspects (Myasnikov). Even the authors that classify the disease in *Laënnec's alcoholic (cirrhosis)* and *post-hepatitis* (post necrotic) *cirrhosis*, admit that there is no clear-cut clinical or pathohistologic difference (Patek, Schiff).

Cirrhosis is as much of interest to the surgeon as to the physician because it is a wide-spread disease and many surgical patients suffer from it. Moreover, certain complications of cirrhosis cannot be controlled by medical treatment and require surgery. Today, these are not considered the only reasons since the fatal course of the disease in most cases (even when correctly treated) demands that new therapeutic methods should be found and opens prospects for surgery that aims at restoring the organ itself.

Pathologic anatomy. In cirrhosis the weight and volume of the liver are abnormal: the liver is either too small (900 gm) or too large (4000 gm); these alterations are conditioned by the proportion of excess fat and the efficiency of hepatocellular regeneration.

Glisson's capsule is always thickened; the surface of the organ is sometimes iregular and nodular and the section reveal fibrous bands including plurilobular islets; in other cases the surface is rough (''portal cirrhosis'') and the sections show fibrous bands delimiting paucinodular islets.

Microscopic examination points to certain general features that make it possible to establish a diagnosis of cirrhosis with all its infinite variety of aspects. The following aspects may coexist:

— atrophic cellular degeneration (Figs 60 and 61) } obligatorily
— fibrosis-sclerosis (Figs 62 and 63) }

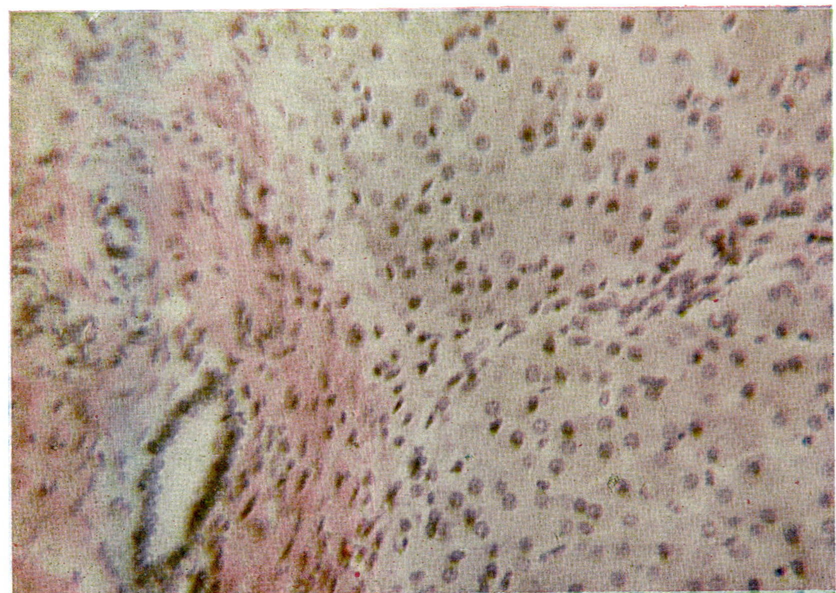

Fig. 60. — Precirrhosis. Granular dystrophy; liver with maintained lobular and trabecular architecture in general. In Kiernan's space note adult connective cells and fibers. Moderate lymphopolyblastic intertrabecular infiltrate. Granular dystrophic lesions in the hepatic epithelia (obj. 3, hematoxylin-eosin).

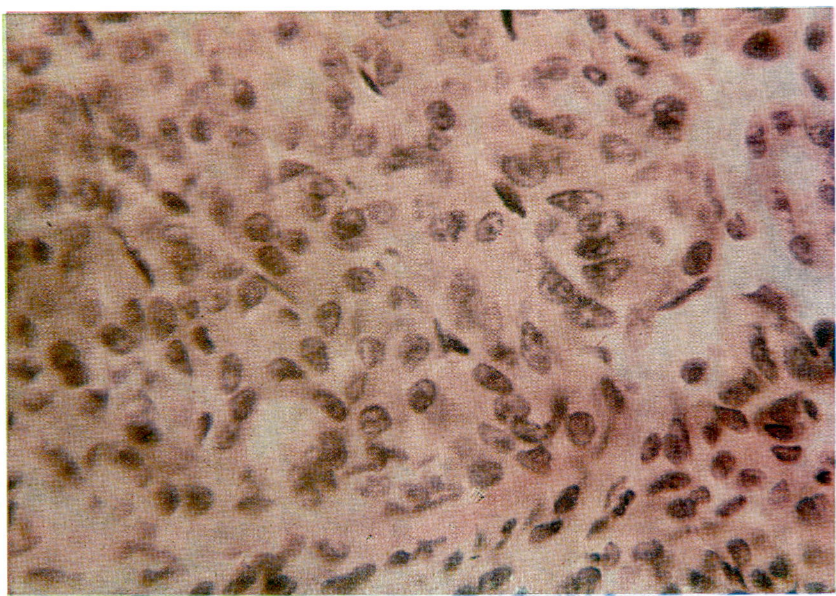

Fig. 61. — Precirrhosis. Accentuated granular dystrophy in the liver cells. Accentuated Kupfferian proliferation (obj. 7, hematoxylin-eosin).

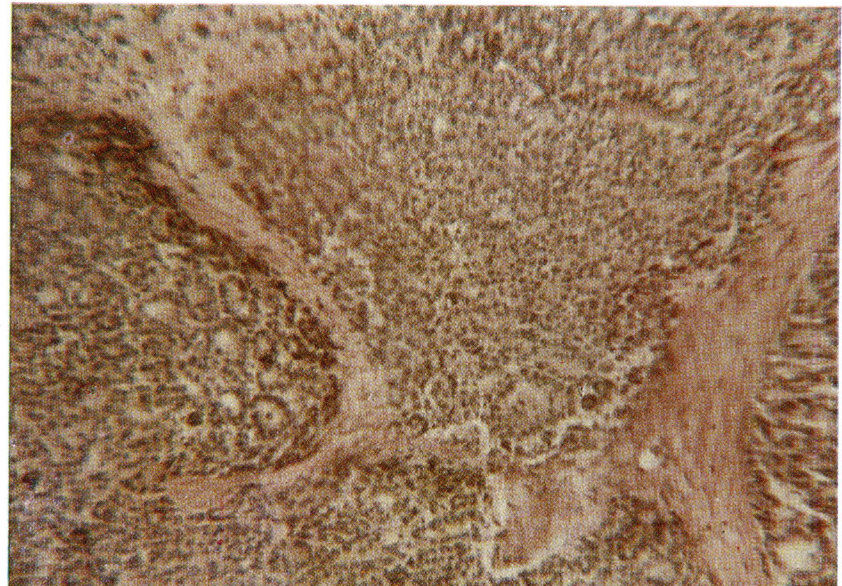

Fig. 62. — Annular cirrhosis. Disappearance of the lobular and trabecular architecture of the liver due to massive proliferation of the connective tissue surrounding the lobe. Rich lymphopolyblastic inflammatory infiltrate in the connective tissue (obj. 3, Van Gieson).

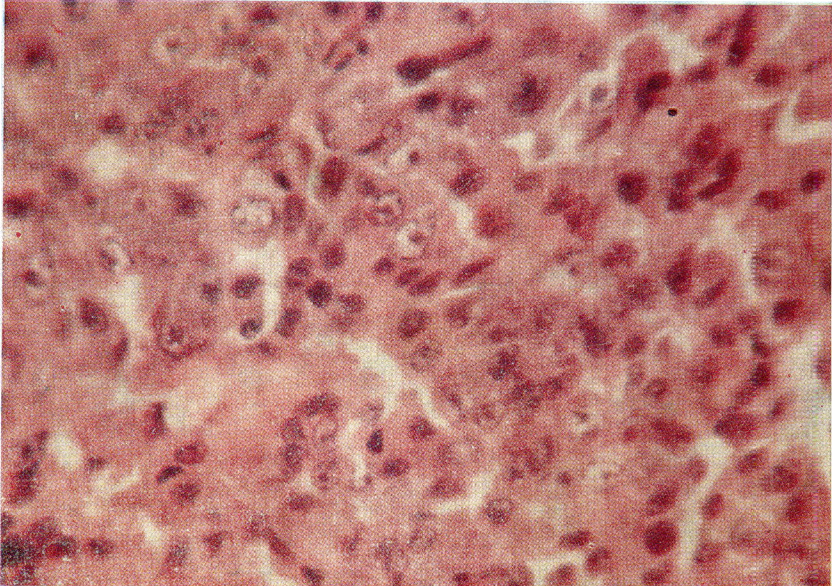

Fig. 63. — Annular cirrhosis. Hepatic epithelium with dystrophic lesions of various degrees (clear intumescence, vacuolar degeneration). In some places note aspects of cellular regeneration (large, binucleate cells) (obj. 7, hematoxylin-eosin).

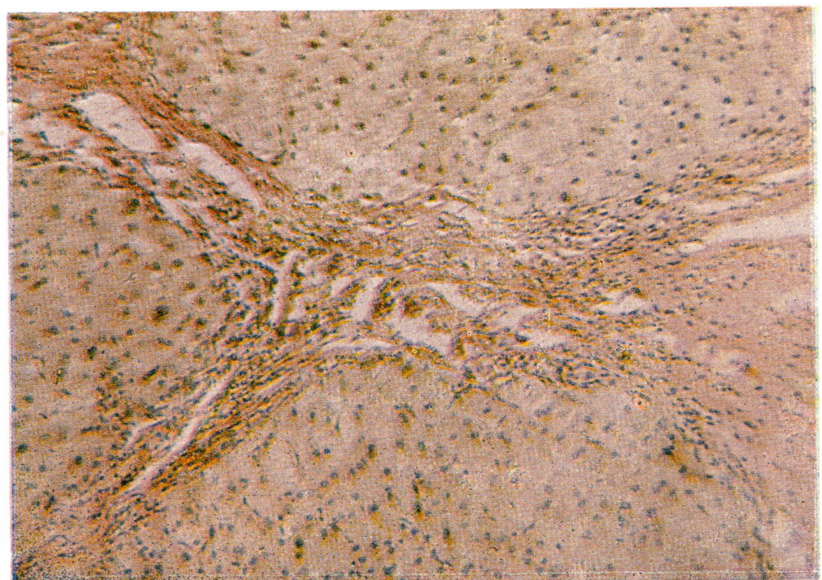

Fig. 64. — Cirrhosis of the liver with steatosis. Disappearance of the lobular and trabecular architecture of the liver due to massive proliferation of the connective tissue surrounding the lobe. Rich lymphopolyblastic inflammatory infiltrate in the connective fibers. Note fatty distrophy lesions (obj. 3, van Gieson).

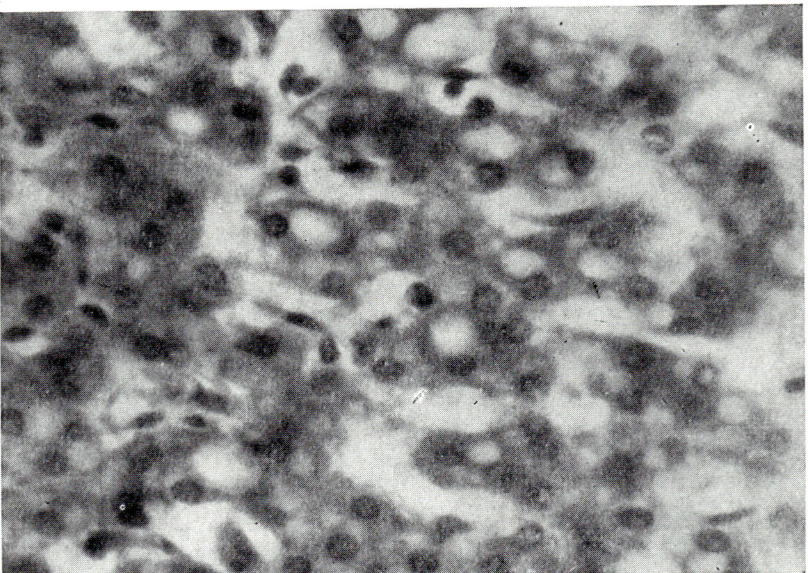

Fig. 65. — Cirrhosis of the liver and steatosis. Accentuated fatty dystrophy lesions of the hepatic epithelium (fat excess, enlarged cells with eccentric nucleus and fatty degeneration (obj. 7, hematoxylin-eosin).

— excess fat (in various proportions) (Figs 64 and 65)

— aspects of cellular regeneration (in various proportions) (Fig. 66).

For a better understanding, we shall divide the material into the classification used by anatomopathologists: atrophic cirrhosis, biliary cirrhosis and fatty cirrhosis.

This division may be used on morphologic bases, but the evolution and prognosis *cannot* be deduced from it.

Atrophic cirrhosis (Laënnec type): small parenchymatous islets are surrounded by fibrous rings (annular cirrhosis). These form part of the lobules and no longer

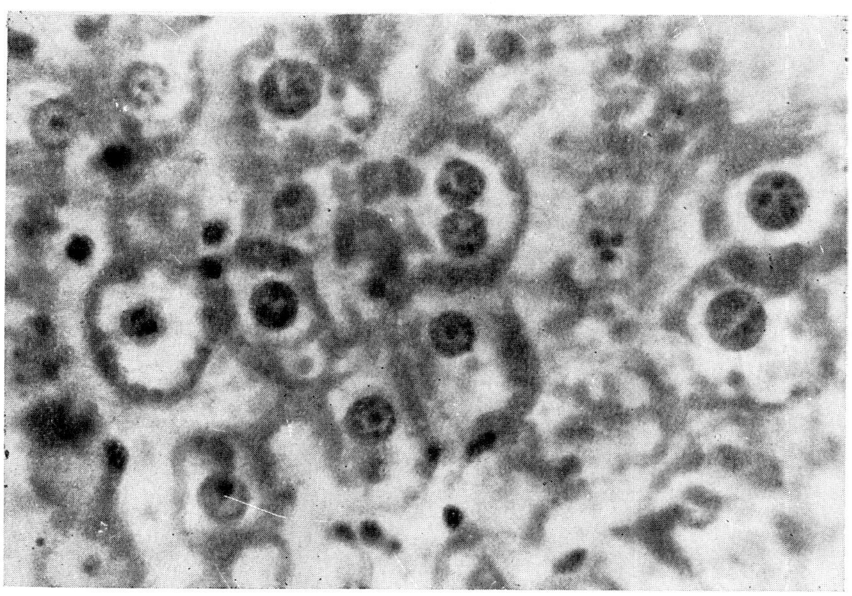

Fig. 66. — Regenerative aspects (binucleate cells).

have a central vein (pseudolobules). In turn, the spaces occupied by connective and vascular tissue are no longer the former portobiliary spaces but also cicatricial zones developing to the detriment of the destroyed hepatic lobules or parts of these lobules (Figs 67 and 68) (E. Crăciun). Here and there a small portion of hepatocellular tissue can be seen in the course of necrobiosis, surrounded by connective stroma in a state of fibrogenetic reaction (granulation tissue), but these aspects are extremely rare. As a rule the slide shows connective-sclerous tissue surrounding small islets of cellulohepatic tissue. However, signs of regeneration may also be detected in these epithelial cell islets: anisokarya, anisokaryochromia and anisokaryotopia (E. Crăciun), but signs of degenerative alterations predominate: glycogenic excess mentioned by Brault, fatty and pigmentary excess (Letulle). Importance is attributed today to the nodular arrangement of regenerative islets (Figs 69 and 70), islets with an abnormal irrigation (predominantly arterial), which compress the surrounding parenchyma and the ramifications of the portal vein, accentuating portal stasis and intrahepatic hypoirrigation. In other words, the reparatory, regenerative hepatocellular process may take on unfavorable morphologic and functional

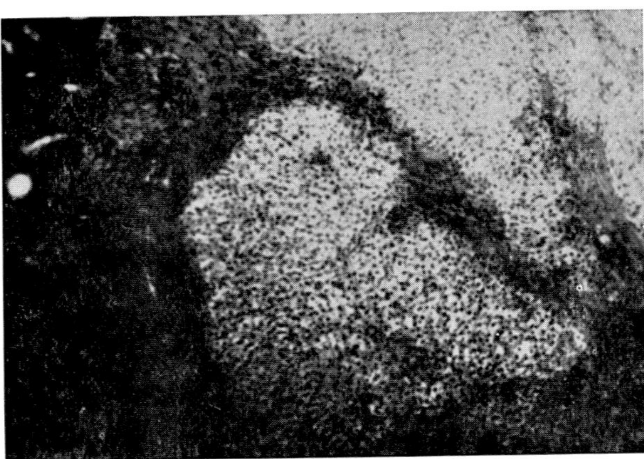

Fig. 67. — Annular cirrhosis: fibrosclerous tissue around the lobe (obj. 3).

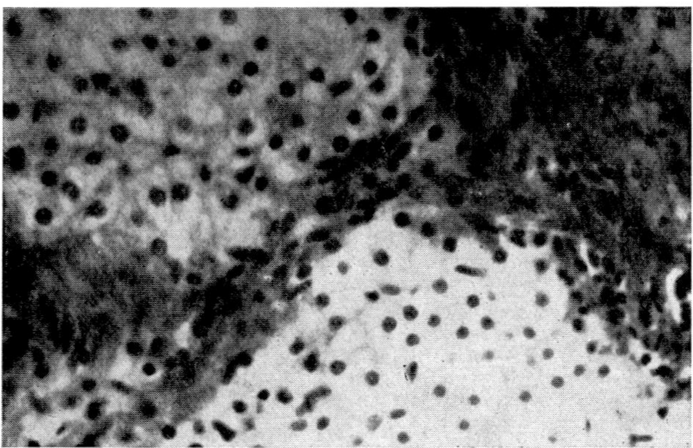

Fig. 68. — Annular cirrhosis: dystrophic cellular lesions and lymphopolyblastic infiltrate in bands of connective tissue (obj. 7).

forms. A much discussed problem is that of the "bile pseudocanaliculi" considered by some as regenerative aspects of the small bile ducts but which must be actually interpreted as aspects of atrophy of the hepatic trabeculae (Letulle), as demonstrated by the presence of glycogen, which is to be found only in the liver cells and not in the cells of the bile ducts (E. Crăciun).

Structural anarchy may develop up to destruction of any systematization of the organ, when it is practically impossible to differentiate the former centrolobular veins from the portal ramifications.

Biliary cirrhosis. The liver is enlarged and its aspect corresponds to some cases labeled "Hanot's hypertrophic cirrhosis". However, Hanot himself admitted,

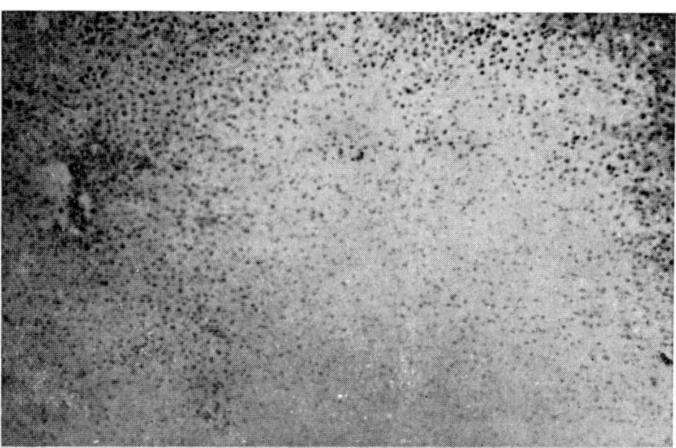

Fig. 69. — Pseudolobular regeneration in cirrhosis of the liver; large sclerosis-free areas (obj. 3).

as a first cause of hypertrophic cirrhosis, inflammation of the intrahepatic bile ducts. Notwithstanding, an "enlarged liver" may mean any type of cirrhosis with a marked excess of fat. It is of importance that in cirrhosis, with a definite cholangitic onset, the microscopic examination shows how the sclerous inflammatory reaction extends from the portal spaces and includes some of the hepatic lobules whereas important signs of active inflammation persist around the bile ducts and the latter show accentuated modifications in the portobiliary space (epithelial atrophy, hyalinization) in contrast to the attenuated alterations of the blood vessels. The liver cells seldom show signs of degeneration but more often of hyperplasia, up to the late stages of the disease when jaundice becomes severe and the liver cell is grossly charged with fats and pigment and the protoplasm is hyalinized (Letulle).

Fatty cirrhosis is an attenuated cirrhotic alteration in a fatty liver (Crăciun). The evident predominant aspect is the excess of fat, the lobular architecture being in general maintained with a certain penetration of the moderately fibrogenetic connective tissue between the cellular cords.

Viewed in their ensemble, these aspects represent a morphologic systematization, grouping together certain cases observed at a given moment of their evolution, especially cases of fatty cirrhosis, as will be seen lower down. From the clinical and surgical points of view, we cannot take into account the morphologic classification alone, as the functional factor is often far more important (the onset of ascites, hepatic insufficiency, etc.). Statistically, it may be admitted that the more important complications necessitating surgery, occurred chiefly in anullar cirrhosis of the Laënnec type (in general small liver). About certain factors, that are known today, and which may cause in some patients only ascites or the rupture of esophageal varices, we shall speak in another paragraph. In order to avoid repetition the data concerning intrahepatic vascular alterations are grouped together under the heading "portal hypertension".

Etiopathogeny. *Statistical data.* Rössle detected hepatic cirrhosis in 1–3% of the routine necropsies; Boles-Klark found 6% cirrhosis in 4000 necropsies

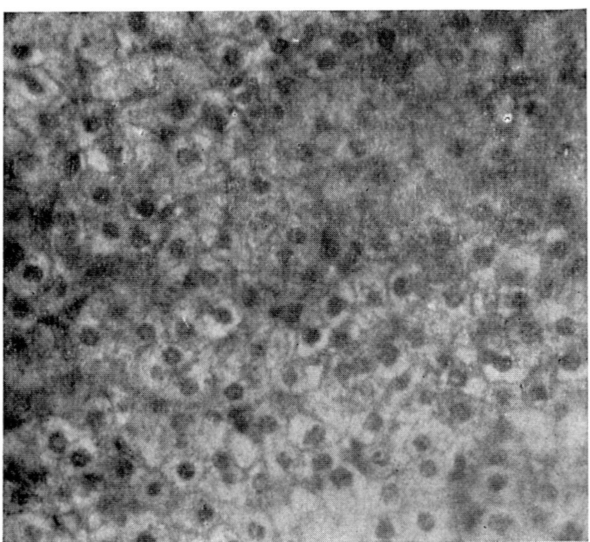

Fig. 70. — Pseudolobular regeneration in cirrhosis of the liver. Large nucleate liver cells next to cells of almost normal aspect (obj. 7).

performed in hospital, and Mallory 5.88% cirrhosis in 9340 postmortem examinations. Davydovskiy and Myasnikov report 0.5—6% cirrhosis in the necropsies performed in the hospitals of the U.S.S.R. However, in Moscow and Leningrad only 0.5% cirrhotics were found (Vinogradov). Much higher proportions are encountered in other regions of the world (Asia and Africa), where certain foods or endemic diseases favor the onset of hepatic cirrhosis.

The data of our clinics show that about 1% of the patients admitted to the hospital come for complications of cirrhosis (this proportion resulted after the clinic was specialized in hepatobiliary diseases). From these statistics we excluded the cirrhotic patients admitted for other surgical conditions.

Age. Cirrhosis generally develops after middle age:

84% between 35—64 years;
66% between 40—59 years.

According to our statistics more than half of the cases occurred in the 26—50 age group.

Sex. Cirrhosis is more frequent in males:

2 males to 1 female: Rolleston;
3 males to 1 female: Ratnoff.

The incidence of different forms is difficult to establish because the various classifications are based upon different criteria; however, it should be emphasized that in surgical departments, ascitic forms or cases of hemorrhage due to portal hypertension are generally encountered, both groups belonging to annular portal atrophic cirrhosis of the Laënnec type.

Pathogeny. We can only outline some of the stages in the evolution of the disease, the pathologic physiology of ascites, portal hypertension and hepatic regeneration being studied in the respective paragraphs.

In cirrhosis, both the epithelial elements and the connective tissue are modified. A correlation evidently exists between the two categories of morphologic changes (epithelial destruction and fibrosclerosis of the stroma). The dynamics of these processes has been differently represented:

— Rokitanski admits initial alteration of the stroma, with inflammatory phenomena; the subsequent retractile sclerosis may be considered responsible for mutilation and atrophy of the parenchyma.

— Ackermann considers that hepatocellular alterations take place first with consequent necrosis of some parts of the lobule and its replacement by juvenile connective tissue (granulation tissue) which will subsequently become sclerous.

— Rössle, taking up again the hypothesis of Siegenbeck (1896) believes that inflammatory interstitial alterations (hepatitis) and degenerative celluloepithelial alterations (hepatosis) are simultaneous phenomena.

Careful follow up of the different experimental models and the clinical cases shows that each of these hypotheses is applicable in certain cases or categories, for instance:

— In clinical biliary cirrhosis (or the experimental model obtained by ligation of the common bile duct in the dog), the inflammatory phenomena are by far the most important and take place in the connective tissue arround the bile ducts, in which stasis and attenuated infections cause the appearance of mononuclear infiltrates, seldom with pericanalicular polynuclears.

— In experimental cirrhosis, obtained by severe metabolic deviations (with a first phase of excess fat) or especially by toxic substances of the carbon tetrachloride type, cellular alteration is at first visible, as in many human occupational toxic hepatitis cases, followed by cirrhosis.

— Simultaneous alterations in the parenchyma and stroma are observed as a rule in human post-hepatitis cirrhosis, the most numerous group encountered in clinical practice and, therefore, the most important (64% according to C. C. Dimitriu et al., 1959; about 50% according to our data). Since the problems set by the pathogeny of human cirrhosis are particularly complex and even the textbooks of internal medecine mention only the numerous factors that "may" interfere in the genesis and perpetuation of cirrhogenic process, we shall only deal with a series of phenomena that are mutually related.

To stress a crucial point, generally accepted today, cirrhosis is not a disease but rather a mode of behavior of the liver with regard to certain nocuous factors, under certain conditions determined by intrinsic functional-metabolic characteristics and by disturbances of the neurohumoral regulatory function. Each link in these complex phenomena actually represents a group of factors that mutually influence one another. Without going into detail, we wish to mention the following:

— in most cases the nocuous factors are extrinsic and clearly defined: a known pathogenic agent (hepatitis virus A, B, or leptospirosis — Myasnikov-Tareev),

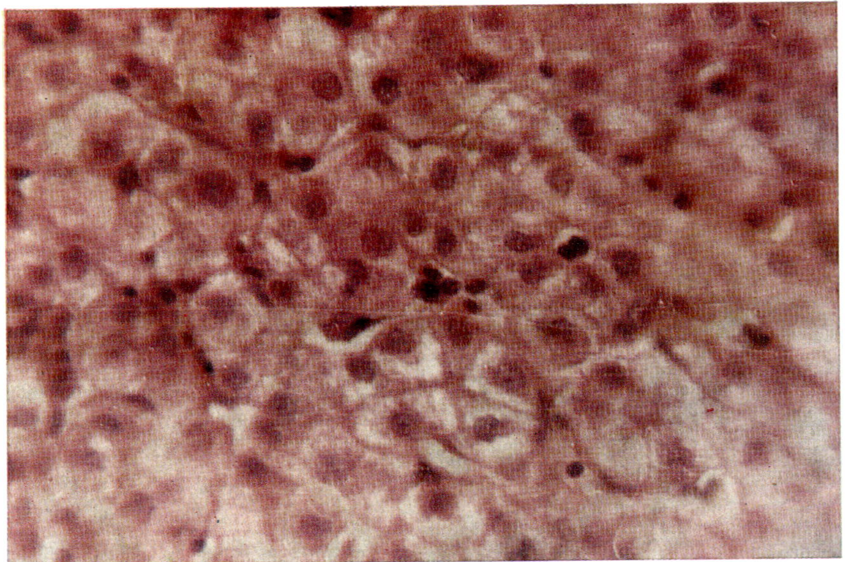

Fig. 71. — Acute hepatitis (obj. 7, hematoxylin-eosin).

less common the toxins of certain repeated inflammatory processes (the microorganisms of repeated cholangitis) and still more seldom certain occupational toxic substances (benzol, carbon tetrachloride).

— Insult, with consequent alteration and necrosis (Fig. 71), is not followed by efficient regeneration or limited replacement, connective healing. The repetition of insult, rather than its initial intensity or duration, determines the diffuse character of reactive hepatocellular and connective inflammatory changes. The regenerative capacity of the liver cell with discrete, diffuse degenerative phenomena (glycogenic or excess fat) is limited and often takes on an unfavorable character. Some diet imbalances, protein deficiencies, excess of fat may be aggravated by repeated ingestion of alcohol. Thus, instead of the formation of hepatic cords (as occurs after experimental resection) *regenerative centers* appear that lead to the formation of nodules, hepatocytic islets with changed vascular connections (linked especially to the arterial network) and hence restricting the functional value of these regenerative nodules. However, without insisting upon the circulatory implication (see portal hypertension) it should be emphasized that in the stroma, fibrogenetic growth and the formation of granulation tissue (particularly rich in lymphoplasmocytes) appears as a reaction to the altered, damaged epithelial tissue and distal to the latter. This would suggest exaggeration of the mesenchymal reactions to certain autoantigens resulting from destruction of the liver cells; the existence of autoantibodies and the importance of immuno-allergic processes in the pathogeny of hepatic cirrhosis opens up a wide field of investigations. This suggestion offers a logical explanation of the character of a self-maintenance phenomenon taken on by human cirrhosis of the liver. In certain stages of the disease (the onset of splenomegaly), diencephalohypophyseal disorders occur, the first manifestation being a decrease in ACTH and cortisone secretion; low elimination in the urine of 17-ketosteroids may account to a great extent for the intensity of the reactional-inflammatory phenomena of the mesenchyma in cirrhosis.

More difficult to investigate, yet fundamentally proved by certain aspects is the relationship between the specific changes in the cirrhotic liver and the neuro-regulating function of the central nervous system. The neurologic syndromes correlated with certain forms of cirrhosis (Wilson syndrome) and the fact that cirrhosis of the liver obtained in the experimental animal is never identical to human cirrhosis (from the viewpoint of morphology, evolution and survival) lend support to the importance of the neurogenic factor. This shows that for cirrhosis to occur, only certain functional deviations in a neuraxon, with a given organizational complexity as exists in the human species, must develop.

In the advanced stages of the disease, the process takes on a predominantly destructive character in the parenchyma and a sclerogenous one in the stroma; to this also contributes the fact that hepatic alteration hinders cellular regeneration everywhere in the organism (deficient mobilization and utilization of non-synthesizable amino acids) on the one hand, and on the other, the intrahepatic vasculo-circulatory alterations (eventually with accentuation of the immunoallergic phenomena) which, by slowing down regeneration, favor enhancement of the connective reaction. However, in the course of the disease, there are numerous periods of stagnation when the equilibrium of the organism may incline towards a stability or even regression of the morphofunctional changes. These are periods in which medical therapy may give good results; it still remains to determine whether it is justified to offer surgery only to the patients in the progressive, decompensated phase of the disease, when the pathologic phenomenon is spontaneously autoaccelerated producing great disturbances (ascites, portal hypertension, hepatic insufficiency) or whether it is preferable to operate in the incipient stages of the disease.

Clinical study. Numerous cases of anatomically established cirrhosis of the liver, discovered incidentally in apparently healthy individuals, as regards the liver at any rate, in the course of a surgical intervention for another disease (or discovered at routine necropsy) leads to the assumption that cirrhosis is latent in many cases. According to some authors these cases represent between half and one third of the total number of clinically manifest cirrhosis (Rolleston-Ratnoff). The duration of the latent phase cannot be precisely determined but varies between 10 months and 3 years (G. Albot). In the latent period the process is complete from the anatomical point of view, but functionally the activity of the liver is still satisfactory, at least when not under unusual stress.

Guy Albot discerns two aspects: *incipient cirrhosis*, clinically and biologically compensated, and incipient clinically compensated but biologically decompensated *cirrhosis*: in the latter case the hepatic functional tests (galactosuria, hippuricuria, the water test, colloidal red reaction, gammaglobulin titration, electrophoresis), indicate certain changes.

However, if it were possible to evaluate retrospectively the behavior of certain undetected cirrhosis patients, marked diminution of their effort capacity, would readily be established as observed by the patient himself. Worthy of note is the slow recovery of these patients after hard work.

The *manifest clinical phase* may be marked by an apparently brutal onset in which the first symptom is a major complication of cirrhosis: in most cases ascites (28%) or upper digestive hemorrhage (10%) and finally jaundice.

In somewhat more than 50% of the cases the clinical phase is revealed by progressive digestive disturbances (often wrongly called dyspeptic), associated with accentuated limitation of the capacity for physical effort and then for intellectual effort (especially after meals). Disturbance in the metabolism of water of the protein balance, portal circulation and abnormality of most of the liver tests, complete the semeiologic picture confirming a diagnosis which at a careful clinical examination may be established correctly.

At clinical examination, the patients will complain of asthenia, a sensation of abdominal distension or even pain. They are pale with reduced subcutaneous cellulo-adipose panniculus or discrete declive edema: cutaneous vascular stars, striae, atrophia can be sometimes observed on the sides of the abdomen.

The liver (visibly modified in size — either smaller or larger) is more consistent and has a sharp edge: the spleen is often moderately enlarged, but seldom reaches or exceeds the umbilicus, maintaining its scalloped contour.

The hematologic tests show a decrease in hemoglobin, with variable anemia, leukopenia, relative lymphocytosis and at times accentuated thrombopenia. The coagulogram is altered by proconvertin and prothrombin deficiency, pointing to hepatic abnormality and to a lesser extent by fibrinogen deficiency. On the other hand, thrombopenia, which is a corollary of splenomegaly may fall very low, altering coagulation.

Among the complementary tests, apart from the biochemical tests mentioned, are the radiologic examinations which permit direct or indirect exploration of the portal area, as well as the recent tests with isotopes (hepatogram). These tests will be mentioned later.

Liver puncture makes it possible to establish a diagnosis when a discrepancy exists between the results of the biochemical tests and the clinical data. In other cases it also makes it possible to follow up the evolution of an incipient cirrhosis under prolonged treatment. It is less conclusive than hepatic biopsy but is also less damaging in the cases in which coagulation disturbances already exist. In spite of its current use in certain medical departments, we should like to express reservations, since it is an examination limited to certain lobules and does not allow a precise, topographic location. It is a cellular rather than a structural examination (C. Nezelof in Guy Albot). C. Nezelof, (well-known specialist in liver biopuncture), has reached this conclusion after more than 500 such examination in a clinic with a hepatobiliary profile. In our opinion, explorative laparotomy under the conditions of modern surgery is preferable, since it offers the possibility of a complete visual and palpatory exploration of the whole organ, as well as the possibility of collecting tissue fragments in which the structure of the organ can be correctly examined. We believe that the hazards of explorative laparotomy are lower than those of biopsy puncture (in recently published statistics, that include 1400 biopsy punctures, there were 4 deaths exclusively attributed to the puncture).

When cirrhosis is confirmed, explorative laparotomy also offers the advantage of being able to perform a palliative operation at least (Talma, Făgărăşanu, etc.).

In the manifest phase, there are three necessary elements:

— disturbance in water metabolism;

— disturbance in portal circulation;

— a variable degree of hepatic insufficiency depending upon the ratio of cellular alteration to cellular recovery.

Any of these three elements in the common picture of cirrhosis may become a predominant complication that threatens or shortens the life of the patient: ascites, portal hypertension, progressive cellular change that exceeds recovery.

The following pages will deal with the surgical approach to these complications.

ASCITES SYNDROME

Ascites means free fluid in the peritoneum: the name comes from the Greek *askites* = pocket or pouch.

Pathophysiology. A small amount of peritoneal fluid is found normally in the peritoneal cavity and its volume is maintained at a constant level by a complex mechanism which equilibrates its production and its absorption.

According to Starling, capillary permeability and osmotic blood pressure play an important part in physiologic production of the peritoneal fluid and in its resorption. Decrease of plasma proteins below 2.59% is followed by a tendency to transudation in all the serous cavities. According to Starling, in the capillary loop, in terms of the ratio of hydrostatic pressure (filtration) to colloidal-osmotic pressure (resorption), a relationship also develops between the respective extent of the transudation zone (near the metartereolar extremity) and of the resorption zone (near the venule extremity). Metartereolar sphincteric rings control the hemodynamic pressure in the capillary loop, playing the role of a protective barrier, which does not allow pressure increase in the arterial wall to influence the capillary directly. On the other hand, in the venule extremity of the capillaries no such sphincters exist, any pressure variation in the venous network (portal) modifying directly and immediately the circulatory regime of the capillaries within the portal area. In other words, increase in portal pressure results in a direct increase in the filtration zone to the detriment of the resorption area in the abdominal viscera, tributary to the portal vein.

This hypothesis is better understood if we bear in mind the role of capillary permeability: under certain conditions increase in the permeability of the endothelial membrane of the capillary may transform the capillary into a transudation element, without resorption.

In the peritoneoportal area we are dealing with, inflammation and irritation of the peritoneum are an important cause of increase in capillary permeability. In the liver as in any tissue or organ, part of the capillary filtrate passes into the lymph: the lymphatics are thus variably stressed according to the volume of fluid that appears around the capillaries, volume which increases with increase in the venous pressure. For the hepatic capillaries, pressure at the venous extremity of the capillary no longer means portal pressure (as in the other intraabdominal viscera), but pressure coming from the inferior cava vein or suprahepatic veins. In these capillaries, any intrahepatic morphologic disturbance, involving the suprahepatic veins, may hinder drainage of the blood toward the suprahepatic veins, with increase in the capillary filtrate. This brings together all the conditions that occur in the Budd-Chiari syndrome (suprahepatic obstruction) and in common cirrhosis.

In such conditions, the liver itself becomes the site of important fluid release or, otherwise stated, the liver is an important source of ascites (Child cited by Kobak; Hyatt, Lawrence, Smith cited by Burlui). These authors maintain that the appearance of ascites droplets can be seen on the surface of the organ.

However, if we reduce the pathogeny of cirrhotic ascites only to the balance between filtration and capillary resorption, we would not take into account the most specific aspect of cirrhosis, i.e. the complexity of the metabolic disturbances and circulatory changes. The hypoalbuminemia of cirrhotics itself is a complex mechanism in which alimentary disturbances, digestive insufficiencies and finally hepatic metabolic deficiency participate, bringing about a subnormal synthesis of albumins in the liver cell, morphologically altered or regenerated but functionally deficient. Hence, hypoalbuminemia, especially total serum albumin (per total plasma volume) measures from the beginning of cirrhosis the deficient functional state of the liver. The corresponding increase in globulins, due to a functional excess of the reticuloendothelial system or to autoimmunization phenomena, may counterbalance the albumin deficiency in grams but does not compensate it in maintenance of the colloido-osmotic pressure (oncotic) because there are fewer larger globulin molecules per gram than small serum albumin molecules.

Disturbance in water-electrolyte metabolism must also be taken into consideration since it is of the greatest importance in postoperative therapy.

Increase in the plasma volume has often been reported in cirrhosis, the blood volume remaining within normal limits by reduction of the erythrocytic volume (Perera, Bateman, Child), as also confirmed by us following radioiodine serum protein determinations. Determination of the volume of extracellular water by radioactive Na suggests a significant increase, but its interpretation is very difficult because sodium metabolism shows accentuated deviations in cirrhosis (Child).

Normally, the liver destroys (metabolizes) the excess of adrenocortical hormone which otherwise would cause excessive Na retention at the level of the renal tubules. The functionally deficient cirrhotic liver leaves certain steroid fractions in excess, which produce a marked retention of Na (probably aldosterone). Actually, sodium retention represents a general metabolic change in cirrhosis even if pathophysiologists, preoccupied by therapeutic prospects, have primarily studied the phenomena taking place in the kidneys. This is also proved by the fact that Na diminishes in the saliva, tears, perspiration, etc. (Child).

Finally, the following facts lend support to this type of secondary cortico-adrenalism (secondary aldosteronism):

— the diurnal-nocturnal cycle of diuresis (Sirota, 1950) is inversed in cirrhosis (Popper, 1952), as has also been obtained experimentally by the administration of adrenocortical extracts (Rosenbaum, 1952):

— refractory ascites can be controlled for a long time by bilateral adrenalectomy.

Anti-aldosterone medication, which appears logical in view of these facts, has proved efficient.

An important role in the disturbance of water-electrolyte metabolism is likewise played by the retrohypophyseal-kidney interrelationship.

In 1948, Vernay showed that following an increase in plasma concentration a retrohypophyseal antidiuretic hormone is secreted (vasopressin): the osmoreceptors appear to be located within the vascular bed of the internal carotid. In the normal human in overhydration, the antidiuretic hormone is not produced, but in cirrhotic patients, in spite of plasma hypotonia accentuated by the water test, this hormone can still be identified in the urine. Among the different hypotheses that try to explain the parallel existence of sodium and water retention, the most satisfactory appears to be that of Eisenmenger: the cirrhotic patient is adapted to a certain level of hyponatremia, any ingestion of salt (retained in the body by hyperaldosteronism) results in a relative increase of natrium in the internal medium, stimulating the osmoreceptors to bring about hypersecretion of the antidiuretic hormone.

As regards the intimate mechanism of diuresis in maintaining the water balance in the body, it is admitted that, normally, a large part of the water and sodium, from the glomerular filtrate, may be resorbed at the level of the proximal convoluted tubules, by participation of carboanhydrase; blocking of this enzyme may produce diuresis with natriuria. On the other hand, at the level of the distal convoluted tubule, a large part of the water and sodium that have not been retained at the level of the proximal convoluted tubule may be reabsorbed under the action of aldosterone. Hence, secondary aldosteronism in cirrhosis may annul the effect of natriuric diuretics. Under the influence of antialdosteronics, it is possible to obtain a natriuric diuretic effect, as will be seen when dealing with the therapy.

In decompensated cirrhosis with ascites, certain respiratory disturbances that are latent in all compensated, chronic hepatic and cirrhotic patients become evident, i.e. hyperventilation, venous pooling (due to intrapulmonary shunts) and arterial hypoxia. (Mihai and Bujor, 1962; Runcan and Racoveanu, 1964; Del Guercio, 1964).

These notions of pathologic physiology help the surgeon to acquire an accurate understanding of the clinical facts and a logical orientation in the pre- and post-operative treatment of patients with ascitic cirrhosis.

Clinical study and medical therapy. As already mentioned, in about 28% of the cirrhotic patients, the first evident sign is ascites: it is admitted that over 50% (78% according to Ratnoff) of the patients with advanced cirrhosis also have ascites. Actually, it is difficult to ascertain or deny the presence of fluid in the peritoneal cavity since fluid up to 1500 ml amounts may not be observed by percussion (Bockus) or may only be detected by percussion in a knee-chest position.

Before being clinically detectable, ascites is preceded by marked gaseous distention, with a sensation of discomfort, more seldom of abdominal pain, more often of permanent fulness. This subjective sensation corresponds to an increase in the circumference of the abdomen and a state of tension of the abdominal wall. The patient observes a diminution in the volume of 24-hour diuresis with an increase in nocturnal diuresis and delay in the increase of diuresis after ingestion of a large amount of water.

It is only by a very attentive follow-up by a specialist, that the "proiuria" phase described by Guy Albot, can be detected. It consists in excess diuresis, exceeding the volume of water ingested, an early phase in disorders of water and electrolyte metabolism which passes as soon as evident decompensation develops (ascites). In the internal medicine textbooks, details are given on the clinical and complementary examination of the ascitic patient.

The patient is pale, with thin limbs due to atrophy of the muscular masses, and has a voluminous abdomen: small, slight supramaleolar edema may also exist (marked ascites).

The aspect of the abdomen is frog-like in the dorsal position or pouch-like when the patient stands erect and the collection of fluid is smaller and globulous in voluminous ascites.

Percussion: mobile, declive dullness with an upward concavity in moderate ascites and subumbilical dullness with reduced mobility in very voluminous ascites (the fluid has no place to move freely in).

The fluid wave sign is present in medium ascites.

Needle biopsy: a serocitric fluid with the character of a transudate (first punctures) or orange with the presence of polynuclears (after several punctures).

Subcutaneous circulation of the portacaval type may be replaced by long venous canals situated in the flanks (of cavocaval type) when large fluid accumulations compress the inferior cava. The volume of the liver and spleen are characteristic of cirrhosis and do not belong to the ascites phase. Hypoalbuminemia with inversion of the albumin-globulin ratio, pointing to cellulohepatic decompensation, is also a clue part of the pathogeny of cirrhosis.

Ascites, which is attenuated or latent in many cases of cirrhosis, may become the dominant symptom, taking on the character of a complication by the accentuated disturbances it gives rise to. According to our findings, about 50% of the cirrhotic patients admitted to the surgical clinic came for ascites, refractory to medical treatment. According to sex, there were two males to one female: the age was greater than 25 years.

Massive ascites (more than 12 liters) results in distension of all the weaker points of the abdominal wall and reveals the presence of latent hernias, especially at the level of the umbilical ring where a swelling may appear, pointing to the existence of a small hernial sac distended by fluid. In some cases the thin wall fissures and a large part of the fluid is discharged, relieving the patient, but aggravation of the evolution soon sets in due to peritonitis caused by infection of the ascites.

In most cases ascitis becomes unbearable because of its volume, hindering respiration and pushing the heart together with the diaphragm upwards. Cirrhotic patients, who in general have difficult respiration owing to pulmonary changes, also have very limited respirations. These aspects of respiratory disturbances are of importance during both the operation and postoperative resuscitation.

A current observation is that of moderate portal hypertension values in ascitic patients; better said, those patients become ascitic who do not die from portal hypertension from the beginning, therefore, in whom the organism is able to compensate the portal hypertension by circulatory means. Hence, ascites occurs as an abdominal sign of liver cell decompensation and of general water electrolyte, hormonal and protein metabolic disorders.

In order to follow up the response of the organism to the treatment of cirrhosis in the ascitic phase, the body weight, diuresis and the water ingested are measured daily. The three resulting curves permit rapid appraisal of the evolution of the case. The water test, performed according to one of the current procedures (Fremont-Smith, Adelkreuz, Adler, Pozzi, Vaquez, Wollheim), but always using the same test in the same patient, gives an exact indication of the behavior of the liver and the entire organism to forced liquid intake. The ascitic cirrhotic patient must, of course, be viewed also from the angle of general or of specific hepatic disturbances (proteinemia, electrophoresis, dysproteinemia, B.S.P., galactosuria, prothrombin, vitamin K utilization capacity, induced hippuricuria, esophageal varices, etc.), but these tests which make it possible to determine the stage and gravity of the cirrhotic disease in general, are comparatively static, and cannot give detailed information of ascitogenesis.

The treatment of cirrhotic ascites is medical and only for a given period or certain phases, is it surgical. The ascitic patient should be treated as any cirrhotic with hypercaloric diet, rest, restriction of the protein intake down to a given limit but not below, marked restriction of fats and a high glucose supply (more than 3000 calories: 150 Gm proteins, 50 Gm lipids and 300 Gm carbohydrates. Flemming-Snell; Vinogradov) with the addition of vitamins. It is essential to reduce salt as the pathophysiologic disturbance begins with salt retention.

Mercurial diuretics (with previous limited ammonium chloride therapy in order not to induce hepatic coma) or carbonic *anhydrase* antagonists (diamox = ederen or chlorotiazide = nephrix) should be resorted to. In this way, prolonged stability of the disease is obtained (Chou Hsüen-Chang, Novello, etc.). If the response to these diuretics is not satisfactory, pointing to the existence of secondary hyperaldosteronism, spirolactone, aldactone or progesterone should be administered as an antialdosteronic (Liu-Hsien) together with chlorothiazide. Clinical practice has convinced us of the necessity of the latter association (antialdosteronic + anticarboanhydrase), especially in the postoperative period, when the treatment must be efficient and sustained. Irrespective of the operation performed, it always implies irritation of large peritoneal surfaces, which accentuates ascites. After any operative intervention, there exists a tendency to retain salt in the organism which aggravates still further the preexisting shift towards ascites; hence, it is rational to expect the reappearance or accentuation of ascites after any kind of operation in ascitic patients. A necessary solution, but not the best is that of repeated peritoneal punctures for partial relief. These abdominal paracenteses avoid evisceration or eventration but accentuate protein depletion and, therefore, favor ascites. Today, these punctures which have become useless are replaced by the logical treatment, that of a diuretic combined with antialdesterone.

In addition, the blood protein level is increased by plasma perfusions of protein hydrolysates in the preoperative and early postoperative period. These data are essential since medical treatment is necessarily applied before any surgical intervention in a patient with a diagnosis of cirrhosis (either for cirrhosis itself or another condition).

Surgical treatment. From the study of the pathologic physiology of ascites, it appears as a consequence of the discrepancy between the production and resorption of the peritoneal fluid. The varied surgical methods proposed and applied act upon one or the other of the two terms and, when *an equilibrium is realized*, then ascites disappears. The effect may be temporary or durable according to the operation, but also to the eventual occurrence of other ascitogenic factors which were not present preoperatively.

Methods favoring resorption or drainage of the ascites fluid. These methods differ from punctures in that the fluid is not lost, of particular importance for the retention of proteins and to a lesser extent for that of salts and water.

The number of surgical procedures applied for the treatment of ascites shows that the problem has not yet been solved; however, we should not share the pessimism of some authors who assert that "a technique for the prevention of ascites has not yet been found" (Child), as some fairly good results have been obtained.

In order to substitute for the exhausting abdominal punctures, different methods have been proposed for "internal drainage of ascites fluid".

Perotte tried to anastomose the medial saphenous vein to the peritoneal cavity, and Marinescu-Voinea fixed a plastic tube with a spongious extremity to the hip joint and left the other end free in the peritoneum. These drainage methods have restricted efficiency, because the great omentum soon covers it, separating it from the peritoneal cavity and hindering drainage.

Capillary drainage of ascites has likewise been proposed with nonabsorbable sutures, passing from the peritoneum into the cellular tissue of the abdominal wall. Fibrous tissue soon develops around the sutures (even when plastic is used although it is well tolerated), covers them, and penetrates within their texture eliminating the capillary spaces; hence, their efficiency is restricted in time.

Omentopexy has been more widely applied.

Its discovery was casual. In 1887, Kummel of Hamburg believed he was operating a hydatid cyst and on opening the abdomen he found voluminous ascites. On closing the abdominal wall he inadvertently fixed the greater omentum between the aponeurotic margins of the wound. After three months ascites had disappeared, the liver was small and large veins had developed around the scar. This case ideally included all the data of the problem and the simplest solution. Actually, the operation became more complicated by the different variants applied, which, however, did not greatly improve the initial method. Today there are three main variants of omentopexy (operation proposed by Thalma who was not a surgeon).

Intraperitoneal omentopexy (Morison-Terrier-Drummond) in which the greater omentum is fixed to the parietal peritoneum, eventually also to the liver (hepatoomentopexy of Burdenko, see Vinogradov). Some surgeons tried to produce a perihepatitis and perisplenitis by local irritation (Morison, 1896). The results were inconsistent. According to Flemming, in a group of 25 operated patients (Bockus):

15 died after 2.10 months } without marked improvement
6 died after 24.6 months }

4 lived up to 7 years postoperatively but with frequent aspirations.

Subperitoneal or properitoneal (Schiassi type) omentopexy is today widely used. The following main stages may be noted:

— horizontal T-incision with the vertical stem along the mammillary line, from the costal margin straight downward and the horizontal branch exceeding the midline above the umbilicus. Section of the planes stops at the parietal peritoneum;

— the musculocutaneous flaps are detached from the parietal peritoneum;

— after incision of the parietal peritoneum along the same line and slow evacuation of the ascites fluid, the greater omentum is extraperitonealized through the transverse aspect of the peritoneal gap. The greater omentum is fixed by mattress sutures closing the gap. In order to favor the utmost induction of adherences, the extraperitonealized omentum is rubbed with gauze moistened in 0.1% mercury bichloride (Fey);

— the abdomen is closed along the vertical line of the incision.

This technique has been modified in order to maintain the strength of the abdominal wall as much as possible:

Fiolle (Marseille) proposed median laparotomy and reflection of the right margin of the incision. In the deep aspect of the abdominal wall thus exposed two transverse, parallel supraposed incisions are cut through the parietal peritoneum and inner layer of the rectus muscle sheath. A flap of the greater omentum is passed below the seroaponeurotic bridge thus formed.

In our clinic this operation has been simplified:

— Median xyphoumbilical laparotomy (with particular attention to paraumbilical ascending veins).

— The aponeurotic sheath of the large abdominal muscles is opened and within the retromuscular pouch thus formed a large part of the greater omentum is introduced and fixed to the muscle by several catgut sutures.

— The abdomen is closed along the *linea alba* with nonabsorbable suture.

This variant of omentopexy has given full satisfaction and marked improvement in many cases, with survival up to 9 years.

In 1950, one of us (Făgărăşanu) modified the technique to favor maximum resorption of the ascites fluid:

— 2—3 long nylon sutures are passed through the mobilized epiploic flap which is fixed in the sheath of the right abdominal muscles, then through the subcutaneous tissue and up to the inguinoabdominal and inguinocrural region, where they are passed through 2—3 lymph nodes.

As shown in a previous work (1957) there was only one death in 20 operated cases and 8 of the patients were even able to take up their former occupation. Some of the patients were followed up postoperatively for four years.

Subcutaneous omentopexy (Narath-Kalb). As its name shows, in this variant the greater omentum (mobilized by right paramedian laparatomy) is fixed below the integument (Fey). As this method exposes the patient to the hazard of eventration it is but little used.

Methods for reducing or removing the production of ascites fluid. As already mentioned, the accumulation of peritoneal fluid depends upon the discrepancy between resorption and the formation of fluid. Fluid may be formed in all cases of portal hypertension and hypoalbuminemia. Thus, if portal pressure or albuminemia is normalized, ascitogenesis may be avoided.

To this end, several methods have been proposed which bring portal pressure down to normal. This will be dealt with in detail in the chapter on portal hypertension. A simple list will be given, mentioning the therapeutic value of these methods only in regard to the aspect of their efficiency against ascites:

— Splenectomy associated to omentopexy (Tansini-Morone);

— Splenopexy associated to omentopexy (Schiassi) in patients in a poor general condition.

As will be seen later on, splenectomy is only indicated after the greatest circumspection; as it does not influence ascites it should be avoided in simple ascitogenic cirrhosis.

Arterial ligation. Apart from ligation of the splenic artery seldom used without splenectomy, the present chapter is concerned with the indications and efficiency of ligation of the common hepatic artery in ascitogenic cirrhoses.

According to Berman and Fields, in atrophic cirrhosis with transitory ascites, ligation of the common hepatic artery should be avoided, since this operation may eventually be used in cirrhosis with persistent ascites. Ligation of the common hepatic artery is indicated especially in cirrhosis with uncontrollable ascites associated with hemorrhage from esophageal varices. This is in agreement with the initial statistics of Rienhof who of 13 cases of ascitogenic cirrhosis operated according to this method had 16% deaths and about 84% improvement.

More recently Léger, taking up again the problem of the indications of ligation of the common hepatic artery in cirrhosis with ascites reached a different conclusion: he observed that in incipient, anascitic cirrhosis, when the operation is better tolerated, more encouraging results are obtained, whereas in the very complex forms (hemorrhage and ascites) results are often unfavorable.

Today, it is no longer agreed that ligation of the common hepatic artery produces marked diminution in portal pressure (which is only a transitory effect), but that it improves the biology of the liver cell by a mechanism that will be discussed in the chapter on portal hypertension. Hence in the last instance, although ligation of the hepatic artery was considered as a weapon against portal hypertension, it actually exercises its effect as a means of reequilibrating the protein fractions, as shown in detail in the chapter on hepatic regeneration. Even if arterial ligation does not constantly give the results expected against ascites (Almeister, 1955), the results should be compared with the natural mortality rate in ascites. It should be recalled that approximately 50% of cirrhotic patients die within the first year after the onset of ascites (Shull and Linton, 1951, in Kobak) and only 17% live for two years (Ratnoff in Bochus). The operative mortality rate is below 50% and lasting results are obtained in at least 30%.

Among the technical variants are the following:

— ligation of the hepatic artery proper below the gastroduodenal artery, associated with ligation of the splenic artery in ascitic cirrhosis without other complications;

— "progressive" (Bergman) or "delayed" ligation (Montegnani).

— dividing of the common hepatic artery with implantation of the central end into the portal vein (portal arterialization) or with implantation of the peripheral end into the portal vein (portalization of the artery).

All these complicated variants, with a high operative risk actually offered only the same results as simple ligation of the common hepatic artery.

It has been demonstrated experimentally that extensive intestinal resection (up to 50% according to Fuller, 1937, and Laufman, 1954) may lower ascites by marked diminution of the portal flow and reduction of the serous surface through which transudation takes place. The method has not been clinicaly applied since it produces major nutritional disturbances in the cirrhotic patient who already has a deficient nutritive balance.

Portal-systemic anastomosis is the most efficient means for reducing the portal blood supply to the liver and for controling portal hypertension. Vascular shunts only improve the condition of patients with cirrhotic ascites and marked portal hypertension in which the mechanical factor is prevalent. Statistically, this is only a minority since in most cases portal pressure is almost normal as numerous spontaneous portacaval anastomoses develop, reducing portal pressure to a great extent. In these patients, if the mechanical factor is not predominant it may be assumed that hyperproteinemia and secondary hyperaldosteronism interfere in the pathogeny of ascites.

Portacaval anastomosis (or its variants) does not improve either hyperaldosteronism or hypoproteinemia (more precisely hypoalbuminemia). On the contrary, it must be kept in mind that immediate operative mortality (32% Welch, 1964) and the quality of the late results depend upon serum albumin levels which reflect one of the aspects of the functional capacity of the liver; the poorest results are obtained in patients with low serum albumin values. Finally, the lowest tolerance to a meat diet after portal-systemic shunt occurs in patients with a reduced hepatic functional capacity, when the portal-systemic shunt is important. Therefore, in cirrhotic patients with massive ascites and almost normal preoperative portal pressure values (showing the development of spontaneous anastomoses), a major shunt of portal blood will take place after the new "efficient" surgical shunt. It is not surprising that postoperatively signs of marked hepatic insufficiency with hepatic coma and exitus occur. From the above data it can be concluded that cirrhosis with persistent ascites is not a rational indication for portal-systemic *anastomosis (Welch,* 1964*) except in the rare cases with evident portal hypertension.*

Cervical lympho-venous anastomosis (Deyni, 1965, Roschke, 1969) is an attempt to do "Portal decompression" via the lymphatic duct, with limited applicability and a difficult technique (Ackeren, 1971).

Hepatic extraperitonealization (Burlui, 1959) was developed in our clinic starting from the observation of Belli and Pisani according to whom ascitic fluid, representing an excess of hepatic lymph, appears in the form of droplets on the peritoneal surface of the liver (see the pathophysiology of ascites).

Technique : Patient in dorsal decubitus.

Right subcostal incision.

The liver is rotated towards the pubis revealing the caudal aspect of the diaphragmatic cupola almost up to the coronary hepatic ligament. An anesthetic solution is injected above the hepatic coronary ligament and then the parietal peritoneum is incised; the serous layer is detached off the diaphragm up to the ventral and lateral costal insertions of the muscle, medially, up to the falciform ligament.

The liver is then rotated in the opposite direction towards the left revealing the upper aspect of the right kidney. After anesthesic infiltration of the posterior parietal peritoneum below the line of reflection of the liver, the serosa is incised and peritoneum detached up to the superior duodenal angle.

The two peritoneal flaps are brought over the inferior aspect of the liver (i.e. with the right lobe extraperitonealized) and are sutured with interrupted catgut sutures, cutting a gap in the flaps at the level of the gallbladder which remains visible within the peritoneal cavity.

In a first lot of four operated patients (cirrhosis with ascites and marked protein water and electrolyte and hepatofunctional disturbances), three patients improved (increase in body weight of more than seven kg, disappearance of ascites) and one died from hepatic insufficiency. Other authors devised an adhesive perihepatitis, applying Eastman's plastic adhesive (Belli, Pisani, 1964). On reviewing the problem of the surgery of cirrhosis with ascites in its entirety the following operations with fairly clearcut indications appear to be applied today:

— Subperitoneal omentopexy for cirrhotic ascites in patients with moderate portal hypertension and advanced hepatic deficiencies;

— Hepatic extraperitonealization for massive ascites without marked changes in the portal pressure.

— Portal systemic anastomosis for the rare cases of ascites with very high portal pressure and moderate hepatic functional deficit.

In general the patient with cirrhosis and ascites is particularly delicate. The peritoneal fluid may form again very rapidly within the first days after the operation, resulting in abdominal distension and sometimes necessitating parancentesis or diuretic therapy of the chlorothiazide type associated with antialdosteronics, as mentioned above (see medical treatment). In the ascitic cirrhotic patient the appearance of visceroviscerál or visceroparietal adhesions should be viewed from another angle than that of other surgical patients.

In some cases, ascites may even disappear with development of adhesions or even after repeated aspirations.

In one case of ascitogenic cirrhosis, repeated paracentesis led to the appearance of a peritoneal plastic process (perivisceritis), gradually followed by diminution, almost up to disappearance of the ascites. Diminution of the fluid was not brought about by hepatic functional improvement as the functional tests showed progressive deterioration and frequent states of precoma developed at variable intervals.

Subsequently, when hypersplenism syndrome necessitated an attempt at splenectomy it was found that the adhesive process *had almost completely eliminated* the peritoneal cavity. The massive vascularization of all visceroviscerál and visceroparietal adhesions (portal decompression pathways) made it extremely risky to mobilize the spleen, totally fixed in its bed, so that splenectomy was abandoned. For another year slow aggravation of the hepatic insufficiency set in, without ascites.

In other cases, we observed the impressive development of the anastomotic vascular network in postoperative omentoparietal adhesions.

For instance, patient *P.C.* (whose clinical case is described in detail in the chapter on portal hypertension) had undergone gastrectomy for upper intestinal hemorrhage three years previously in another surgical department. In the course of laparotomy for splenectomy we found very numerous adhesions joining the greater omentum to the abdominal wall along the line of the former xypho-umbilical incision. These adhesions included enormously dilated veins in continuity with the subcutaneous large veins. Involuntary injury to one of the subcutaneous branches produced more major hemorrage than laparotomy in the usual cases. This is readily explained if we bear in mind that in this patient portal pressure (intraoperative splenomanometry) reached 70 cm of water (Claude manometer) and, therefore, the increase in venous pressure was readily felt in the subcutaneous veins communicating directly with the epiploic veins.

Subsequent findings have confirmed the trust put in omentopexy with regard to the role it plays in portal systemic shunt with increasingly larger vessels as time elapses after the operation.

The fragility of these patients is also apparent from analysis of the lethal cases in hospital, since besides death following the Talma operation of hepatic extraperitonealization, there was also a case of death after simple explorative laparotomy. This is not surprising since there was also a fatal case in the preoperative period (hepatic coma after paracentesis): hence, surgery should be recommended with the greatest precaution since any operation is followed by a critical period and the life of the ascitic patient is threatened by the brutal onset of hepatic coma. In our clinical group almost 30% of the patients were treated medically alone as it was considered that the functional state of their liver was too low to tolerate an operation.

PORTAL HYPERTENSION SYNDROME

Pressure in the portal vein depends upon the blood supply to the liver (hepatic artery plus portal vein) and the blood flowing from the liver (hepatic veins), not taking into account the small amount of water subtracted per minute for bilisecretion. These two kinds of circulation are connected by a network of hepatic sinusoids and intrahepatic venovenous shunts: the existence of a sphincter at the two extremities of the sinusoid has likewise been mentioned.

Under these conditions, it is not surprising that any morphologic alteration of the evacuation pathways or of the intrahepatic vascular network should produce portal *stasis* and implicitly an increase in portal pressure. Therefore, the portal hypertension syndrome may have various causes. In general, the question is simplified by grouping the anatomical aspects into three large categories, according to the site of the obstruction:

— suprahepatic obstruction of the Budd-Chiari type not so often encountered (in about 30% of the cases):

— intrahepatic obstruction (especially various forms of cirrhosis) a very frequently encountered type (almost 70%).

— subhepatic obstruction (thrombosis of the portal trunk or larger branches) seldom encountered in practice.

It should be stressed from the beginning that pressure in the portal vein is not stable and may oscillate in the same individual within fairly large limits in terms of the physiologic phase (digestion or rest), being also influenced both by neurohormonal factors and by blood pressure variations. On the other hand, the "normal" level of portal pressure often varies from one individual to another and marked deviations have been recorded according to the method used. Hence, the attempts at determining portal pressure within the limits of the portal area, only possible in pathologic cases with venous ectasis (esophageal, hemorrhoidal, paraumbilical varices, etc.) will only give relative information because at these levels a fall in pressure takes place due to discharge into the tributary veins of the cava system. Moreover, determination of the pressure in the portal area by no-blood methods (Bean) also gave approximate values. Therefore, the best method is that of determining the pressure as close as possible to the portal trunk:

— determination of intrasplenic pressure (M. Avrutszky, Le-Go, Lebon), which always give lower values than in the portal trunk (Léger):

— direct portal manometry: during the latter years this method has become available to all surgical departments since it has been simplified by the use of a manometer with a water column (normal saline-Moreno), considering zero level on the anterior aspect of the lumbar vertebrae (in the patient in dorsal decubitus). This method gives "normal" average values of about 215 mm normal saline $\pm$ 49 mm (limits within which 67 of 100 nonhepatic laparotomized patients are situated). Portal pressure can also be determined with the aid of a polythene catheter introduced into an ileal venule up to the porta with an electromanometer (of the Alvar or Galileo type).

From the experience of most surgeons in the treatment of portal hypertension it results that hemorrhagic accidents may occur and be repeated at values of over 300 mm of water.

However, it should not be forgotten that portal pressure has variable causes and is consequently unstable. This accounts for certain apparent paradoxes in the cases with typical portal hypertension accidents in which subsequent determinations showed values without significant deviations from the normal. This also explains certain dramatic accidents occurring in the evolution of cirrhosis. Actually, the main reason for a fall in portal hypertension is the development of a portal-systemic anastomosis whose site is fairly well known. According to Pick (1909) and McIndoe natural anastomoses may be divided into hepatopetal and hepatofugal types (Fig. 72).

The hepatofugal collaterals are the most important pathways for the discharge of portal stasis and may be grouped into three categories:

a) at the two points of transition between the glandular epithelium and the pavement epithelium (cardia and anus),

b) along the round ligament (fetal vascular remains),

c) retroperitoneal veins (Retzius). Branches sometimes arise between the splenic pedicle and the left renal vein (branches that can be cut during a splenectomy with a single ligature on the splenic pedicle).

Today, esophageal varices are interpreted in different ways. Although they are generally considered as a consequence of portal hypertension, not all authors agree that they represent a natural and important route of portal discharge. Some workers consider them as a kind of reservoir rather than a shunt in view of their reduced output. At any rate, esophageal varices should be considered as a stigmatum of portal hypertension, as esophageal varices due to other causes (congenital) are so seldom encountered. Esophageal varices evolve parallel to portal pressure values and are attenuated when a natural portacaval shunt develops lowering hypertension or when an efficient surgical portal-systemic shunt is carried out.

Esophageal varices — more precisely esocardiofundal varices — may be the site of massive, sometimes fatal hemorrhage. The latter are the first symptoms of cirrhosis in 10 per cent of the cases, but if the entire evolution of cirrhosis is taken into consideration then up to 25 per cent of the patients present gastrointestinal hemorrhage and 25 per cent die from hemorrhage. In 80 per cent of the cases of cirrhosis a vascular fistula at the level of the esophageal varices is the causative factor of the hemorrhage (Bochus). According to our data, hemorrhage is encountered in about 30 per cent of the patients with portal hypertension. As regards the intimate mechanisms which produce the vascular fistula, the idea of mechanical rupture of the thin varicose wall under the action of high venous pressure is now considered obsolete. As a matter of fact, this hypothesis could not account for the high incidence of esofundal venous fistulas in comparison to the extreme rarity of intraperitoneal rupture of the epiploic veins, enormously dilated at times.

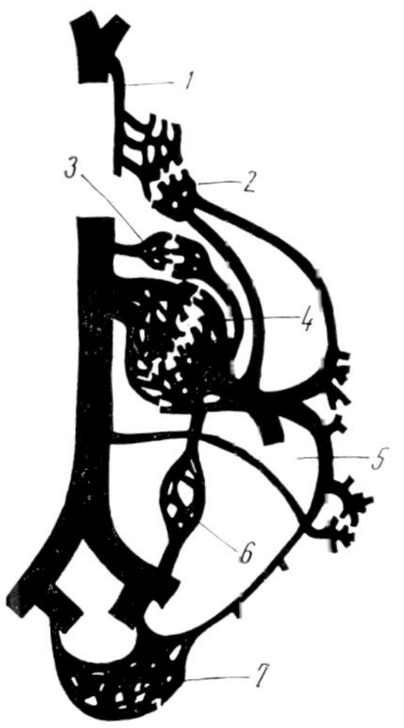

Fig. 72. — Communications of the portal system with the vena cava system.

1 — azygos vein; *2* — esophageal plexus; *3* — phrenic vein; *4* — hepatic capillaries; *5* — Retzius vein; *6* — Sappey's vein; *7* — hemorrhoidal vein.

Today it is admitted that the existence of turgescent varices at the level of the cardia hinders the normal function of the sphincterovalvular apparatus of the cardia with consequent esophageal reflux and peptic esophagitis. The latter produces ulcerations in the esophageal mucosa, which is more vulnerable at the site of a varicose distention. By an analogous mechanism, i.e. low resistance of the mucosa that covers vast blood pools, the occurrence of venous fistulas at the level of the gastric fundus is readily explained (another frequent site of hemorrhage). Finally, it is worthy of note that no direct correlation exists between the extent of the esophageal varices and gravity of the cirrhotic lesions in the liver; indeed, varices express the existence and the relative value of portal hypertension which partly depends upon the gravity of the intrahepatic barrier (respectively cirrhosis) and especially upon the development of the spontaneous collaterals in the portal systemic system. This explains why large esophageal varices are found especially in non-ascitic patients rather than in ascitic patients: ascites represents a later period and until then numerous other pathways of discharge of the portal bed have had time to develop, partly reducing portal hypertension and attenuating the varices.

From the very beginning portal hypertension influences the volume of the spleen which is enlarged due to its role of elastic reservoir. Initially, this splenic dystention is fairly variable, reflecting variations in portal pressure, but later on, splenomegaly exhibits a relatively constant value, that is a slow but progressive increase. The difference between the two types of splenomegaly is represented by interstitial fibrosis which occurs with time in the spleen during stasis. This explains why lowering of portal hypertension by broad portocaval shunts does not remove splenomegaly with its entire sequence of symptoms which will be dealt with later on.

Without going into the details of pathophysiologic hematology and without anticipating the symptomatology, we shall mention the inhibitory effect of hypersplenism upon several hematopoietic factors. Three aspects are directly slowed down and result in oligocytemia, granulopenia, and thrombopenia. The latter phenomenon is actually the most striking, the most constant and severe because it interferes with the mechanism of coagulation (thrombokinase and accelerator deficit) in patients in whom the so-called liver cell deficit leads to a high degree of hypoprothrombinemia. This confers upon hemorrhage from esophageal varices a particularly severe aspect in a region in which the clot is formed with difficulty in the presence of gastric hydrochloropepsic action (± reflux), in patients with delayed coagulation and from vessels whose amuscular walls are incapable of vasoconstriction, in areas with a high intravaricose pressure.

Thus, splenomegaly, a mild symptom in the course of cirrhosis, relic of the unavoidable initial portal hypertension phase, becomes a sign characteristic of a group of patients with particular clinical and evolutionary characteristics necessitating individualized therapy.

The pathophysiology of portal hypertension in cirrhosis of the liver. The normal hepatic artery brings about 24% of the afferent volume of blood supplied to the liver. The arterial blood ensures a certain level of oxygenation of the liver cells and, in addition confers upon the hepatic gland a certain degree of turgescence, thus regulating the portal output by the resistance offered by the sinusoidal bed. Therefore, a given volume of blood from the portal bed is evacuated transhepatically more rapidly at lower arterial pressures. Herrick (1907) showed that in cirrhotic patients an appraisable part of the arterial blood is regurgitated in the portal rami within the liver. Determinations performed by the same author in the normal and cirrhotic liver showed that perfusion through the hepatic artery at a pressure of 130 mm Hg induces in the normal liver a portal pressure of only 13 mm Hg (about 170 mm water) and in the cirrhotic liver a pressure much above 30 mm Hg (410 mm of water). Therefore in the cirrhotic patient a precapillary, intrahepatic arteriovenous shunt occurs partly explaining portal hypertension and hypervolemia (Schiff). These considerations justify to a certain extent ligation of the hepatic artery.

Portal hypertension is also explained by diminution of the intrahepatic vascular network due to morphologic alterations in the structure of the lobuli with destruction of a large portion of the trabeculosinusoidal complex, as described in the paragraph on the pathologic anatomy of cirrhosis.

In the liver, a number of venovenous shunts (portal vein, hepatic vein) develops offering to the blood a direct pathway across the liver, which is, however, nonfunctional from the metabolic point of view.

The original branches of the portal vein (abdominal visceral veins) are turgescent, hypertension influencing the capillaries, which offer a wide area favoring filtration and a restricted zone of active resorption. Hence, in terms of colloid osmotic pressure, massive filtration of the peritoneal fluid may occur, accounting to a great extent for ascitogenesis (in which hypoproteinemia has a more important role than increase in portal hydrostatic pressure).

Moreover, the functional value of certain capillaries with a specific role in resorption in the gastrointestinal tract diminishes, explaining gaseous distention, preascitic abdominal distension and the existence of soft diarrheic stools in cirrhotic patients.

Under the influence of the permanently increased portal pressure certain portal collaterals develop, forming a connection with the vena cava area, where hydrostatic pressure is almost equal to 0 mm Hg. The most important portal systemic communications occur in the anal (symptomatic hemorrhoids), cardioesophageal junction (esophageal varices) and more seldom the periumbilical or splenorenal region.

Under the influence of the permanently increased portal pressure, the spleen likewise increases in volume: therefore, splenomegaly secondary to cirrhosis. Splenomegaly is soon followed by "hypersplenism" in which the most severe aspect is thrombopenia.

Although subjected to a marked mechanical trauma, hemorrhoids are seldom the cause of hemorrhage in the course of the portal hypertension syndrome, and periumbilical varices cause hemorrhage only exceptionally. The common site (80%) of hemorrhage in cirrhosis are the cardioesophageal veins. We have already spoken about the probable mechanism of production (reflux, esophagitis, ulcerations).

Thrombopenia and hypoprothrombinemia secondary to cellulohepatic alterations bring about important changes in the speed of coagulation and other properties of the clot.

The gastric or esophageal coagulum is permanently subjected to the hydrochloropeptic action of the gastric juice (esophageal reflux).

Under the action of intestinal proteolytic bacteria, the products of protein disintegration (ammonia, ammonia compounds) reach the liver with a limited ureogenetic capacity (see Physiology: Hepatic coma). Part of these compounds pass through the direct, non-functional hepatic portavenal pathways through the liver and another part bypass the liver, at a distance, through the natural portal-systemic anastomoses. This explains the increase of ammoniemia concomitant to severe disturbances in the function of the central nervous system (portal encephalopathy, hepatic coma). The ammoniemia level will probably be considered as an "indicator of the degree of shunting in the liver under conditions of massive resorption of toxic intestinal products", rather than as directly responsible for the production of severe neuropsychical disturbances. This would also explain the relative inadequacy of the treatment of hepatic coma with substances that lower ammoniemia without saving the patient (glutamic acid).

In spite of the tendency to hypocoagulability in the cirrhotic patient with portal hypertension, important thrombosis of the original branches of the portal vein (especially the splenic vein) or even of the portal trunk may occur. This apparent paradox is accounted for by *blood stasis* in the dilated veins in which the very direction of circulation is reversed in certain areas. As the portal trunk has no valves, the direction of the circulation is dictated only by the gradient of hydrostatic pressure. Normally, the circulation is constantly hepatopetal but with increase in the resistance of the intrahepatic vascular network, during the period of maximum stress (after meals, for instance) a certain volume of blood will be evacuated from the portal trunk by some of the natural orthosystemic anastomoses described: within this area a hepatofugal flow occurs. In addition, part of the supply of blood regurgitated by the hepatic artery into the intrahepatic portal branches will appear in the portal trunk through which it flows in a hepatofugal direction (reverse of the portal flow). In the periods and at the sites of equilibrium of the portal circulation, zones of turbulence appear and variable speeds of the blood column, factors which favor thrombosis. To these are added certain endothelial alterations due to deficiencies or to the presence of microorganisms that readily cross the mucosa of the gastrointestinal tract, whose resistance is diminished against a background of blood stasis.

The consequences of thromboses differ according to their site and two locations are of particular interest to the surgeon.

Thrombosis of the splenal vein may occur at an early date concomitant to development of the first natural portal-systemic anastomoses. This accentuates splenomegaly and the onset of a severe hypersplenism syndrome concomitant to the stress exercised upon the cardioesophageal network. These are the patients with large esophageal varices, marked splenomegaly and less advanced cirrhosis. It is very important to detect these cases since they are not improved by portacaval shunts and, on the other hand, splenorenal anastomosis cannot be performed. The indications for splenectomy will be discussed lower down.

Portal trunkular thrombosis occurs much later when the numerous bypasses of the portal bed have already developed: it is much better tolerated than portal thrombosis in the normal human. With time, the thrombus again becomes permeable and forms the so-called "pseudoangioma of the lesser omentum". Preoperative recognition of these cases avoids useless laborious dissection of a portal vein that can no longer be used for anastomosis and which is surrounded by a "sponge" of varices.

Clinical study of the portal hypertension syndrome. Clinical study of the portal hypertension syndrome reveals all the signs of cirrhosis and the semeiologic manifestation of morphofunctional disturbances, connected with the permanent, accentuated increase of portal pressure.

It should not be forgotten that portal hypertension is a connex phenomenon that forms an integral part of the clinical and pathophysiological picture of cirrhosis of the liver. In this chapter, however, we shall only deal with particularly important aspects of the constant increase in portal pressure. In our Surgical Clinic, of 108 operated cases of cirrhosis of the liver, 31 (20.5%) presented one of the manifestations of portal hypertension. Within this relatively small group, the proportion between the sexes was almost equal with a slight predominance of males (4:3). Most of the patients belonged to the 26—50 year age group (more than half the cases). At times the accidents characteristic of hypertension occurred in apparently healthy states representing about 10% of the manifestations which made evident a cirrhosis that was latent until then.

Dyspeptic disturbances, inherent to cirrhosis, are more accentuated since, apart from gaseous distention, flatulence and a tendency to diarrhea, there is also pyrosis that marks the presence of esophageal reflux. The entire contour of the anus is marked by the constant presence of internal and external hemorrhoids.

The sensation of abdominal discomfort is not only due to distension of the intestinal loops but also to a gradual increase in the volume of the spleen. The patient complains of discomfort or even sharp pain in the left hypochondrium, especially in the first period when the spleen is still elastic and overdistended during each phase of increase of portal pressure. Subsequently, when the enlarged spleen is progressively fibrosed, the pain is replaced by a feeling of subcostal weight on the left side. The clinical examination initially detects splenomegaly by increased dullness on percussion (in this phase portal hypertension is attenuated), then the spleen can be gradually palpated over larger areas, sometimes to the level of the umbilicus or the midline; however, the spleen never reaches the size observed in leucosis. An important feature of splenomegaly in the portal hypertension syndrome is the existence of scalloped margins that can be readily felt on palpation in the patient without ascites (when portal hypertension is very high). For some time the spleen is mobile, but when perisplenitis develops, it is fixed by adhesions, a fact of importance to the surgeon, but difficult to appraise clinically because in such cases the spleen is immobilized in a single block with the diaphragm during respiration.

Gradually, the hypersplenism syndrome develops and is at first manifested by coagulation disturbances. In women metromenorrhagia develops or gingival bleeding so common in cirrhotic patients of both sexes. Subsequently, thrombopenia below 75,000 or 50,000 with periodical variations accounts for the large ecchymoses that appear at the site of slight injuries and finally even for spontaneous orthostatic purpura, manifested by small petechiae on the lower half of the legs in a standing position. Marked changes in the number of thrombocytes were found in almost 80% of our patients with portal hypertension syndrome and cirrhosis. These cases of accentuated thrombopenia are more seldom encountered in the course of common cirrhosis where the incidence is 24% (our statistics).

At this stage of evolution, the patient is particularly delicate and the natural progressive evolution of errosive esophagitis results in fistulization of the esophageal varices. Upper gastrointestinal hemorrhage is very seldom slow and prolonged, manifested only by an unexplicable melena (5% of our cases); in most cases a large amount of blood appears in the form of a dramatic hematemesis, refractory to the current treatment of rest and coagulants (the cause of 50% of the upper gastrointestinal hemorrhage according to Schiff, 1966).

The anemic patient (due to hepatic insufficiency and hypersplenism) may reach a state of severe anemia within one or two days, when he does not die within the first hours. Agitation justified by the severity of the hemorrhage, becomes gradually more accentuated (after 48—72 hours) when the products of ammonia disintegration appear in the intestine. From one day to another, a state of confusion may develop, then a stupor alternating with agitation or convulsions that characterize hepatic coma and precoma, i.e. portal encephalopathy. We have outlined the evolution of the symptomatology of the cirrhotic patient with portal hypertension and a common evolution, with a complete clinical picture. But not all cases can be included in this picture.

For instance, there are cases in which hypersplenism, justified by marked early splenomegaly, (thrombosis of the splenic vein) is not followed by evident development of esophageal varices. Instead of the dramatic picture of intestinal hemorrhage, we may encounter in these cases accentuated anemia, thrombopenic purpura, refractory metrorrhagy, etc. This aspect was met with in over 25% of our cases with portal hypertension. In other patients upper intestinal hemorrhage occurs very early when cellulohepatic insufficiency is not yet very accentuated and, therefore, is not complicated with portal encephalopathy, the patient surviving numerous such hemorrhagic accidents (each accident being equivalent to temporary portal decompression). In some cases with an insignificant hydrochloropeptic secretory capacity of the gastric mucosa (cirrhosis, secondary aldosteronism, etc.), the mucosa with venous stasis is readily erroded and gastric or duodenal ulcers develop, refractory to the medical treatment and with a marked tendency to hemorrhage (the ulcer disease as a secondary phenomenon was encountered in two of our patients with resection for bleeding ulcer). Finally, in some patients the only clinical manifestation of portal hypertension is the presence of bleeding hemorrhoids. The endoscopic aspect of this form should be known: internal and external hemorrhoids are to be found all around the anal canal and numerous venous ectases are visible throughout the rectal mucosa. When these "symptomatic hemorrhoids" are not detected, surgery may intercept one of the important routes of the portal network thus laying increasing stress upon the other collaterals and eventually giving rise to hemorrhage from the esophageal varices. Even simple anorectal compression with gauze strips may cause severe, fatal hematemesis (case 8, J.W. Pate, 1962). Still more dangerous is Whitehead's operation. The logical treatment in such cases is that of portal hypertension and not of the anorectal complication.

Without giving a description of the different types of collateral circulation (portacaval and cavacaval) we shall emphasize some of the particular developmental forms of the subcutaneous veins starting from the umbilicus, veins upon which one may sometimes perceive thrills and murmurs that give a clear image of the output of these portal shunts.

Finally, in a small proportion of the patients with high portal hypertension and hypersplenism, certain conditions may lead to the formation of ascites (in only 16% of our cases). This confirms once again the fact that in the pathogeny of ascites, proteinemia alterations, secondary to accentuation of the hepatic insufficiency are of greater importance than the high level of portal pressure.

Of importance for a closer understanding of the portal hypertension syndrome are the complementary examinations: visualization of the esophageal varices and portal trunk, determination of the parameters of portal circulation and hepatic function tests.

In the following pages, we shall deal with the current methods verified in practice and accepted by most workers.

Complementary examinations. Varices may be examined by endoscopic means (esophagoscopy), but it is generally resorted to only for therapeutic purposes (Crafoord method) or for manometric puncture (with fairly high risk). Direct visualization in specialized centers appears to be a highly accurate method for the detection of esophageal varices (Greene).

Cardioesophageal varices may become clearly visible when filled with contrast medium in the course of splenoportography. As a rule, the latter is resorted to in order to confirm a collection of abnormal findings and not before the patient has been suspected as having portal hypertension.

Esogastric barium meal. An innocuous and particularly useful routine examination is that of the esophageal barium transit time, when accurately performed. Either a barium meal or fluid barium can be used. The patient's posture should bring the esophagus as close as possible to the screen, dissociating it from the spinal shadow (right oblique anterior and left oblique posterior, D. Negru). The patient should also be examined in supine and standing position (Fanardjian). During passage of the barium meal, particular attention should be paid to distension of the esophagus (which should be normal) and the appearance of filling defects (usually round or ovoid) which generally appear at different levels of the esophagus, replacing the long strips of the normal mucosa relief. After passage of the barium meal, small droplets of the opaque medium remain suspended upon the esophageal varices (Figs 73, 74 and 75). According to whether large amounts of barium are used, which fills the esophagus up to a high level, or whether small, repeated portions of barium are swallowed at a time, specific images are obtained of a "distensible cylinder with scalloped margins" (Berg) or "the passage of opaque

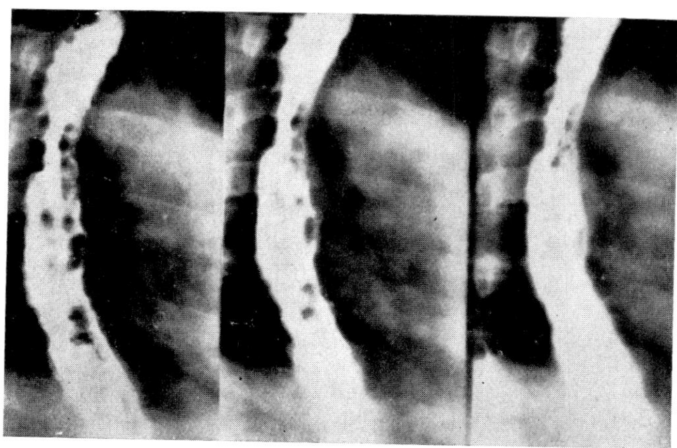

Fig. 73. — Splenomegalic cirrhosis; portal hypertension. Esophageal varices (serial images).

medium through the venous ectasic prominences" (Wolf). Varices are more frequent in the lower third of the esophagus and continue with venous ectasia of the large gastric fundus, revealed in the Trendelenburg position which also shows the existence of esophageal reflux. Sometimes varices may be observed the whole length of the esophagus.

Radiologic examination of the esophagus gives a large amount of morpho-functional information and is, moreover, a routine method readily accepted by the patient and which can be repeated at various intervals, presenting a dynamic image of the evolution of the varices, in respect to the portal hypertension syndrome they reflect. Some authors have used this method in emergency conditions in order to elucidate as rapidly as possible the etiologic diagnosis of hematemesis. However, it should be mentioned that a conclusive image of varices allows for a correct diagnosis whereas a negative image does not exclude portal hypertension, which may fail in the bleeding patient with peripheral hypotension and minor distension of the esophageal varices. Hence, a premature roentgenogram in the course of upper digestive hemorrhage may lead to erroneous conclusions; for this reason it is our practice to wait until the patient's general condition and other signs have pointed to arrest of the hemorrhage and circulatory reequilibration.

Direct examination by laparoscopy is not a routine examination and will not be discussed here. Radiologic examination of the portal tree with contrast medium will now be discussed.

Splenal and portal venography or portal venography is carried out according to whether introduction of the radioopaque substance is into the spleen or a portal branch. The two methods are not mutually exclusive and both have their advantages and drawbacks.

Splenal and portal venography was first suggested by Sousa-Pereira in 1949, then experimentally performed by Abeatici and Campi who, together with Lucien Léger reported the first clinical applications in the human, in 1951.

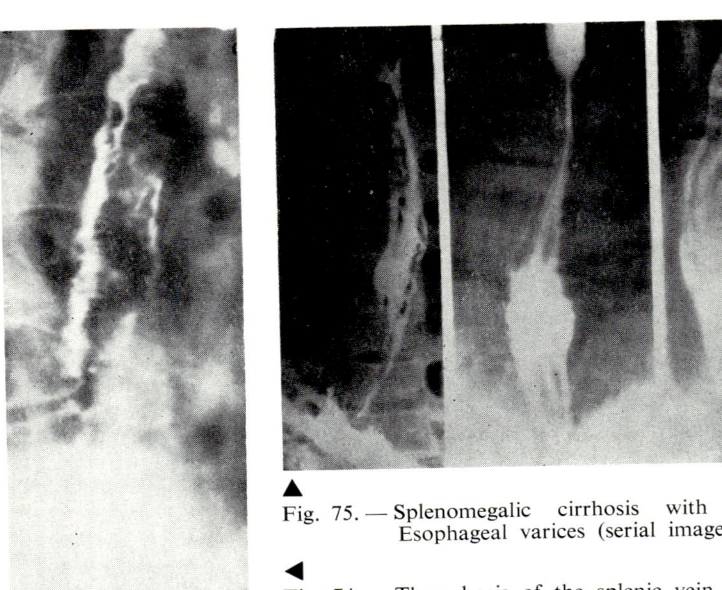

▲ Fig. 75. — Splenomegalic cirrhosis with hypertension. Esophageal varices (serial images).

◀ Fig. 74. — Thrombosis of the splenic vein. Splenomegaly with hypersplenism. Esophageal varices.

The following is the technique of Léger:

Sensitivity to iodine is tested for by instilling a drop of radioopaque solution on the conjunctiva.

Nargenol (or Romergan) is injected one hour before the venography.

Local anaesthesia is used and spleen is probed with a 20 cm long needle, having a diameter of at least 1.5 mm. The site of the puncture varies according to the size of the spleen. In large splenomegaly, the puncture is done below the costal margin but in lesser splenomegaly it may be necessary to puncture an intercostal space under radiographic control. The correct intrasplenic position of the needle is indicated by its movements with respiration, by blood oozing from the needle and by a stable radioopaque spot around its tip after injecting 2—3 cm of 70% Diiodine.

The patient holding his breath, 20—40 ml warm radioopaque solution is rapidly injected (a few seconds), and the first film is taken after the injection is finished, then a new view every second (if the apparatus permits) (Abeatici, Campi). Firică et al. (1957) recommend injection through the same needle, immediately after the radioopaque substance, 10 ml 0.75% novocaine which increases the patient's tolerance to iodine.

Many authors have made a contribution to splenal and portal venography which has now become a routine examination in many medicosurgical centers. The value of the time factor in the interpretation of morphofunctional information offered by splenal and portal venography results from the work of these authors. As remarked by Gvozdanovici (1955) neglect of the time factor accounts for the discrepancy met with in the literature; the author used a radiology apparatus permitting rapid change of the films.

In 1951—1952, Daniel and Prichard (in Child) showed experimentally the advantages of serial portal venograms which reveal the filling time of the portal vein, of the sinusoids and of the hepatic veins. The most conclusive views are obtained with the angiocardiography apparatus, at two seconds intervals or with radiocinematography with special light amplifying screens. But useful pictures can also be obtained with a device for changing the films every three seconds, adapted to the roentgen apparatus. One or two images taken approximately at the end of the injection and after five or six seconds gives only part of the information obtained by the serial method.

Roentgenograms, taken at a well chosen moment and individualized according to the calculated importance of the circulatory disturbances may give images suggestive of esophageal varices, especially in those with a very slow blood flow. The following are the characteristic aspects of splenal and portal venography (Firică):

Normal splenal and portal venogram: on the spleen a dense central opacity appears, representing the pool of iodate substance around the tip of the needle. Sometimes the contour of the spleen is finely outlined showing subcapsular diffusion of the substance. The spleen occasionally appears as a hypertranslucent area against the dense opacity of a "negative image"; this indicates either cleavage of the spleen with discharge of the opaque substance in the peritoneum or a technical defect (the needle has passed completely through the spleen). From the spleen, the splenic vein runs transversely; it is as a rule large, of uniform size and with certain tortuosities.

The splenoportal junction is clearly visible, the column of the opaque substance continuing to progress without reflux into the other branches. Normally at this level the density of the opacity is strongly diluted. When the rate of the injection or the concentration of the substance are insufficient the dilution may be so great that the opacity disappears, simulating obstruction of the lumen (false image).

The portal trunk is slightly oblique with respect to the spinal column. The normal diameter of the portal vein (depending upon the size of individual) is of about 20 mm.

The intrahepatic branches of the porta are clearly visualized, especially in portal venograms performed with a Bucky diaphragm, but even the portal venograms performed in the operating theatre with a portable apparatus clearly show the division of the porta in the hilus and continuation of its branches in the right half of the liver. In the left half, the portal branches are as a rule narrower and even the main left branch after bifurcation of the porta usually appears shorter in the front projections (an optical effect of perspective, this branch lying in an almost sagittal direction).

Pathologic splenal and portal venograms: we shall concentrate especially upon the morphologic changes in comparison to the normal aspect described, since evaluation of the various "moments" of the venogram is not yet currently applicable owing to the practical difficulty of recording so many films. A correctly applied technique and 3 images (at 3—5—7 seconds or 3—6—9 seconds after the beginning of the injection) will reveal the morphologic changes.

In hepatic cirrhosis with portal hypertension:

Early in the disease, the vascular image is clearly outlined in the region of the porta and its branches (due to increase in the size of the vessels and sluggishness of the circulation). The portal trunk runs almost parallel to the spinal column (wrongly considered as "verticalized") (Fig. 76).

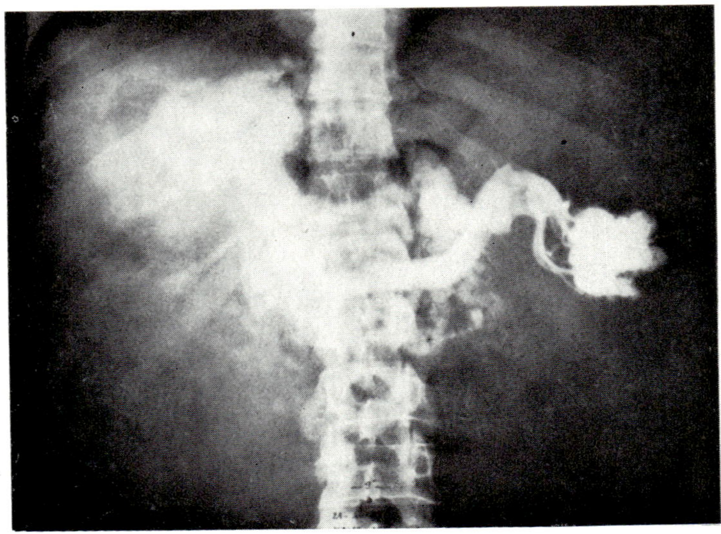

Fig. 76. — Splenal and portal venography in cirrhosis with portal hypertension. Note marked sinuosity of the splenic vein and reflux in the afferent left gastroepiploic veins.

In a more advanced phase always accompanied by clinical symptomatology, reflux appears in the other original branches of the portal trunk with regional changes in the direction of the blood flow, and a relative lucency of the intrahepatic portal arborizations (reduced number of branches per cm^2).

In terms of the evolutionary special findings we may often see, starting from this stage, the outline of the natural portal bypass and filling of the first esophageal varices (Fig. 77 *a*, *b*,).

Finally, in the very advanced stages, rough changes of the porta and its intra- and extrahepatic branches appear. A wide range of suggestive images exists: from massive reflux into another route of the porta (lower mesenteric vein, eventually gastric coronary vein) to integral evacuation of the opaque substance from the splenic vein, retrograde through the left gastroepiploic vein into the blood pools of the esophageal varices which can be followed up to the mediastinal and azygos veins or abdominoparietally (Fig. 78 *a*, *b*, *c*). The opaque substance suddenly stops at the head of the thrombosis (in the portal trunk or splenic vein). If the porta is still patent up to the hilus, only a few small branches arise from the two main branches (slightly opacified due to retrograde flow, probably of arterial origin) (leafless tree image).

In the last two stages, often accompanied by hemorrhage or the portal hypertension syndrome, the course of the splenic vein is modified and two segments appear at a right angle, the juxtasplenic segment becoming paramedian following lowering of the splenic hilus and the juxtaportal one remaining transverse but with marked tortuosities.

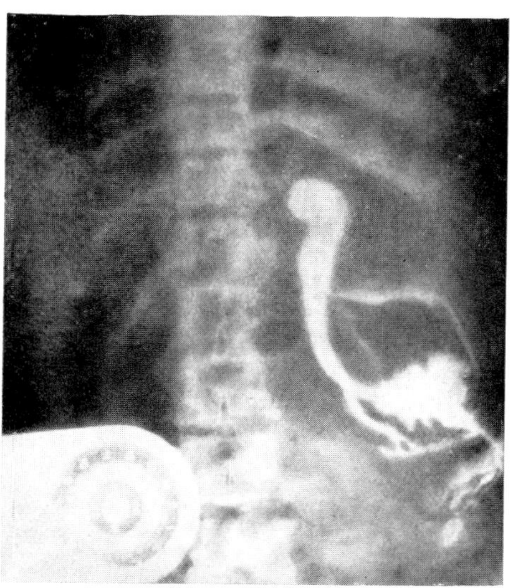

a

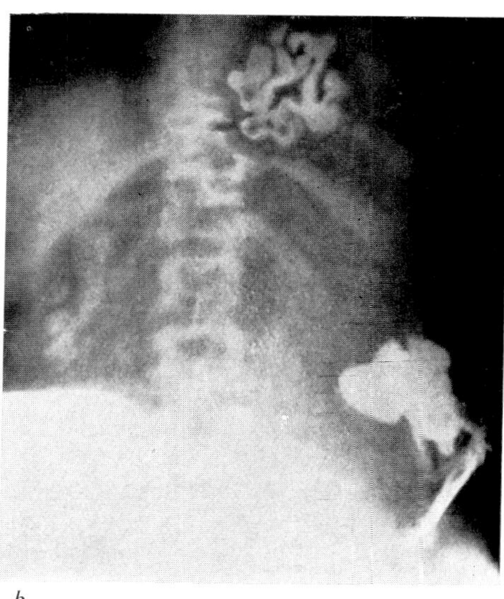

b

Fig. 77. — Splenal and portal venography. Successive images in cirrhosis of the liver with portal hypertension (esogastric varices, splenomegaly and hypersplenism).

a) At 2.5 sec. angulated, ectatic splenic vein apt for portarenal anastomosis; *b)* at 9 sec.: the opaque medium slightly outlines the liver and is denser in the gastroesophageal veins.

Apart from this information obtained in cirrhotic patients, splenal and portal venography makes it possible to identify isolated thrombosis of the splenic vein (Fig. 79), compression of the portal trunk (with intact normal intrahepatic ramifications) and finally even suprahepatic obstructions.

Owing to the informative material supplied, splenal and portal venography is now currently used in many medical departments and may be repeated several times preoperatively. It also permits determination of portal pressure and is seldom complicated by severe hemorrhagic accidents that demand emergency splenectomy.

Portal venography. As splenal and portal venography does not give conclusive images of the portal trunk in cases of splenic thrombosis and cannot be repeated after splenectomy or splenorenal anastomoses, other techniques have been developed suitable to all patients irrespective of the condition of the splenoportal junction.

Portal venography was developed by several investigators almost at the same time (1950—1951); important contributions were made by Child, Moore, Prichard and Bridenbaugh, Rousselot, etc.

Portal venography is performed as follows, in the operating theatre, under anesthesia: the peritoneal cavity is opened by minimal laparotomy, a loop is exteriorized (preferably the ileal loop), and a polyethylene catheter is introduced into a suitable vein. The loop is replaced into the abdomen after carefully fixing the catheter to the vein. The catheter should be introduced as

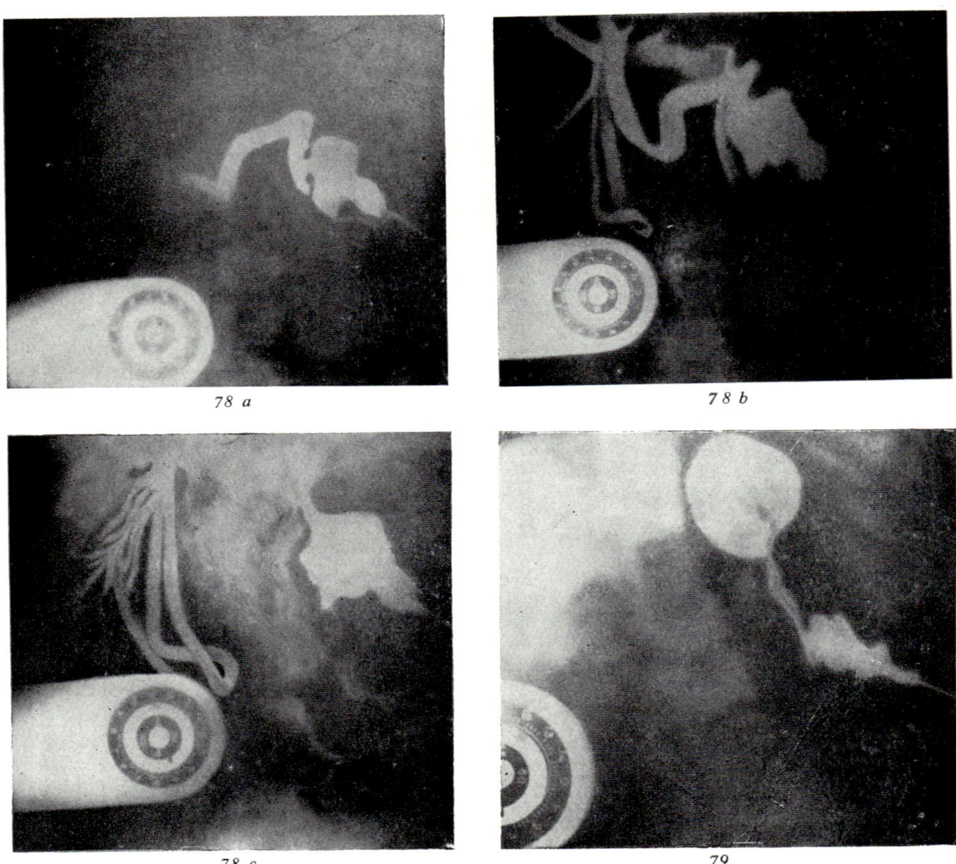

78 a   78 b   78 c   79

Fig. 78. — Splenal and portal venography. Successive images in splenomegalic cirrhosis with hypersplenism (natural portal-systemic shunts).

a) At 2 sec.: double angulated splenic vein, with verticalized juxtasplenic portion; *b)* at 7 sec.: large portal vein with rare ramifications (tree with shedded leaves); *c)* at 11 sec.: evacuation of the opaque medium especially through the umbilical vein and veins of the abdominal wall.

Fig. 79. — Splenal and portal venography in thrombosis of the splenic vein, at its origin. At 12 sec.: evacuation of the opaque medium especially through the gastric veins.

high as possible into the superior mesenteric vein. Rapidly inject 40 ml of a 60—70% iodate radio opaque solution, then record the radiographic images as with splenic and portal venography. Under experimental conditions, the left gastroepiploic vein was successfully used by us (1957). Together with Prichard and Bridenbaugh, we also were aware of the important contribution made by the introduction of serial portal venography.

This technique accurately reveals reflux in the inferior mesenteric vein (more frequently than splenal and portal venogram). Portal venography alone demonstrates the state of the portal tree in patients with thrombosis of the splenic vein, but is far from supplying the valuable information given by splenic and portal venography in esophageal varices.

Thus, these two methods are often complementary to one another and both the clinical examination and the radiologic aspects may be required in order to obtain a clear-cut image of the case studied. Morphological rather than functional relations are supplied by double venography, i.e. routine splenal venography and simultaneous portal venography (the latter performed by catheter inserted into the residual umbilical vein, as proposed by Bayley in 1964 and Burlui in 1965).

A secondary aspect in connection with the study of "portal visualization" is peritoneoscopy (laparoscopy), which may incidentally demonstrate a suspicion of portal hypertension and cirrhosis when the slightly granular aspect of the liver is corroborated with the existence of distended omental veins. This, however, is no merit of the method but negligence on the part of the physician who has overlooked many of the current tests (neither has he inquired in detail into the past history of the case) and has passed on prematurely to a complementary method that could have been avoided. The existence of portal hypertension should be diagnosed without resorting to laparoscopy, which cannot establish the characteristics of the evolutionary stage.

Hemodynamic studies. The chapter on the specific methods used for examining a patient with portal hypertension cannot be brought to a close without mentioning the procedures used for determining the *parameters of portal circulation*. Our approach would be scientific if we could evaluate the stage of the disease by means of precise data; portal output, intrahepatic capillary resistance or speed of flow through the portal vein, as possible in other segments of the circulatory system. These data may be correctly determined in experimental investigations, but in the clinic we must be content with approximate data obtained by indirect methods, because the direct ones can only be applied intraoperatively (a single, comparatively late moment in the course of the disease, under non-physiologic conditions).

Transhepatic portal output can be appraised by means of the values of the parameters listed above.

— Portal pressure is measured directly intraoperatively or by splenic puncture in the course of a splenic and portal venography and also indirectly and approximately by Iversen's equation: portal pressure $\geqslant$ (serum oncotic pressure — ascites oncotic pressure) + ascites hydrostatic pressure.

However, this equation is only applicable to ascites cases and does not keep account of water electrolyte changes brought about by secondary aldosteronism in the ascitic patient.

— In varices of the natural portal-systemic derivations (esophageal varices, hemorrhoids), the pressures listed are always below the portal pressure determined intraoperatively.

— Increase in portal pressure has also been deduced from the high values found in the hepatic veins, by catheterization of the cava veins.

— The speed of portal circulation can also be appraised radiographically by means of a radiocinematography apparatus in the course of any of the portography methods. A simplified technique is that of the *portal time* and *hepatic time*, which reveals fairly accurately slowing down of the portal circulation (the appearance of intrahepatic ramifications 6 sec. after beginning the injection).

Finally, a still more approximate method for determining the speed of portal flow has been proposed, that of comparing the time interval between the moment in which certain substances are introduced into the lumen of the gastrointestinal tract and also into the peripheral veins (Sherlock) and the moment they reach the gustatory or olfactory receptors, or the ether rectum-lung interval (Newman).

The transhepatic output was initially appraised with bromsulphalein (a method criticized by Cohn) and somewhat more correctly with colloidal radioactive gold (Velter, 1954) or radioactive chrome phosphate (Nardi, 1955), methods restricted to investigations in research institutes.

From the foregoing data, it may be seen that determination of the hemodynamic parameters in the portal circulation is far from offering the clinician the positive, accessible information supplied by radiologic or direct examination corroborated with the clinical and laboratory findings (confirming the existence of cirrhosis).

The diagnosis may be placed into two main categories:

a) Evident cases: clear history, complete symptomatology including signs of cirrhosis and the symptoms characteristic of portal hypertension (splenomegaly, esophageal varices with upper gastrointestinal hemorrhage, thrombopenia).

b) Cases with incomplete symptomatology.

— Gastrointestinal hemorrhage in apparently normal subjects; dysproteinemia test on admission, detection even of a moderate splenomegaly, electrophoresis, and after a few days barium swallow and, eventually, esophagoscopy, may elucidate the nature and mechanisms of the hemorrhage.

— Thrombopenia with apparently isolated splenomegaly and, eventually, metrorrhagia in women. The same tests and sigmoidoscopy may evidence portal hypertension against a background of cirrhosis, at the beginning of the clinical period.

— Bleeding hemorrhoids with exaggerated secondary anemia: the existence of thrombopenia, a characteristic sigmoidoscopia appearance, bring into consideration the diagnosis of cirrhosis with portal hypertension, which may be confirmed by biologic tests (electrophoresis, dysproteinemia, BSP, Quick test).

The main complementary examinations are esophagoscopy, roentgenography with barium swallow for esophageal varices, and splenic and portal venography to determine the extent of the circulatory disturbances in the portal tree and the site of the obstruction. In rare cases only can the clinical diagnosis be established without biopsy. As a rule, physicians prefer needle biopsy, and surgeons biopsy in the course of laparotomy, when faced with the question of portal hypertension necessitating surgery or with another surgical condition. We are against laparoscopy with or without puncture biopsy, for the reasons discussed before.

A diagnosis of portal hypertension should be carefully weighed since it may lead, when too readily accepted, to regretable errors of diagnosis and therapy. Certain conditions whose symptomatology has findings in common with portal hypertension should not be ignored:

— Hiatal hernia with cardioesophageal ulcer: a radiological examination must be done in the Trendelenburg position in order to reveal the presence of the hernia, esophageal reflux and any ulceration; in case of a hiatal hernia, the esophageal mucosa will only show linear folds without varicose nodules as observed in portal hypertension.

A small localized esophageal neoplasm appears on the radiologic image as a gap along the longitudinal lines of the esophagus and in serial radiographies, the esophageal wall at that level has a limited distensibility (it is not supple as in varices). The clinical context is altogether different.

— Acute hemorrhage due to upper gastric fundal ulcer may be discovered after hematemesis which is the first symptom. The past history of the case (the absence of hepatitis), blood dysproteinemia tests, the absence of splenomegaly, establish the diagnosis within the first hours. After a few days (if hemorrhage has not required an emergency laparotomy) the examinations may be completed by barium meal. If the unfavorable evolution of the case requires laparotomy and no lesion is found on the serous aspect of the stomach (the lesion may be recent and affecting only the mucosa), the absence of macroscopic hepatic changes will be noted intraoperatively, as well as the normal volume of the spleen and epiploic veins. Gastrotomy will reveal the acute ulcer that may be centered around a bleeding vessel of the submucosa.

— Long-standing ulcer disease with gastroduodenal hemorrhage may sometimes give rise to difficult problems of diagnosis since it is frequently accompanied by dysproteinemia, by changes in the hepatic tests (BSP, Quick, galactosuria) and finally even by hepatic histologic or cytologic changes. Apart from the evidently intricate forms (cirrhosis + ulcer disease) which concern the physician, we shall deal with the hemorrhagic forms of long-standing ulcers in which we must establish whether the hemorrhage is due to the ulcer and there is only a cellulohepatic involvement or a portal hypertension syndrome that favors the progress of the ulcer, as noted in two of our cases. This problem may sometimes only be elucidated intraoperatively by determination of portal pressure with a simple catheter with normal saline, puncturing an important afferent vein rather than the portal itself.

— Regional portal hypertension, with strictly local causes is more frequent within the area of the splenic vein and its collaterals (pancreatic compression, thrombosis of the splenic vein, etc.) and demands careful study and double venography (splenal and portal venography and then portal venography through the collaterals). If an obstruction of the splenic vein exists and the portal vein is intact and the liver tests good (with eventual checking by biopsy) we may exclude thrombosis of the splenic vein as an epiphenomenon of cirrhosis with portal hypertension establishing a correct diagnosis of "thrombosis or compression of the splenic vein, autonomic phenomenon". The treatment will be surgical, splenectomy being advocated.

— Mention has already been made of the particular features of splenomegaly in leukosis and splenic tumors (loss of the scalloped aspect of the anterior margin of the spleen).

Treatment of the portal hypertension syndrome in cirrhosis. Since the hypertension syndrome in the course of cirrhosis appears as a phase in the evolution of the basic disease, a medical and dietetic treatment should be maintained. Portal pressure, both normal and pathologic is a variable parameter and only when it persists above 30 cm of water are the consequences harmful. This accounts for clinical cases in which the accumulation of several factors increasing portal pressure may bring about (in a cirrhotic patient) a dramatic hemorrhagic accident although the surgeon has not modified the anatomic status of the portal tree (case 9, J. Pate). This helps us to understand the paradoxical evolution of certain atypical cases; on the other hand, statistics show that 70% of the patients die within the first 12 months from their first hemorrhage (30% in the first month). These figures point to the necessity of active surgical treatment which may save the life of a large number of patients.

It is difficult to give the operative indications in cirrhotic portal hypertension since various therapeutic methods have been applied to very different cases and the differential characteristics of the clinical groups are not always described in detail neither are the results sufficiently objective.

In the present stage of our knowledge it is, however, possible to sum up the most important methods used. These methods and operative procedures fall into four main categories, according to the fundamental object in view:

— methods for reducing the arterial blood flow to the viscera in the portal area;
— methods favoring outflow of the blood from the portal tree;
— isolation of the esophageal varices from the portal area;
— direct treatment of esophageal varices.

Several attempts have also been made at a neurosurgical treatment of the portal hypertension syndrome:

— resection of the autonomic ganglia (Wanke) is a complex operation also influencing the other viscera and is only exceptionally applied;

— hepatic periarterial sympathectomy (Mallet-Guy) has given encouraging results in prolonged hepatic jaundice but its efficiency must still be demonstrated in cirrhosis of the liver. The same is true when the method is completed by decortication of the common bile ducts (Stucke).

Surgical indications will be discussed with reference to the treatment of:

— hemorrhage from esophageal varices;
— portal hypertension with hypersplenism;
— portal hypertension in cases with a satisfactory hepatic function;
— portal hypertension in cases with hepatic functional imbalance.

Methods for reducing the arterial blood flow to the viscera of the portal area: ligation of the celiac branches, separate or in pairs according to the importance of the blood output, has been recommended.

The gastric coronary artery has the smallest output of the three subdivisions of the celiac trunk. Ligation of the gastric coronary artery *(gastrica sinistra)* together with the two gastric epiploic arteries was attempted by Flerow in 1926. He also added ligation of the lower mesenteric vein and reported successful prevention of hemorrhage. Walters only ligated the gastric coronary artery. We consider of greater importance the diminution of gastric acidity obtained after partial devascularization of the stomach than reduction of the arterial supply to the portal bed. Moreover, it does not appear advisable to ligate the inferior mesenteric vein which serves as a secondary route of decompression of the portal region, as revealed by numerous portal venograms.

In two emergency cases of portal hypertension syndrome with upper gastrointestinal hemorrhage, arterial ligation was performed.

— In one patient ligation of the coronary artery *(gastrica sinistra)* and gastroduodenal artery was carried out. The result was comparatively good with mild hematemesis on day 15 after the operation. The postoperative course was rendered more difficult by the onset of postoperative ascites which at that period was treated by repeated paracenteses. The patient recovered surgically and was discharged.

— In the second patient, an intraoperative thrill was detected in the splenic vein, suggesting an arteriovenous fistula. The splenic and the pyloric artery were ligated. The postoperative course was favorable although the patient had been suffering from liver disease for a long time and had several preoperative hematemeses, with alteration of the liver function (64% prothrombin index; 24% gammaglobulin, positive Gross and Takata-Ara tests) and accentuated thrombopenia (65,000). Full recovery was obtained.

Therefore, in our clinic, arterial ligation is only used exceptionally as a rapid and nontraumatizing operation, reserved for specific severe states.

Ligation of the splenic artery was proposed by Blain who considered that the output of the splenic artery represented up to 40% of the arterial supply to the viscera of the portal distribution. This method has recently been used by Raitzev and Komiliadze but is not widely used since the spleen which has not been removed receives sufficient blood through the collaterals of the splenic artery distal to the ligature; thus the spleen continues its inhibitory action upon certain hematopoietic aspects. Consequently, the course after ligation of the splenic artery with conservation of the spleen is not advantageous in the forms with established hypersplenism, although it may be favorable in some forms without hypersplenism. Hollman and Gerbode reported on the progressively improved course of the disease in two patients followed during 12 years. Maintenance of the spleen actually represents maintenance of its venous connections that are also shunts of the portal venous bed.

Splenectomy implies ligation of the distal extremity of the splenic artery; from this point of view it does not differ much from ligation of the splenic artery at its origin. However, it presents the advantage of removing the immediate cause of the "secondary hypersplenism", and is followed by striking hematologic improvement. This also explains the favor it enjoyed after Spencer Wells performed it for the first time in 1866 for "splenic anemia".

However, in most cases of cirrhosis with portal hypertension and hypersplenism, hematologic improvement was counterbalanced by aggravation of the portal hypertension syndrome sometimes followed by hemorrhage that was more important than before the operation. This is accounted for by the current splenectomy technique with ligation of the pedicle before bifurcation of the artery in the splenic hilus. This ligature, more readily performed than separate ligation of the vascular branches in the hilus, has an unfavorable effect in that it suppresses some of the dilated venous collaterals forming part of the natural portal systemic anastomoses and subsequent obliteration of other splenic collaterals due to unavoidable thrombosis below the ligature. It is known that, distal to any ligature, thrombosis develops in terms of the rate of the blood flow and that within the portal area in cirrhosis with portal hypertension the circulation is slowed down. Hence, the conditions favor thrombosis of the splenic vein after ligation with its severe effects.

This shows the major importance of adopting a splenectomy technique with ligatures applied near the splenic parenchyma in the hilus, on each separate branch. Portal hypertension brings into relief the enormously dilated veins with thin walls, rendering isolation of the vessels very difficult, but an attentive technique may

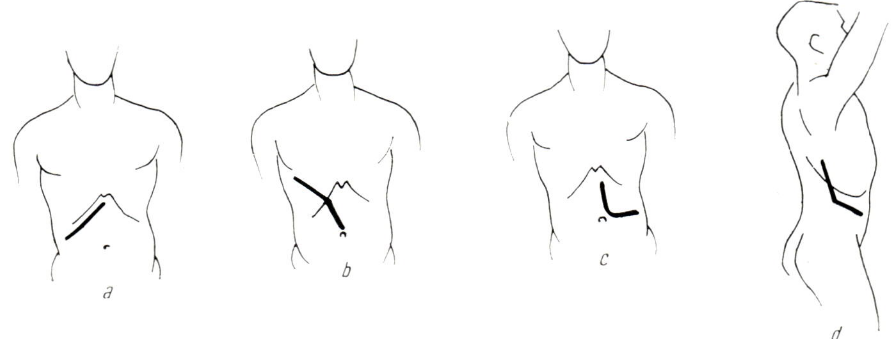

Fig. 80. — Types of incision.

a) Right subcostal incision for exploration of the liver, eventually followed by extraperitonealization of the liver or omentopexy; *b)* right anterolateral thoracoabdominal incision permitting portalization of the hepatic artery or arterialization of the porta; *c)* left costal xyphoumbilical abdominal incision, which we prefer to the more difficult splenectomy that can be followed by splenorenal anastomosis, periarterial neurectomy of the hepatic artery or omentopexy; *d)* right posterolateral thoracoabdominal incision; broad route of access for portacaval anastomosis.

result in perfect isolation and ligation of the vessels in the immediate proximity of the capsule, in the hilus. This requires sectioning of the anterior peritoneal leaf of the gastrosplenic mesentery which extends towards the left in front of the splenic pedicle, up to the hilus. This must be done with the greatest precaution in the immediate vicinity of the spleen so as not to injure the afferent veins from the stomach, coursing in the splenic omentum.

In splenomegaly, in cirrhosis with portal hypertension and marked hypersplenic syndrome, the following operative technique is applied (Fig. 80).

The patient lies in a supine position with a roll below the left shoulder and hip. A splenal and portal venography and splenomanometry are carried out. A broad V incision is performed with one arm oriented along the xyphoumbilical line and the other from the umbilicus to the left, tenth rib. This incision which can readily be transformed into a laparophrenothoracotomy has always given sufficient exposure without it being necessary to continue towards the thorax. At any rate simple median supraumbilical laparotomy, recommended in the past by Toma Ionescu, should be avoided as the exposure is not sufficient to be able to control hemorrhage often caused by detachment of the phrenosplenic adhesions (well vascularized in patients with portal hypertension).

The spleen is examined and the opportunity of sectioning the splenoparietal adhesions (between two forceps or ligatures) as a preparatory stage for freeing of the spleen appraised, or a previous exposure of the vessel in the hilus *in situ* is performed (in more difficult cases with a large adherent spleen). When the perisplenic adhesions are highly vascularized representing a single portacaval shunt, the surgeon will have to consider whether removal of these shunts without their replacement by previous or concomitant portal-systemic anastomosis would not aggravate the patient's condition still further by increasing portal hypertension. In favorable cases the most important, natural, portal systemic communicating vessels arise from the splenic vein immediately after its origin in the hilus and while the splenoparietal adhesions are still poorly vascularized.

When the spleen can be mobilized, it can be partly rotated in the wound with the greatest precaution and after sectioning the peritoneal leaf on the anterior aspect of the hilus, the vessels are identified and isolated from below upwards with a blunt curved forceps. Slight traction is applied to the vessels in order to lengthen them and obtain another 4 to 5 mm at their entrance into the capsule, so as to have sufficient space to apply two fine Kocher forceps or two Halstead forceps between the ligature and the spleen. The vessel is then severed between the two forceps: one remains close to the spleen if it cannot be replaced by a ligature, and the other on the stump of the first ligature is gently unclamped and the quality of the ligature checked. As each separate vessel is ligated, it is not necessary to use powerful clamps (Mikulicz, etc.). Particular attention should be paid to the upper polar branches which sometimes arise further along the splenic vessels at the site of their angulation caused by lowering of the splenic hilus. The venous branch coursing through the upper pole must be found and ligated only after being sure that the splenic vein *in toto* has not been caught up in the ligature which would jeopardize the first part of the procedure. In order to obtain better access to the upper pole of the spleen, the peritoneal leaf that covers the posterior aspect of the splenic pedicle (dependant upon the pancreaticosplenic omentum) is severed, when this is not done at the beginning of the operation. If the splenoparietal adhesions could not be divided between ligatures or clamps at the beginning of the operation, this must be done step by step freeing the spleen in the hilus, and permitting its mobilization. The phrenosplenic ligament, broadened by intimate contact of the enlarged spleen with the diaphragm, contains several veins that cannot be spared; hemostasis should be carried out with the greatest attention. The large veins in the gastrosplenic ligament should at any rate be spared (short gastric vessels).

If the ligature slips and the operative field is flooded with blood, the forceps should not be applied haphazardly when, in the best of cases, the splenic vein itself may be clamped together with the tail of the pancreas, but the splenic pedicle must be caught up tightly between the fingers and, after aspiration, gently let go in order to see exactly the lumen of the branch from which the ligature had slipped and, after applying the forceps visually, to ligate it again. In general, hemostasis leaves a clean, bloodless field at the end of the operation. The spleen, with the vessels in the sectioned hilus, divided adhesions and peritoneal reflections of the incised pedicle, is cut adrift and the ligatures are carefully checked. Drainage is not indicated when hemostasis was done with great care. The abdominal wall is closed; a roll of cotton tied with quill sutures should be applied the whole length of the incision, especially in patients with accentuated thrombopenia and insufficient coagulation. Bleeding along the parietal part of the incision is as a rule efficiently checked by correct suture of the muscular layers and rapid application of the roll of cotton. It is useless to try and perfect hemostasis of the wall by increasing the number of ligatures as this lengthens the operation, increasing the loss of blood and hazard of fibrinolysis and necessitating rapid transfusion.

Therefore, there is a fundamental difference between the technique of splenectomy performed in the cirrhotic with portal hypertension (and hypersplenism syndrome) and that carried out for rupture of the normal spleen or splenomegaly in patients without portal hypertension against a background of cirrhosis. In any situation apart from cirrhosis, rapid splenectomy may be done by single ligation of the splenic vessels before they divide in the splenic hilus, while in cirrhosis each blood vessel must be ligated separately after it branches off in the hilus (Fig. 81).

Moreover, in comparison to splenectomy in the hilus, performed on a normal spleen for esophagoplasty with gastric tube (Gavriliu and Heimlich), splenectomy in the cirrhotic patient is infinitely more difficult due to ectasis and friability of the veins and to the impossibility of mobilizing and exposing the spleen from the beginning (a hemorrhagic maneuver, dangerous and illogical in the

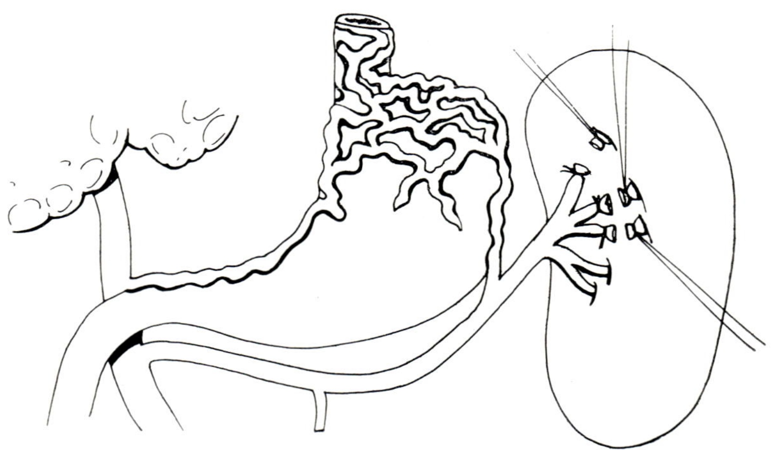

Fig. 81. — Splenectomy in the hilus, in portal hypertension.

cirrhotic), as with the normal spleen in which numerous pancreaticoparietal veins serve as pathways of portal decompression.

Ligation of the hepatic artery was proposed by Rienhoff (1951), who hoped to lower the portal output to the level of the functional possibilities of the hepatic sinusoids. He considered that a vascular shunt is a complicated and risky operation, in contrast to the easy technique of ligating the hepatic artery. A further, more recent argument, exists; suppression of the arterial blood supply will reduce hepatic "turgescence" and, therefore, the resistance of the sinusoids to the portal flow, i.e. it will reduce portal pressure, favoring transhepatic circulation. Experimentally, in the isolated organ the transhepatic output of portal and arterial perfusion is smaller than the sum of the output obtained with successive arterial and portal perfusions (Inquimbert, 1966). It is not proved that an efficient lowering of portal pressure is obtained and, on the other hand (as also recognized by Child), the supporters of vascular shunts cannot even pretend that portacaval communications improve intrahepatic circulation that may follow upon ligation of the artery.

However, there is no general consensus concerning ligation of the hepatic artery. In normal human beings, only ligation of the common hepatic artery (before emergence of the gastroduodenal artery) is compatible with life, whereas in cirrhotics, Rienhoff shows that the main hepatic artery can also be ligated without vital hazard, and that only at this level has ligation of the artery therapeutic significance. The results of ligation of the main hepatic artery in the dog (death from activation of latent microbism and development of Welch's bacillus) should not be identified with the benign results of its ligation in the normal human individual. Notwithstanding, Lowe (Child) reports 5 deaths after ligation in the hepatic artery in man (with the development of bacteria producing gas in the

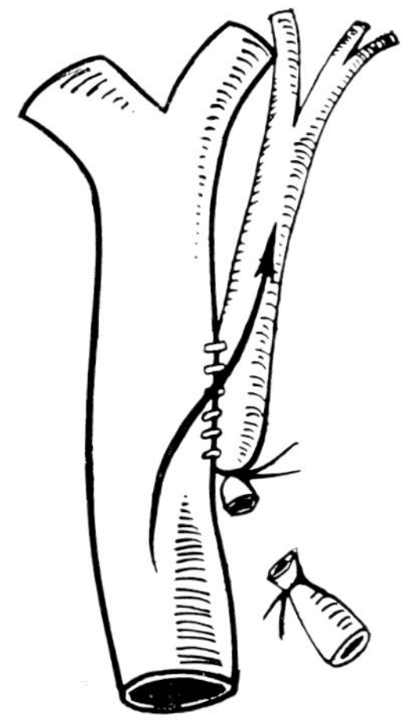

Fig. 82. — Portalization of the hepatic artery. Saegesser operation (author's drawing).

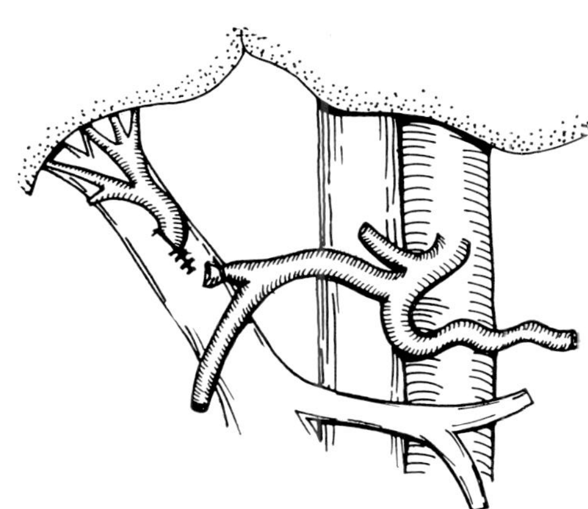

Fig. 83. — Portalization of the hepatic artery.

liver), in 27 clinical cases. In addition, in 1933, Graham and Cannell found 15 deaths in a series of 27 cases occurring more rapidly the further the artery was ligated from its origin.

Since it is not possible to appraise preoperatively to what extent ligation of the main hepatic artery will be tolerated in each case of cirrhosis, ligation of the common hepatic artery, as recommended by Léger, appears preferable, especially as the fall in portal pressure is temporary. In view of this finding and of the progressive improvement of the liver tests in the surviving patients, the question of ligation of the common hepatic artery no longer appears pertinent in the therapy of portal hypertension, but should be raised in cases of hepatic insufficiency. To a still greater extent are the other variants questionable: implantation of the proximal (Mallet-Guy) or distal end of the hepatic artery (Saegesser) in the porta (with uncertain permeability effects) (Figs 82 and 83).

Methods favoring evacuation of the portal blood. Several techniques have been proposed for obtaining portal decompression through portal-systemic shunts. These anastomoses or shunts may be carried out directly, or the surgeon may create the conditions in which they will develop subsequently.

In the first category:

portacaval (truncular) anastomoses
splenorenal anastomoses
mesenteric-caval anastomoses } radicular
omphalocaval anastomoses

In the second category:

omentopexy (Schiassi, Făgărăşanu, etc.)
thoracalization of the spleen (Turunen)

— *Portacaval anastomosis* was proposed by van Eck as far back as 1887, but was first applied only in 1945 by Blakemore and Lord (Guy Albot) and is

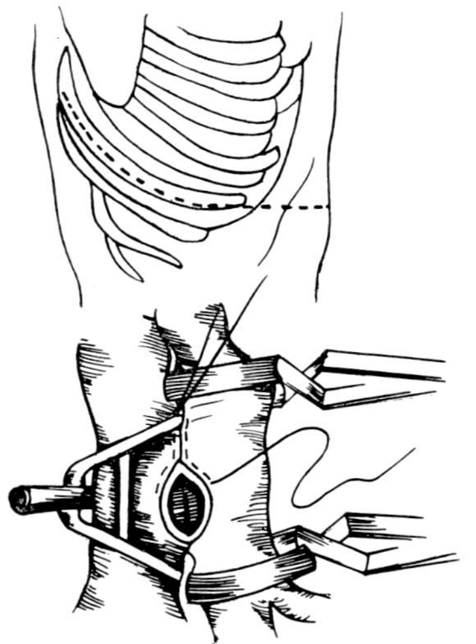

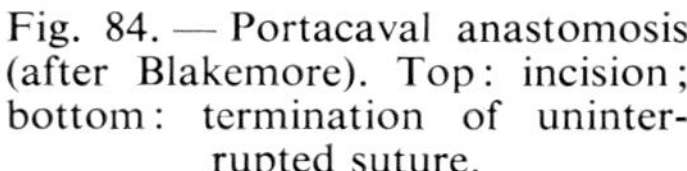

Fig. 84. — Portacaval anastomosis (after Blakemore). Top: incision; bottom: termination of uninterrupted suture.

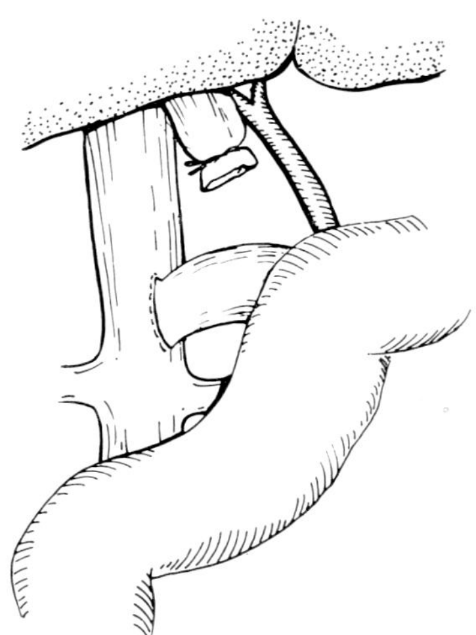

Fig. 85. — End-to-side portacaval anastomosis (drawn after Child).

now used by many surgeons (F.G. Uglov, DeBakey, etc.). Right subcostal or right transverse incision exposes the hepatic pedicle and can easily be transformed into a thoracophrenolaparotomy. The latter, recommended by Blakemore, permits cranial rotation of the liver and offers better access to the portal vein and lower cava vein (Fig. 84).

Exposure of the portal vein is difficult because of ectasis of the lesser omentum veins and because of thickening of the tissue around the porta (periphlebitis). There are cases in which the porta cannot be exposed; it is then freed along the lesser omentum, from the duodenum to the liver hilus, separating it carefully from the common hepatic duct and hepatic artery. An attempt is made to bring it, with the aid of elastic loops, towards the vena cava; when this is not possible a technical artifact will be necessary.

The posterior parietal peritoneum is then incised in order to reveal the inferior vena cava; this is easier than the preceding maneuvre but more difficult than in the normal subject. The end-to-side (Fig. 85) or side-to-side (Fig. 86) anastomosis is chosen according to experimental criteria and especially to anatomic conditions. The side-to-side shunt does not exclude the liver from the portal circulation; the end-to-side shunt gives certain shifts in aminacidemia and BSP tests and inhibits hepatic regeneration. When the two veins can readily be approximated, a side-to-side shunt will be performed, whereas when the distance between

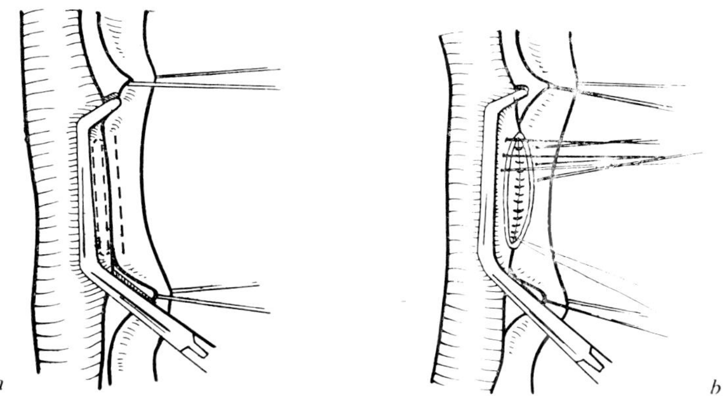

Fig. 86. — Side-to-side portacaval anastomosis with a singular vascular clamp.

a) Lateral clamping of the vena cava; application of the stay-sutures on the vena porta. Incision (. . .) on the porta and excision of a narrow band; *b)* side-to-side suture with interrupted suture.

the two veins is greater, an end-to-side shunt with section of the porta is carried out or an intermediary graft is used (bridging). Bridging between two vessels with partial shunt leads to obstruction, therefore either lateral shunt is performed or, after section of the porta below the hilus, an end-to-side shunt either directly or with a vascular graft. Although end-to-side anastomosis is more readily performed, it must be carried out very rapidly because only an arrest of the portal circulation of 20 minutes can be tolerated at normal temperature; in case of thrombosis death is inevitable.

Special forceps are used for anastomosis (lateral clamping forceps of the Blakemore or Potts type) as well as needles and special silk or plastic material (orsilon, nylon, dacron, relon) for vascular suture.

Different opinions have been sustained concerning the use of anticoagulants. In general, particular attention is paid to correct suture techniques without excessive trauma of the margins of the vascular orifices, since thrombosis generally occurs within the first two days when the use of anticoagulants presents the highest risks.

The operation is considered successful when portal pressure falls below 30 cm water, which may be obtained by end-to-side shunt and by side-to-side shunt with an opening equal to the diameter of the porta. Thrombosis occurs more often following anastomosis with a graft.

Splenorenal anastomosis was adopted as a necessary solution by Blakemore in a case of thrombosed, useless portal vein. This is, as a matter of fact, the fundamental reason for the method but the technique has been developed very much.

Initially, Blakemore recommended direct end-to-end anastomosis of the splenic vein (after splenectomy) with the left renal vein (after nephrectomy). This demanded

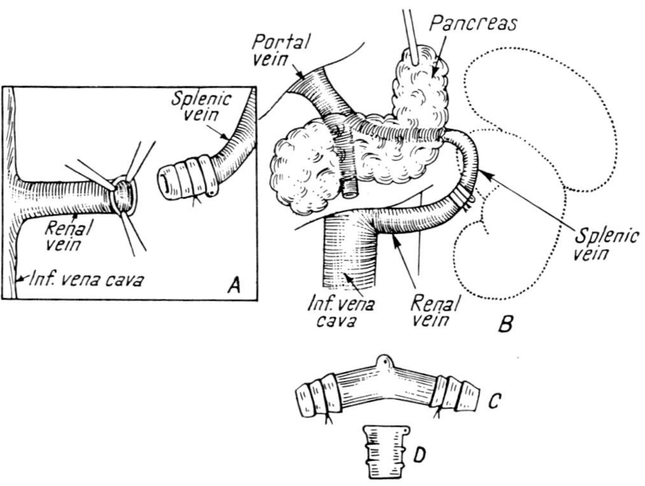

Fig. 87. — Splenorenal anastomosis (Blakemore), with vitallium ring and right nephrectomy (after Child).

the great sacrifice of the left kidney and seldom freed the renal splenic veins over a sufficient area to obtain their apposition, even with the aid of a vitallium ring (Fig. 87).

Soon afterwards Rousselot, based upon the anatomofunctional findings of Ashworth, Baxter, Lichtman who reported on the high incidence of renal alterations in cirrhotic patients, modified the procedure. Rousselot recommended conservation of the kidney with limited lateral clamping of the renal vein or even total clamping (maximum 45 minutes according to Santy, Marion) and end-to-side implantation of the splenic vein (after splenectomy) into the renal vein. Similarly, Rousselot showed the advantages of exposing the splenic vein up to the dorsal aspect of the pancreas and, therefore, of interposing a venous autograft on the renal vein (Fig. 88). The submesocolic route of approach for splenorenal anastomoses, described more recently by L. Léger (1968) may offer real advantages for performing the anastomosis, even in the side-to-side variant proposed by D.A. Cooky (1968).

According to Poilleux, the two blood vessels to be anastomosed, and eventually the intermediate graft, should have a diameter of more than one centimeter so as not to risk thrombosis of the anastomoses. Patsiora, a supporter of splenorenal anastomosis, modified the technique using the upper polar branch of the left renal vein and facilitated the suturing, which is sometimes very difficult, by means of a vascular suturing device.

This anastomosis can only be performed immediately after splenectomy. When this moment has been exceeded, the splenic vein becomes thrombosed over variable extents and can no longer be used. However, even when the patient has undergone splenectomy some time ago and the portal vein is thrombosed, a

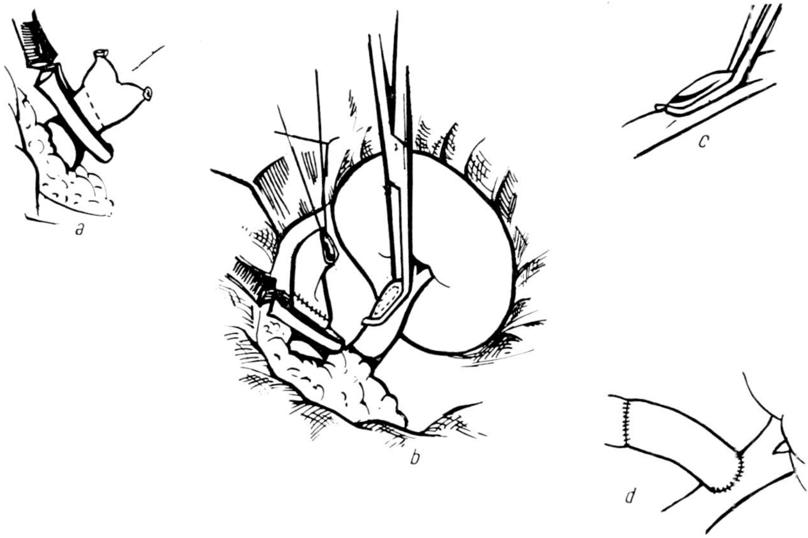

Fig. 88. — Rousselot technique of splenorenal anastomosis with venous graft.
a) Clamping of the free end of the splenic vein, with ligatures applied in the course of splenectomy; *b)* partial, lateral clamping of the left renal vein and elliptic excision of a portion of the vein; *c)* suture of the venous graft to the sectioned end of the splenic vein and preparation of the anastomosis between the graft and the renal vein; *d)* result: end-to-side splenorenal anastomosis and venous graft.

portacaval shunt can be carried out as shown by Blakemore, exposing the venous pool of the upper mesenteric confluent in the splenic vein and interposing a venous graft between it and the cava.

In carefully diagnosed cases oblique laparotomy can be performed from the umbilicus to the 8th-9th rib and continued along the rib when a left laparo-phrenothoracotomy is necessary.

Splenal and portal venography, performed if possible percutaneously, immediately before the operation, will show the caliber of the splenic vein and whether it is patent or not. When these aspects show that the splenorenal shunt is possible, splenectomy is rapidly carried out according to a simplified technique (ligation of the vessels before they branch off close to the hilus), without attempting to spare the venous collaterals as described in the splenectomy technique applied in cirrhotic patients with hypersplenism.

The splenic vein is freed up to the dorsal aspect of the pancreas severing the branches that restrict its mobilisation.

The posterior parietal peritoneum is incised over the left renal pedicle and the renal vein is carefully isolated and raised on elastic loops. After preparing the vessels for the anastomosis, eventually lengthening the splenic vein with a venous graft, the renal vein can be clamped laterally or even crosswise and longitudinal phlebotomy of the renal vein of the same size as the lumen of the splenic vein will be performed. Anastomosis must be done rapidly, eventually by posterior basting suture at a distance, before carrying out the anterior suture. The forceps are removed from the renal vein (within less than 45 minutes) and from the splenic vein, completing the anastomosis by one or three separate sutures if necessary for it to be tight. If the suture is well done it has every chance of remaining patent when:

— its diameter is equal to that of the splenic vein;

— the splenic vein at the site of the anastomosis is of about 10—17 mm in diameter; the splenic vein is not under tension or bent.

This anastomosis will be efficient against hemorrhage from the esophageal varices when pressure in the portal vein falls below 30 cm of water.

Another form of radicular portal systemic shunt is the *mesenteric-cava anastomosis* performed in man by Bogoraz. This operation was experimentally carried out for the first time in 1907 by I. Jianu. It is not, however, widely applied because the upper mesenteric vein has a relatively small diameter exposing it to the severe hazard of thrombosis, with inevitable death, but it is the only solution in patients in whom the anatomic situation prevents the other kinds of anastomoses described and when portal systemic shunt is indispensable. Attempts have also been made, but with frequent early thrombosis, to anastomose the lower mesenteric vein to the left renal vein.

Mention should be made of the omphalocava anastomosis used in cirrhosis of the Cruveilhier-Baumgarten type (Léger, Vaillant).

Progressive portal systemic shunts: with all the operative procedures described the surgeon creates, from the beginning, a portal systemic communication that may remain as such or may gradually narrow down due to thrombosis.

In contrast are the techniques favoring the development of vascularized adhesions. Neovessels develop in these adhesions with progressively enlarging diameter and represent an important route of portal systemic communication, which is not exposed to thrombosis. In this category are:

— Omentopexy of the Schiassi and Făgărăşanu type.

— Thoracalization of the spleen (Turumen).

Properitoneal omentopexy has been described in the paragraph on the surgical treatment of ascites. This procedure is particularly benign, the operative risk minimal and its efficiency remarkable if the clinical course permits an interval of 4—6 months, necessary for the development of veins with a sufficient output to drain the portal system.

In 3 cases we had the occasion to reoperate, one to several years after omentopexy, for various indications and found numerous blood vessels of fairly large calibre, forming veritable angiomatous pools in some places, coursing from the omentum into the abdominal wall; their total area exceeded by far the largest portacaval anastomosis that can be realized between the two veins. However, in the cases with a rapid course the repetition of hemorrhage may lead to death long before sufficient neovessels have developed following omentopexy. Therefore, it is a benign operation with actual but delayed efficiency, a characteristic that should not be overlooked when the indications are established. In 10% of the cases of the portal hypertension syndrome with hypersplenism we consider it necessary to combine splenectomy with omentopexy of the Schiassi type. In 5% of the cases of portal hypertension admitted, hypersplenism was less important than the portal hypertension and in these cases Schiassi omentopexy was performed as a method of progressive portal systemic shunt. The mildness of this operation performed in patients with deficient functional tests is demonstrated by the absence of mortality (which was 9% in splenectomies, in the same syndrome complicated by hypersplenism).

Thoracic transposition of the spleen was performed as a treatment of portal hypertension for the first time by Turunen and Nylander in 1952 (the first cases were published in 1955). The patients followed up to 5 years after the operation, exhibited numerous splenothoracic neovessels with disapearance of esophageal varices. The authors based their operation upon the intraoperative finding of numerous, richly vascularized adhesions between the spleen and thoracic wall in a patient with diaphragmatic hernia and displacement of the spleen into the left pleura. Freedlander (1960) carried out an experimental study on the development of neovessels over the thoracalized spleen in the dog and found that the portal vein can be brusquely ligated with 50% survivals after thoracic transposition of the spleen. This encouraged Freedlander to apply the operation clinically to three patients.

Foster and coworkers took up this experimental study again and in 1961 published favorable conclusive results. The thoracalized spleen rapidly forms vascular connections with the veins of the thoracic wall and mediastinum, the blood passing from the spleen into the intercostal veins and azygos veins. Up to 75% of the dogs with thoracic transposition of the spleen survived following brusque ligation of the porta.

However, as in the portal hypertension syndrome the spleen has a nocuous effect upon hematopoiesis (hypersplenism), conservation of the spleen, even with partial vascular connections with the systemic veins, does not avoid thrombopenia. Therefore attempts are made today at a fairly difficult technique, that of segmentary resection of the spleen and thoracic transposition of the remaining spleen.

Thoracic transposition of the intact spleen is, however, a relatively simple operation with an actual but delayed efficiency making it preferable in patients with a general deficient state, inapt for vascular anastomosis, while the complicated modifications of the initial technique render the operation just as complex as splenorenal anastomosis the decompressive effect of which is immediate (therefore immediate efficiency for equal hazard).

Lagache (1965) emphasizes that the late results are poor.

General considerations of portal-systemic shunt. The enthusiasm raised by the technical success of portal-systemic shunts and the first spectacular clinical results (disappearance of esophageal varices and of hemorrhage from esophageal varices) was at a given moment dampened by the unfavorable results obtained by some surgeons (postoperative deaths, late neuropsychiatric accidents, etc.).

At present, sufficient material has been accumulated to be able to draw conclusions concerning portal-systemic shunts and also, to some extent, concerning delayed portal-systemic shunts.

Any portal-systemic shunt, when patent and fairly large and efficient may be compared to Eck's fistula from which it derives and which will consequently shunt the portal blood from the liver, lower metabolic efficiency and, what is more important, decrease or annul the antitoxic role of the liver.

The liver of the patient with portacaval shunt still receives blood from the hepatic artery which will allow delayed interference in the metabolic cycle of substances resorbed from the intestine via the porta. Therefore, ligation of the hepatic artery in end-to-side portacaval shunt is forbidden and should be avoided in all forms of shunts.

Diminution of the portal supply to the liver lowers hepatic regeneration. This explains why the hepatic tests are not improved after a shunt or are even deteriorated when already altered preoperatively; from this point of view, splenorenal anastomosis is less harmful: Linton (1965) had 57% survivals of over 5 years with this technique and only 36% survivals of over 5 years after portacaval shunt.

Therefore, it may be concluded that shunts can be performed in patients in whom the mechanical phenomena of portal hypertension threaten the patient's life, cellulohepatic insufficiency being attenuated. The high mortality rate (up to 8% according to Saegesser in patients with less than 3% proteinemia, agrees in this sense.

As jaundice and ascites, even attenuated, point to marked cellulohepatic involvement, immediate portal-systemic shunt should be avoided in these patients and omentopexy or thoracic transposition of the spleen recommended.

Portal-systemic shunts (immediate communications) are more efficient in portal hypertension without cirrhosis (due to extrahepatic obstruction), but this will not be dealt with here.

Methods for isolating cardioesophageal varices. Cardioesophageal varices represent the ectatic segment, with thin walls and disproportionately large lumen, of a venous system that receives portal pressure directly through its intraperitoneal extremity and has an insufficient distribution into the cava and azygos veins through its cranial extremity. Interruption (or reduction) of the communication of these varices with the portal system has two results:

— it removes the cause of distension of the varices, the cause of continued hemorrhage (whose complex mechanism has already been described);

— it removes a shunt of the portal network, therefore it raises to a variable degree pressure in the portal area.

The first is favorable and sometimes essential for saving the patient's life; the second is unfavorable for long-history cases.

This clearly shows that isolation of the esophageal varices is only a temporary measure that may save the patient's life for the moment and permit the application of a rational treatment of portal hypertension. Among the methods used are:

— Total gastrectomy, proposed and carried out by Wangensteen (1945), taken up by Phemister (1947) as esogastrectomy with lengthening of the vertical extension, and still more completely by Merendino (1955) as partial esogastrectomy with interposition of the jejunal loop and pyloroplasty. Macpherson (1966), correlating the high mortality rate with the frequent reappearance of hemorrhage, considered that esogastrectomy is not an elective procedure.

— Sectioning of the esophagus (Tanner);

— Subtotal resection of the esophagus (Cooley — DeBakey);

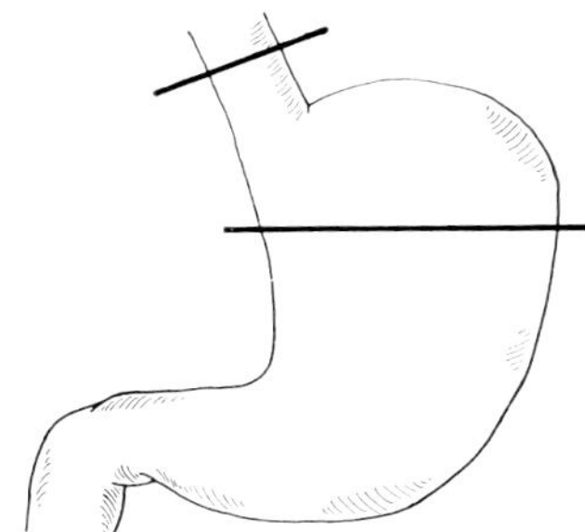

Fig. 89. — The limits of upper polar gastric resection.

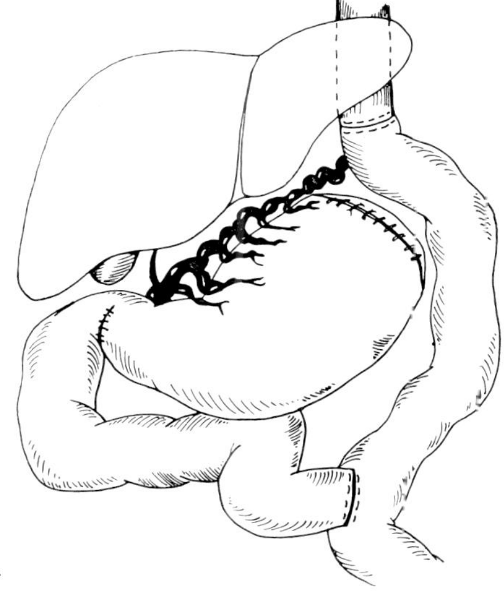

Fig. 90. — Upper polar gastric resection for azygoportal disconnection in esophageal varices. Note sutures: pyloroplasty; end-to-end esojejunal anastomosis; end-to-side jejunojejunal anastomosis. ▶

— Resection of the cardia (Phemister), upper polar gastrectomy (Figs 89 and 90).

These operations efficiently remove esophageal acidopeptic reflux and the communication between the portal territory and the veins upon which the varices develop (eventually also resecting the segment of the digestive tract with the varices), but are excessively complex, with high hazard and, therefore, inapplicable in patients with a general condition deteriorated by recent hemorrhage. When the patient has regained balance by an adequate conservative treatment, it is better to avoid such methods with a strictly temporary solution.

Gray (1950), who attributed to the acidopeptic mechanism a role in the genesis of ulceration of the varices, performed vagotomy, gastroenteroanastomosis and ligation of the visible ectatic veins. Whitesell recommends partial gastric resection, splenectomy, vagotomy, hoping that removal of acidopeptic secretion will render esophageal reflux less harmful and that splenectomy might eventually reduce portal pressure and certainly correct thrombopenia. The operation in itself may be considered an acceptable hazard, but it still remains to be seen how long the results last. In a patient with gastric resection (performed in another clinic) for hematemesis attributed to the ulcerous disease, hypersplenism with accentuated enlargement of the spleen subsequently developed against a background of posthepatitis cirrhosis. Anemia was aggravated by a new hemorrhage. Splenectomy for hypersplenism was followed by very favorable results. In this case, Whitessell's procedure (except vagotomy) was almost completely performed in two stages.

Methods for direct treatment of esogastric varices. As upper digestive hemorrhage due to abrasion of the cardioesophageal varices threatens the patient's life and the conservative treatment is often inefficient, several direct operative methods have been proposed, with an immediate effect upon the bleeding vessel.

— Endoscopic methods: injection of sclerosing substances (sodium morrhuate) into the varices by means of esophagoscopy (Crafoord, 1939, Auvert and a few other specialists) is an extremely benign method, but demands great skill and special instruments and can only be practised by specialists with experience in endoscopy.

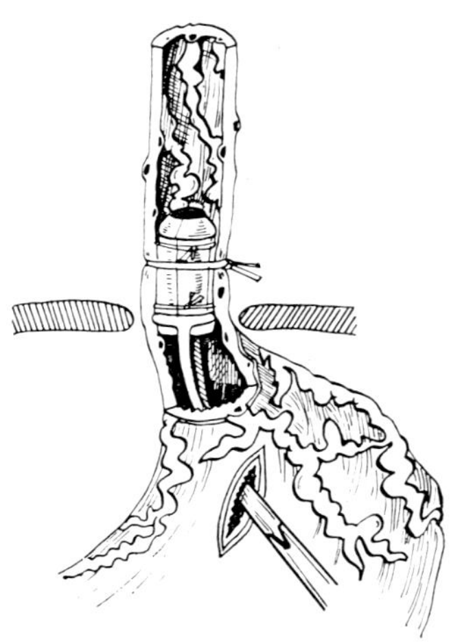

Fig. 91. — Vossschulte's operation, in portal hypertension with esophageal varices.

— *Ligation of the esophageal varices by thoracotomy.*

— Nissen applied three coils of perforating ligatures on the ectatic veins visible upon the outer aspect of the esophagus.

— Crile, Linton (1953), Boerema (1960) and in Romania Burlui preferred to expose the varices by a long, longitudinal esophagotomy (from the cardia to the arch). However, some surgeons specializing in surgery of the esophagus consider that such a long longitudinal suture exposes the esophagus to fistulas (Gavriliu).

Several authors with a basic experience in portal systemic anastomosis (Linton, Blakemore, Warren) during hemorrhage may resort to one of these methods of direct transthoracic treatment of the varices, as a preparatory stage. However, there is no general agreement and other surgeons (Child) prefer to start directly with portal systemic anastomosis. We cannot bring to a close the direct operative treatment of varices without mentioning tamponade of the mediastinum (Garlock and Som), performed by transthoracic approach; its purpose is to compress the esophageal varices (immediate hemostatic effect) and facilitate by its irritative action the development of numerous esomediastinal neovessels, which subsequently permit better discharge of the esophageal veins. The method is not widely used. The method has been simplified and extended by Heimlich, who provided tamponade of the entire esophagus through a small incision in the neck.

— Of particular interest is the method proposed by Vossschulte, which is efficient (at least temporary) and reduces the operative time to a minimum. Supraumbilical laparotomy exposes the anterior aspect of the stomach; lesser gastrotomy is carried out below the cardia and the special prosthesis devised by the author is introduced into the cardia and lower esophagus (Fig. 91). The prosthesis is a small plastic cylinder with 3 longitudinal segments and is fixed to the cardia by a circular ligature. Gastrorrhaphy is followed by closure of the abdomen. At the level of the ligature, the esophageal wall becomes necrosed within a few days and a ring of fibrous tissue develops, separating the esophageal veins from the portal system (gastric veins). After about 14 days, the prosthesis falls apart into the 3 segments in the stomach, from where they are readily eliminated by natural pathways.

Viewed together, these direct methods of treatment of esophageal varices, which represent at most a single stage with temporary results, appear to be major, complex operations unduly severe with respect to the duration and quality of the result, except for Heimlich's posterior mediastinal packing. Consequently, only ligation of the varicose veins on the outer aspect of the esophagus, as the complementary stage of a limited operation, appears justified: vagotomy with pyloroplasty or gastroenteroanastomosis, with or without splenectomy and omentopexy, combining median laparotomy with well directed phrenotomy. This is true, however, only for those patients in which the conservative treatment was inefficient, the general condition deteriorated by hemorrhage and no direct method for modifying portal pressure can be used. These limitations also account for the restricted use of this method in practice.

After a review of each method and what it offers, we can now briefly outline the therapeutic indications in the different forms and phases of the portal hypertension syndrome.

Emergency treatment of hemorrhage from esophageal varices. The medical treatment may sometimes be sufficient.

To arrest the hemorrhage, coagulants are administered by intramuscular route (Manetol, Clauden-Hemophobin and vitamin K, 2—4 vials daily, 20 — 40 mg). Thrombin is administered by oral route in order to obtain a local effect; it is dissolved in a little water or normal saline and given every 3 hours in small amounts. When the hemorrhage continues and causes excessive hematemesic vomiting that prevents the formation of a thrombus at the site of the vascular abrasion, mild, continuous gastric aspiration can be accomplished with an Einhorn tube, by suction drainage. This procedure has the advantage of removing the acidopeptic gastric secretion (C.C. Dimitriu), whose unfavorable role during esophageal reflux has already been discussed.

Our experience has convinced us of the utility of adding to these measures repeated injections with pituitary extract, that transiently lowers portal pressure, explained by Clark and Wiggers as due to a diminished supply in the affluent portal flow consequent to long-standing splanchnic arteriolocapillary vasoconstriction. Recently, Papahagi and coworkers, on discussing the therapeutic method used in the Clinic of the Emergency Hospital checked the favorable effect of the treatment with pituitary extract in hemorrhage from esophageal varices.

In many medical departments, trust has been put in intragastroesophageal compression of the varices, although failures increased to 25—55% of cases (Schiff, 1966). Several types of balloon catheters exist, permitting introduction of the tube at the desired site and compression of the varices. The Sengstaken-Blakemore type of three-way balloon catheters are introduced into the stomach, with the end balloon close to the cardia and the proximal one in the lower third of the esophagus. Distension of the two balloons fixes the catheter and compresses the varices. Better and more certain results are obtained by exercising slight traction upon the catheter, which ensures permanent application of the balloon below the cardia. Aspiration of gastric content through the tube excludes errors of diagnosis, since in gastric ulcer intragastric hemorrhage will continue. Similar results are obtained with a two-way catheter with a single balloon (Startsev type). Any correctly applied catheter, immediately, mechanically arrests the hemorrhage, but it is very difficult to control it completely by this procedure. Esophageal compression must be interrupted every few hours, since the risk of devitalizing the portion of the esophagus upon which maximum compression is exercised (juxtacardial), is very great. Cases of death due to ulceration of the supracardial esophagus have been reported. Another form of conservative treatment, with temporary effect in most cases, is gastric cooling, used in preoperative preparation. Initiated by Wangensteen et al., it consists of introducing into the stomach a two-way catheter through which a fluid flows at low temperatures (even below 0°C/132° F) for a restricted time. The fluid may be free in the gastric cavity (open system) or enclosed in a plastic balloon covering the end of the catheter (closed system). An efficient system was devised by Mateescu et al. Local hypothermia, especially when combined with general hypothermia, rapidly lowers gastric acidopeptic secretion, portal pressure and consequently hemorrhage. The effect is temporary but arrest of the hemorrhage may allow a thrombus to develop. However, this method has also resulted in severe accidents, for instance explosion of the stomach which has become friable, and must still be improved upon. It is considered indispensable in profuse hemorrhage, as it permits reequilibration and recovery of the blood volume, and the patient can be prepared for emergency surgery.

— Circulatory hydration and reequilibration is only carried out as long as the hemorrhage lasts, after which small amounts of fluid are ingested, then semi-fluids (whipped cream, purée) and much later minced boiled meat, etc.

— The blood volume lost is totally replaced on the first day, under protection of endoesophagogastric compression, or by small or massive blood transfusions (fractional restitution) when hemorrhage cannot be controlled by the balloon catheter. Pressure instability, with a tendency of the maximum to fall below 10 cm Hg and a small difference between the two pressures of less than 3 cm Hg, after interrupting the blood perfusions, shows that hemorrhage continues and resuscitation has failed. When parenchymatous (kidney-liver) and encephalic deficiencies due to hypoirrigation with prolonged hypoxia develop, the therapeutic failure is complete.

— Hepatic coma (or more precisely portal encephalopathy) is prevented by aspiration of the blood from the stomach since its breakdown in the intestine results in massive resorption of toxic bodies and ammonia, followed by hepatic coma. Maintenance of the blood pressure at a constant level of over 100 mm Hg maximum, and optimal oxygenation by nasal intubation helps to overcome hepatic hypoxia. As it has been demonstrated that the action of the intestinal proteolytic flora leads to the appearance of encephalotoxic ammonia bodies, even more than simple breakdown of the blood under the action of human digestive enzymes, broad spectrum antibiotics must be administered orally.

— Emergency surgery is not obligatory in all cases of hemorrhage from esophageal varices; it is reserved for failure of correctly applied medical treatment after 8—24 hours. This is justified both by the efficiency of the medical treatment in numerous cases and by the difficulty of applying the surgical treatment to a patient with shock, hemorrhage and portal hypertension (F.G. Uglov).

The following conditions must be met:
— The operation should not exceed the patient's resistance;
— It should be adequate to the results expected;
— It should offer a chance of reducing portal hypertension;
— It should be compatible with the functional state of the liver.

Various, divergent treatments have been proposed. In Romania, Papahagi et al., in 12 emergency cases of portacaval anastomosis had 4 postoperative deaths (33%) and of the 8 survivors 4 presented transitory postoperative hepatic coma.

Account must be kept of the fact that after anastomosis, the products of blood proteolytic breakdown, under the action of the intestinal microbial flora, will lead to more intense, rapid cerebral morphofunctional alterations (portal encephalopathy) than before shunting when the portal blood passes through the liver, whose antitoxic function is limited.

Under the four conditions listed above, grouped into clearly individualized forms, the following treatment may be established (table 2):

Table 2

Dominant character	General state	Hepatic tests	Treatment
Portal hypertension	Satisfactory (A)	Satisfactory	Stable shunt in agreement with the state of the porta and splenic vein.
	Unsatisfactory (B)	Satisfactory	a) Median laparotomy and phrenotomy. Stage I. — Ligation of the inferior esophageal varices (outer aspect) — ligation of 2 gastric pedicles (lowers acidity) or vagotomy + pyloroplasty. — Schiassi omentopexy. b) After reequilibration. Stage II: stable shunt in agreement with the state of the porta and splenic vein.
Hepatic insufficiency	Satisfactory (C)	Unsatisfactory	a) Stage I — as above b) Stage II — Surgery stimulating hepatic regeneration.
	Unsatisfactory (D)	Unsatisfactory	a) and b) as above, or only stage I as above (cases on the borderline of surgical indications).

In the above paragraphs account has not been kept of the intricate phenomena of hypersplenism, whose treatment will now be dealt with.

Treatment of the portal hypertension syndrome with hypersplenism. The clinical aspects of hypersplenism secondary to splenomegaly in the cirrhotic with portal hypertension have been discussed, showing the vital danger of digestive hemorrhage in these patients with thrombopenia and bone marrow inhibition. Consequently, in these patients therapy is centered upon removal of the cause of hypersplenism, i.e. upon splenectomy which is categorically indicated. On exposing the splenectomy technique, stress was laid on the special aspects of splenectomy in the cirrhotic with portal hypertension. All the details are of primordial importance when splenectomy is not combined with portal-systemic shunt.

In the cases in which an accentuated hypersplenism syndrome coexists with severe manifestations of portal hypertension but with hemodynamic reequilibration and fairly good liver functional tests, a splenorenal shunt is indicated immediately after splenectomy. This variant, warmly recommended by Rousselot, amongst others, is seldom applicable since it can only be carried out *when all the conditions specified here are met*. In most cases hypersplenism is far too important or else the hepatic alterations are too accentuated to permit a surgical shunt. In such cases it is more prudent to end splenectomy by a properitoneal omentopexy, which will permit progressive attenuation of portal hypertension. Applying this procedure, we obtained good results, without any risk. The same attitude has been adopted by T.P. Makarenko and L.E. Ponomarev (1960).

Our experience (Făgărăşanu-Bujor, 1964) helped us to establish the details of the postoperative therapeutic management of cirrhotics with splenectomy but *without surgical portal-systemic shunt*.

The pathophysiologic basis of the therapy may be briefly outlined as follows:

Splenectomy, especially followed by splenorenal shunt, a difficult operation, may be complicated by fibrinolysis (fibrinopenia and excess plasma fibronolytic activity). Correct treatment implies the use of fibronolysis inhibitors (epsilon-aminocaproic acid) (Grassi-Rousselot, 1964).

After splenectomy, thrombosis in one of the collaterals of the splenic vein may develop immediately, due to ligation of the vein at a badly selected site. It has already been shown why the original branches of the splenic vein must be ligated in the hilus.

Within a few days, following removal of the medullary inhibitory effect, the deficits of the figured elements of the myeloid series gradually improve, with hypercorrection phases. Of particular importance is the increase in thrombocytes, which augment within a few days (4—8 days) from very low values (sometimes less than 40,000) to very high ones (400,000—800,000 and even 1,200,000). A concomitant imbalance occurs between the coagulating and anticoagulating factors, favoring thrombosis. As in the splenic vein a recent thrombus, however small, develops close to the ligatures, and all the more so when applied to the splenic vein itself, after it arises from the joint branches, this will be the site of extensive thromboses (Patsiora). Clinically, this is manifested by a febrile state, resistant to antibiotics — which is not of microbial origin (leukocytosis likewise being due to removal of splenic inhibition). At first the patients tolerate the febrile state caused by the evolution of thrombosis in a venous segment with a slow circulation. With time, however, the temperature rises (on day 10—12 after the operation) and the patient's general condition deteriorates, probably due to spread of the thrombosis over portions closer to the porta or even lengthening of the thrombus into the portal lumen, and progressive accentuation of hepatic insufficiency aggravated by metabolic stress due to prolonged fever. These febrile states appear after splenectomy in most cases (82% of our cases) if special precautions are not taken to prevent thrombosis during increase of the thrombocytes.

Between the 9th-20th day after the operation, fever gradually falls in at most 15—30 days. The fact that in most cases the patients bear up with the febrile episode does not imply that "survival" should be taken for a "good result". On the contrary, it is admitted that the liver tests often point to lowering of the functional capacity of the liver (already altered by cirrhosis), neither should it be forgotten that nothing can protect these delicate patients against their accentuated hepatic insufficiency. In the fatal cases after splenectomy for hypersplenism — portal hypertension, death was always preceded by high fever, which rose gradually and on the 4th-9th day became complicated with irreversible hepatic coma (9% of the splenectomized patients). Therefore, the pathophysiologic phenomena during postsplenectomy fever lower the quality of the operative results: actually the patient who is no longer anemic and thrombopenic acquires in exchange a greater hepatic functional deficiency and, in addition, thrombosis may block several natural shunts, hence increasing ascites either transiently or permanently. Therefore, the benefits of splenectomy can only be felt when the entire cycle of harmful phenomena are removed.

Since not only the numerical increase of thrombocytes but also the tendency to consecutive hypercoagulation is the first event in this cycle, a careful study was carried out on the post-splenectomy thrombocyte curve, and certain of the coagulogram parameters (tolerance to heparin, coagulation in Lee and White tube, Howell time, prothrombin time and determination of Quick's coagulation factors), as well as the temperature curve.

At a level of 300,000 thrombocytes/mm^3 (direct count) a frequent shift was noted towards hypercoagulation in the heparin tolerance test.

At this moment, adequate treatment with anticoagulants may prevent fever irrespective of the high thrombocyte count, which may reach up to 600,000—900,000. After a steady increase, the number of thrombocytes falls again to about 400,000—300,000 and the intensity of the anticoagulant treatment can be gradually lowered. These phenomena should be followed up within the first 21 days after the operation as we may thus have the satisfaction of obtaining a course without incident and with maximum benefits, provided splenectomy is performed with all the precautions previously mentioned. This therapeutic attitude, recently established, makes it possible to obtain the best results after splenectomy with minimal hazard, when the indications are correct.

The anticoagulant therapy is started as soon as the thrombocyte count rises to 3—400,000 and a tendency appears to a shorter coagulation time or a shift towards hypercoagulation of the heparin tolerance test.

In the first days heparin is prescribed (15,000 IU/24 hours) in 6 doses, administered intravenously at 4 hours. The efficiency of the therapy is checked by following up the coagulation time which must exceed by one third the upper normal threshold of the method used (coagulation time in the test tube 8—12 minutes), therefore to reach a coagulation of about 16 min. Moreover, the temperature must also be within normal limits. A tendency to low-grade fever and a coagulation time within normal limits shows that an insufficient heparin dose is being used;

the total heparin dose should be increased to 20,000—30,000 IU/24 h, and in no case are the injections to be done at an interval longer than 4 hours.

As a rule, the therapeutic effect is felt within 48 hours and can be maintained with a dicoumarin anticoagulant administered *per os* (long-standing effect). The drug is changed after 1—3 days parallel administration of both drugs (in our cases we used Thrombostop*): heparin is administered in the same doses together with 3 tablets Thrombostop one day, then daily three tablets Thrombostop (6 mg) with decreasing doses of heparin until within 2 or 3 days of mixed treatment normal coagulation values are obtained, and the prothrombin time and prothrombin index points to a decrement of about 75% of the circulating prothrombin. After a further 2 days of dicoumarin treatment the latter values should show a decrement of about 50%, but not below 30%. The treatment is continued for some time with smaller doses (2 tablets a day), following up the temperature curve, thrombocyte count and prothrombin index. In rare cases, lowering of the temperature to normal is not obtained with dicoumarin and the heparin treatment must be started again; however, particular attention should be paid to the patients with a latent fibrinolysis syndrome (partial lysis of the clot at 24 hours) in whom spontaneous hypercoagulation is more dangerous than pharmacodynamic hypocoagulation. As the tendency to thrombosis due to hypercoagulability is a complex biologic phenomenon, the moment at which one may interrupt the anticoagulating treatment cannot be established on the basis of the thrombocyte count. We may initially have clear indications to begin the treatment at 300,000 thrombocytes/mm^3 and to stop it when, after an increase up to 600,000—800,000, the count returns to 400,000. Therefore, it is not the *number* of thrombocytes which is decisive but the *tendency* to hypercoagulation (prothrombin time during the dicoumarin treatment, heparin tolerance test after interrupting the treatment). Tetracyclin or chloramphenicol should not be associated with the dicoumarin treatment since these drugs exercise a mutual potentiation effect that may lead to a dangerous fall in prothrombinemia, arrest vitamin K synthesis in the intestine owing to intestinal sterilization and prothrombin synthesis in the liver, owing to the action of dicoumarin.

In order to illustrate the application of this anticoagulating therapy after splenectomy, here is the description of two clinical cases:

Case 1. Patient *U.G.*, male, 38 years, was admitted to the Surgical Clinic from January 14 to March 3, 1963 with a diagnosis of cirrhosis with hypersplenism (referred to us from the Medical Clinic). In the past history: infectious hepatitis with a long period of jaundice (90 days).

The patient complained of postprandial distention, asthenia, repeated bleeding from the nose and gingivae. He was pale, with a reduced subcutaneous celluloadipose layer and petechiae on the legs. The abdomen was slightly painful in both hypochondria. The liver whose upper limit could be detected at the level of the 6th rib exceeded by three finger breadths the costal margin and had a sharp anterior edge. On pressure the liver was tender and hard. The spleen, percussable over a wide area exceeded the costal margin by the breadth of a hand.

Preoperative tests showed slight hepatic involvement (thymol 16 M.L. units, Gross 0.9—1.16; prothrombin time 78%) and signs of hypersplenism, manifested by thrombopenia (69,000) and leukopenia (3800), a tendency to hypocoagulability (heparin tolerance 0.34 and the aspect

* Sintrom, acenocumarolum.

of the thromboelastogram), and in addition latent fibrinolysis (partial lysis of the clot at 24 h). Fibrinemia being 326 mg%, fibrinogen was procured and splenectomy was performed with all the precautions mentioned above.

Postoperatively, after 24 hours, fibrinolysis became manifest (total lysis of the coagulum in 24 hours) and epistaxis was severe.

On the second and third day, the patient received daily perfusions with fibrinogen which were interrupted when fibrinemia attained 400 mg% (postperfusion febrile reactions). The thrombocytes increased slowly and steadily. As soon as heparin tolerance showed a shift towards hyper-

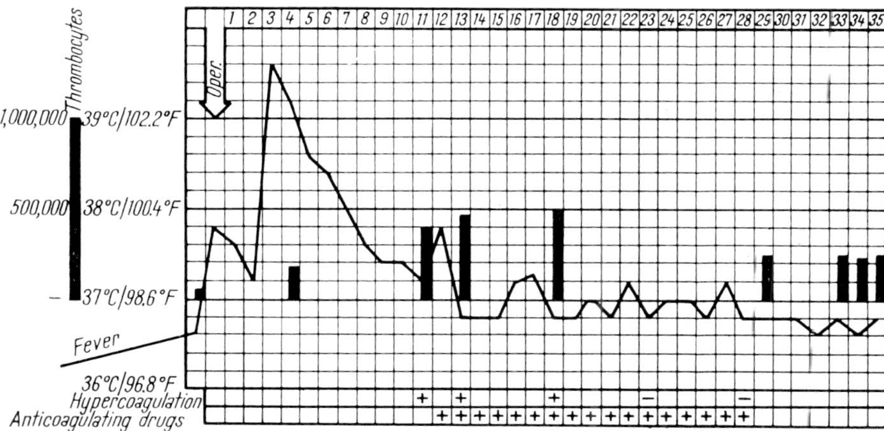

Fig. 92. — Effect of the anticlotting treatment in postsplenectomy hyperthermia in the cirrhotic with hypersplenism.

coagulation (day 12), the thrombocyte count being over 400,000 (as against 69,000 before the operation), an anticoagulating treatment with heparin was instituted, according to the scheme discussed beforehand. Hypocoagulability was maintained until the thrombocytes fell to about 200,000 (day 29), when the heparin tolerance test showed that there was no more risk of thrombosis. Thus postsplenectomy hyperthermia was avoided under anticoagulant treatment in spite of the numerical increase of the thrombocytes (Fig. 92).

Case 2. Patient *P.C.*, male, aged 24, was admitted to the Surgical Clinic from March 23 to April 30, 1963 with a diagnosis of cirrhosis and hypersplenism.

The patient, referred to us from a Medical Clinic had suffered in the past from malaria and gastric resection for hematemesis attributed to ulcer, three years previously.

The patient complained of asthenia, fits of dizziness after a recent hematemesis and enlarged volume of the upper abdomen.

After gastrectomy, performed 3 years previously he felt much better for one year, then gradually lost his power to work, parallel to an increase in the size of the abdomen.

Two months before admission during an intense physical effort, he had a marked hematemesis, fainted and only recovered very slowly and incompletely.

Clinical findings: the patient was thin and pale, with a broadened chest at the base, evidently enlarged abdomen, and superficial collateral circulation of the cavacaval type. The liver of apparently normal consistency exceeded the costal margin by four finger breadths. The spleen, very much enlarged, extended to the midline and descended below umbilical level; it was hard, with an apparently maintained mobility and scalloped anterior border. Slow recovery of the red blood cell count (3,410,000) and hemoglobin titer (55%), accentuated thrombopenia (65,000), leukopenia (3700), next to the macroblastosis aspect of the myelogram, demonstrated the presence of hypersplenism. On the other hand, the absence of hepatitis in the past history and the dysproteinemia, aldolase, transaminase, B.S.P. tests and proteinogram (beta globulins 13% and gamma globulins 16%) were against the preoperative diagnosis of cirrhosis (confirmed, however, intraoperatively). Doubts were raised concerning the cause of portal hypertension (preoperative splenomanometry 42 cm) when faced with a splenal and portal venography that revealed ectasis of the splenic vein and portal trunk without evidence of the intrahepatic portal branches.

Splenectomy was indicated in view of the hypersplenism, and certain data were to be completed intraoperatively.

The operation was performed under orotracheal anesthesia on April 3, 1963. Splenomanometry showed 70 cm of water and splenal and portal venography indicated an important natural ascending colateral splenosystemic shunt. The xyphoumbilical incision brought to view an intense adhesive process, that had developed after gastrectomy and was richly vascularized due to portal hypertension. The liver was small, especially the left lobe which was retracted and covered by the gastric stump, together with the transverse mesocolon and efferent loop. Through a gap, opened with difficulty, the surface of the left lobe dotted with nodules and its sharp border, could be felt.

The enlarged spleen occupied the whole, left, subphrenic recess and adhered to the neighboring structures in the flank. Splenectomy with ligation of the splenic vessels in the hilus and minute hemostasis of the splenoparietal adhesions, was difficult. The postoperative evolution was closely followed: thrombocytes increased from 65,000 to 130,000 on day 1, then to 204,000 on day 3 when low-grade fever became more accentuated. On day 5 the temperature rose to 38°C/100,4°F, there was a shift of the heparin tolerance test from hypo- to hypercoagulability, also indicated by rapid coagulation (Lee and White). These were accounted for by increase of the thrombocytes to 515,000 mm^3. A mixed anticoagulant treatment was applied: heparin (30,000 IU/24 h) and Thrombostop (3 tablets/day according to the indicated scheme). From day 5 onwards, the *temperature fell sharply and constantly remained below 37°C/98.6°F.*

On day 8, Thrombostop alone was administered, the prothrombin time being maintained at 50—60%, coagulation time at the upper threshold, although the thrombocytes increased to 658,000 and even to 876,000 (day 12).

On day 14, the thrombocytes began to decrease (774,000) and attained 654,000 on day 19. Insufficient anticoagulant doses resulted in temporary reappearance of the tendency towards hypercoagulation, but this was corrected by increasing the doses, after which the prothrombin index fell to 38%.

The protective anticoagulant treatment was brought to a close after 3 days of heparin on day 23; there was no febrile reaction (Fig. 93). The surgical results were satisfactory and the patient was discharged with a final diagnosis of clinically compensated atrophic cirrhosis with splenomegaly and secondary hypersplenism (variable portal hypertension).

This therapeutic scheme is, of course, reserved for the patients for whom it was initially devised: cirrhotics with portal hypertension and hypersplenism due to splenomegaly. It should not be applied mechanically after any splenectomy performed in other categories of patients, since hypercoagulation, the risk of thrombosis and fever seldom exist in non-cirrhotic patients. It is now pertinent to define our management of Banti's syndrome and Banti's disease, as splenomegalies with hepatic involvement, closely resembling the hypersplenism of portal hypertension in cirrhosis.

Management of Banti's syndrome. Banti's disease (1894), with a clinical course in three stages (anemia with splenomegaly, to which a hemorrhagic syndrome and finally, in the last phase, ascites is added), is an entity in view of the evolutive splenomegaly, with characteristic periarteriolar sclerosis, in patients without a

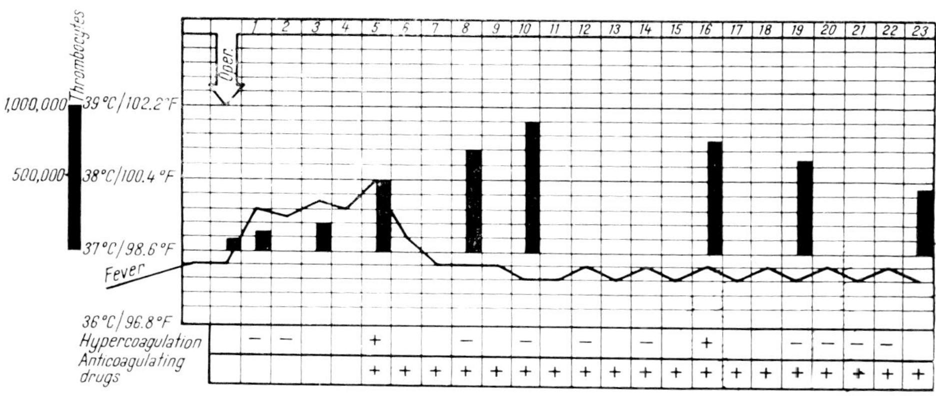

Fig. 93. — Effect of the anticlotting treatment in postsplenectomy hyperthermia in the cirrhotic with hypersplenism.

history of hepatitis and at first with far more accentuated structural lesions in the spleen than in the liver, where they are notwithstanding present. Some authors contest its existence as a separate entity (Hegglin), but hepatologists such as N. Gh. Lupu, recognize the absence of any specificity of the Gandy-Gamna nodules and, discarding the term of fibroadenia, sustain the existence of Banti's disease, characterized pathohistologically by pre- and centrofollicular arteriolar sclerosis. It is a rare disease.

Forms of isolated splenomegaly without characteristic splenic lesions, but with an analogous clinical course, are frequently encountered, with attenuated or no hepatic functional changes, without hepatitis in the antecedents and in which the pathoanatomic changes are predominant in the spleen and altogether attenuated in the liver. These clinical aspects are usually grouped under the name of Banti's syndrome and represent a fairly large number of patients with splenomegaly in our clinic. Over an eleven year period, these cases of isolated splenomegaly (Banti's syndrome for the sake of convention) represented up to 15% the total number of cirrhotic or hepatosplenic patients admitted for surgery.

The term of Banti's syndrome is provisional; the future will show whether, as believed by some authors (Léger and others) splenic alteration actually brings about hepatic alteration, or whether it is a question of attenuated cirrhosis of the liver, complicated at an early date by thrombosis of the splenic vein and marked splenomegaly or a cirrhosis well compensated both clinically and biologically, and complicated much later by splenomegaly, likewise due to the same process of thrombosis of the splenic vein.

When splenomegaly entails phenomena of hypersplenism and especially when regional phenomena of portal hypertension exist, due to isolated thrombosis of the splenic vein, then splenectomy is indicated. Splenography, the aspect of the blood vessels in the portal area observed in the course of splenectomy and the histologic aspect of the liver (incidental biopsy) will show whether it is a question of attenuated cirrhosis with marked splenomegaly or isolated enlargement of the spleen. Only then can one decide upon the splenectomy procedure to be applied — single ligation of the vessels between the hilus and tail of the pancreas for isolated splenomegaly, or separate ligation of the venous branches in the hilus of the spleen in the portal hypertension syndrome with hypersplenism.

Postoperatively, the coagulants (permitted on the day of the operation) will be stopped after 24 hours and the temperature, thrombocytes and coagulogram atentively followed. If the case has been correctly interpreted as splenomegaly alone, it is seldom necessary to administer an anticoagulant treatment (only 60% of the patients present transitory fever). Therefore, in Banti's syndrome both the course of the disease and the therapy are simpler; the results are always favorable (removal of hypersplenism) without hazard of lowering the functions of the liver.

The treatment of portal hypertension with insufficient hepatic function. These patients represent the great majority (up to 70%) of all the cases of portal hypertension admitted to hospital. The accentuated degree of the hepatic functional deficit is manifested by certain clinical signs even before obtaining the laboratory data: diminution of muscular mass, asthenia — adynamism, ascites, subclinical icterus or even mild jaundice.

In these cases, a portal-systemic shunt (trunkular or radicular) will bring about many untoward side effects:

— Mortality rate far exceeding that of 10—15% given by cases with optimal indications (sometimes up to 80% — Saegesser);

— Accentuation of jaundice;

— Unfavorable shift of hepatic tests;

— A marked tendency to edema and ascites (Child).

Of greater importance is the repeated postoperative appearance of portal encephalopathy, because a large amount of blood bypasses the liver and reaches the brain with toxic factors of intestinal origin. Several such cases, after a number of reversible comas ended in death (Payne, 1955; Lan Hsi, 1957; etc.) Consequently, the methods that reduce portal hypertension gradually should be given preference. Still under discussion are ligation of the common hepatic artery (Léger), thoracic transposition of the spleen (Turunen), properitoneal omentopexy (Schiassi), eventually associated with splenectomy when marked phenomena of hypersplenism are associated. In a recent clinical and experimental study, L. Léger examined the technical possibilities of carrying out thoracic transposition of the spleen and the results that can be obtained in this category of delicate patients. In comparison to the thoracic approach, eventually with pneumopexy (Castellani) or polar resection (Castellani-Bourgeois), he prefers to operate by abdominal approach (laparophrenotomy) with simple transposition. Léger pertinently notes that this intervention has been developed as less traumatic and, therefore, any needless complication impairs its essentially benign character.

We do not believe that simple transposition is more efficient than omentopexy, or easier to carry out in order to create a portal-systemic shunt, and at any rate is far less efficient against secondary hypersplenism than splenectomy with omentopexy, and with almost equal hazards. In order to arrest hemorrhage immediately, Turunen, and, later, other authors, proposed to associate ligation of the cardioesophageal varices with gastrolsophagotomy. As stated by Léger, the frequency of suppuration after this intervention will be higher following the association of contamination (gastrotomy). At any rate, the patient should be closely followed through the whole postoperative course because hepatic coma or death may occur at any moment within the first 7 days. Moreover, peritoneal irritation due to the operation, accentuates the tendency to produce ascites, necessitating either complex diuretic treatment or repeated punctures. In order to emphasize the difficulties that can be met with in the postoperative management of such patients it is sufficient to show for instance, that in case of a high degree of hyperbilirubinemia, progesterone cannot be used as an antialdosteronic drug because it may have an unfavorable effect upon blood bilirubin; in the prevention of hepatic coma, daily injections of Glutacide* should be complemented by tetracycline *per os* in order to restrict the production of toxic ammonia bodies to the greatest possible extent.

We recommend, in addition, a hypercaloric diet, with limited protein ration (obligatorily starting on day 3) and vitamin therapy. Only in this way can surgical recovery be obtained and the patient will then be able to benefit progressively by the gradual lowering of portal hypertension. This group of patients who are actually on the borderline of indications for surgery particularly require close medico-surgical attention in the hospital and must also be carefully followed at home.

The results may be considered satisfactory when portal hypertension falls, ascites disappears, the evolution of cirrhosis becomes stable and the patient partially recovers his capacity to work. These results, which are far from spectacular, should however be set up against inevitable death that follows within the first year after the first hemorrhage or the appearance of ascites.

Management of the portal hypertension syndrome in patients with satisfactory hepatic function. This is as a rule a smaller group (about 30%) made up of two totally different categories of patients.

— Patients in the early stages of cirrhosis, with manifest portal hypertension.

— Patients in the late stages of cirrhosis, well compensated both metabolically and clinically.

The first category represents an ideal indication for trunkular or radicular portal-systemic anastomoses, according to the results of venography (portal venogram, splenal-and-portal venogram).

Operations may be planned with very low risk, and when the correct medical treatment is applied simultaneously the results will be optimal. According to Child-Auvert the mortality rate is 10–17%, at any rate higher than in shunts for extra-hepatic block, where it is only 7% (Blakemore) or even 4% (Linton). The results are evidently good when portal pressure falls below 30 cm of water (Blakemore).

* Glutaminol

However, it is fairly difficult to determine portal pressure correctly at the end of a complicated operation when a series of factors of error may interfere (arterial hypotension, etc.). Castenfors (1956) introduced a polyethylene catheter into the afferent branch of the portal vein to follow variations in portal pressure during the first days after operation and repeated portal venography every few days. In spite of the interesting information obtained, the complicated course of the only case known is not in favor of this method.

A portal-systemic gradient of less than 50 mm implies a risk of subsequent thrombosis of the anastomosis (Matzander, 1964).

Recently, an attempt was made to use the hepatic blood output (correlated to hepatic vascular resistance) in order to establish indications for portacaval anastomoses: an output of more than 800 ml/minute is considered a contraindication (J.-N. Maillard, 1966).

In the second category, in patients with proteinemia over 0.3 gm% the same operative procedures are indicated, with individualization of the method according to the permeability of the portal trunk or splenic vein; results are, however, foreshadowed by the risk of postoperative decompensation of the liver functions.

In order to ensure more ample participation of the liver in general metabolism after end-to-side portacaval anastomoses, arterialization of the portal stump through the repermeabilized umbilical vein appears to offer a solution that is often efficient (Burlui, 1968).

This likewise points to the importance of following the hepatic tests, not only the rather unspecific serum protein electrophoresis or dysproteinemia tests, but especially BSP, hippuric acid synthesis, alkaline phosphatase, prothrombin index, induced galactosuria and water test.

No general consensus exists concerning the indications for surgery in patients with esophageal varices but without hemorrhage. It must be borne in mind that the first hemorrhage brings about death of the patient in very many cases. In the statistics of Welch (1956), 38 of 50 cirrhotics with hemorrhage died after the first hemorrhage. Blakemore, moreover, adds: "the first hemorrhage may decompensate cirrhosis". Therefore, portal hypertension in a cirrhotic, important enough to determine the appearance of varices should be considered, especially in the presence of esophageal reflux (hemorrhage risk 5-times increased: Lataste, 1968), as a *future operative indication.* This point of view, adopted by physicians, will help the surgeons to obtain very good results with portal-systemic shunts.

EXPERIMENTAL AND CLINICAL ATTEMPTS AT STIMULATING HEPATIC REGENERATION IN CIRRHOSIS

In hepatocellular pathology the term of regeneration is frequently used and has led to the concept of a particular capacity of the liver to build up again after various insults or resections. We shall not attempt to establish to what extent the liver of gasteropodae or even of rodents possess this property, but must emphasize the fact that in mammals closer to the biology of humans and in man himself there cannot be a question of regeneration of the liver, as an organ. In a cell, regeneration occurs in the portions damaged by various functions or toxic substances. When only a small portion of a lobule is destroyed, the cells are partially replaced by fibrous, cicatricial tissue and partially by juvenile, "lobule regenerating" cells. Otherwise stated, when a cell is destroyed, it definitely disappears, and *another new cell* takes its place. When a lobe is removed by anatomic operation, the remaining lobes increase in size, due to hypertrophy of the remaining lobes combined with compensatory hyperplasia, as demonstrated by our experimental investigations carried out in 1957—1958. This has nothing in common with a true regeneration because the liver with an anatomic resection remains with a reduced number of lobes (dogs, humans). Any assertion to the contrary is not based on fact.

Therefore, the term of regeneration in hepatocellular pathology only has the significance of a *recovery* after destruction.

In the course of cirrhosis altered cells, that will be replaced by fibrous sclerous tissue, and new "regeneration" cells coexist. According to Nezeloff (in G. Albot), the following are the features of cellular regeneration in cirrhosis:

The cells are small and irregular, the protoplasm intensely basophil and granular, with a rich, dense chondriome. The protoplasm is rich in glycogen and pyroninophil substances. The nucleus is large with a dense chromatin and at times without any nucleoli. In man, division is usually amitotic. The binucleate cells may attain a proportion of 50% (as a rule 25% according to Pfuhl). It is sometimes difficult to assess in the cirrhotic liver whether it is a question of regeneration or cancerization, becauses in 48% of the cases hepatic cancer coexists with cirrhosis (Girard, 1964).

Distribution of the regeneration cells: they are usually to be found at the periphery of the lobule and are *rare*. In pathologic cases they form a crown at the periphery of the lobule and often join forming pseudoadenomatous nodules, especially in nodular hepatitis and cirrhosis, or they are disseminated throughout the whole microscopic field, giving it a mottled aspect.

Newly formed bile canaliculi develop, either by differentiation of the proximal cells of Remak's cords, or by regenerative neoformation.

Intrahepatic vascularization appears early and is deeply modified in cirrhosis. According to some data, still under discussion, the early structural changes in cirrhosis can be more readily understood if we admit that in man lobulation with the cellular cords centered around the central vein is an effect of the normal difference between pressures in the intrahepatic branches of the portal vein and those in the central, original branches of the hepatic veins. The difference in pressure guarantees the flow through the sinusoids which cross the spongy "plates" together with the liver cell cords. Increase in the pressure of the hepatic veins or decrease in portal pressure will center lobulation around the portal axis instead of around the central vein (Elias-Sokol, 1953). Hence, the liver appears to have a remarkable plasticity in the arrangement of its cells.

In cirrhosis, an early change occurs in the relationship between the cellular cords and the pathways with a maximum blood output.

As early as 1861, Frerichs observed a diminution of the capillary bed, and subsequently Sabourin reported numerous intrahepatic arterioportal anastomoses, in cirrhotics. A characteristic aspect was revealed by Kretz (1905) by celloidin injection into the blood vessels: the portal branches often discharge directly into the original branches of the hepatic veins. Thus important zones of the parenchyma are bypassed by the circulation in the cirrhotic liver. The Kretz specimens clearly revealed arterioportal anastomoses. On comparing these aspects with eccentric location of the "central" vein in the cirrhotic lobule which still maintains an almost normal configuration, Richard Kretz concludes that *regeneration in the cirrhotic has an asymmetrical character* (Child). Finally, Steinberg and Martin (1946) demonstrated the nonhomogeneous character of the blood supply to the areas with regeneration nodules by means of a modern technique. In contrast to the homogeneous aspect of the normal hepatogram with thorium dioxide, in the rat with experimental cirrhosis of the liver, a nonuniform distribution appears, due to regeneration nodules which are free of any vessels or very poorly vascularized. The more recent theory of Rappaport and Gotvin (1963) concerning the morphofunctional hepatic units (simple acini, complex acini, acini clusters) directed towards the portal and arterial branches with the original suprahepatic veins (called "central veins" until now) located at the periphery, rationally explains the onset of the first toxic degenerative lesions around the "central" vein, which is actually in the peripheral zone. This also readily explains why the regeneration nodules have more chances of developing along the arterioportal axis (zones of optimal nutrition), but cannot account for the predominantly arterial and deficient portal supply of these nodules.

This theory was confirmed by the findings of other authors who showed that the poor vascular network of the regeneration nodule is often dependent upon the arterial flow and upon the vessels supplied by the portal vein.

The poor vascularity and the arterial blood supply explain to a great extent the unquestionable metabolic properties of the regeneration nodules in their totality; a curious exception is the macroinsular development of spontaneous regeneration in human cirrhosis (Ioniță, Bujor, 1966).

In their ensemble, these unsatisfactory aspects of the most frequent modes of hepatic "regeneration" in cirrhosis (with the formation of regeneration nodules), show us why therapy should not only favor "regeneration" of the cirrhotic liver but should also try to determine the most useful form of regeneration that can be obtained.

Surgical methods. It should be initially stated that very few of the therapeutic methods used in the different syndromes of cirrhosis (ascites, portal hypertension) pretend to favor "hepatic regeneration". The following methods will be discussed: ligation of the bile ducts; ligation of the common hepatic artery; arterialization of the portal vein; hepatic periarterial neurectomy; hepatic resection.

Ligation of a bile duct. Léger (1957) and Schalm (1960) drew attention to a number of structural changes, stasis, fibrosis, aspects of biliary cirrhosis with accentuated cellular multiplication below the ligature (after some time lesions of the biliary cirrhosis type become predominant) and a certain stimulation of cellular regeneration on the opposite side. Although useful since it creates a period in which hepatic regeneration is accelerated in the liver, the method is not yet applied clinically since it is not always easy to ligate a fairly large bile duct without damaging the neighboring vessels, nor has it been proved as yet that the final changes of the biliary cirrhosis type that appear on the side of the ligature do not give rise to drawbacks that diminish the benefit of the first postoperative period.

Ligation of the common hepatic artery, a technique and probable mechanism of action in the portal hypertension syndrome we have already discussed, is considered by some a satisfactory means of stimulating reparatory processes in the cirrhotic liver. Léger reports on the favorable course in one case, with slowing down of connective tissue proliferation occurring 19 months after ligation when the cellular biopsy aspect was almost normal. However, Trapani, using the same method under biopsy puncture control, only employs the following histologic arguments: "attenuation of the cellular degenerative phenomena and of perivascular infiltration".

Therefore, ligation of the hepatic artery appears to be an especially advantageous method for realizing better portal circulation in the hepatic liver, excluding exaggerated reflux of the arterial blood in the portavenous anastomoses that bypass the functional parenchyma.

The operation is comparatively easy to perform and mild which renders it acceptable for patients with altered hepatic functions; in comparison to other techniques it has the advantage of having been thoroughly evaluated in the clinic.

Portal arterialization. In order to have a clear idea of what this method actually offers, it is necessary to recall some of the results obtained in experimental surgery.

After hepatic resection any diminution of the blood supply to the liver will reduce or even arrest recovery of the weight of the liver.

Eck's fistula, which removes the portal supply (70% of all the blood supply to the liver) annuls recovery of the weight of the liver after resection.

After hepatic resection in which the entire portal supply is replaced by the inferior vena cava supply (portacaval transposition — Child) the liver recovers only 50% of its weight (not 100% as with an unmodified portal circulation).

After 14 days an arterioportal shunt in the normal liver produces portal hypertension (Cohn, Parsons — 1950) and after a longer period necrosing arteriolitis develops (Cohn, Rather — 1953). The technique of implantation of the hepatic artery in the portal vein (Mallet-Guy) appears to have been applied for the first time by Narath (1961); the technique is difficult and the shunt seldom remains patent.

Eck's fistula (sectioning of the porta) and arterialization of the juxtahepatic portal vein may be assumed to offer optimal supply of oxygenated blood under pressure to the liver and, moreover, to reduce portal hypertension.

This technique was experimentally tested with variable success by Julian (1949), B. Fischer and C. Russ, A.N. Morris, H.H. Miller (1951), Jamison (1951) (Figs 94 and 95), Burlui (1968) in readily performed variants (with a graft between the aorta and portal stump in the hilus) (Figs 96 and 97). This operation appears to be fairly well tolerated by the patients, but the regeneration it leads to exhibits certain particular features (vacuolized cells-Fischer). Long-standing hyperoxygenation of the liver cell may be harmful, because such cellular alterations also appear after keeping a dog for a long interval in an atmosphere too rich in oxygen (Paine, 1944).

Likewise of interest is the observation of Strikler (1952) in a case of arterioportal fistula which resulted in the development of portal hypertension, with varices and ascites. Similarly, it should be expected that prolonged portal arterialization, even under protection of an end-to-side portacaval anastomosis should lead to cardiac alterations (ectasis of the right atrium), as demonstrated experimentally by Jamison (1951).

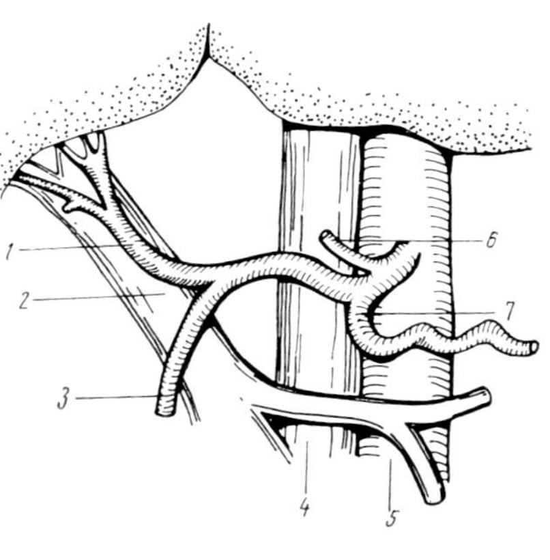

Fig. 94. — Vascular relationships that determine arterioportal anastomosis procedures.

1) Hepatic artery proper; *2*) vena porta; *3*) gastroduodenal artery; *4*) inferior vena cava; *5*) aorta; *6*) left gastric artery (stomach coronary); *7*) — splenic artery.

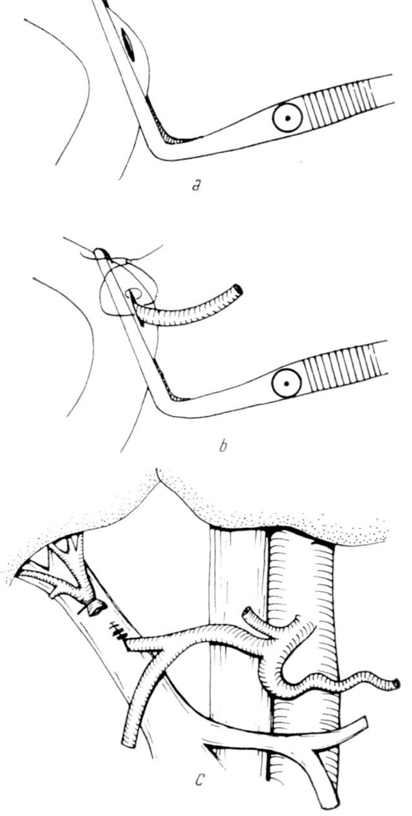

Fig. 95. — Arterialization of the portal vein (implantation of the proximal end of the hepatic artery proper in the portal vein). ▶

Therefore, following the results of experimental investigations a therapeutic scheme in two stages can be drawn up:

Stage I: end-to-side portacaval anastomosis shunting the portal blood into the lower cava; total arterialization of the portal stump in the hilus with aortic blood (interposed graft) or through the repermeabilized umbilical vein; subsequent investigations will determine the bore and patency of the anastomosis.

Stage II (after recovery of the liver tested by functional tests and liver biopsy): section of the aortoportahilar graft near the aorta (with closure of the aortotomy), severing of the portal vein close to the anastomosis with the inferior vena cava (the buttonhole is closed) and joining of the portal trunk thus released with the previous (or a new) graft implanted in the portal stump, in the hilus, hence returning to normal integral perfusion of the liver with portal blood, at a moment when the liver has favorably recovered and can fully take over its metabolic task and blood transit.

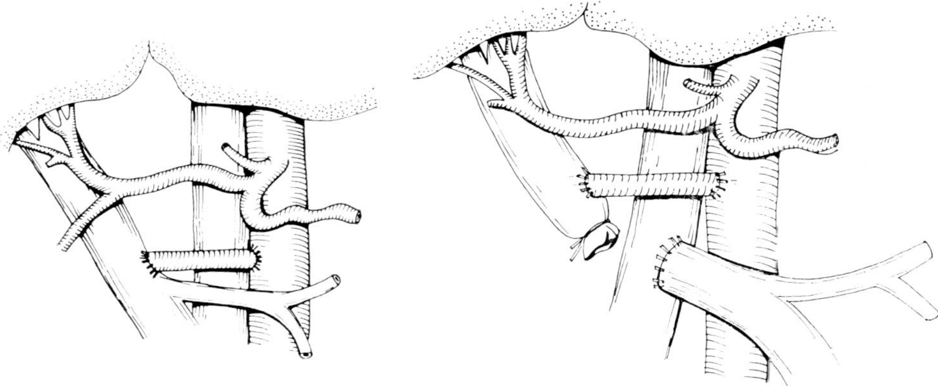

Fig. 96. — Arterialization of the portal vein (experimental variant difficult to calibrate).

Fig. 97. — Juxtahepatic arterialization of the porta, with a graft; improved variant in which the porta-caval anastomosis reduces the effect of the arterio-venous fistula.

However logical this scheme appears, it should be checked experimentally in the normal and cirrhotic liver, as certain points cannot be foreseen, such as the aspect of the intrahepatic blood network after prolonged perfusion under aortic pressure and the extent to which the eventual intrahepatic vascular changes are compatible with taking up again of the circulation at the normal transhepatic rate of flow under normal portal pressure after stage II. At any rate, man cannot be expected to tolerate ample hepatic arterialization as would result after stage I, since in Fischer's (1955) experiments only 5 dogs survived of 85 subjected to hepatic arterialization (stage I of our scheme).

Therefore, although extremely interesting, portal or rather hepatic arterialization is far from having exceeded the experimental stage and one cannot yet establish how much it will really be used in the surgery of cirrhosis of the liver.

Hepatic periarterial neurectomy was introduced in the therapy of certain hepatopathies by Mallet-Guy who opposed this method to ligation of the hepatic artery in cirrhosis. Mallet-Guy had the merit of overcoming the fear and lack of confidence with which interventions on the hepatic plexus were viewed since Heller (1942). By his clinical and experimental studies, he promoted investigations on various problems in different countries, among which Romania (Constantinovici, 1961; Firică, 1962; Burlui, 1963; Făgărășanu, 1965; Nana, 1966; etc.).

Mallet-Guy started from the idea that in ligation of the hepatic artery two simultaneous acts are performed, i.e. interception of the periarterial plexus (underestimated by his predecessors) and interruption of the patency of the artery (not always without risk). In view of the advantages of section of the nervous plexus and disadvantages of severing of the artery, neurectomy with a patent artery appeared the logical solution.

Technically, the operation is simple and almost always implies only slight trauma.

The route of approach may be a median xyphoumbilical laparotomy (preferable, we believe, to the Rio-Branco incision recommended by Mallet-Guy); transverse laparotomy of the Sprengel type or a wide, V-shaped, left xyphoumbilical-costal incision has offered the possibility, in complex cases, of associating hepatic periarterial neurectomy to other procedures (splenectomy, cholecystectomy, etc.).

The periarterial plexus should be intercepted, in our opinion, at the level of the common hepatic artery, on the upper margin of the pancreas, both for reasons of neurovascular topography (Mallet-Guy, 1955—1956) and for the exceptional event of injury to the hepatic artery, its ligation at this level being less risky than at the level of the hepatic proper, as may happen when neurectomy is performed in the hepatic pedicle by the Stucke technique (neurectomy associated with decortication of the common bile duct).

In order to expose the artery, both the lesser omentum *(pars flaccida)* and the posterior parietal peritoneum must be incised over the upper border of the pancreas. The artery can readily be recognized on inspection and by palpation. It is often covered by a voluminous lymph node (prolonged hepatitis or chronic hepatitis with incipient cirrhosis). Ablation of this node is often necessary. We would recommend uptake of the artery, surrounded by its venous plexus, on a blunt Deschamps needle, underrunning a heavy traction suture which allows for rapid action in case of vascular damage.

After incision of the neurofibrous tissue on the anterior aspect of the artery, the artery is exposed and isolated over a distance of 10—15 mm by raising with the forceps the margins of the enveloping sheath. Examination of the resected neurofibrous tissue (Fig. 98 *a,b*) will show the importance of the nervous trunks and frequency of neuritis and perineuritis lesions (Fig. 98). This operation does not imply for us a periarterial sympathectomy alone but is actually a neurectomy, with resection of the anterior hepatic plexus, composed of efferent fibers of the celiac plexus, vagal and orthosympathetic fibers.

The effects of hepatic periarterial neurectomy are very complex and not yet clearly defined; they have been frequently investigated in experimental and clinical studies. We cannot assert that the problem is fully elucidated, but great importance may be attributed to the circulatory effect which, in our opinion, may be considered as chiefly responsible for the trophometabolic effects obtained (in opposition to the authors of the method).

Increase in the transhepatic blood supply was demonstrated experimentally by Mansouri (1959), Bielicky (1865) immediately after the operation; in the human clinic shortening of the plateau time in scintigraphy (^{131}I rose bengal) led to the same conclusion.

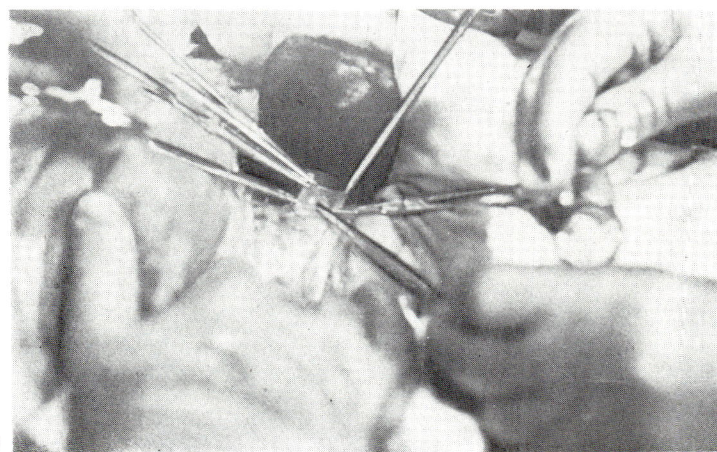

a

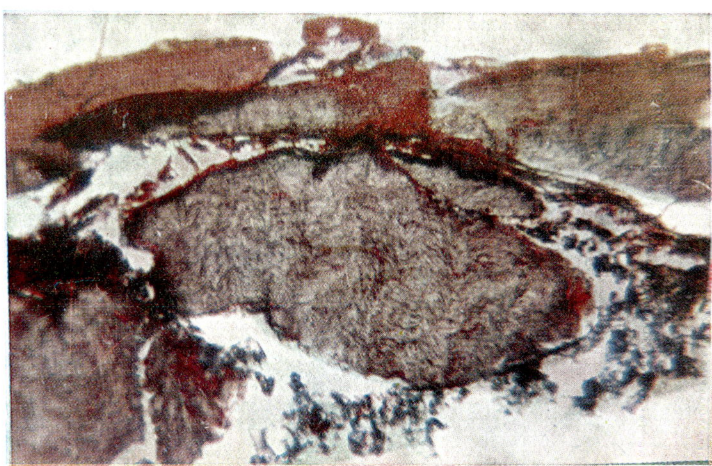

b

Fig. 98. — *a)* Hepatic periarterial neurectomy: freeing the artery from the neurofibrous sheath; *b)* hepatic periarterial neurectomy: nerve in the periarterial plexus with visible neuritis and perineuritis lesions.

The activity of the hepatic parenchyma, more amply supplied with blood, is manifested by displacement and broadening of zone I (permanent metabolic and cytogenetic activity) radially along the sinusoid capillary towards the centrolobular vein. Simultaneously, the intermediary zone II is displaced and the rest and maximum fatty deposition zone (zone III) is narrowed, with rare aspects of cellular multiplication (Lenart, 1962, 1964; Mallet-Guy, 1962). The fact that steatosis can be avoided or arrested in experimental toxic hepatitis and the human clinic (even

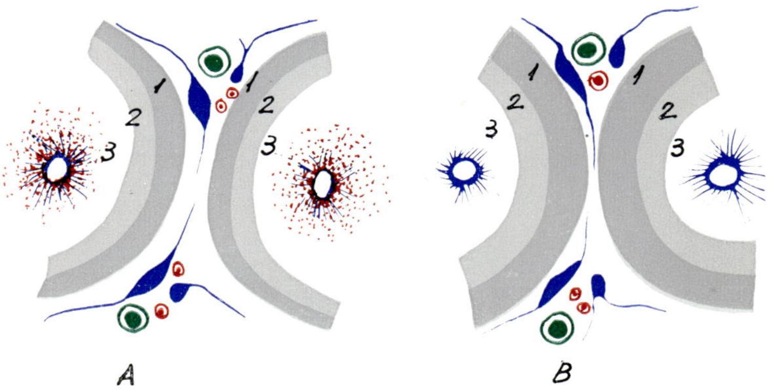

Fig. 99. — The effect of periarterial neurectomy of the hepatic artery in cirrhosis.

A) cirrhosis with steatosis (red-centrolobular excess fat): *B)* cirrhosis after periarterial neurectomy; *1.* zone of maximum activity; *2.* zone of medium activity; *3.* zone of minimum activity: disappearance of steatosis, activation of the liver cells, persistence of sclerosis.

in cirrhosis with steatosis) has been noted by several authors (Dudfield, Făgărășanu, Nana, etc.) (Fig. 99 *a*, *b*).

Two aspects still widely discussed now remain to be taken into consideration.

The antiinflammatory action of hepatic periarterial neurectomy has been reported in experimental investigations carried out by several authors who approached this problem. In the human clinic, disappearance of the inflammatory lesions has been observed. The mechanism of this unquestionable morphologic event has not been satisfactorily explained.

The contributing (not stimulating) effect of regeneration of the liver cells has been sustained bringing as an argument broadening of the acinolobular zone I, rich in ribonucleic and deoxyribonucleic acids, without it being possible, however, to prove a clearcut difference between multiplication of the hepatocytes, before and after hepatic periarterial neurectomy. Notwithstanding, it should be mentioned that Nana et al. (1966) found definite signs of hepatic regeneration in toxic hepatitis induced in animals with previous hepatic periarterial neurectomy.

Finally, we should like to recall the spectacular disappearance of prolonged jaundice (hepatocellular or due to cholangitis) observed by several authors (Mallet-Guy, 1959; Czizewsky, 1965, etc.).

The clinical results may be appraised on the basis of a collective statistics of 200 hepatic periarterial neurectomies (of which 52 of our own) performed in

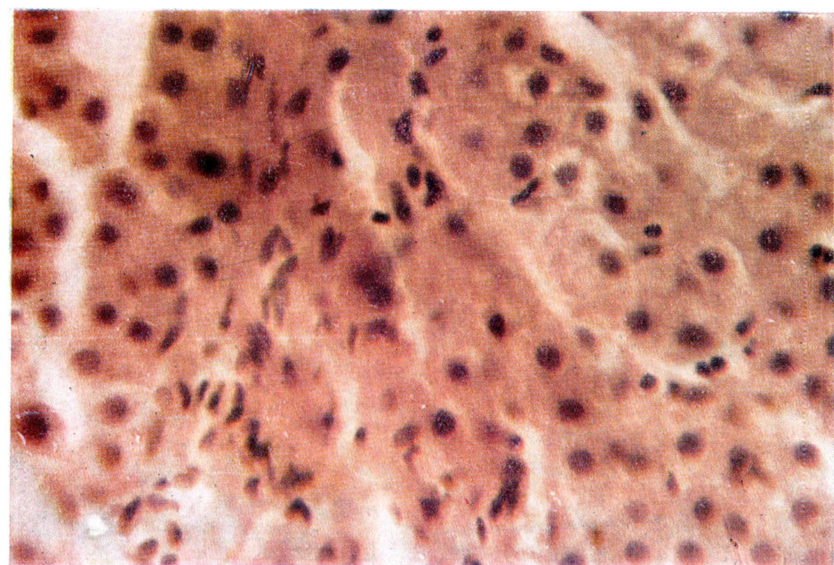

a

b

Fig. 100. — Chronic hepatitis. *a)* Intraoperative biopsy (obj. 7, hematoxylin-eosin). *b)* biopsy puncture 30 days after periarterial neurectomy of the hepatic artery (obj. 7). Note disappearance of the intercellular inflammatory dystrophic lesions. Fibrosis is maintained unmodified.

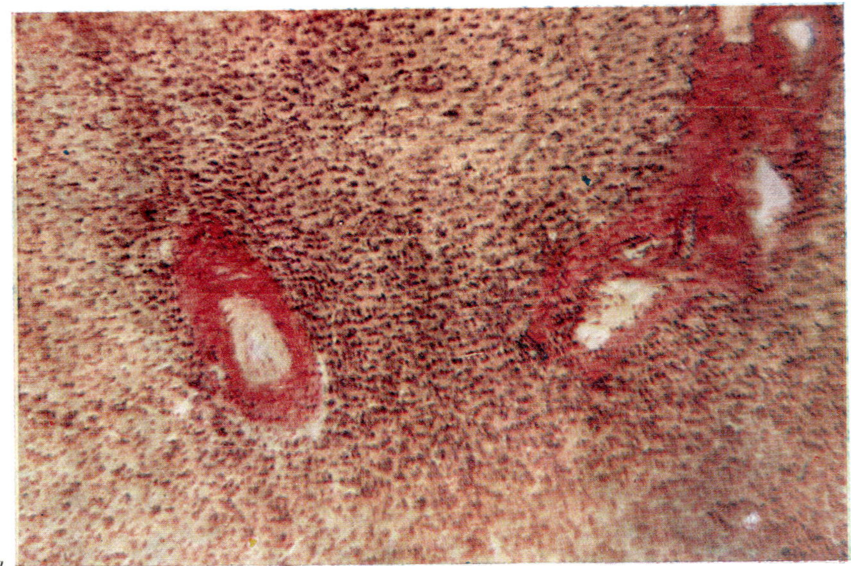

a

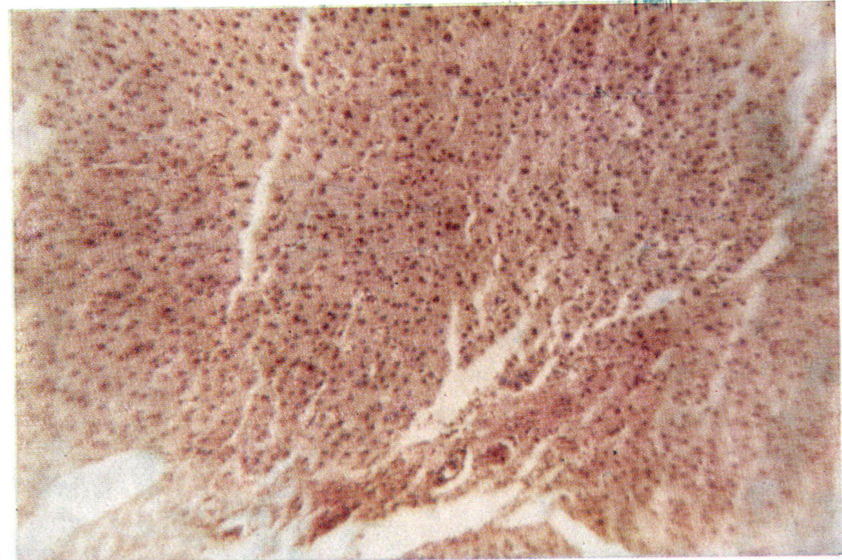

b

Fig. 101. — Cirrhosis. *a)* intraoperative biopsy (obj. 7; *b)* biopsy puncture 30 days after periarterial neurectomy of the hepatic artery. Marked improvement of the epithelial lesions, disappearance of the perilobular inflammatory lesions. Frequent regenerative aspects.

Romania, in our and another 6 surgical clinics (Th. Firică, A. Nana, D. Burlui, T. Georgescu, D. Gerota, N. Costescu); particular attention shall be paid to the forms in which cellular regeneration was of major importance.

In acute hepatitis, surgery was justified by the misleading clinical aspect, neurectomy bringing to a close an explorative laparotomy that invalidated the diagnosis of obstructive jaundice. Although the operation was successful in 3 cases (of which one of our own), it must be considered as an exceptional indication since the hazard of postoperative aggravation cannot be foreseen.

In prolonged chronic hepatitis or hepatitis with relapses — 111 cases (of which 18 of our own), neurectomy gave good clinical results, followed up by scintigraphy or biopsy, in 81% of the cases and only 16% failures and 3 deaths. This is probably the best indication.

In chronic hepatitis, with relapses and the onset of cirrhosis — 50 cases (of which 15 of our own) — only 60% were successfully operated, as demonstrated by frequent biopsies (Fig. 100 *a*, *b*) and scintigraphy, as against 35% failures and 3 deaths. Of importance is the parallel diminution of the surface of the zones with degenerative alterations of the hepatocytes. The fibrosclerosis lesions are not modified. Neurectomy is indicated in such cases.

Under the term of "posthepatitis syndrome" (36 patients) we have grouped together 17 cases of cholangitis, dyskinesia (one case of our own) which do not offer sufficient material for discussing hepatic regeneration and 19 cases of cirrhosis, accepted as being of posthepatitis origin.

Success was obtained with neurectomy in 12 of 19 cases of cirrhosis (of which 17 of our cases), with disappearance of steatosis, diminution of hepatocyte alterations and frequent regenerative aspects, confirmed at biopsy (Fig. 101 *a* and *b*) and scintigraphy. With broadening of the morphologically normal areas, the strips of sclerosis appear comparatively smaller, but actually remain the same size. In such cases, neurectomy may be useful but in 32% of the cases it has no effect and may even be harmful in cases of centrolobular sclerosis (Haeffner, 1962).

Comparison of the experimental and clinical data shows that hepatic periarterial neurectomy presents minimal hazard, but the effects are complicated.

It is clearly indicated in chronic hepatitis and plays a preventive role in cirrhosis. As a therapy favoring regeneration, it is useful in incipient cirrhosis, especially in steatosis, but in advanced cirrhosis it should be indicated with many reserves and must be contraindicated in cases with predominant centrolobular lesions.

Hepatic resection in cirrhosis. As the forementioned methods are either uncertain (ligation of the arteries or of the bile ducts) or too complicated even when they become of clinical interest (hepatic arterialization), it now remains to investigate stimulation of the cirrhotic liver after hepatic resection.

The phenomena that occur in the *normal* liver after hepatic resection are dealt with in the chapter on Physiology.

Some time ago Mann-Fisback observed that after hepatic resection, the cirrhotic liver shows a much slower tendency to "regeneration" than the normal liver which, notwithstanding, implies tissue recovery even in cirrhosis.

A recent attempt has been made to apply hepatic resection in cirrhosis. A first, apparently paradoxical, justification of this method (resection of an already deficient organ) is the finding, also checked by us, that after resection, the liver shows a tendency to recovery *en masse* and not a tendency to the formation of pseudoadenomatous nodules. The cells of the liver which has reached its initial weight after a few months, take on an aspect that is absolutely similar to that observed at biopsy, preceding hepatectomy (also confirmed in our cases). Hence, it was hoped that in the cirrhotic liver, resection will bring about substitution of the predominantly lobular regeneration by a uniformly dispersed one throughout the whole parenchyma; the appearance of "pseudoadenomatous nodules", of low metabolic efficiency and which accentuates the vascular shunts, would thus be avoided.

Even if in the modern concept the hepatic lobule is a formation possessing certain plasticity, and whose plates with their cellular cords have a given orientation determined by circulatory conditions (in opposition to the classically admitted fixed hexagonal lobe), it appears increasingly certain that different topographic zones have a particular metabolic role (Rappaport). Vasilescu and coworkers (1963), using modern methods of infracellular research, confirmed the varied metabolic role of the cells close to the central vein, participating in lipid metabolism, as compared to the cells neighboring the supralobular portal branches and their first intralobular divisions, participating especially in carbohydrate metabolism. It is certain that only a harmonious blending of the activity of the two groups of cells ensures an optimal metabolic rate of the liver in its entirety. Therefore, it is important to enhance the tendency to diffuse recovery throughout the whole mass of the parenchyma, both close to the central veins and to the portal rami, as offered by hepatic resection.

Several investigators have dealt with this problem (Mancuso, Ardey and Costa, Reifferscheid, Puchetti, etc.), obtaining interesting clinical results, but unfortunately also some tragic issues.

The study of resection of the liver in the normal dog showed the existence, immediately after resection, of an initial period of functional stupor, when the liver has a lower metabolic rate than expected in view of the amount of remaining parenchyma, and this period of severe functional deficit is the more to be feared in cirrhotics with their marked hepatic deficit.

Hence, further experimental studies appear necessary in order to establish recovery of the cirrhotic liver after major resections and the optimal extent of the resection in terms of the gravity of the hepatic alterations and the actual efficiency of inducing diffuse and not nodular recovery, before its more widespread use in the clinic. T. Maros et al. (1963) followed up experimentally the favorable effects of hepatic resection on cirrhosis induced by tannic acid in the rat.

This question is also being followed up in our clinic and includes the study of hepatic recovery after resection (in 1957 starting with the normal liver as previously described), experimental cirrhogenesis, recovery of the cirrhotic liver after resections of varied extent.

In experimental cirrhogenesis, the use of different hepatotoxic substances (which also exercise a general action upon the organism) is, we believe, inadequate since they produce gross lesions whose mechanism differs from that of human cirrhosis. In general, gross necrosis followed by death or hepatic sclerosis is obtained, totally different in character from those observed in the human liver. We, therefore, adopted in our experiments the technique of Cameron: ligation of the common bile duct which is followed by biliary stasis; after 4—8 weeks, the lesions found in the liver are very close to those observed in various evolutive phases of human cirrhosis.

In the second stage of our experiments, the microscopic aspects of liver cirrhosis were characteristic already four weeks after ligation of the common duct. In the third stage the biliary obstruction was removed by cholecytogastrostomy, followed by resection of 40% to 50% of the parenchyma. Although fairly complex, this operation is well tolerated by part of the animals and the results may be considered encouraging.

Clinical application of hepatectomy implies a close cooperation between physician and surgeon and, here too, as with portal systemic anastomosis, a careful selection of the patients will either ensure the success of the method or compromise it.

On reviewing the surgical methods for stimulating recovery of the cirrhotic liver it may be stated that there is as yet no widely applicable method. Ligation of the common hepatic artery can only be carried out in the cases in which shunting of the portal flow is not indicated, reserving hepatic periarterial neurectomy for patients with incipient lesions, especially those with steatosis.

Once hepatic arterialization (wrongly named "portal"), has exceeded the experimental stage it might be applied in cases of medium hepatic alteration when the patient may be expected to stand the complex operation with hopes of survival. Surgery will probably have to be carried out in two stages.

Hepatic resection, today a promising method, is on the point of being codified for its application in cirrhotic patients, and will probably be the ideal solution for patients with incipient or stable cirrhosis.

✦

The preceding pages have analyzed the different aspects in the evolution of cirrhosis, that determine the patient to come to the surgeon, and the actual extent to which the surgeon may really be of help.

These aspects, studied separately, actually coexist but with different degrees of gravity. Surgery is prevalently addressed to the most threatening clinical aspect, the complication that has brought the patient to hospital. This does not always mean treatment of cirrhosis but rather a chance of saving the patient's life.

These methods, useful against some aspects of the symptomatology, may not favor the stability of the disease from other points of view. For instance, portal systemic anastomoses, that save the patient in portal hypertension accidents have an unfavorable effect upon regeneration of the liver, antitoxic action and, in general, the metabolic efficiency of the cirrhotic liver. Hepatic extraperitonealization, which is definitely efficient against ascites, does not improve portal hypertension. Omentopexy, efficient against ascites and with time against the more important accidents of portal hypertension, does not offer the liver a good chance of recovery.

Isolation of cardioesophageal varices, by any type of esogastric resection, and their ligation, may be efficient against recurrent hemorrhage but harmful from the point of view of portal hypertension.

Only the methods that have in view stimulation of the recovery of the cirrhotic liver in its entirety, will be able, if successful, to attenuate or remove the elements that stand at the basis of cirrhosis. However, these methods too imply moments of increased hazard (any more important hepatic resection initially increases portal pressure which is already high in the cirrhotic patient). This emphasizes once again the importance of further investigation of this method.

Therefore, cirrhosis of the liver, a complex disease, cannot be solved by any simple procedure. In the future, attempts will be made not only at dealing with one of the complications of the disease, but with the disease itself, implying detailed study of complex techniques.

Pre-, intra- and postoperative cooperation between physician and surgeon is of outstanding importance. The large number of patients and the gravity of the disease are sufficient reasons for new endeavours to be made to improve the medicosurgical treatment of cirrhosis of the liver.

REFERENCES

1. Albot G., Poillieux F., *Le foie et la veine porte*, 1955, Masson, Paris, p. 257.
2. Belli L., Pisani F., Forti D., Parmeggiani A., Minerva chir. 1965, **19**, *18*, 644.
3. Biellicki V., Oleszkiewicz L., Szydlowski Z., Rev. int. Hépatol., 1965, **15**, *4*, 613.
4. Bockus L. H., *Gastroenterology*, vol. III, W. B. Saunders, Philadelphia, 1953.
5. Burlui D., Rațiu O., Albu E., Chirurgia, 1961, **10**, *4*, 615.
6. Castenfors H., Nordenstrom B., Acta chir. scand., 1956, **110**, 464.
7. Child G. Ch., *The hepatic circulation and portal hypertension*, Philadelphia, W.B. Saunders, 1954, p. 111.
8. Chou Hsuen Chang, Huangsfu Ming, Chin. med. J. 1962, **81**, 246.
9. Crăciun E. C., *Introducere în morfologia patologică*, Ed. medicală, Bucharest, 1959, p. 262.
10. Czyzewsky K., Oleszkiewicz L., Rev. int. Hépatol., 1965, **15**, *4*, 651.
11. Dimitriu C. C., Buligescu I., Safirescu Gh., Panaitescu Gh., Viața med., 1959, **6**, *12*, 1093.
12. Dudfield Rose J., Tomlinson B. E., Rev. int. Hepat., 1965, **15**, *4*, 658.
13. Dimitriu C. C., *Tratamentul complicațiilor în hepatitele cronice și în cirozele hepatice*, Ed. medicală, Bucharest, 1961, p. 628.
14. Făgărășanu I., Burlui D., J. Med. Latinas, Madrid, 1957, **5**, 159.
15. Făgărășanu I., Ionescu-Bujor C., Alexe Fl., *Ciroză și regenerare hepatică (contribuții experimentale)*, Communicated Soc. Surg., Bucharest, 4 Jan. 1964.
16. Făgărășanu I., Ionescu-Bujor C., Alexe Fl., Florea C., *Mecanismul și tratamentul hipertermiei postsplenectomie la bolnavii cirotici cu hipersplenism*, Communicated, Session X.I.M.F. XI, 1964.
17. Făgărășanu I., Ionescu-Bujor C., Rev. int. Hépatol. 1965, **15**, *4*, 626.
18. Făgărășanu I., Constantinescu Frida, Ionescu-Bujor C., *Modificări morfologice reparatorii hepatice după neurectomie periartera hepatică*, Communicated, National Conference of Morphology, Bucharest, 15—18 May 1966.
19. Făgărășanu I., Bucur A., Bratu V., Bujor C., *Circulatory effects of perihepatic artery neurectomy in chronic hepatitis and pre-cirrhotic conditions scanned by means of the scintigram and of hepatic rheography. Recent Advances in Gastroenterology*, vol. III, Tokio, 1966.
20. Fanarjan V. A., *Radiologia tubului digestiv*, Ed. medicală, Bucharest, 1954, p. 46.
21. Firică Th., *Hemoragiile digestive superioare*, Ed. I.M.F., Bucharest, 1957, p. 235.
22. Firică Th., Roman St., Aluneanu Ileana, Chirurgia, 1957, **6**, *5*, 690.
23. Fischer B., Russ C., Fedor E., Wilde R., Surgery, 1955, **38**, 181.
24. Foster H. J., Stoney S. W., Scott H. W. Jr., Surgery, 1961, **49**, *2*, 223.
25. Gavriliu D., *Chirurgia esofagului*, Ed. medicală, Bucharest, 1957, p. 221.
26. Girard M., Plauchu M., Révillard J. P., Lyon méd., 1964, **211**, *21*, 1415.

27. GROSSI G. E., ROUSSELOT L. M., PANKE W. F., Amer. J. Gastroenterol, 1964, **91**, *2*, 117.
28. GROZDANOVICI V., HAUPTMANN E., Surg. Gynec. Obstet., 1956, **102**, *1*, 101.
29. GUERCIO (DEL) L. R. M., COMMARASWAMI R. P., FEINS N. R., WOLMAN S. B., STATE D., Surgery, 1964, **56**, *1*, 57.
30. INQUIMBERT PH., BERAUD C., TRAISSAC F. J., Arch. franç. App. digest., 1966, **55**, *3*, 247—248.
31. IONESCU-BUJOR C., VELICAN N., BERONIADE V., FLOREA C., CONSTANTINESCU C., *Modificări morfofuncţionale după hepatectomii tipice, (studiu experimental)*, communicated, Institute of Therapeutics, Bucharest, 8 Feb., 1959.
32. IONIŢĂ C., IONESCU-BUJOR C., VASILESCU G., *Regenerare hepatică insulară în cursul cirozei hepatice umane.*, Med. int., 1966, *6*.
33. KOBAK W. M., Surg. Gynec. Obstet., 1956, **102**, *6*, 521.
34. LAGACHE G., MARTINOT M., COMEEMALE B., VEYSSIERE G., Arch. Mal. Ap. digest., 1965, **54**, *6*, 692.
35. LAN HSI, CH'UN YAO CHUAN WEN, CHEN CHAC-EU, Surg. Gynec. Obstet., 1957, **104**, *2*, 252.
36. LEFFMAN H., PAYNE TH. J., Amer. Surgeon, 1955, **21**, 488.
37. LÉGER L., FERRON A., Presse méd., 1957, **44**, 1039.
38. LÉGER L., DETRIE PH., BAKALOUDIS P., Chir., 1964, **87**, *1*, 5.
39. LETULLE M., *Anatomie pathologique*, vol. III, Paris, Masson, 1931, p. 1706.
40. LINTON R. R., Surg. Gynec. Obstet., 1965, **121**, *1*, 117.
41. LIU HSIEN, TANG MING KUEI, CHENG-CHIA-SHUN et al., Med. J., 1962, **81**, *8*, 543.
42. MAC PHERSON A., INNES H., Lancet, 1965, 1/7393, 999.
43. MAKARENKO T. P., PANOMAREV L. E., Vestn. Khir., 1950, **85** *10*, 24.
44. MATZANDER U., Chirurgie, 1964, **305**, *5*, 466.
45. MANCUSO M., GRAND (DEL) G., Surg. Gynec. Obst., 1956, **102**, *3*, 258.
46. MĂNESCU GH., SIMIONESCU N., GOLDSTEIN MAIA, Chirurgia, 1962, **11**, *4*, 549.
47. MAROS T., SERES STURM, RACZ L., KOVACS V. VIRGINIA, Chirurgia, 1963, **12**, *2*, 207.
48. MIHAI C., IONESCU-BUJOR C., PETRIC MIA, HULUBEI P., VASILESCU V., Z. ges. inn. Med., 1962, **17**, *24*, 1118.
49. MORENO H. A., CHIESA D., AFFANI J., Surg. Gynec. Obstet., 1957, **104**, *1*, 25.
50. NANA A., MIRCIOIU C., NEUMANN E., URAY Z., STOILA C., ŞUTEU D., Lyon chir., 1966, **62**, *2*, 217.
51. NEGRU D., *Radiodiagnostic clinic*, H. Welther, Sibiu, 1944, p. 513.
52. PAPAHAGI E., CIUREL M., POPOVICI Z., CIOBANU N., *Asupra anastomozelor porto-cave de urgenţă*, communicated Soc. Surg. 17 Jan. 1964, 4 March 1964, Bucharest.
53. PATE W. J., STORER H. E., Surg. Clin. Amer., 1962, **42**, *5*, 1339.
54. PATSIORA M. D., Khirurghiya, 1954, *1*, 149.
55. PUCHETTI V., GALANTI G., Chir. Pat. Aper., 1960, **8**, *11*, 2.
56. RAPPAPORT, GOTVIN, Rev. int. Hépatol., 1963, **13**, *5*, 291.
57. REIFFERSCHEID N., Arch. klin. Chir., 1959, **290**, 315.
58. RENÉ L., ALLIBERTO B., Lyon chir., 1962, **58**, 1.
59. RUNCAN V., *Probleme de hepatologie*, Ed. medicală, Bucharest, 1964, p. 118—244.
60. SAVY PAUL, *Traité de thérapeutique clinique*, vol. I, Masson, Paris, 1942, p. 768.
61. SCHALM L., Lyon chir., 1962, **58**, 1.
62. SCHIFF L., *Bolile ficatului*, Ed. medicală, Bucharest, 1966, p. 255—709.
63. SCHIFF L., Amer. J. digest. Dis., 1966, **11**, *1*, 68.
64. STUCKE K., *Leber Chirurgie*, Springer, Berlin, 1959, p. 200—232.
65. UGLOV F. G., Vestn. Khir., 1960, **84**, *6*, 147.
66. TRAPANI A., INFRANZI A., Surg. Gynec. Obstet., 1957, **104**, 252.
67. VAILLANT I., GOYER B., GRASSIN P., J. Chir., Paris, 1964, **87**, *4*, 463.
68. VASILESCU V., TOADE V., Viaţa med., 1963, **10**, *3*, 145.
69. * * * *Medicina internă*, vol. VI, Ed. medicală, Bucharest, 1959, p. 252—264.
70. * * * *Mnogotomnoe rukovodstvo pokhirurghii*, vol. VIII, Medghiz, Moscow, 1962, p. 277.
71. WELCH H. F., WELCH C. S., CARTER J. H., Surgery, 1964, **56**, *1*, 75.

CHAPTER 5

INTRAHEPATIC LITHIASIS

Incidence. Since the introduction of peroperative cholangiography and radiomanometry, an increasing number of gallstones have been detected in the intrahepatic ducts. Up to the moment when these new methods of exploration were applied, this form of hepatic lithiasis was considered very rare. Even today, the incidence of gallstones in the intrahepatic ducts varies within broad limits, according to different authors, from 0.38 to 18%, linked to the intraoperative methods of exploration used. In the Far East, hepatic lithiasis is very frequent, owing to the high number of parasitic diseases in this geographical area, and especially to cholangitis secondary to the infections caused by parasites and their eggs.

In our practice we encountered 48 cases of hepatic gallstones in 2000 hepatobiliary operations performed during 12 years, starting in 1954, when intraoperative cholangiography began to be systematically applied (2.4%). However, this does not represent the actual proportion of hepatic gallstones, since in the cases of wide choledochoduodenostomy hepatic calculi might have been overlooked and subsequently evacuated through the anastomosis. The same may be said of operations with sphincterotomy and even with choledochotomies with T-tube drainage; many of the "residual" stones detected at the postoperative cholangiography may certainly have been hepatic calculi that afterwards passed into the common duct. We consider, however, that the incidence of hepatic gallstones in our geographical regions cannot be higher than 4 to 5% (3.2% Mirizzi; 7.2% Hausen; 7.6% Best; 8.3% Beer; 16% Wolgnzev; 18% Kourias). The Scandinavian authors (Lund, Norman) found a much higher proportion, which can only be explained by a special tendency of the population in those parts towards the formation of gallstones, or possibly by intraoperative maneuvers that favor passage of the stones from the common duct into the higher bile ducts (the cherry stone phenomenon of Caroli; the "mouse" calculi of Mirizzi).

History. We owe the first necroptic observations to Morgagni, then to Courvoisier (1891), who reported on the first 50 cases. In 1904, Beer accumulated 150 cases. More recent general studies were published by Rufanov (1936), whose work has become classical, by Santy and Mallet-Guy (1936), Sorlin (1936), Best (1944) and, in recent years, after the introduction of cholangiography, an increasing number of papers have dealt with this problem (Sénèque, Mouchet, Kourias, Glenn, Florent, Cormier, Mirizzi, Champeau, Hepp, Couinaud, Schmidt, Richard, Bové, Huang Ch'Iang, etc.).

Ton That Tung, Mirizzi, Cl. Olivier, Caroli and Corcos devote a whole chapter to this problem in their monographs.

In Romania, I. Porumbaru (1963) and D. Gerota (1965) reported the first cases.

Classification. There is no general consensus concerning the term hepatic lithiasis; some authors consider this term to include all the gallstones within the hepatic duct system, both intraparenchymatous and extrahepatic, whereas others prefer to designate the latter variety as lithiasis of the hepatic duct (Hepp, Lortat Jacob).

On the other hand, a sharp distinction exists between hepatic lithiasis in the eastern and western European regions and America, and hepatic lithiasis in the Far East.

The hepatic lithiasis proper of our regions may be intraparenchymatous, a rare variety, or intracanalicular.

It has justly been shown and we, too, have observed countless times that gallstones in the hepatic duct and its primary branches are often produced by intraoperative maneuvers and especially by rapid injection of the contrast medium for cholangiography, which may force the mobile stones from the common duct towards the common hepatic duct or its original canals (Figs 102 and 103).

Intrahepatic lithiasis "nostras" presents several anatomoclinical forms

— primary single stone (metabolic);

— secondary hepatic lithiasis due to cholangitis, parasites migrating in the upper hepatic ducts, or congenital or acquired stenosis of these ducts;

— associated hepatic and extrahepatic lithiasis. Gallstones in the common duct may be accompanied by stones in the gallbladder and intra- and extra-hepatic bile ducts (petrification of the bile ducts) (Fig. 104).

In several cases, however, the gallbladder may be free of stones, while calculi may be found in the common duct, common hepatic duct and its intra-hepatic branches (Figs 105, 106 and 107). Lithiasis of the gallbladder accompanied by gallstones in the intrahepatic ducts without involvement of the common duct seldom occurs.

The absence of calculi in the gallbladder may be readily explained by their passage into the common and the hepatic ducts through a distended cystic duct (migration lithiasis), whereas an anomaly of the cystic duct that strangles and compresses the hepatic duct (Fig. 108), or an abnormal vessel, or even more frequently congenital or acquired stenosis of the hepatic duct or one of its branches, almost always stands at the basis of the concomitant existence of stones in the gallbladder and hepatic ducts, without participation of the common bile duct.

In some of our cases, a biliobiliary fistula explained the passage of one or several calculi from the gallbladder towards the upper bile ducts (Fig. 109).

Primary solitary gallstones of the intrahepatic bile ducts are extremely rare. Caroli only found conclusive evidence in 20 cases published in the literature, including one of his own and one belonging to Mircea Petrescu (1932).

Hepatic lithiasis is as a rule, especially in the Far East, secondary to cholangitic infection and parasitoses. But this form of secondary lithiasis may also be encountered in southeastern Europe owing to the frequent displacement of the population, inherent to and facilitated by today's civilization.

Among our patients there was a 14-year-old Korean girl with clinical signs of hydrops of the gallbladder. Surgery disclosed a hydrops without any gallstones, and in the common duct, common hepatic duct and the two primary hepatic ducts, 9 calculi measuring 20 mm one above the other, the whole length of these ducts. Hydrops of the gallbladder was accounted for by displacement of one of the calculi lying crosswise in the adherent portion of the cystic duct and compressing it from within. Examination of the stones, with their concentrical layers of

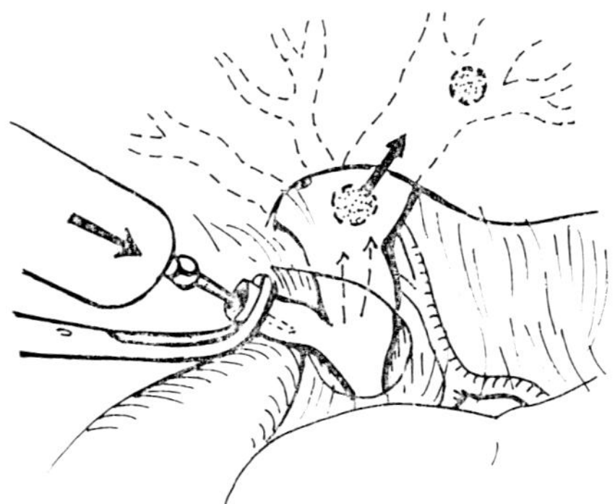

Fig. 102. — Scheme representing a peroperative cholangiography done with a syringe in a case of hepatocholedochal gallstones. The contrast medium forcefully introduced may force the hepatic calculi into the intrahepatic ducts ("mouse" calculi — Mirizzi).

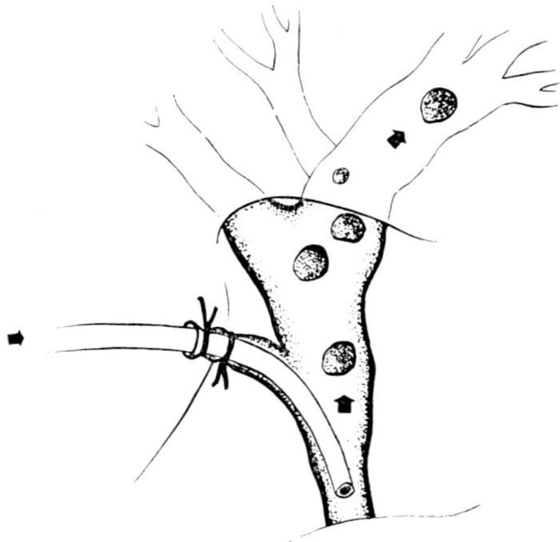

Fig. 103. — The same may happen when washing the lower common duct or on introducing the contrast medium too quickly through a polythene tube.

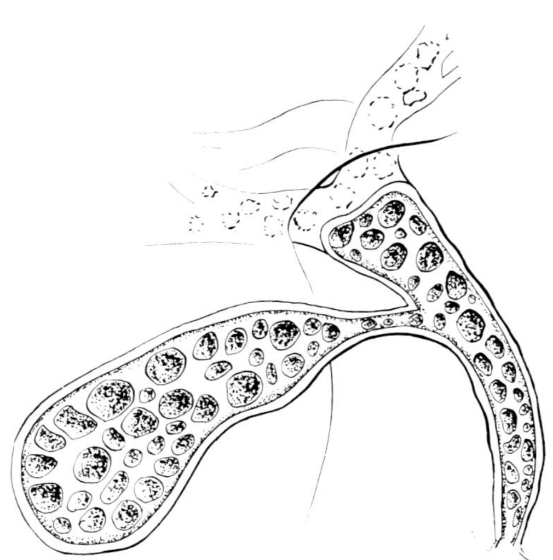

Fig. 104. — Intra- and extrahepatic lithiasis following migration of the stones from the gallbladder into the bile ducts (modified after Mirizzi).

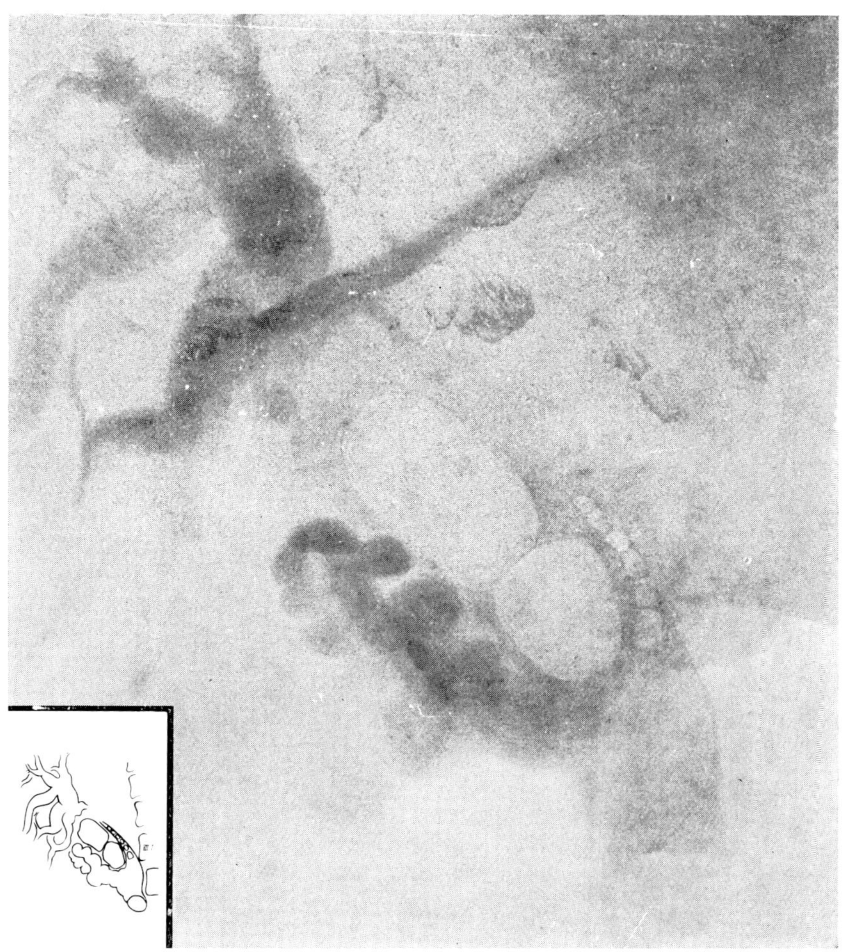

Fig. 105. — Case *N.F.* Obstructive jaundice; cholangitis. Peroperative cholangiography: scleroatrophic gallbladder does not contain calculi. Lengthened, dilated cystic duct following evacuation of the stones into the common hepatic duct. Lower common duct and hepatic duct contain numerous calculi; choledochoduodenostomy after evacuation of the stones by choledochotomy.

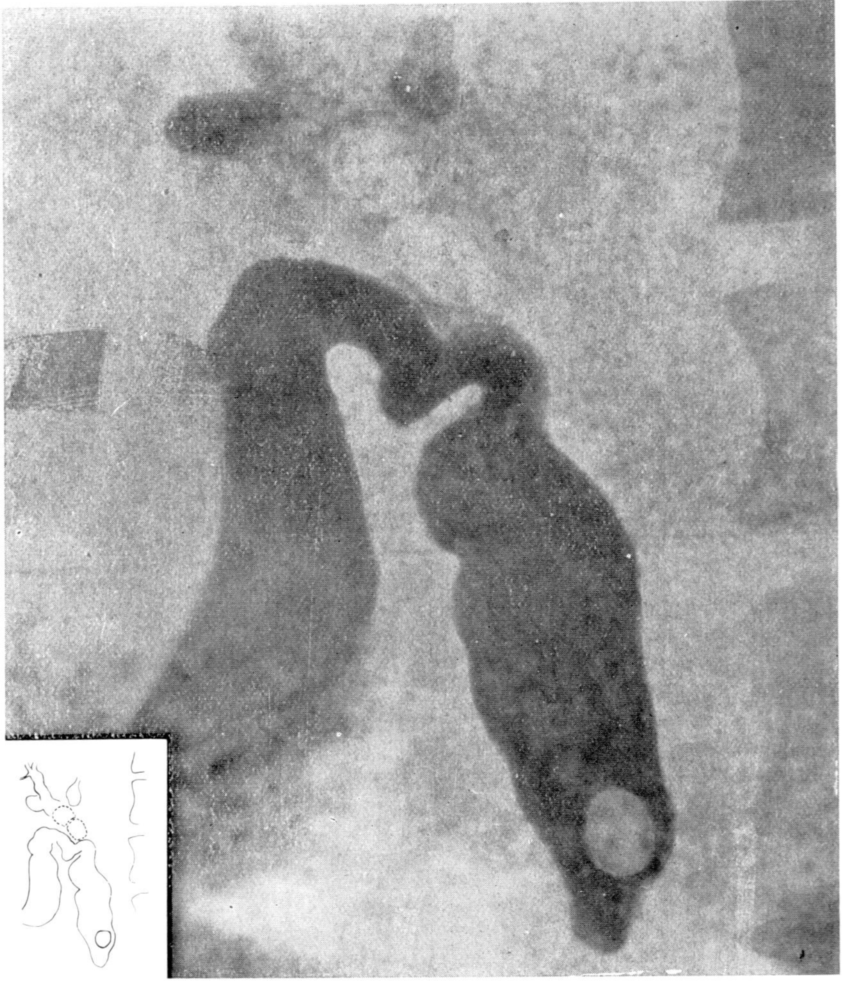

Fig. 106. — Case *C.V.* Choledochal and intrahepatic calculosis. Gallbladder with thickened walls but without any stones; very dilated cystic duct, proof of the migration of the calculi from the gallbladder into the common hepatic duct. Confluence of the hepatic ducts and common hepatic duct does not appear on the peroperative cholangiography because of the stones that block it.

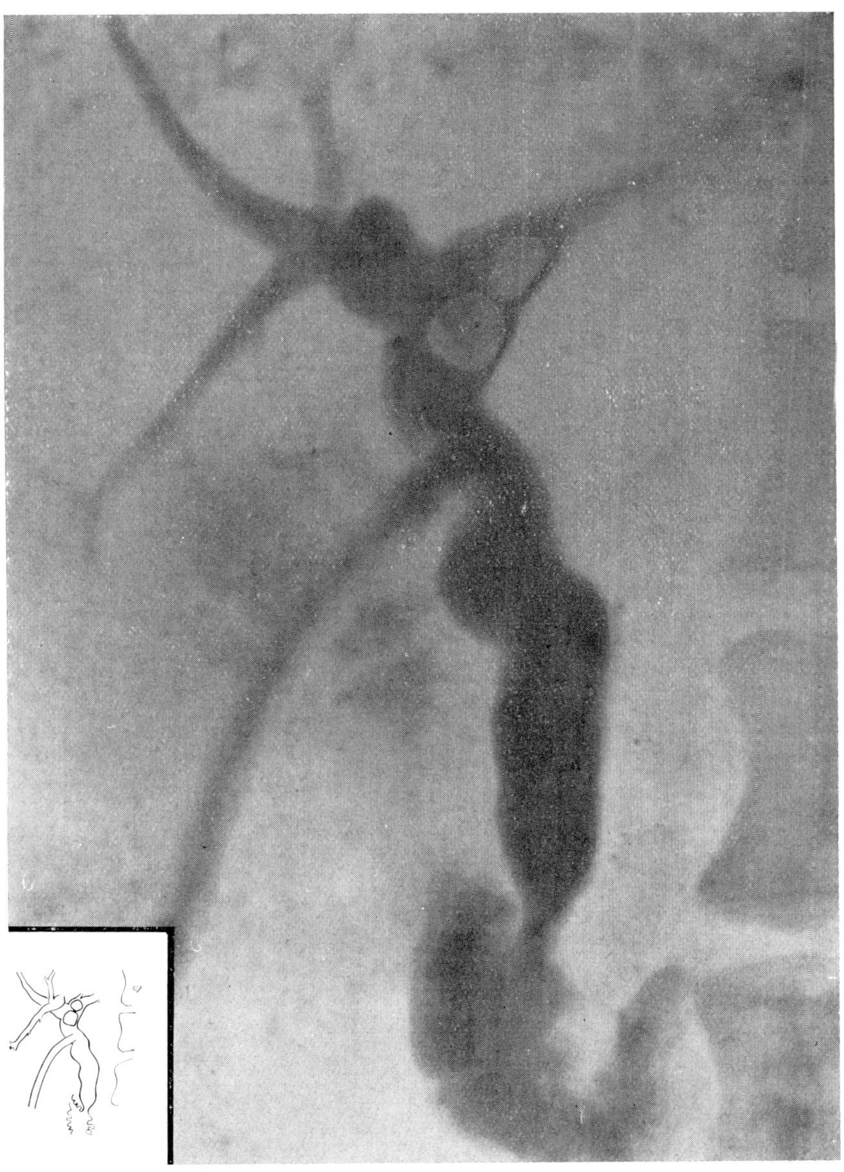

Fig. 107. — Case *C.V.* After extraction of the calculi from the lower common duct, a new cholangiography through the T-tube shows the presence of two gallstones that block the left hepatic duct and confluence of the hepatic ducts.

cholesterol, bile pigments and salts, revealed the presence of a center formed of parasitic remains (Fig. 110).

Apart from congenital stenosis, traumatic scar stenosis is in most casas the cause of stasis, infection and precipitation of cholesterol crystals, bile salts end pigments that generate intrahepatic calculi. In three of our cases of scar sten-

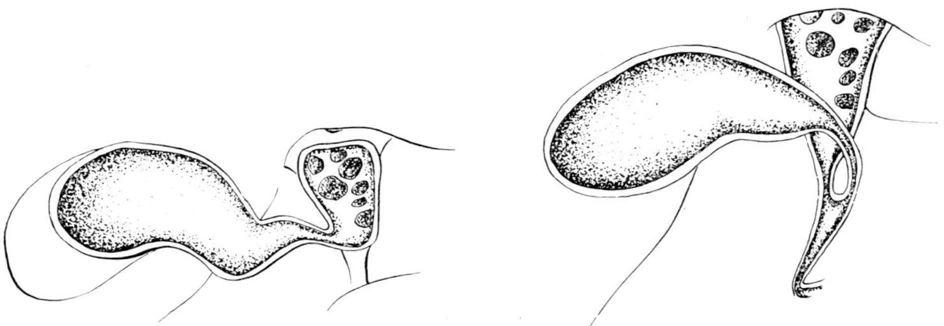

Fig. 108. — Certain anatomic arrangements of the cystic duct predispose to intrahepatic calculosis by the stasis it favors (modified after Mirizzi).

osis of the common hepatic duct, hepatic calculi were found close to the hilus (Fig. 111).

On the other hand, the anatomy of the left hepatic duct, that forms an angle of up to 90° with the main bile duct, accounts for the stasis and frequent predisposition of this duct to hepatic calculosis.

Hepaticojejunal anastomosis may also be the cause of gallstones in the intrahepatic bile ducts, even when the anastomosis is not obstructed. A recent case confirms this finding, made by previous authors.

The patient *V.E.*, with hepaticojejunal anastomosis for scar stenosis of the hepatic duct close to the hilus, came back a year later with an attack of cholangitis and subclinical icterus. Surgery revealed a patent anastomosis, but numerous gallstones obstructing the passage of the bile into the jejunum. The intrahepatic bile ducts contained numerous pigmented calculi of different size (Figs 112, 113 and 114).

Hepatic calculosis is seldom observed after hepaticoduodenal anastomosis, probably because this procedure is seldom applied; the cases operated by us, some of which were followed up for 7 years, evolved without any infectious incident, whereas hepaticojejunal anastomosis was followed by ascending infection and intrahepatic lithiasis, although the anastomosis was done *en Y*.

In one case of hepatocholangiogastric anastomosis (personal procedure), obstructed several months after surgery, jaundice and fever reappeared. The reoperation revealed enlarged intrahepatic bile ducts and the presence of hepatic calculi. Dilatation of the hepatic stump in the hilus permitted broad hepaticojejunal anastomosis with lasting favorable results.

In another case, passage of the hydatid vesicles and membranes into the hepatic ducts following incision of a dead hydatid cyst led to the appearance of

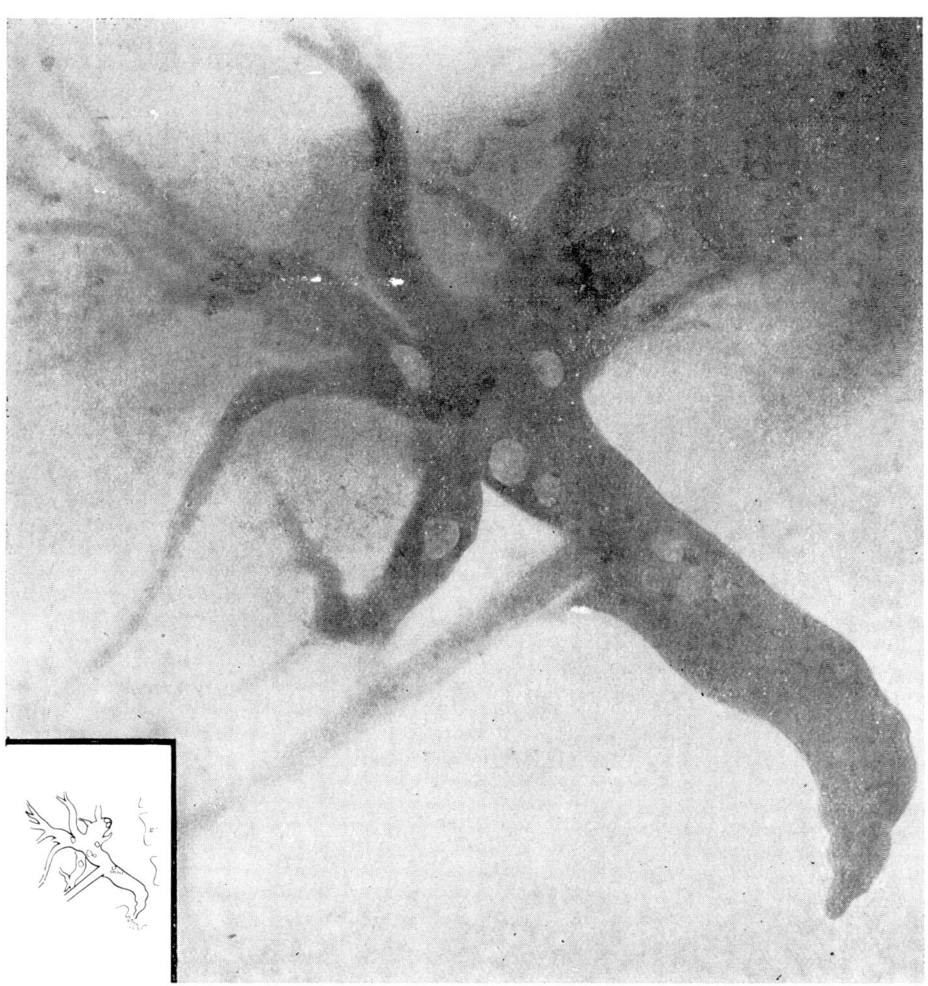

Fig. 109. — Case *G.P.*, aged 60. Lithiasis of the gallbladder, common bile duct and intrahepatic ducts. Peroperative cholangiography reveals a cholecystohepatic fistula and Oddi stenosis: cholecystectomy, choledochotomy with extraction of the calculi, transducdenal sphincterotomy.

hepatic and choledochal gallstones and to the necessity of an extensive sphinctero-tomy that permitted evacuation of the calculi and dead vesicles from the hepatic and common ducts, and recovery. This kind of parasitic calculosis of the intra-hepatic ducts occurs far more frequently in our regions than lithiasis caused by distomiasis or ascariasis that are very frequent in the Far East (Fig. 115).

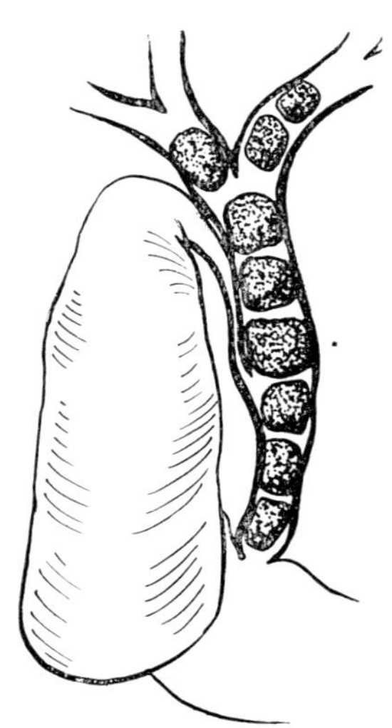

Fig. 110. — Case *H.S.Io.*, aged 14. Hydrops of the gallbladder; intrahepatic calculosis. Schematic representation of an intraoperative cholangiography that revealed 9 stones about 20 mm in size, of which one situated crosswise compressed the cystic duct.

Clinic and diagnosis. The diagnosis of primary hepatic lithiasis has seldom been established before operation, but may be suspected when intravenous cholangiography, morphine tomocholangiography or hepatic scintigram with rose bengal ^{131}I are performed.

In a first phase, the clinical picture is dominated by pains typical of gallbladder colic, which, however, may sometimes be dull and continuous.

The second phase sets in with its train of symptoms: fever, and chills, preceded by pain.

In the third phase, jaundice may develop when the gallstones occupy a single segment or the parenchyma. This can only be explained by cellular alterations caused by infection and perhaps by spasms of the hepatic ducts which are free of calculi.

As a rule, however, jaundice appears in the diffuse, petrified forms or after displacement of a gallstone towards the confluence of the hepatic ducts, or when it is impacted within the papilla.

Enlargement of the liver may be observed, but is not obligatory. In general, the clinical signs are those of gallstones of the common duct.

The diagnosis is difficult to establish before surgery, but when the radiologist or the surgeon's attention is drawn towards a possible hepatic lithiasis, the current roentgenogram, intravenous cholangiography or tomocholangiography after morphine may facilitate the presumptive diagnosis in some cases, until checked intraoperatively.

In one of our cases, the diagnosis was made before surgery, owing to intravenous cholangiography (Figs 116 and 117).

Preoperative cholangiography can only offer sufficient diagnostic elements when the intrahepatic ducts are clearly visualized. In such cases, the radiologic diagnosis can be established on the basis of the following signs: the intrahepatic bile ducts are irregularly distended, exhibiting one or several filling defects; one or more ducts may appear to be amputated, ending in a cup-like or "lobster claw" extremity. In other cases, the main bile duct appears to be very dilated, without the presence of calculi. This should draw our attention to the possible existence of hepatic gallstones. In other cases, the intrahepatic ducts are visualized before the main bile duct, pointing to an obstacle in the way of the opaque medium.

Transparietocholangiography may be necessary in cases of stenosed or unaccessible bile duct.

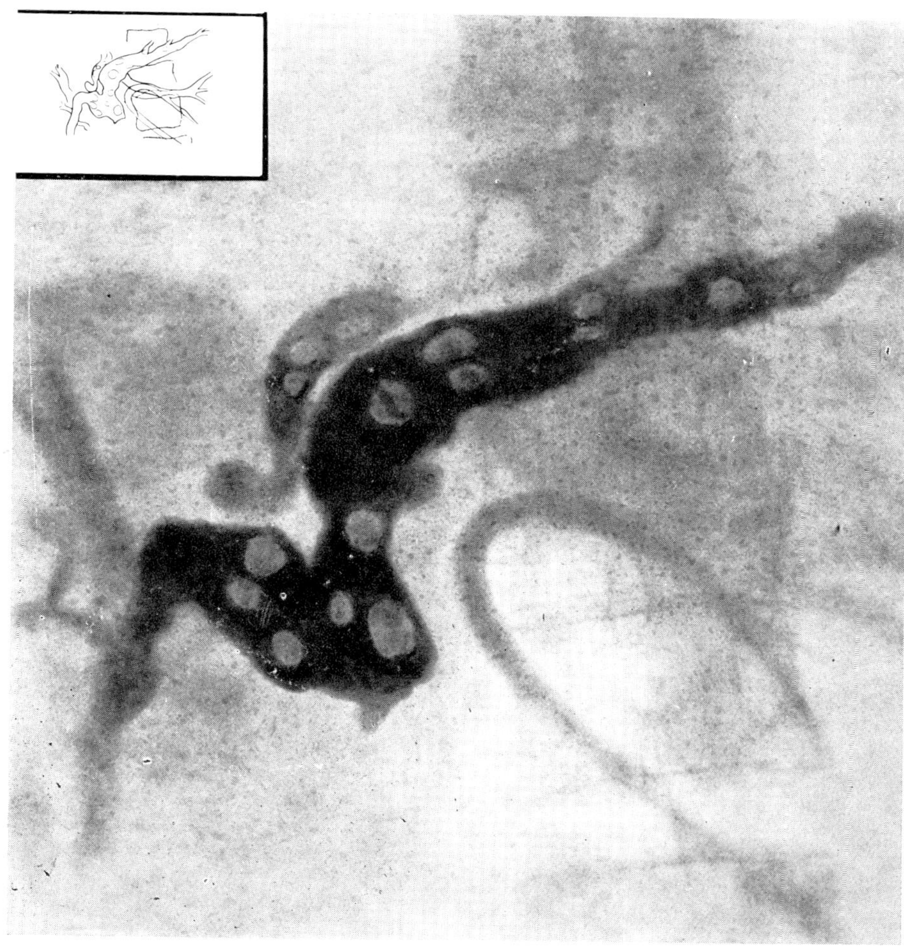

Fig. 111. — Case *F.A.* Intrahepatic lithiasis in a case of cicatricial obstruction of the extrahepatic bile ducts. Peroperative cholangiography following exposure of the duct in segment III in the fissure of the round ligament, in view of a biliointestinal anastomosis (hepatocholangiogastrotomy, personal procedure).

Laparoscopic cholangiography (Royer) is considered theoretically useful, but has not yet been applied (Caroli).

Radioisotopic exploration of the liver damaged by the presence of gallstones, especially in a single sector or lobe, with alteration of the respective liver parenchyma, may give precious information for the preoperative diagnosis and the choice of surgical therapy, particularly when the question of hepatectomy arises.

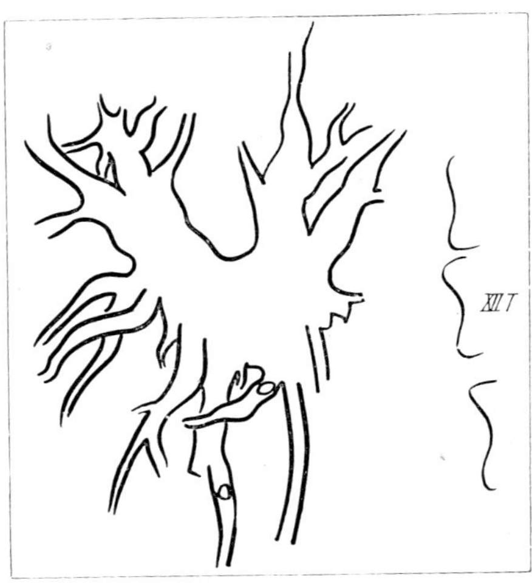

Fig. 112. — Case *V.E.* Tight cicatricial stenosis of the hepatic duct in the hilus, after cholecystectomy. Cholangitis, subclinical icterus. The bile ducts appear enormously dilated on the peroperative cholangiography. On opening the confluence of the hepatic ducts, exposed by detachment of the hilar plaque, stasis bile with microcalculi was evacuated. Hepaticojejunostomy *en Y*-loop, with polythene splint for calibration, removed after 2 months.

The intraoperative diagnosis must be based on visual inspection of the liver, manual exploration of the liver and extrahepatic bile ducts, essential and valuable maneuvers, sometimes sufficient to establish the presence of large hepatic calculi or petrification of a liver lobe. In such cases, the affected lobe, as a rule the left because lithiasis of the left hepatic duct is more frequent, appears modified both on visual and on manual examination. By bimanual examination, the existence of calculi may be detected, the affected lobe giving the impression of a bag full of hazelnuts. In some cases, the gallstones impacted in the left hepatic duct were palpated and extracted after detachment of Glisson's capsule (Champeau) (Fig. 118).

Intraoperative cholangiography is essential for detecting hepatic calculi, but repeated films are necessary, with good filling of the upper bile ducts.

Pressure must be avoided and the opaque medium instilled very carefully, so as not to force the gallstones from the common duct into the hepatic canals. Mirizzi, who calls these mobile gallstones "mouse" calculi, a suggestive expression, recommends extreme care during injection of the contrast substance.

Radiomanometry plays a part especially in detection of the gallstones migrating towards the papilla and determination of the functional state of the sphincter of Oddi. Therapeutic indications can only be reasonably established after using this means of exploration. In the absence of radiomanometry, the surgeon must be content with the results of peroperative cholangiography; after removal of the gallstones, if instrumental exploration of the Oddi region and cholangiographic

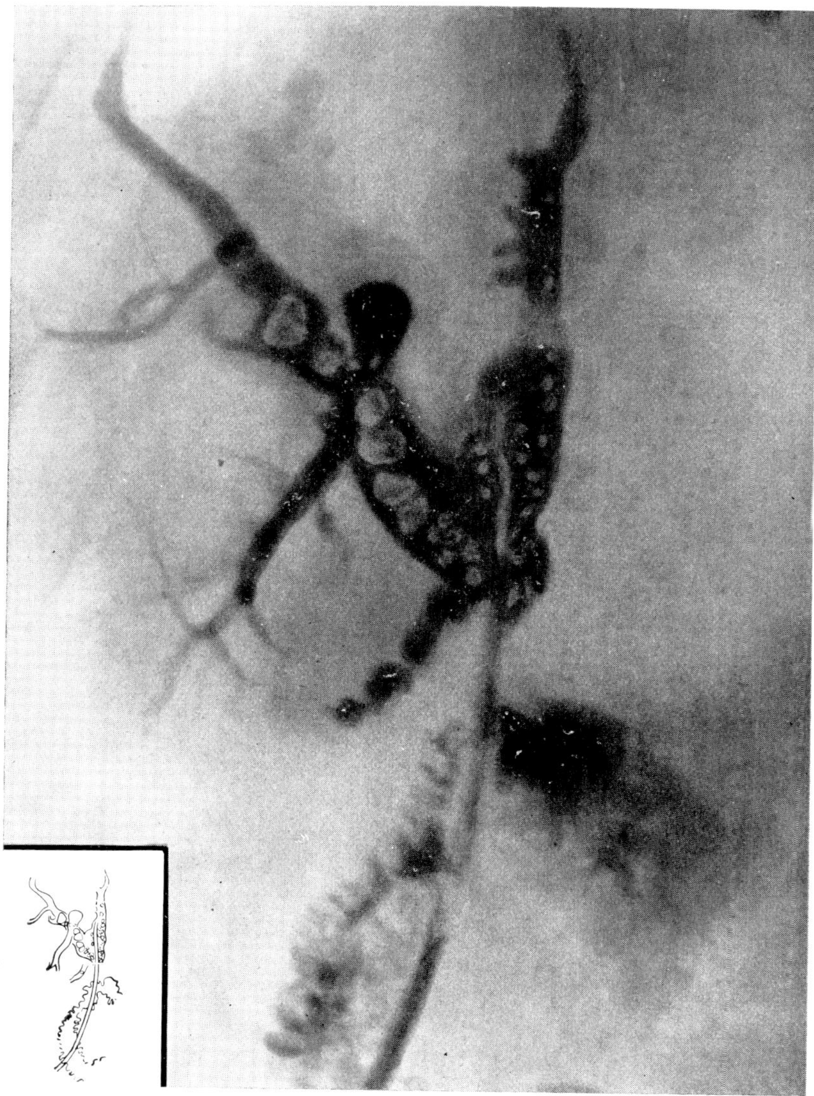

Fig. 113. — Case *V.E.* Secondary intrahepatic lithiasis after hepaticojejunal anastomosis *en Y*-loop. The patient returned one year after the primary operation, with jaundice and fever. At the second operation, the hepaticojejunal anastomosis was found to be patent, but the hepatic ducts were full of pigment calculi, bile mud and septic bile. The calculi were evacuated by enterotomy of jejunal loop *en Y*, without touching the anastomosis which permitted easy passage of the forceps used for removing the stones.

control have shown that no gallstone blocks the papilla, but that the opaque medium passes with difficulty or not at all into the duodenum, the diagnosis is sclerosing odditis. In this case, it will be necessary to perform sphincterotomy or choledochoduodenostomy when the common duct is very distended and existent chronic pancreatitis nodules compress the lower portion of the common duct.

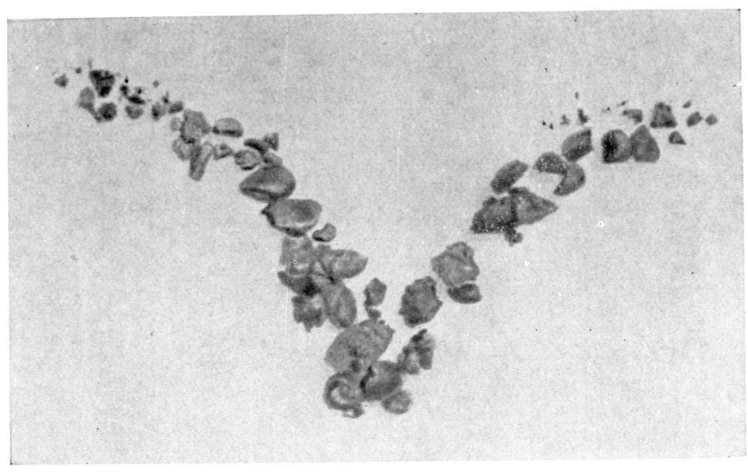

Fig. 114. — Case *V.E.* Intrahepatic bile calculi extracted through the hepaticojejunal anastomosis.

Pathologic anatomy. Visually, the hepatic parenchyma may not be modified when there are few intrahepatic gallstones and the bile ducts are not infected. In long-standing forms, with repeated attacks of cholangitis, the parenchyma exhibits signs of cholostatic cirrhosis, or when the gallstones or strongly dilated bile ducts are in the immediate vicinity of the external capsule, it may take on a whitish, mammillated aspect, giving the impression of neoplastic metastases.

Hepatic abscesses may develop around the gallstones within the parenchyma or around the stones within the dilated, infected intrahepatic ducts. These abscesses may sometimes be considered as a common, suppurated cholangitis; evidence of the gallstones, the true cause of these abscesses, will only be found following their incision.

The bile ducts may exhibit one or several stenoses that account for stasis and the underlying dilatations that form veritable pouches full of biliary mud, gallstones and pus.

The main bile ducts may be distended even when they do not contain calculi, which is of importance for the diagnosis of this kind of lithiasis.

Destructive lesions generally involve the left lobe of the liver, because the left hepatic duct drains with greater difficulty as it joins the common duct at an angle of almost 90°.

The healthy parenchyma becomes functionally hypertrophic when lithiasis or cholangitis are not generalized. In the latter case, the parenchyma may undergo

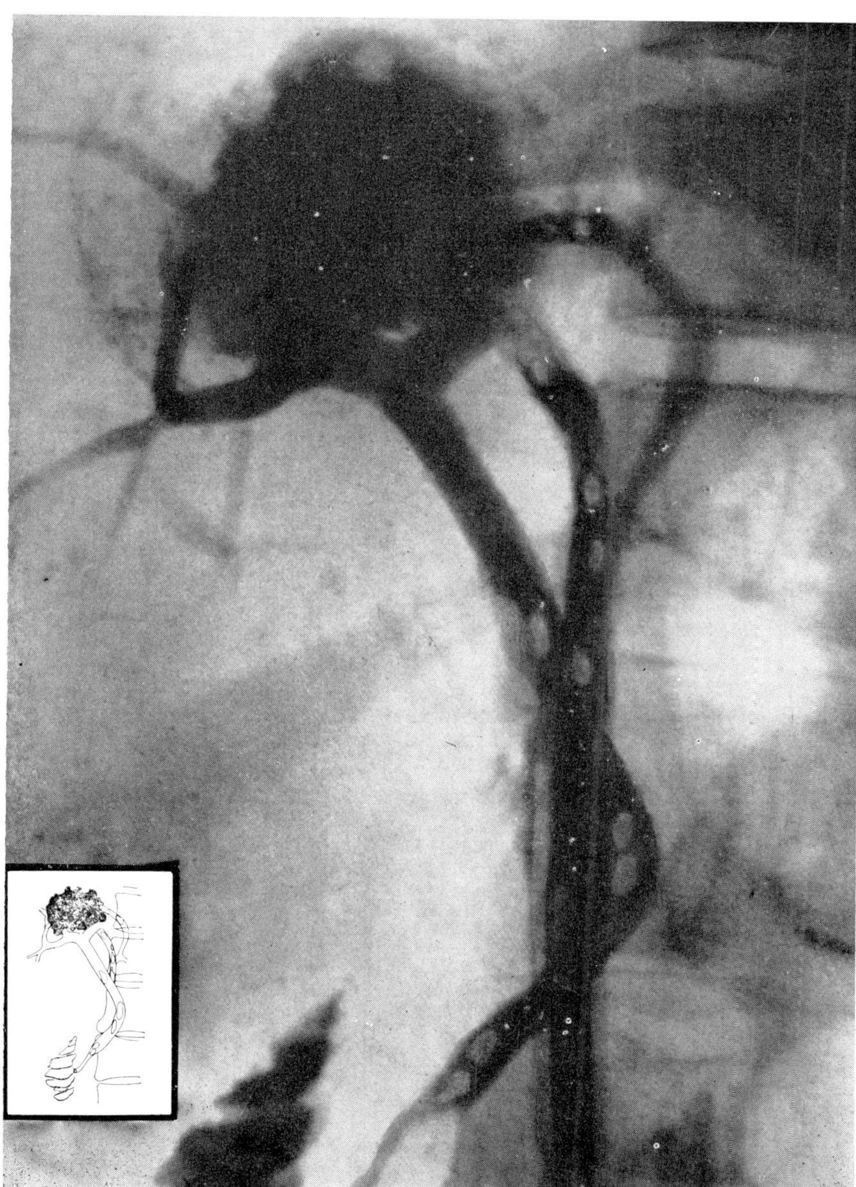

Fig. 115. — Case *P.A.* Hydatid cyst opening into the bile ducts; jaundice a few weeks after surgical removal of the cyst. Cholangiography through the external biliary fistula showed the presence of calculi and hydatid membranes in the intrahepatic bile ducts, common hepatic duct and papilla. Transduodenal sphincterotomy. Recovery.

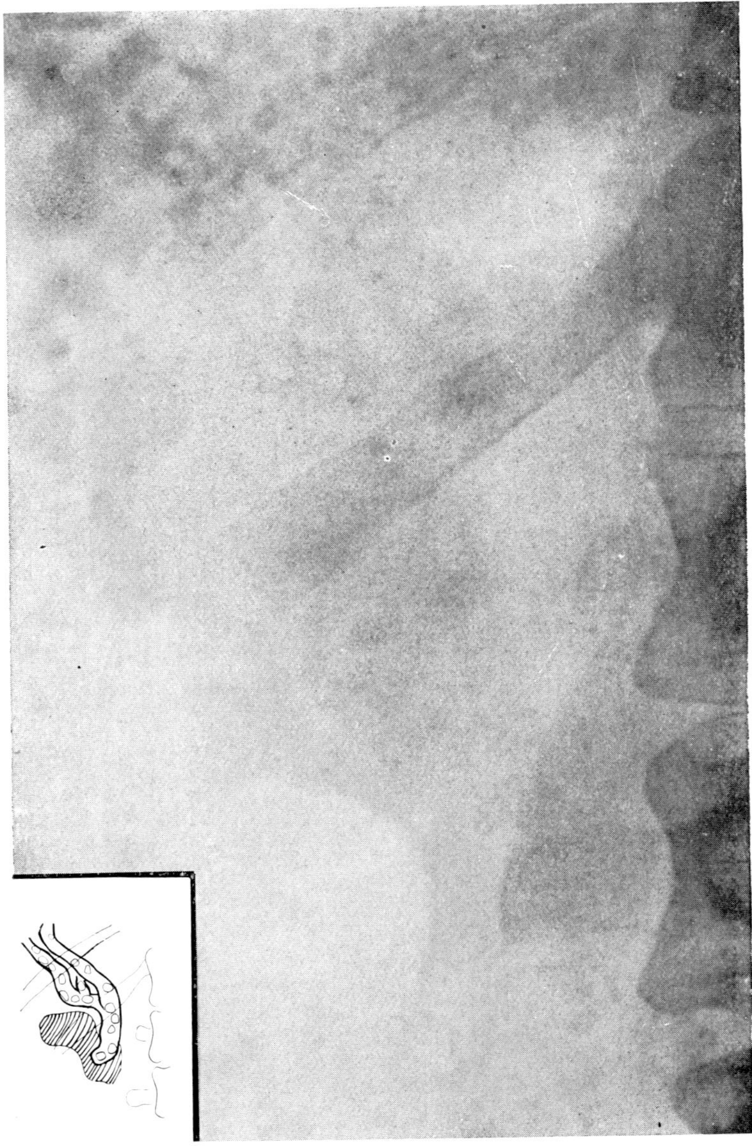

Fig. 116. — Case *C.G.* Intra- and extrahepatic gallstones with cholangitis and jaundice. Preoperative cholangiography with biligraphin. In this case, intrahepatic lithiasis was diagnosed preoperatively.

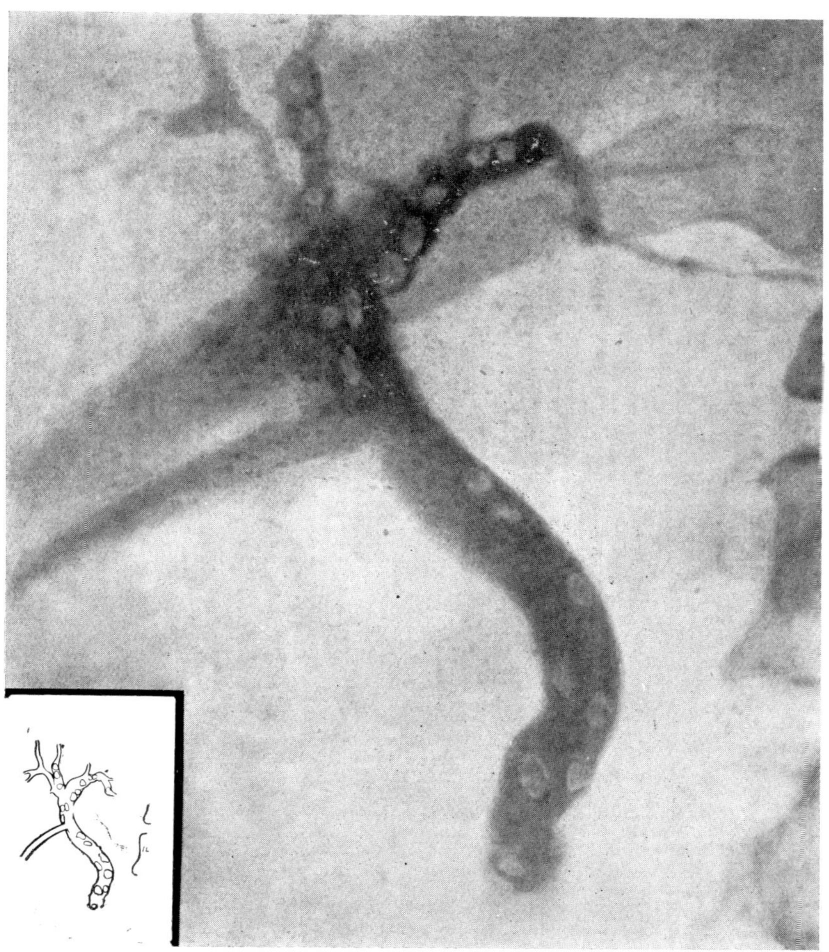

Fig. 117. — Case *C.G.* Peroperative cholangiography confirms the findings obtained with biligraphin. The gallstones occupy both the common duct and intrahepatic ducts. Note moderate dilatation of the common hepatic duct.

severe alterations that explain the hepatic insufficiency and fragility of these patients.

Gallstones may be single or multiple, sometimes causing the transformation of a lobe, usually the left one, into a bag full of stones. The gallstones may take

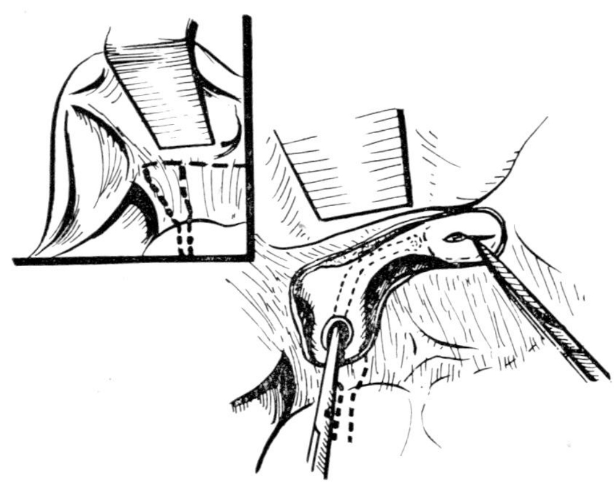

Fig. 118. — Detection of a gallstone impacted in the left hepatic duct, following detachment of the hilar plate (Champeau). After extraction of the stone by direct incision of the duct above it, the operation may be ended by T-tube drainage or anastomosis of the left hepatic duct to Y-jejunal loop (according to Hepp-Couinaud).

on two completely different forms, whose aspect is of the greatest diagnostic and prognostic importance.

In migration lithiasis, formed of vesicular calculi that pass into the hepatic and the common bile ducts, the aspect of the stones is characteristic of and very similar to that of the stones in the gallbladder: the facets are as a rule formed of cholesterol, sometimes with a superficial layer of bile pigments deposited after infection of the bile ducts.

Locally developed calculi are generally friable, made up of pigment, mixed with biliary mud or biliopurulent magma.

Their arrangement varies. When they occupy a single duct, a large stone may be impacted at the level of a bifurcation or stenosis; a sequence of other smaller stones may succeed it, filling the whole canal. Removal of the head gallstone brings about evacuation of the other calculi, which explains the possible onset of jaundice after mobilization of the head stone when all the calculi are not removed during the intervention.

Evolution and complications. Hepatic lithiasis that accompanies lithiasis of the extrahepatic ducts, diagnosed in time, has a good prognosis when all the calculi are evacuated from the hepatic ducts together with those from the common duct.

However, this possibility is very rare. Cholangiography and morphine tomocholangiography make it possible to establish the preoperative diagnosis in some cases. At any rate, peroperative cholangiography is the best means for revealing hepatic calculi, their site, number and possible anomalies of the bile ducts, scar stenosis, etc. The subsequent evolution depends upon a good intraoperative diagnosis.

This evolution may be favorable even when complete evacuation of the intrahepatic ducts is not certain in spite of multiple maneuvers and attempts, but the operation is completed, for the sake of caution, by extended sphincterotomy in the cases in which cholangiography reveals a sclerous papilla, or by choledocho-duodenostomy when the common duct is very distended.

In secondary hepatic lithiasis, due to congenital or acquired stenosis of an intrahepatic duct or confluence of the two primary hepatic ducts, the prognosis is more severe, as in these cases biliary stasis leads to infection, and repeated attacks of cholangitis maintain a latent septic state, although most or all the gallstones have been removed from the bile ducts.

In such cases, cholestatic cirrhosis develops in the infected lobe, with atrophy of the parenchyma. When an intrahepatic duct is completely obstructed, abscesses appear due to cholestasis and infection. In some cases, abscesses located at the periphery of the parenchyma open into the peritoneum, producing severe, fatal peritonitis.

Secondary infected lithiasis predisposes to frequent relapses even after surgery with evacuation of the calculi, when normal drainage of the bile is not ensured.

Reinterventions, that are often necessary, present an increasingly weaker patient, less able to withstand a long and traumatizing operation because of the severe alterations of the whole hepatic parenchyma, resulting in hepatic insufficiency.

Spontaneous migration of hepatic gallstones may be observed after an intervention in which calculi were removed from the hepatic and common bile ducts, mobilizing a large stone that blocked one of the intrahepatic ducts. In these cases jaundice may develop after the operation, or repeated transient jaundice be observed in the subsequent follow-up of these patients.

Postoperative cholangiography, which should be performed in all cases in the course of drainage of the main duct, may reveal a calculus or calculi that have migrated into the lower common duct or the papilla.

Involvement of the papilla and Oddi region, chronic pancreatitis and especially enlargement of the main bile ducts are frequently noted, but are not obligatory. In one of our cases with numerous calculi in the intrahepatic bile ducts and the hepatic and common ducts, the latter were but slightly dilated (Figs 116 and 117).

The sphincter of Oddi may be scleroatrophic even in cases with a long-standing development, as in one of our operated cases (Figs 124 and 125) in which good postoperative results were obtained by sphincterotomy that allowed return of the enormously dilated bile ducts to their normal size.

Treatment. Medical treatments have been attempted, but with few chances of success; they may, however, be useful as a preparatory therapy prior to surgery. Best recommends a cholagogue, antispastic medication and a fatty diet on the eve of the operation in order to favor descent of the gallstones from the hepatic branches into the main bile ducts. Mirizzi justly observed that this method may induce painful attacks, whose intensity and development is hard to foresee. In impacted stones this treatment is unsuccessful, and surgery alone can clear the obstructed bile duct.

In general, the surgical treatment of hepatic lithiasis closely resembles that of gallstones of the common duct.

Choledochotomy is imperative in all cases and is sufficient in most of them.

The incision of the common duct must be transverse, in the immediate vicinity of the first portion of the duodenum, so that it may be used at any moment for choledochoduodenal anastomosis.

In the majority of our cases, hepatic calculosis was accompanied by lithiasis of the main duct, and the first operative stage consisted in extraction of the stones from the hepatic and common ducts. After determining the patency of

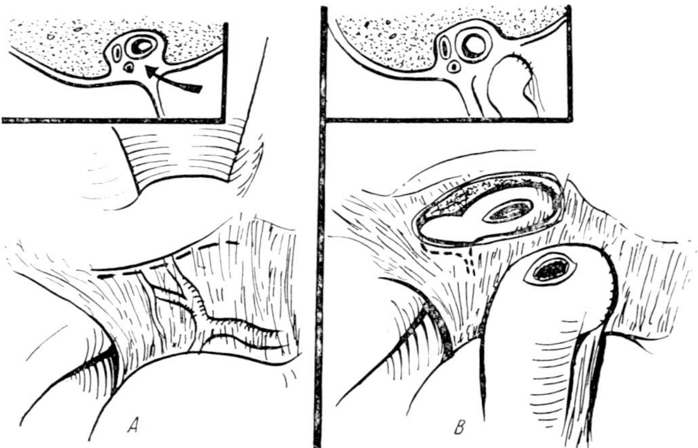

Fig. 119. — Exposure to the left hepatic duct in the hilus following detachment and lowering of the hilar plaque. The duct can be then easily anastomosed to a Y-jejunal loop (according to Hepp-Couinaud).

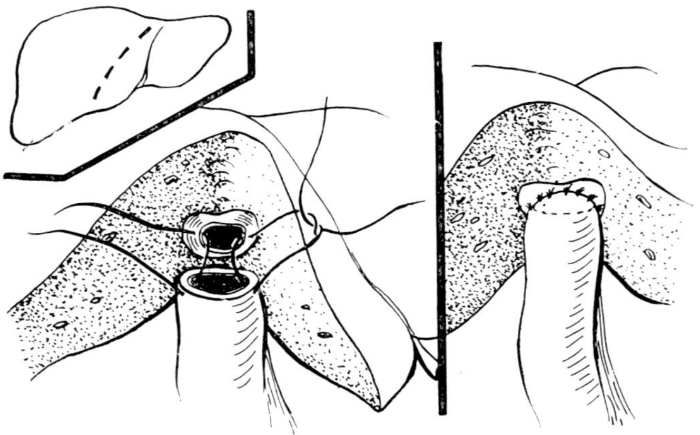

Fig. 120. — Exposure of the confluence of the two intrahepatic ducts by hepatotomy along the long fissure. End-to-end anastomosis to a jejunal loop can be easily performed. The broad route of access permits extraction of the calculi from both hepatic ducts (Champeau).

the papilla, the second and most important stage follows: extraction of the gallstones from the intrahepatic ducts.

To this end, the common calculi forceps will be used, as well as various malleable scoops. Instrumental extraction is, however, difficult and often insufficient, and irrigation of the ducts with warm saline is resorted to, or suction of their content with the aspiration apparatus, to which a bevelled rubber tube is fixed.

Each of the three branches of the hepatic tract must be investigated separately. For stones in the hilar portion of the left hepatic duct, exposure of the origin of this duct by turning down Glisson's capsule and incision of the wall of the hepatic duct may facilitate extraction of a gallstone, that could not be extracted through the choledochal incision.

The cranioventral branch of the right hepatic duct may be explored and existing stones extracted with a malleable scoop. Approach of the dorsocaudal branch is more difficult because of its bent, down- and backward curved position.

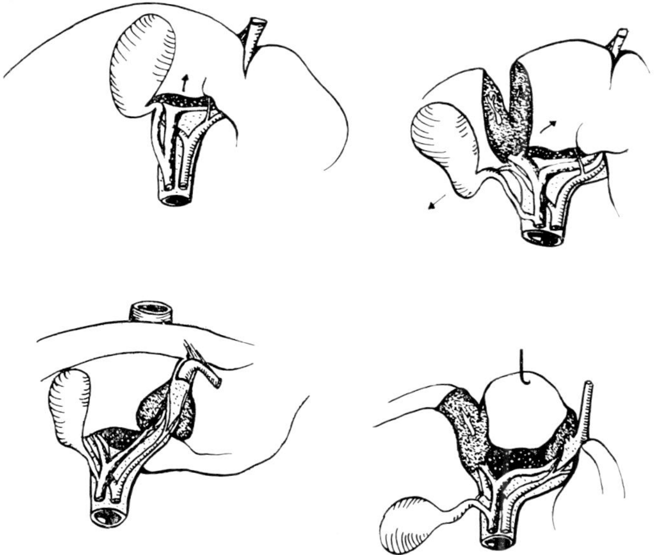

Fig. 121. — Broad exposure of both hepatic ducts and their confluence by mobilization of segment IV. After detachment of the hilar plate, two sections in the liver parenchyma, one along the large fissure and the second along the lateral fissure, parallel to the round ligament close up to Rex' recess, frees the quadrate lobe (segment IV) which can be easily raised in order to expose to view all the elements of the hilus (after Champeau and Vialas).

In difficult cases, Champeau's maneuver, exposing bifurcation of the hepatic duct by hepatotomy along the large fissure, may be indicated since it permits direct exploration of both hepatic ducts.

Another technique, recently described by Champeau, consists in mobilization of the IVth segment by cross incision of Glisson's capsule and two anteroposterior incisions, one along the round ligament up to the notch in the anterior border of the liver, the other along the large fissure. In this way the quadrate lobe can be easily mobilized, exposing both hepatic ducts and the origin of the segmentary ducts over a large area (Fig. 121).

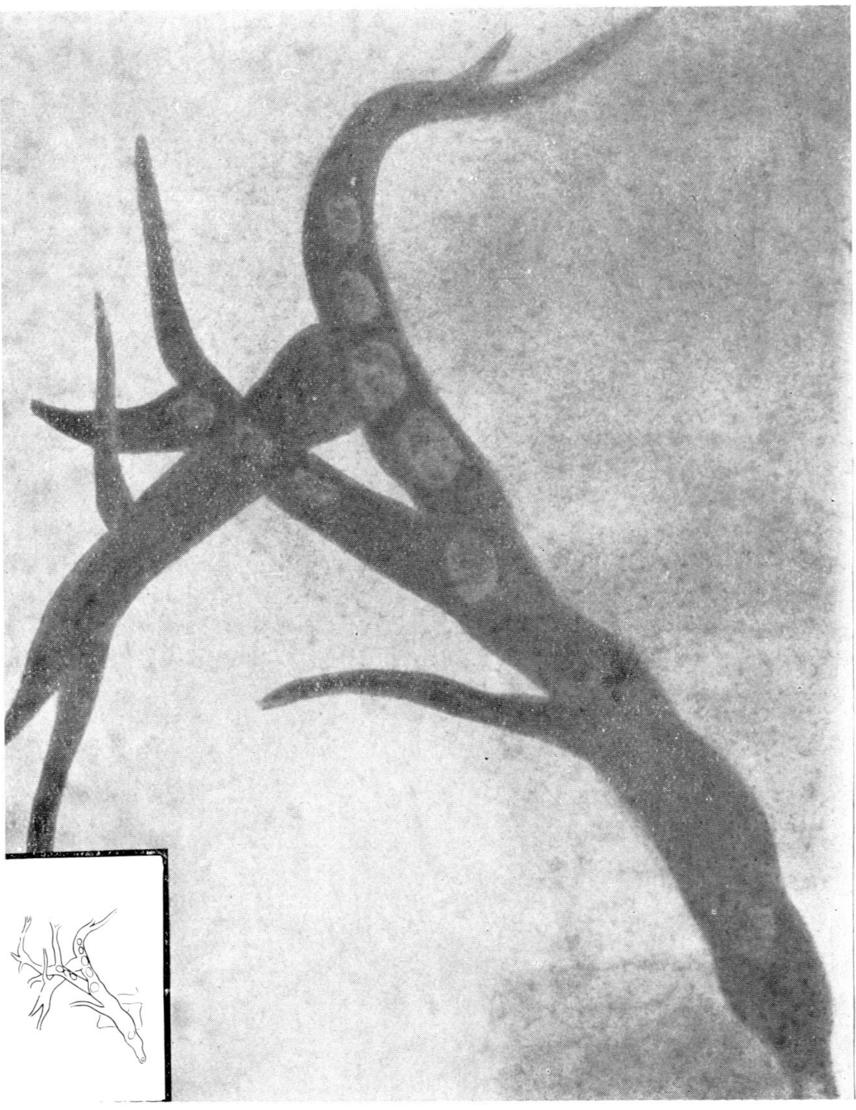

Fig. 122. — Case *I.F.* Intra- and extrahepatic lithiasis. Hydrops of the gallbladder. After cholecystectomy and choledochotomy with extraction of a large number of stones, peroperative cholangiography revealed the presence of gallstones in the common bile duct and intrahepatic ducts.

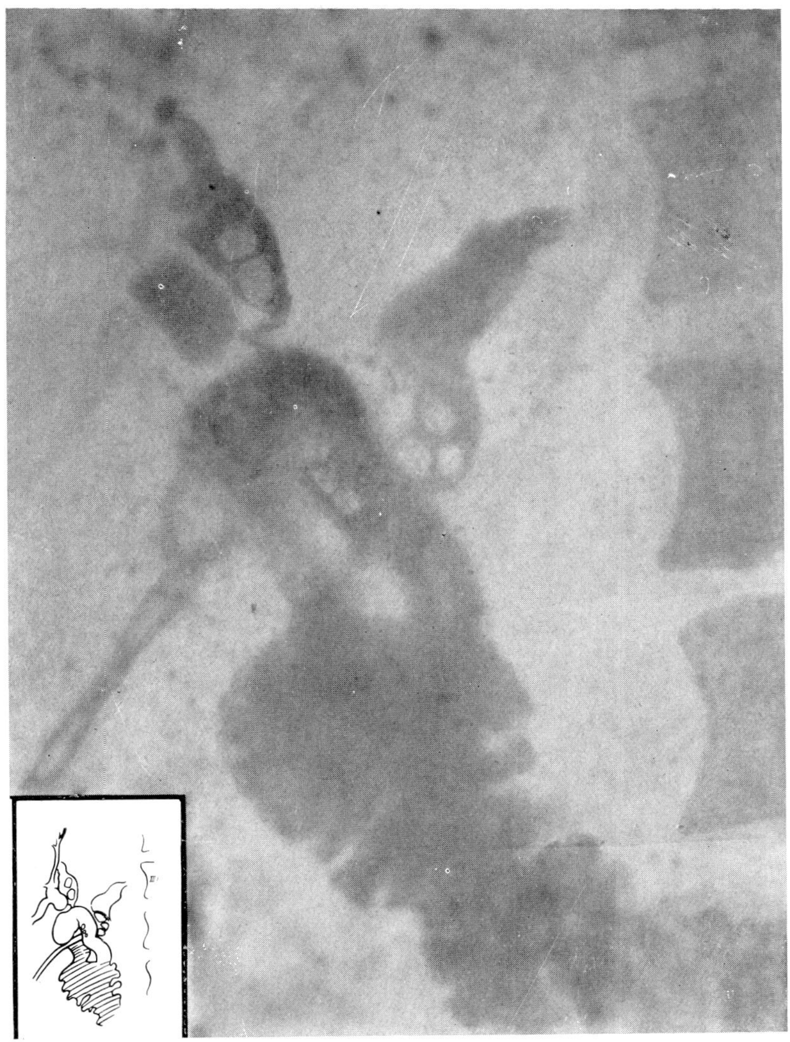

Fig. 123. — Case *I.F.* Intra- and extrahepatic lithiasis. Cholangiography through the T-tube shows the presence of residual intrahepatic and choledochal calculi. Sphincterotomy, T-tube drainage, Pribram washings.

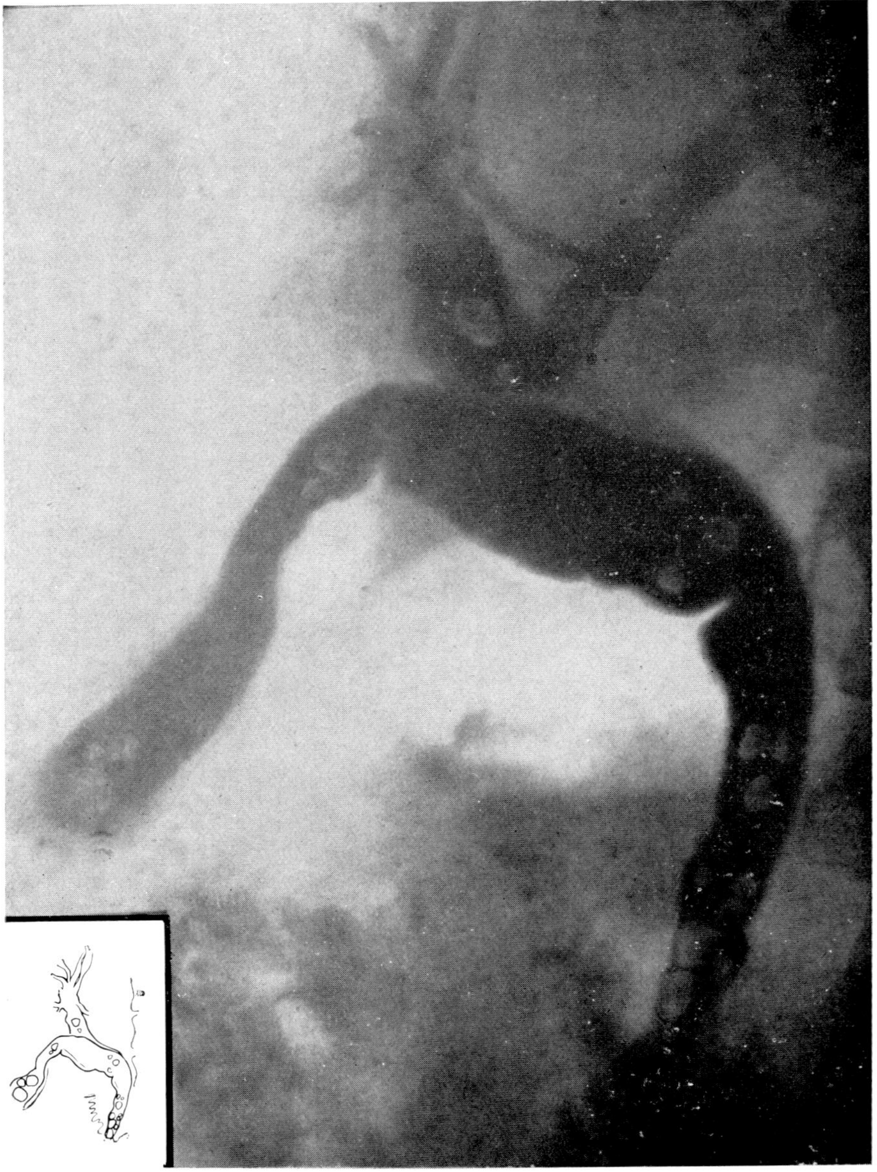

Fig. 124. — Case *A.L.* Peroperative cholangiography through the gallbladder. Numerous stones in the gallbladder; enormously dilated cystic duct; stones in the hepatic common duct and confluence of the hepatic ducts. All the bile duct system is very dilated. Vater's ampulla obstructed by a gallstone. Jaundice.

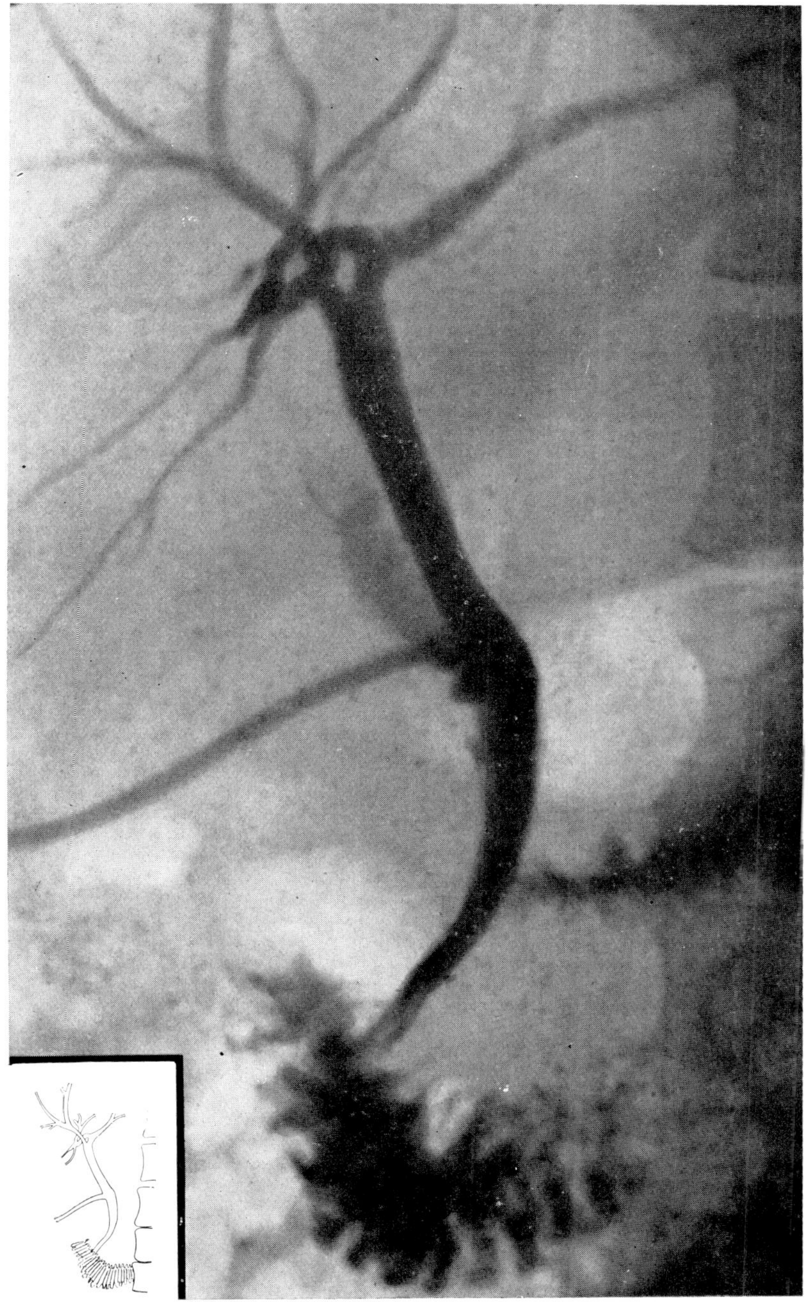

Fig. 125. — Case *A.L.* The same patient as in Fig. 124. Postoperative cholangiography. The bile ducts are free of calculi and have returned to normal dimensions after choledochotomy with T-tube drainage and transduodenal sphincterotomy.

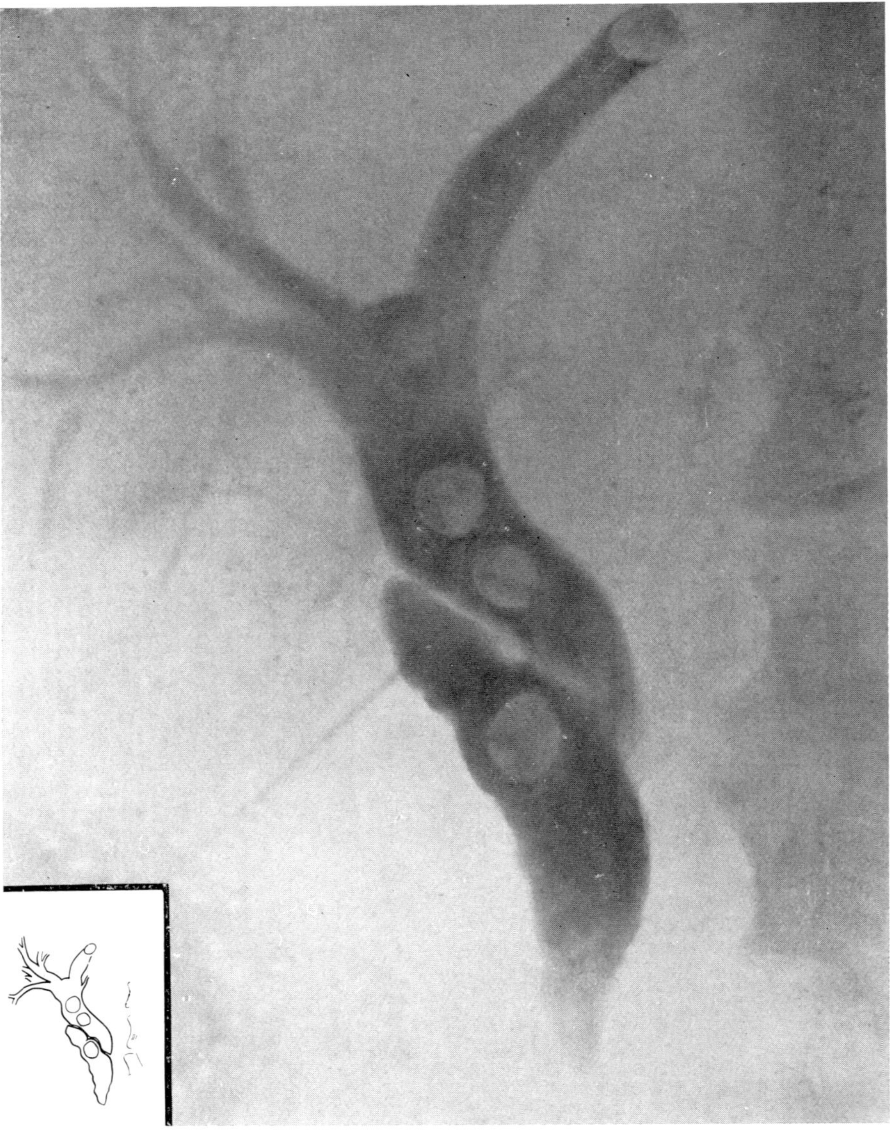

Fig. 126. — Case *F.M.* Intra- and extrahepatic lithiasis. Three large calculi occupy the common bile duct and common hepatic duct. One calculus is impacted in the left hepatic duct, which appears to be amputated. After extraction of the calculi by choledochotomy, end-to-end choledochojejunostomy was performed (the duodenum being improper for anastomosis) because of the sclerosis lesions of the odditis region, visible on the cholangiography.

For the calculi situated close to the surface of the hepatic parenchyma, direct hepatotomy may give very good results, especially when the gallstone is situated in the parenchyma or when an impacted stone produces a hepatic abscess.

If extraction of the stones is done by simple choledochotomy, drainage with a T-tube is imperative. Through this tube it is possible to irrigate the ducts with ether oil according to the Pribram method, a procedure that has given good results in the hands of Kourias. We, too, have used it with excellent results when the bile ducts were severely affected, and continuous or interrupted instillations with wide spectrum antibiotics, resulting in their sterilization, were followed by successful application of this method (case *I.F.*, Figs 122 and 123).

In many instances, however, simple drainage of the common duct cannot ensure the evacuation of the gallstones remaining in the upper ducts. Hence, in all the cases in which the common bile duct is dilated, and this is the rule, *choledochoduodenostomy* should be the treatment of choice. In some of our cases, peroperative cholangiography revealed the presence of stenosing odditis. In such cases *broad sphincterotomy* is preferable (Figs 124 and 125). In one case in which the intrahepatic bile ducts were packed full with gallstones and dead hydatid vesicles, sphincterotomy gave a long-lasting recovery.

In our opinion, *T-tube drainage and the Pribram method combined with sphincterotomy may give even better results than choledochoduodenostomy performed upon an insufficiently dilated common duct.*

This method has the drawback of not being applicable to patients with a general precarious state for whom prolonged trauma is contraindicated.

When the patient's general condition is good, but removal of the stones is not complete, biliointestinal anastomosis on a Y-shaped jejunal loop is indicated in all the cases in which a hilar or inscisural approach was necessary for relief of obstruction of the intrahepatic ducts (Figs 118, 119, 120).

Controlled hepatectomy is indicated in all the cases in which a segment or lobe is transformed into a veritable bag of stones. The results obtained by Huang Chi Ch'Iang, Ton That Tung, Gerota and more recently Guillemin, illustrate the value of this method when partial ablation of the liver is indicated.

Controlled hepatectomy is seldom applied in this form of hepatic lithiasis, but 18 cases have been reported in the literature: one case of Rozanov (1936), another of Caroli and Couinaud for Western hepatic lithiasis, two cases operated by Huang Chi Ch'Iang, 13 cases operated by Ton That Tung (Hanoi) for Far Eastern hepatic lithiasis, one case communicated by Guillemin (Lyon) and one published by Gerota (Bucharest).

Although seldom practiced, controlled hepatectomy is the only satisfactory means of treating hepatic gallstones that completely jeopardize the liver parenchyma of a segment, lobe or half the liver.

REFERENCES

1. BEER E., Arch. klin. Chir., 1904, **74**, 115.
2. BERMAN I., PFEFFER R., Amer. J. Surg., 1967, **114**, *6*, 969.
3. BEST R. R., Surg. Gynec. Obstet., 1944, **78**, 425.

4. Bove P., Oliviera M., Speranzini M., Gastroenterology, 1963, **44**, *3*, 251.
5. Burlui D., Ratziu O., Presse méd., 1969, **77**, *46*, 1671.
6. Cachera A., Caroli J., Bolgert M., *Maladies du foie, des voies biliaires du pancréas*, Flammarion, Paris, 1951.
7. Caroli J., *Les ictères par rétention*, Masson, Paris, 1959.
8. Caroli J., Corcos V., *Maladies des voies biliaires intrahépatiques segmentaires*, Masson, Paris, 1964.
9. Celice J., Grossiord A., Castaigne P., Bull. Mém. Soc. Méd. Hôp., Paris, 1964, **62**, 296.
10. Champeau M., Arch. Mal. Appar digest., 1960, **49**, 81; Mém. Acad. Chir., 1966, **92**, 1415.
11. Chiray M., Albot G., Thiebault F., Demartial L., Ann. Anat. path., 1938, **15**, 88.
12. Cormier J., Albot G., Bydlowski, R., Arch. Mal. Appar. digest., 1962, **51**, 737.
13. Couinaud C., Ann. Chir., 1963, **17**, *19*, 1249.
14. Couinaud C., Ann. Chir., 1963, **17**, 19.
15. Firică Th., Crișan L., Rădulescu M., Bărbat N., Kelemen V., *Considerații asupra intervențiilor chirurgicale pe regiunea oddiană* in *A IX-a Sesiune științifică I.M.F. București, 22—23 Nov. 1963*, p. 10.
16. Florent R., Charpin R., Presse méd., 1961, **69**, 1435.
17. Fogarty T. J., Krippaehne W., Dennis D., Fletcher W., Amer. J. Surg., 1968, **116**, *2*, 177.
18. Futorian E., Subin B., Khirurghiya (Moscow), 1961, **10**, 37.
19. Gerota D., Florea P., Stăncescu M., Popa Gh., Georgescu P., Chirurgia, 1965, **14**, *3*, 219.
20. Glasianov G. G., Khirurghiya (Moscow), 1961, **12**, 115.
21. Glenn F., Moody G., Ann. Surg. 1961, **153**, 711.
22. Glenn F., Moody F. G., Ann. Surg., 1961, **153**, 711.
23. Graham H. F., Ann. Surg., 1932, **96**, 154.
24. Guillemin G., Girard M., Cuilleret J., Dargent D., Lyon chir., 1966, **61**, *5*, 769.
25. Hardy J. D., J. Pediatrics, 1961, **59**, 265.
26. Hepp J., Couinaud C., Presse méd., 1956, **64**, 947.
27. Hepp J., Isserlis G., Ann. Chir., 1959, **13**, 1065.
28. Hepp J., Pernod R., Hautefeuille P., Ann. Chir., 1963, **17**, *17—18*, 1121.
29. Huang Chi Ch'Iang, Chin. Med. J., 1959, **79**, 40.
30. Huang Chi Ch' Iang, Huang Wen, Liu Ting Chien, Yang Chiang-Fei, Chin. Med. J., 1962, **81**, 287.
31. Huart P., Autret J., Ton That Tung, Bull. Soc. Méd. Chir. Indochine, 1937, 903.
32. Jud E. S., Burden V. C., Surg. Gynec. Obstet., 1926, **42**, 322.
33. Kourias B., Mém. Acad. Chir., 1950, **86**, *9*, 274.
34. Kourias B., *La lithiase intrahépatique*, Soc. Chir., Lyon, 10 March 1966.
35. Léger L., Zara M., Arvay D., Presse méd., 1952, **60**, 936.
36. Lewisohn J., Ann. Surg., 1916, **63**, 535 ; Ann. Surg., 1922, 283.
37. Maki T., Arch. Surg., 1961, **82**, 599.
38. Mallet-Guy P., Froment R., Dancez R., Rev. Méd. Chir. Mal. Foie, 1936, **6**, 97.
39. Mirizzi P. L., *Lithiase de la voie biliaire principale*, Masson, Paris, 1962.
40. Mirizzi P. L., *Chirurgie du système du canal hépatique. Lésions bénignes*, Masson, Paris, 1962.
41. Mouchet A., Marquand J., Mém. Acad. Chir., 1960, **86**, 380.
42. Olivier Cl., *Chirurgie des voies biliaires extra- et intrahépatiques*, Masson, Paris, 1961.
43. Pap S., Zbl. Chir. **88**, *22*, 553.
44. Pedinielli M., Mém. Acad. Chir. Paris, 1957, **83**, *31*, 951.
45. Petresco M., Ann. Anat. Path., Paris, 1932, 663.
46. Porumbaru I., *Litiaza intrahepatică*, Communicated at the Society of Surgery, Bucharest, 2 July 1963.
47. Puestow C. B., Surg. Clin. North Amer., 1934, **14**, 947.
48. Richard C. A., Lortat-Jacob J. L., Fekete F., Maillard J. N., Ann. Chir., 1962, **16**, 1017.
49. Rufanov G., Ann. Surg., 1936, **103**, 321 and 580.
50. Santy P., Mallet-Guy P., Lyon Chir., 1936, **33**, 257.
51. Sénèque J., Chatlin C., Mém. Acad. Chir., Paris, 1960, **86**, *10—11*, 310.

52. SEROR J., Mém. Acad. Chir., 1961, **87**, 823.
53. SHULMAN A. G., Surg. Gynec. Obstet., 1957, **104**, *4*, 504.
54. SORLIN L., *La lithiase des voies biliaires intrahépatiques*, Thesis, Lyon, 1934, p. 35.
55. SOUPAULT R., SULTAN R. A., Ann. Chir., 1959, **13**, 1049.
56. STAFFORD F. S., ISAACS J. P., Ann. Surg., 1958, **147**, 812—816.
57. TON THAT TUNG, *Chirurgie d'exérèse du foie*, Hanoi, 1962.
58. ŢURAI I., PAPAHAGI E., CIUREL M., ROSEALA E., CONSTANTINESCU M., DRAGNEV D., *Experienţa noastră în reintervenţiile pe căile biliare*. Communicated at the Interregional Meeting of Surgery, Bucharest, 28—29 May 1962.
59. VACHELL H. R., Stevens W., Brit. Med. J., 1906, **1**, 434.
60. VU THI CHIN (Nyguyen Dinh Nam), *La lithiase biliaire au Nord-Vietnam*, Thesis, Hanoi, 1952.

CHAPTER 6

LIVER ALTERATIONS DUE TO DIAPHRAGMATIC HERNIAS AND RELAXATIONS

DIAPHRAGMATIC HERNIAS

- Embryonic hernias of the liver

DIAPHRAGMATIC EVENTRATIONS

- Total diaphragmatic eventrations
Partial diaphragmatic relaxation
- The cervicodiaphragmatic syndrome (I. Făgărăşanu and N. Dobrovici Syndrome).

The left half of the diaphragm comes in contact, along its abdominal aspect, with the stomach, spleen, left liver lobe and left angle of the colon, organs situated in the left hypochondrium, whereas the right half of the diaphragm comes in contact along its abdominal aspect with a single organ, the liver.

A large gland, weighing about 1500 gm, with an elastic but fairly firm consistency, the liver may readily mask some of the congenital or acquired defects of this mobile partition which separates the abdominal from the thoracic cavity. It is perhaps for this reason that the defects of the right diaphragm are known to a lesser extent and considered in general rare, or at least rarer than the defects of the left diaphragm.

On the other hand, the defects of the left diaphragm are more difficult to bear, their clinical symptomatology drawing the physician's attention to this region of the body. In such cases, the clinical diagnosis is completed by radiologic examinations which reveal the presence of a congenital hernia, an acquired, a traumatic or non-traumatic hernia, or partial (paresis) or total eventration of the dome.

Displacement of the abdominal organs from the left hypochondrium towards the thorax, where they are drawn up by the difference in pressure between the two cavities, brings about a complex, acute or at times attenuated symptomatology, which is however annoying enough to draw the doctor's or the radiologist's attention.

With defects of the right diaphragm, the liver alone is involved, and the symptomatology widely differs.

DIAPHRAGMATIC HERNIAS

Embryonic hernias of the liver. In large, embryonic congenital defects, communication between the abdomen and right hemithorax is open because of total or partial aplasia of the diaphragm, the pleura continuing the peritoneum without any partition or a hardly perceptible one. In these embryonic malformations in which the pleuroperitoneal folds have not developed and joined together because of the absence of coalescence between the *septum transversum*, pleuropericardial lamina and Uskow's pillar, the organs of the abdominal cavity occupy the thoracic cavity, compressing the lung, preventing normal hematosis and displacing the mediastinum. The newborn child is asphyxiated and generally dies at birth or within the first few days, when the gases swallowed into the stomach and intestine increase compression of the intrathoracic organs (Potter). These are true congenital intrathoracic hernias, without a sac.

On the right side, the only organ that can be drawn up into the thoracic cavity is the liver, which may be found in such cases occupying the right hemithorax together with the lung. The liver is rotated with its lower aspect turned forward. This is also observed in eventration of the right diaphragm; the dorsopetal liver described by Didanski may be accounted for by this acquired or congenital diaphragmatic defect.

If the defect is partial and the congenital hernia is reduced to the right posterolateral portion, part of the right lobe of the liver may protrude into the thorax. This is compatible with a normal development of the newborn child and the diaphragmatic defect with partial hernia of the liver may pass unobserved for several years, until radioscopy or radiography performed for an altogether different purpose reveals the bilobate aspect of the right liver, partly protruding intrathoracically, as in the case reported by Chester.

DIAPHRAGMATIC EVENTRATIONS

Diaphragmatic eventrations, more frequently known as *fetal hernias*, are as a matter of fact diaphragmatic relaxations, paresis or eventration.

According to appearances, these cannot be of congenital origin, but are acquired at a given moment in life; the serous, peritoneal and pleural leaves are in apposition over their entire diaphragmatic surface, the two cavities thus being completely separated from each other. Moreover, traces of degenerated muscular fibers and fibrous tissue were found on the histologic sections. This finding invalidates the hypothesis of the congenital origin of these defects. The name of fetal hernia does not appear appropriate, neither is the term of congenital hernia with sac, as the sac is actually only the diaphragm, which has no muscular elements but is reduced to a fibroconnective partition lined by a serous membrane on both aspects. This defect, which we prefer to call *diaphragmatic relaxation (relaxatio diaphragmatis)*, may involve both the right and the left diaphragm, but is considered more frequent on the left side, the same as congenital hernias. They are almost always acquired, their congenital origin being very difficult to demonstrate. For the same reasons as mentioned above, we believe that total or partial diaphragmatic eventrations are just as frequent on the right side, but the defect is more readily masked by the liver.

In *total diaphragmatic eventrations* the liver may be drawn high up in the thoracic cavity, the diaphragmatic dome bulging up to the level of the 3rd and even 2nd rib. In such cases, intraoperative findings show a liver turned with its lower margin frontwards, above the costal margin (sometimes 4—6 finger breadths). This anatomic position of the liver may give rise to serious problems in the course of procedures on the gallbladder, bile ducts or hepatic parenchyma, as encountered in a recent case.

Didanski described two morphologic types, related to the constitutional type: the *ventropetal liver*, characteristic of the longiline type, with the convex aspect coming in contact with the abdominal wall and the posterior aspect facing backward, and the *dorsopetal liver*, characteristic of the breviline type in which the convex aspect is turned more towards the spinal column and dorsolumbar region and the inferior aspect faces forward. This rotation of the liver described in the dorsopetal type by Didanski corresponds to our findings in patients with total, right, diaphragmatic eventration.

These relaxations may have several pathogenic causes: surgical (phrenicectomy) or acquired lesions of the right phrenic nerve, degenerative lesions of the diaphragm due to pleurisy (tuberculous, etc.), subdiaphragmatic infections followed by pus collections, perihepatitis, etc.

In case of injury of the phrenic nerve or one of its roots, which may result in total or partial diaphragmatic relaxation, the lesions must be looked for in the cervical region, at the origin of the phrenic nerve roots.

In other cases, neuritis of the phrenic nerve may be caused by a tumor at the base of the neck or disease of the pleural cupola, generally of tuberculous origin.

Total relaxation of the right diaphragm, followed by rotation of the whole liver towards the thoracic cavity has not formed the subject of special investigations, since both clinicians and surgeons have been preoccupied by the surgical solutions rather than by finding a pathogenic explanation of these abnormal cases.

Partial diaphragmatic relaxation (eventration) is more frequent and important than the former. Only part of the diaphragm is deprived of active muscles, the other part being completely normal. The relaxed part is transformed into a fibroserous membrane sharply delimited from the remaining diaphragm.

This aspect has led several authors to consider partial eventrations as diaphragmatic hernias with a sac, the healthy part of the diaphragm giving the impression of a hernial ring around the sac. Histologic examinations demonstrated the presence of atrophic, degenerated muscular fibers, therefore not a hernial sac, but part of the diaphragm that has lost its contractility due to regional atrophic degeneration of the diaphragmatic musculature.

The organs of the abdominal cavity, i.e. the liver in case of the right diaphragm, pushed upward by abdominal pressure and drawn by the pleural vacuum, mould the thoracic cavity and give the convex side of the liver a hemispheric, mammillated aspect, sharply delimited, and which has been described by radiologists under different names: "cupola", "brioche", "sunrise", "mosque window". For many years it was considered as a pathognomonic sign of hydatid cyst of the convex aspect of the liver.

These images, that usually appear on the anterointernal part of the right diaphragm, at times along the midline but never at the periphery of the diaphragmatic muscle, close to the insertion of the ribs, raise serious problems of differential diagnosis. This detail is worthy of note, since it is of the greatest importance in the pathogeny of these partial relaxations, which affect the convex aspect of the liver.

The diaphragm receives both a peripheral innervation through the intercostal nerves (the 6th, 7th and 8th pair) and a central one through the phrenic nerve which has its roots at the level of the conjugate foramina of vertebrae C3—C4, C4 — C5, C5 — C6. Moreover, it also receives additional connections from the brachial plexus; when the latter is sectioned it produces total unilateral diaphragmatic paralysis, the dome is entirely raised and immobile. Its stimulation produces a converse aspect that corresponds to hypertonia. Phrenic and intercostal nervous stimuli govern the function of the diaphragm. These stimulations may be synergic, in which case contraction or relaxation takes place only in segments, in a reduced number of muscular fibers. When this asynergic stimulation occurs within the phrenic nerve, as for instance after partial section of the nerve or of one of its roots, after alcoholization or congealing, crushing, etc., the activity of some of the nervous fibers is totally abolished and the radiologic image will show partial diaphragmatic protrusions that correspond to paresis or paralysis of the muscular fibers depending upon these nervous fibers.

These findings, checked by us in experiments on rabbits and dogs, led us to assume the likelihood of such pseudocystic images induced by injuries or rheumatic lesions in the cervical region (diskarthrosis, spondylarthrosis, etc.), or by injury of the phrenic nerve along its pathway to the diaphragm, by a disease at the base of the neck such as an osteoma of the cervical column, or a cervical rib, etc., or bacillary or tumoral lesions of the pulmonary or pleural apex, lesions that alter the structure of the phrenic nerve.

Our first two cases, diagnosed as "hydatid cyst" in view of the pseudocystic radiologic image obtained and in which the true cause was only detected intraoperatively, i.e. diaphragmatic paresis with a pseudohernial sac, determined us to seek for the existence of cervical or apical lesions in all such cases. Similarly, a pneumoperitoneum which might reveal the persistence or disappearance of the assumed cystic images following gaseous detachment of the liver from the diaphragm, appeared to be absolutely necessary before any surgical intervention.

In this way we were able to detect, together with N. Dobrovici, numerous cases in which the pseudocystic image of the right diaphragm corresponded to cervical spondylodiskarthrosis, with posterior osteophytes that damaged one or two roots of the phrenic nerve and could be detected on the right sideviews of the spinal column, in which the conjugate vertebral foramina clearly appear like so many "keyholes" (Fig. 127).

In some cases, the radicular or trunkular neuritic lesions were caused by the existence of cervical ribs or by osteochondroma of the spinal column. In another case, sclerous pleuropulmonary bacillary lesions of the right pulmonary apex encompassed the phrenic nerve, accounting for the phenomena of diaphragmatic paresis.

In many of these cases in which pneumoperitoneum was systematically performed, the polycyclic image disappeared over the convex aspect of the liver but persisted at the level of the diaphragm, following insufflation with oxygen or carbon dioxide in the abdominal cavity. This sign is sufficiently conclusive to invalidate the diagnosis of hydatid cyst or hepatic tumor of the convex aspect of the liver (Fig. 128).

The cervicodiaphragmatic syndrome. These findings, evidence of which was supplied by us (I. Făgărăşanu and N. Dobrovici), represent a true cervicodiaphragmatic syndrome. The coexistence of certain articular or bony lesions, chiefly of rheumatic origin, at the level of the cervical column, with partial relaxation of the diaphragm and in which pneumoperitoneum supplies evidence of the disappearance of the hepatic tumor, are the main elements of this syndrome, also checked by other authors following our publications.

The diagnostic value of this syndrome has been repeatedly verified. However, in some cases the hepatic pseudocystic image did not disappear at the pneumoperitoneum, and explorative laparotomy was performed. Puncture of the liver at the level of the cysts showed in some cases the absence of any cyst or tumor, persistence of the bulging being due to increased hepatic consistence caused by sclerogenous hepatitis or edema induced by cholostasis or blood stasis, etc. Of late, the use of hepatic scintigrams also eliminated this error coefficient, as for instance patient *M.I.*, aged 53, who was referred to the clinic with a diagnosis of hydatid cyst. The cervical roentgenogram and hepatic scintigram pointed to right

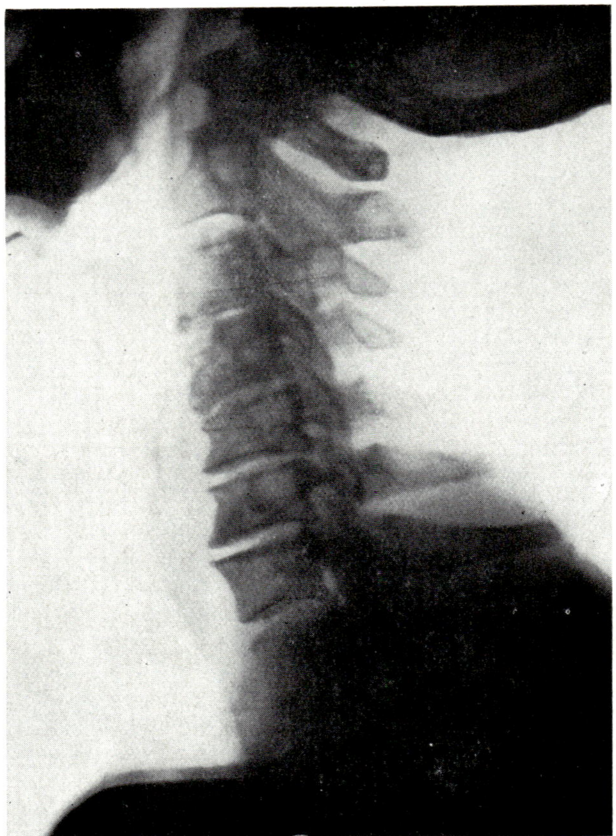

Fig. 127. — Case *M.I.*, 53 years. Roentgenogram of the cervical column, left side view. Spondyldiskarthrosis with posterior osteophytes at C_4 — C_5 and C_5 — C_6 level.

diaphragmatic relaxation (Fig. 129) due to cervical spondylarthrosis. The patient was not operated.

The *positive diagnosis* of hepatic pseudocysts, also called "phantom cysts", for which many surgeons, and we too, have interfered uselessly, should be based upon elimination of the diagnosis of echinococcosis by laboratory tests — eosinogram, Casoni test —, etc. These two laboratory tests are not, however, pathognomonic and may be positive in cases without hydatid cyst, or negative in cases with hydatid cyst. In more than 50% of the cases of false images studied by us, eosinophilia exhibited increased values, which are also encountered in other parasitic diseases, such as helminthiasis and trichinosis, and in skin diseases — eczemas, psoriasis, pemphigus — , or allergic diseases, serum diseases, asthma, etc.

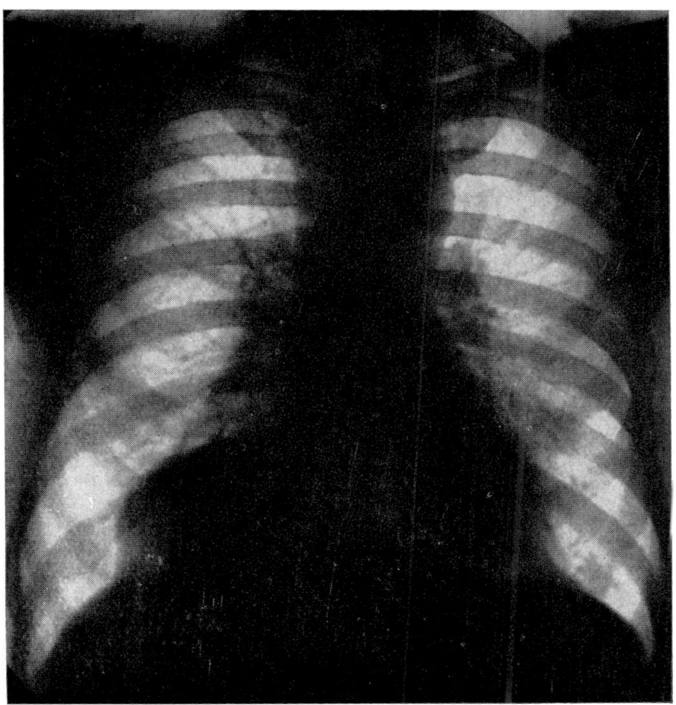

Fig. 128. — Frontal view of the diaphragmatic region shows a double swelling that does not disappear after institution of the pneumoperitoneum (partial paresis of the right diaphragm, confirmed by hepatic scintigram).

The Casoni test is considered as specific in the diagnosis of hydatid cyst, but the results obtained by us were inconclusive, being positive in cases in which no cyst was found at the intervention.

The radiologic examination alone is not able to show whether the defect of the diaphragm is due to a cyst, or whether a false image has been obtained. Pneumoperitoneum gives a more precise answer but is not infallible, since it may point to the existence of a cyst that is only the cast of the liver upon the partial diaphragmatic eventration, which may persist even after gaseous insufflation.

When hepatic scintigraphy does not clearly outline the existence of a cyst or a tumor, then explorative laparotomy should be resorted to as the only means of establishing the diagnosis.

The differential diagnosis should have in view diseases of the right lung, diaphragm, pleura, pericardium and liver. In some cases this is more difficult when a pseudocystic formation is not envisaged and a radiologic examination of the cervical columm (front and side views) and diaphragmatic region are not performed, together with pneumoperitoneum.

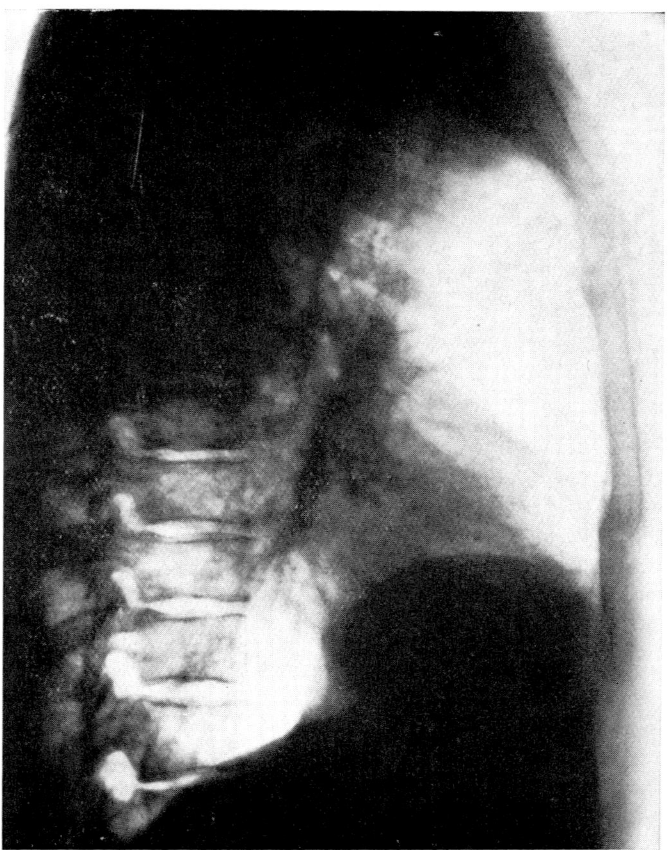

Fig. 129. — Side radiography of the patient from figure 128.

In one of the cases treated by us, a diagnosis of hydatid cyst of the lower lobe of the right lung had been made. Thoracotomy performed in a thoracic surgical department revealed the absence of a pulmonary cyst, but as bulging of the diaphragm appeared to indicate a cyst of the upper aspect of the liver, the patient was referred to us for an abdominal intervention.

The laboratory tests being uncertain (6% eosinophilia, slightly positive Casoni test), laparotomy was performed. No cyst or tumoral formation was found, only partial diaphragmatic eventration. This case is demonstrative of the difficulties encountered in establishing the differential diagnosis, especially when pneumoperitoneum, cervical radiography and scintigram of the liver are not systematically performed.

In conclusion, a protruding right diaphragm cannot be considered as a certain sign of hydatid cyst of the liver or of the lung, demanding a thoracotomy.

Pneumoperitoneum should be applied whenever we are not absolutely certain of the existence of a hydatid cyst. The diagnosis only appears certain after several images of hydatid cyst of the liver are obtained, or when the presence of a hydatid cyst is found in another region or organ, or in cases of recurrent cyst, when a new cyst should immediately be suspected. In long-standing, infected cysts with a perihepatic reaction, the adhesions between the liver and the diaphragm prevent the gases from penetrating below the latter, rendering the pneumoperitoneum inoperative.

Partial paresis or relaxation of the right diaphragmatic muscle are in most cases caused by pseudocystic images. These relaxations are due, as already shown, to neuritic lesions of the right phrenic nerve or its roots, caused by injury to the spinal column or rheumatism (spondylosis, spondylodiskarthrosis with posterior osteophytes, fragmentary fractures of the cervical vertebrae, etc.) or other diseases of this region, such as osteochondroma, hypertrophy of the transverse process of the 7th cervical vertebra, lesions of the pulmonary apex or pleural cupola, of tuberculous origin in most cases.

These defects of the right diaphragm are of particular diagnostic interest. They seldom give rise to disturbances that necessitate special surgical interventions, as those occurring on the left side which may cause accentuated displacement of the stomach, distorsion *(volvulus)* with its severe consequent gastrointestinal disturbances.

Attention has been drawn to these diaphragmatic defects because they may influence the morphology of the liver and because they should be taken into consideration on establishing the differential diagnosis.

In total relaxation of the diaphragm, its plication (V. Buţureanu) or a nylon network sewn over the margins of the chest wall may bring the liver into its normal position (B.V. Petrovskiy). In partial relaxation, repair of the defect by endothoracic approach is often useless.

REFERENCES

1. Balgairies E., Aupetit J., Amondru C., Grailles M., J. Radiol. Electrol., 1957, **38**, *3—4*, 213.
2. Constantin I., J. Radiol., 1950, *7—8*, 513.
3. Charpin J., Taranger J., Presse méd., 1951, **59**, *5*, 93.
4. Curtillet E., Aubaniac R., J. Chir., Paris, 1950, **66**, *4*, 257.
5. Drouet P. L., Faivre G., De Ren G., Lamy P., Antoine V., J. Radiol. Electrol., 1951, **32**, *9—10*, 845.
6. Drouet P. L., Frank V., Lamy P., Arnoult G., J. franç. Méd. Chir. thor., 1954, *4*, 358.
7. Dorfman L. L., Nikiforova E. I., Vestn. Rentghenol. Radiol., 1956, **31**, *4*, 71.
8. Debray G., Hardouin J. P., Rev. Prat., 1956, **6**, *23*, 2517.
9. Făgărăşanu I., Bujor C. I., Lonchiar L., Florea C., Chirurgia, 1961, **10**, *2*, 191.
10. Făgărăşanu I., Bujor C. I., Aloman D., *Aspecte clinice şi terapeutice ale herniilor diafragmatice*, Communicated at the Society of Surgery, 8 Dec. 1963.

11. Făgărășanu I., Bujor C. I., Bucur A., *Masele plastice în tratamentul operator al herniilor și eventrațiilor* in *Probleme de Chirurgie și Ortopedie*, Ed. Acad., Bucharest, 1964, p. 41—51.
12. Făgărășanu I., Bujor C. I., Lonchiar L., *Procedeu personal pentru cura operatorie a herniei hiatale*, Communicated at the Society of Surgery, 17 Jan. 1961.
13. Făgărășanu I., Dobrovici N., Med. int., 1957, *1*, 36.
14. Făgărășanu I., Bujor C. I., Lonchiar L., Presse méd., 1962, *12*, 585.
15. Făgărășanu I., Dobrovici N., Probl. Terap., vol. V, 1957, p. 89.
16. Jmur V. A., Buianov V. M., Vestn. Khir., 1959, *4*, 71.
17. Laurence G., Rev. Prat., 1956, **6**, *23*, 2561.
18. Laurence G., Rev. Prat., 1956, **6**, *23*, 2497.
19. Petrovskiy B. V., Babichev S. I., Nicolaev N. O., Khirurghiya, 1958, *12*, 26.
20. Quénu J., Moreaux J., Rev. Prat., 1956, **6**, *23*, 2547.
21. Roux M., Robin V., Le Bihan V., J. franç. Méd. Chir. thor., 1955, **9**, *2*, 181.
22. Roche J., Conos B., Dreiger Ch., Dufer V., J. franç. Méd. Chir. thor., 1954, *2*, 147.
23. Rațiu O., Vasilescu D., Teju Gh., Chirurgia, 1959, **8**, *2*, 271.
24. Thomeret G., Rollin G., J. franç. Méd. Chir. thor., 1954, *2*, 155.
25. Țurai I., Papahagi E., Maximilian V., Ciochină C., Ștefănescu V., Jercan Albu M., Petrescu C., Chirea B., Rosala E., Chirurgia, 1959, *4*, p. 489—498.

CHAPTER 7

HYDATID CYSTS OF THE LIVER

The problem of hydatidosis has increasingly been dealt with in the medical literature during the last few years. The incidence of the disease has increased in several countries and has become a problem not only in South America, Australia and North Africa, but also in Europe, especially in the countries of the Mediterranean Sea and the Balkans.

Important foci were detected in South America, Canada, Alaska and the Mediterranean Basin. In Uruguay the annual incidence is of 1520 cases and in Chile (Neghume et al., 1956) of 8.7 cases per 100,000 inhabitants.

T. Simitsch analyzed the incidence of hydatidosis in several eastern and southern European countries and found an incidence of 7.3 per 100,000 inhabitants in Greece (Marecas, 1957), 3.37 per 100,000 in Yugoslavia (Simitsch, 1957), 2.88 per 100,000 in Bulgaria (Matof, 1955), and a very low incidence in Poland (Stefanschi, 1956 — cited by Lupaşcu-Panaitescu, 1968).

In Romania, cases of hydatidosis were already reported in the middle of the last century, but no conclusive statistics existed for a long time. The number of cases during the last years ranged from 1735 cases in 1935 to 806 cases in 1956 and 750 in 1968, according to Gh. Lupaşcu and D. Panaitescu. During the last 10 years (1958—1968) there were 7609 cases with an annual average of 738.4 cases or 5.6 per 100,000 inhabitants.

In some areas the incidence is very high. Teodorescu (1958) found at necropsy in the hospital of Constanţa 12 undiagnosed hydatid cysts in 1866 post-mortem examinations. A comparatively high incidence was also reported among animals. The numerous cases reported in the regions of Cluj, Suceava, Bacău, Craiova, Galaţi and Constanţa are related, according to Lupaşcu, to the increase in the number of cattle in these regions.

In view of the wide spread of the disease, the International Association of Hydatidosis of Montevideo (Uruguay) initiated several world congresses, starting in 1951 in Alger, then Santiago de Chile, Madrid, Athens and Rome.

The conclusions of these congresses may be summed up as follows: in spite of the progress made, especially in the surgical treatment, hydatidosis still remains a severe parasitic disease that raises many problems.

It is true that in most cases the location of the hydatid cyst in humans may be considered as benign due to the progress of surgery, but the proportion on invalidity among the operated patients is still very high and hydatidosis still is a complex problem today and the subject of numerous investigations.

✦

According to most statistics, human hydatidosis appears to be localized in two thirds of the cases in the liver. In Romania, too, the hepatic localization of the hydatid cyst is the most frequent, but an increase has been observed in the pulmonary locations. Both older (Iacobovici, 1933 and 1942) and more recent statistics (Nana, Făgărăşanu, Buţureanu) report a proportion of 40 to 56% hepatic localizations, and in several regional statistics (Teodorescu in Constanţa and Anastasiu-Mocanu in Galaţi) proportions of 58% and respectively 52% were found.

The problem of the diagnosis and treatment of hydatid cysts will be dealt with in this chapter on the basis of our experience in 315 cases of hepatic cysts followed up over a 10-year period.

HISTORY

Although described many centuries ago by Hippocrates (463—357 b.C.), Aretacus (9—79 A.D.), Galenus (130—200 A.D.) and many others, the etiology of the hydatid disease remained unknown up to the end of the 18th century. In 1781, Pallas suggested that the disease in humans was transmitted by animals. The next year, Goeze, who carried out a detailed microscopic study, established the parasitic origin of the disease.

The hypothesis of Pallas was confirmed 40 years later, in 1821, by Bremmeser (Vienna) who identified the hydatid cysts found in man to those observed in animals.

The experimental stage continued with Von Siebold who was able between 1852 and 1854 to follow up the developmental stages of one of the phases of the disease and obtained experimentally the adult echinococcus incriminated as causing the disease. However, the whole evolutionary cycle of the parasite was not demonstrated until ten years later. In 1862, Leuckhard and Heubner gave a detailed description of the entire cycle, and reproduced the larval form in suckling pigs. During the following years the double developmental cycle of *Echinococcus granulosus* was established: the adult form in dogs and other carnivorous animals and the larval, cystic form in herbivorous animals, especially domestic, and in man. However, clinical experience was often contradictory.

Some doctors reported on dissemination of the disease following rupture of the cyst (J. Hunter, 1786; Budd, 1857); others, based upon clinical and parasitologic facts, rejected this hypothesis. Budd is the first who considered that certain hydatid cysts were secondary to an initial cyst in the liver. At that time, Davaine and Neiser considered this hypothesis incompatible with the known fact on the evolution of cestodes.

Others, among whom Cruveilhier, brought clinical arguments against the possible dissemination by rupture of the hydatid cyst and discharge of the fluid, which implicitly resulted in death.

R. Bright (1861) raised the question of the risk of puncturing the cyst because of the hazard of intraabdominal dissemination. Seven years later, the Danish surgeon I. Finsen communicated 11 cases of relapses following interventions for hydatid cysts opened in the course of the operation and recommended isolation of the cyst by suture before the puncture. Volkmann showed that seeding was the greatest risk.

The end of the 19th century must be considered as a turning point in the clinical understanding of the disease. In 1897, at the Congress of Surgery held in Moscow, Bobrov and Tokarenko approached the problem of hydatidosis from several angles. A year later, the works of Bobrov were confirmed by one of his coworkers, Alexinski, who demonstrated the possibility of producing multiple hydatid cysts in the peritoneal cavity not only by daughter cysts but also by proligerous capsules and scolices, representing the asexuate cycle of the echinococcus.

At the beginning of the 19th century, Devé, likewise on the basis of experimental findings, showed the possible vesiculous transformation of the scolices, i.e. the so-called hydatid sand. He coined the notion of "secondary echinococcosis" and broadened the sphere of research by furnishing interesting data concerning migration of the parasite, with hydatid allergy and anaphylaxis.

After the works of Devé, the progress made in this disease referred especially to the diagnosis and clinical aspects.

Of particular interest among the older observations are those of Bühl (1852) who described a tumor process, as a rule hepatic, with a malignant, invasive, necrosing course that he called alveolar echinococcosis. Virchow assumed the parasitic origin of the disease. Although more than a hundred years have elapsed since then, our knowledge of the disease has shown no outstanding progress. Some consider it a common echinococcosis with a different mode of evolution, under different climatic conditions; Rausch, Schiller and Vogel sustain that it is due to an echinococcus transmitted by the fox.

In three cases treated by us, the invasive and necrosing character of a formation with microvesicles led us to suspect an alveolar echinococcosis. No anatomopathologic or parasitologic evidence was found in the disease. The formations found in the left lobe were accompanied by cysts in the right lobe (2 cases) and quadrate lobe (1 case).

Anaphylactic studies have thrown a new light on some of the clinical aspects and accidents of echinococcosis. The wide scale use of radiology led to the discovery of some direct and indirect signs which facilitate the diagnosis. The modern approach in the hydatid disease is linked to the progress made in radiology.

In 1912, Tomasso Casoni developed a biologic method of diagnosis of human hydatidosis. No further progress was made in this direction, in spite of the various tests devised (flocculation, hemagglutination, complement fixation).

Today the treatment of hydatid cysts is predominantly surgical. The first cases of surgical interest were published by Bertherard (Algeria) over a hundred years ago and by Vincent some 30 years later, who obtained the first conclusive results in hepatic hydatid cysts.

At first, before broad operations of the liver were carried out, surgery consisted in puncture and evacuation of the cysts (Murlati, 1864; Ette, 1833); following the use of Delbeau's tube (1856), Heidelberg and Verneuil introduced through the tube or the puncture needle an irritating substance after evacuation of the cystic contents.

Surgery proper started with Kircher, one of Lindemann's coworkers who operated hydatid cysts in a single stage after its isolation from the peritoneal cavity by suture. This method stands at the basis of the intervention of Lindemann and Landau known under the name of marsupialization. The same procedure was recommended by Volkmann.

Attempts were then made to solve the question of the remaining cavity. Bobrov, then Thornthon, tried to suture the remaining pouch and abandon it in the peritoneal cavity. The method developed in 1890, without drainage, with or without capitonnage (Bond, 1891).

Gradually the question of cystectomies and pericystectomies was approached more daringly, and cystic or hepatic resections were performed.

An important contribution was brought by Romanian surgery in the problem of hydatid cysts of the liver. G. Severeanu successfully operated hydatid cysts of the liver and lung and published interesting reports.

Toma Ionescu likewise dealt with this problem and discussed 80 cases in 8 different papers. In 1900, at the International Congress of Medical Science held in Paris, he read a joint report on the "Surgical Treatment of Hydatid Cysts of the Liver". At that time he already practiced suture of the cystic cavity and marsupialization, and later on developed a series of techniques in which the elements of modern surgery can be discerned.

Iacobovici published interesting statistics in 1910—1913 and then again in 1933—1942, discussing 66 cases of hepatic cysts and referring to the casuistics of the Clinic of Surgery, Cluj, including 325 cases of echinococcosis, of which 48% had hepatic localization. The techniques used did not differ much from those described in the world literature. Buţureanu published statistics of 150 cases, of which 66 hepatic localizations, and Teodorescu 264 cases, over a three year period, of which 90% had hepatic localization.

The variety of surgical approaches is very great and should be based on a close understanding of the pathologic physiology of hydatidosis and of hepatobiliary physiology. Only in this manner can we expect to select the most adequate method not only for survival of the patient, but also for preventing late sequelae connected with the subsequent course of the parasitic disease, or the hepatobiliary consequences of the intervention. Hence we consider it of interest to start with the peculiarities of the parasitic disease itself.

BIOLOGY OF THE PARASITE

The hepatic hydatid cyst is a localization of the hydatid disease in the liver, as encountered in humans and animals produced by the tumor, vesicular development of the larva of *Echinococcus granulosus* Goeze 1782; *Taenia echinococcus* Von Siebold 1835; *Echinococcus echinococcociferus* Wieland 1861.

We do not intend to go into the details of the double life of these cestodes which takes place in two different animal species. This parasite belongs to the *Platyhelminthes phylum*, Cestoda order, and is an entozoon parasite.

Normal evolution. The host of this entozoon is as a rule the dog, more seldom the fox, wolf or cat.

The host harbours in its large intestine hundreds of these minute cestodes, formed of 3—4 segments not exceeding 3—6 mm in length. It has no digestive system of its own and the food passes through its cuticula. The last segment that reaches maturity measures about 2 mm; it breaks off and is eliminated with the feces. This proglottis contains 400 to 800 embryophore eggs placed within a striate cuticula, the *oncosphere* or *hexacanth embryo.*

The latter resists for a long time under unfavorable conditions and may reach the intestine of the intermediary host by direct or indirect contamination (polluted drinking water or infested vegetables).

The list of intermediary herbivorous animals is very long: sheep, oxen, pigs, donkeys, horses, goats, etc. Once it has reached the intermediary host, the embryo migrates by blood route and reaches different organs. The hexacanth embryo is only released in an alkaline medium, as proved by Devé, Martin and Rosse, therefore after leaving the duodenum-jejunum and not under the action of the gastric juice as believed at first.

The echinococcus penetrates within the thickness of the intestinal mucosa, where it casts off its six hooks, passes into the lumen of several veins and is then carried by the blood flow to the portal vein, similar to a microscopic embolus, and transplanted as a rule into the liver, since the liver is essentially a filter. In other cases, due to its malleability it manages to pass through the liver and is borne by the blood flow, or the lymph according to others, to other organs.

In the organ it has reached, the embryo undergoes a cystic degeneration and is transformed into an echinococcal vesicle or hydatid cyst, which is at first sterile but subsequently becomes fertile by internal budding of the germinal layer, an asexuate, agamic evolution taking place. The buds become brood capsules with minute scolices within them.

The formed cyst is like a pouch full of fluid, with a fine cuticula, formed of overlying concentric, highly elastic lamina, impermeable to microbes and large albumin molecules, but permeable to crystalloids and the toxalbumins produced by the cyst. This cuticula is lined by a brood capsule that is granulous and only slightly resistant. The clear hydatid fluid that fills the cyst is sterile as long as the cuticula remains intact. Once infected, it is an extremely favorable medium for the development of microbes, readily producing suppuration of the cyst. When the hydatid, which is at first only a cavity full of fluid, reaches the size of a pigeon's egg (5—6 months), proligerous vesicles attached to the walls fall into the cavity and form hydatid sand. According to some authors, the large number of daughter cysts reflects suffering of the cyst. When the resistance of the host organism is greater, more daughter cysts are formed and for this reason hydatid cysts are more frequent in the liver than in the lungs.

When a dog ingests the viscera of an animal containing fertile hydatid cysts (with proligerous vesicles), the scolices come out of the vesicles and fix themselves on the villi of the small intestine of the dog where the echinococcus develops, thus bringing to a close the "large cycle" (Devé). Therefore, from the dog intestine it passes into the herbivorous animal in the form of a hexacanth embryo and reaches the viscera where it becomes a hydatid cyst; from here the scolices again reach the dog and the cycle rebegins.

Lesser evolution. Devé also demonstrated the existence of a lesser echinococcal cycle following rupture of the hydatid cyst and release into the organism of hydatid sand containing hexacanth embryos, which produce secondary echinococcosis, hence a seeding starting from the first localization. This sometimes renders difficult location of the initial cyst, especially as the secondary cysts may be the source of further seedings. Rupture of a hydatid cyst in the liver into the vena cava may give rise to multiple pulmonary embolisms.

This secondary seeding is one of the causes of the polymorphism of the disease. From a single voluminous intravisceral cyst, up to the numerous minute vesicles of the bones, the most unexpected and varied localizations may be observed with functional consequences.

Involution of the cyst. Involution of the cyst, once it has reached the stage of maturity, may occur. Pressure falls, the membrane detaches from the adventitia and a space is formed. The membrane withers, fissures, the daughter cysts flatten out, the fluid becomes turbid and thickens into magma. The cyst is no longer fertile and is reduced under pressure of the neighboring tissues that tolerate it as a foreign body. However, in this stage several of the scolices still maintain their vitality in some of the daughter cysts.

Calcification of the cyst. The hydatid may at times be calcified and, according to some authors, this represents a spontaneous recovery. However, in some cases calcification represents a source of severe complications. This must be kept account of in the operative approach, since such an empty cavity will not heal spontaneously. An older calcified cyst with a fissure into the bile ducts may have severe consequences upon the hepatic tissue, giving rise to actual cirrhosis of the liver due to cholostasis. If we also bear in mind the possible existence of still viable scolices in some of the daughter cysts, then the danger of such calcified hydatid cysts in the organism clearly appears. Calcification is a relatively long-standing process that begins by calcium depositions in the adventitia, which appear to favor the development of bile canaliculi fissures. These calcifications are not exclusively found in the liver, they also appear in other organs but are more frequent in the liver.

The hydatid fluid is richer in calcium than plasma (150—880 mg/liter as against 100 mg/liter) and hence in case of fissure the problem of perihydatid deposition naturally arises, the more intense the denser the tissues of the host organ. Therefore, a more accentuated tendency exists to calcification of the cysts in the liver.

Calcium impregnation of the pericystic adventitia may also exist in some younger hydatids, but a calcified cyst presupposes an older hydatid cyst with several successive layers of lime salts. Among our patients we found 8% calcified cysts (28 cases). All the patients were over the age of 35.

Frequency of hydatid cyst localizations in the human organism. Man only casually forms part of the cycle of the parasite. He is the victim of direct or indirect contamination, especially from dogs. The hexacanth embryo measures about 28 microns when it passes through the intestinal wall. The hepatic capillaries measure about 20 microns and hence the hepatic filter is the first to stop them. Devé demonstrated that the embryo is, however, very malleable and can become thinner, crossing the barrier into larger vessels and reaching the right heart and lungs. A new barrier then arises, that of the pulmonary capillaries which do not exceed 8 microns at this level.

Extrahepatic routes of dissemination are likewise possible, either by portacaval anastomoses or by lymphatic pathways. It is generally accepted that in 60% of the cases the site of the cysts is the liver, in 30% the lung, and in 10% the remaining organs; an important site is the brain, preceded only by the spleen and followed by the kidneys, pointing to the existence of a correlation between the site of the cyst and the richness of the vascularity. Cysts have not been reported on the walls of the gastrointestinal tract, with exception in one of our cases in which a cyst was found in the small intestine, as confirmed on examination of the wall sections.

SPECIFICS IN THE DEVELOPMENT OF THE HYDATID CYST IN THE LIVER

As long as the cyst is not infected, it progressively grows by centrifugal expansion to the detriment (condensation) of the host organ tissues. This condensation gives rise to the pericyst which is formed of three layers when it is to be found within the depth of the parenchyma. The inner layer is a sclerohyaline mass with fibrinoleukocytic deposits, then there is a connective layer and a layer of cells of the involved parenchyma, more altered the closer they are to the hydatid. When the process takes place towards the outer surface of the organ, no traces of the affected parenchyma tissue will be found, the pericyst being formed by connective tissue, Glisson's capsule and the peritoneum. It is the only area in which the pericyst resembles a "membrane". A massive vascularity surrounds the hydatid.

The liver appears to favor development of the cyst, but at a given moment opposes considerable resistance, far greater than that of the lung for instance. The initial infestations often exhibit a very slow evolution. Two of our patients were infested in childhood together with their brothers and sisters, but the disease became apparent only at the age of 24 and 29 respectively.

This latent evolution may sometimes be deduced when the patient comes from an endemic region he has long ago left and lives in an area where the disease is very rare. Some specialists, such as Devé, uphold that "infestation occurs before the age of 15 in one of two cases, and before the age of 30 in two of three cases". This also throws a light upon the incidence rate in terms of age. The highest frequency in our statistics was found in the 21—37 years age-group, followed by a second peak between the ages of 40 and 50. This is in agreement with the data of the Ministry of Health that shows the highest incidence between the ages of 20 and 40.

There are cases, however, in which the hydatid cyst develops very rapidly. One patient was operated 30 days after excision of the cysts by abdominal approach, in a first stage; the cyst left for the second stage had to be approached by transthoracic route, as the cyst had almost doubled its size in the meantime.

The variety of the anatomoclinical forms of the hepatic hydatid cyst is brought about by the location within the liver, the relationships with the bile ducts, vena porta, hepatic arteries and neighboring organs, and the evolutive stage of the parasite.

Relationship of the hydatid cyst to the bile system is one of the main problems to which this disease gives rise, with its anatomic, physiologic and clinical implications, which must be taken into consideration on studying the therapeutic solutions.

In the course of its excentric development in the liver, the parasite comes into conflict with the blood vessels, parenchyma and intrahepatic bile ducts. The bile canaliculi resist better to the pressure exercised by the cyst than the liver cells proper. The most severe and irritating consequences are linked to involvement of the bile ducts, located either in the immediate vicinity of the cyst or distally, at the level of the secondary or main bile ducts.

In the course of the development of the hydatid, the intrahepatic bile ducts are gradually included in the fibrosis process. The bile canaliculi are concentrated at the margin of the cyst, forming a pericystic network. The bile canaliculi and adventitia of the cyst being mutually conditioned (Bourgeon), the structural changes of the adventitia are directly related to the morphofunctional state of the compressed bile ducts and the state of the latter is linked to the degree of organization of the adventitia. The pericyst or periparasitic zone of visceral origin ceaselessly evolves, thickens, is infected, undergoes sequestration, is calcified. One may sometimes assist to the seeding of a new parasitic colony, a local secondary echinococcosis, as observed by us in 4 cases.

Case 117. Patient *C.M.*, aged 47, was admitted for recurrent hepatic hydatid cyst. He had been operated four times in other surgical departments, the last cystotomy with drainage of the remaining cavity being performed five months previously. Presenting signs: parietal fistula in the right hypochondrium through which bilious magma was discharged.

On opening the cyst, the pericyst was found to be lined by multiple hydatid cysts of various size, that did not exceed 2 cm in diameter (relapse — *in situ*). Pericystectomy up to the healthy tissue. Plombage with omentum. Recovery after 14 days.

According to most authors, intracystic pressure ranges between 75—100 cm^3 of water, being 6- to 7-fold that in the bile ducts.

As long as the parasite does not develop too much or its site of development is chiefly cortical, the signs of involvement are very few. Gradually, however, the pressure exercised by the growing cyst renders the wall of the neighboring bile canaliculi more fragile and, owing to dissociation of the surrounding tissue, fissures develop, especially when the layer of tissue is very thin between the parasite and the canaliculus. At the level of the bile canaliculi, encompassed in the adventitia and which come in contact with the brood capsules, a zone of necrosis develops, partly due to compression and partly to trophic alterations of the bile duct walls. When the cyst exceeds 4—5 cm in diameter, fissures begin to develop. In spite of them, the periparasitic space only virtually communicates with the lumen of the bile duct, since the hydatid under pressure covers the fissure or even small ruptures. Sometimes, as observed on examining the slides after cystoresection, multiple fissures of the same duct may exist plugged by the hydatid membrane. Herniation of the brood capsule into the bile ducts occurs and part of the hydatid fluid passes into the bile tree. At the moment in which the pressure falls in the cyst, the space becomes infected and the brood capsule suffers. At first, partial detachment occurs and then the membrane perforates. Fissuring must not be taken for rupture. In the former only part of the hydatid fluid passes into the bile ducts, whereas rupture also implies passage of the solid component parts of the cyst into the bile ducts. As long as intrahydatid pressure is high, the hydatid fluid empties into the bile ducts and, conversely, when pressure falls below that in the bile ducts, bile and microbes penetrate into the cyst. This phenomenon takes place because in the immediate vicinity of the fissure the brood capsule detaches itself from the adventitia, creating a zone of negative pressure that aspirates the bile from the bile duct. This is one of the most severe complications of the disease, connected, on the one hand, to the parasite and production of daughter cysts, infection of the parasite, etc., and, on the other, to the defense reactions of the organism, thickening of the pericyst to which phenomena of compression are added and a fairly marked and extensive inflammatory sclerosis.

This is of the greatest importance for the clinical study and selection of the surgical approach. Devé's work, a corner stone in our understanding of the intrahepatic development of the parasite and its treatment, pointed out the close relationship between it and the bile ducts.

CLINICAL STUDY

Hepatic hydatidosis is an essentially benign disease, but certain forms may produce severe complications, of which many are fatal.

Description of the classical symptomatology has been increasingly abandoned of late. A description of the evolution in two phases: a pretumoral and tumoral phase is artificial. Neither are Chauffard's painful form or Dieulafoy's biliary form fully satisfactory. Separation of the symptomatology into intra- and extrahepatic cannot be upheld, in view of the mutual dependence of these symptoms. Consequently, the symptomatology should be appraised bearing in mind the extent to which development of the hydatid cyst will influence the bile ducts. Applying this classification to our statistics there were 35% simple forms and 65% biliary forms.

Simple, uncomplicated cysts are abdominal tumors localized in the liver, i.e. a left, right or total hepatomegaly. The tumor appears either on the convex or the posterior aspect of the liver and forces the liver parenchyma down and forward. A compensatory hypertrophy may develop at times, or the liver may exhibit regular, round renitent swellings. At times, the clinical examination may reveal a fluid wave symptom. Devé has described the hydatid "fremitus" sign both in cysts under normal tension and in those undergoing alterations. These signs must be correlated with the laboratory tests, radiologic findings and other complementary data.

Latent, asymptomatic cysts also exist. In three of our cases, small young cysts were found in the depth of the hepatic tissue or cysts in the course of involution, but not yet calcified, incidentally detected in the course of an intervention.

Case 165. Patient *V.M.*, aged 24, admitted for repeated jaundice and duodenal ulcer syndrome, confirmed at the radiologic examination. Hepatic tests: normal. Eosinophilia 10%. In the course of the operation for duodenal ulcer, a hydatid cyst was found in the left hepatic lobe, measuring 2 1/2 cm in diameter. The cyst was sterilized and emptied. Removal of operculum. Postoperative course: without complications. The patient was discharged on the 12th day after the surgery.

In most instances, uncomplicated cases gradually become complicated, although some authors have reported on spontaneous recovery due to death of the parasite, followed by involution and shrivelling of the cyst. Infection may result in death of the parasite, but complicates the course of the disease. Death of the parasite is not known to be caused by any other factor. It is worthy of note that death of the parasite and even calcification of the cyst cannot always be considered as recovery. The cyst may remain latent, as shown by its casual discovery in some cases at a radiologic examination, surgery or autopsy. These hydatid cysts never give a symptomatology that induces the patient to consult a doctor.

However, we were several times obliged to operate for dead, calcified cysts because of the perihepatic discomfort they gave rise to.

In some instances, autopsy revealed shrivelled up hydatid cysts which would give evidence for eventual spontaneous recovery. This is a rare occurrence that cannot be kept account of, but surgery may be put off until the cyst is exteriorized.

As a rule, the uncomplicated forms are characterized by slow increase in the size of the cyst, which may suddenly turn into a rapid evolution and complications. In one of our patients the cyst developed very slowly for many years, probably since childhood, and then, after the age of 30, showed a very rapid growth.

It does not appear clinically justified to differentiate sharply uncomplicated from complicated forms, especially as the clinical complication does not always correspond to the anatomic one.

Biliary forms. Evidence of fissures or rupture of the bile ducts is seldom found immediately, and in most cases there is a discrepancy between the clinical signs and the anatomic lesions.

Complications generally mean the slow, progressive evolution of simple cysts. This determined us not to draw a clear-cut borderline between our clinical study of the symptomatology and the chapter on complications. This stands particularly true for the biliary forms of the hydatid disease. Biliary complications of the hepatic hydatid cyst were found in almost 65% of our cases. Olivieri reports 90% biliary complications.

A description will now be given, according to Olivieri, of the fissure syndrome, opening and migration, considered as the main clinical forms.

a) **Fissure syndrome.** The symptoms of a hepatic hydatid cyst often become evident as soon as the so-called fissure syndrome develops. A painless cyst will suddenly become mildly painful (rather a tenderness on moving the body); with pain in the right hypochondrium, thoracic pain without irradiation or pain occurring rhythmically with alimentation. Pain may appear when the cyst develops up to a given size and produces the beginning of a fissure. This pain, by its diaphragmatic or epigastric symptomatology, may sometimes point to the direction in which the cyst is developing.

The fissures are caused by alternate distension and retraction of the cyst due to infection; they rapidly become larger. The surrounding wall, the pericyst, becomes rigid and the lumen of the fissured bile duct gapes, preparing a large opening for discharge of the cyst contents into the bile system, as already described by Devé. When the cyst comes in contact with one of the larger bile ducts or one of the two hepatic ducts, the fissure becomes complicated by broad opening of the cyst and rupture into the bile ducts.

b) **The syndrome of opening into the bile ducts** was observed by us in 15% of our cases. Pain is often added to fever and jaundice or subclinical icterus in some cases. To this corresponds the so-called "accordion" hydatid liver. The attacks of pain are sometimes very sharp and fever develops, taking on the aspect of fever observed in influenza or intestinal involvement and refractory to broad-spectrum antibiotics.

In the absence of fever, the attacks of pain may be accompanied by the retention of bile, with colored urines and subclinical icterus of the mucosa and skin. As the damaged bile ducts adhere intimately to the pericyst, radiology may furnish in this phase pathognomonic data. The thick resistant wall of the cyst prevents flattening, even after evacuation of the contents, and the cavity contains air, infected bile and flattened daughter cysts; the parasitic membrane is detached and floats within the cyst.

c) **Migration syndrome** was encountered by us in 3% of our cases. Hepatic colic, fever and jaundice definitely coincide with the moment in which the tumor palpably flattens. The radiologic signs are likewise evident. Everything points to emptying of the cyst into the bile ducts.

Migration due to rupture outside the hepatobiliary system will be studied in another chapter.

Of particular importance in the migration system is the site of the cyst in the liver. Rupture into the gallbladder or common bile duct is the most frequent form of the migration syndrome. In two cases operated in our Clinic, the symptomatology took on the aspect of lithiasis of the common bile duct and discovery of the hydatid during the operation came as a surprise.

Case 219. Patient *G.M.*, female, aged 63. The onset of the disease dated back 14 years. The patient was admitted with jaundice, cholangitis phenomena, large tumor in the right hypochondrium, painful on palpation. Intraoperative cholangiography revealed rupture of the cyst into the intrahepatic bile ducts. The dilated common duct contained daughter cysts. Right non-anatomic hepatectomy and choledochotomy were performed for removing the daughter cysts. The postoperative course was favorable. Recovery on the 20th day after the operation.

Whether we have to do with a fissure syndrome or with an opening into the bile ducts, the existence of infection must always be assumed. It is not always blatently manifest, but is present in all cases of lesions of the bile ducts; 83% of our patients had a subfebrile state before operation (this does not include the cases of manifest infection or pyopneumocyst).

The opening and migration syndrome raises problems of jaundice or subclinical icterus. Even if obstruction of the bile ducts is eliminated by migration of the hydatid, jaundice may be caused by prolonged spasm of Oddi's sphincter, irritation of the common bile duct, the existence of parahydatid lithiasis of the common bile duct (4 cases in our statistics) and finally compression of the cyst upon the hilus. In these cases, jaundice runs a progressive course, in most cases without signs of cholangitis.

COMPLICATIONS

a) **Infection.** Apart from biliary involvement, the most dreaded complications from the surgical point of view, other factors must also be had in view and the most frequent is infection. According to V.S. Semenov, suppuration appears in 23.4% of the cases; according to Mirer in 12.4%; Cijov reports 47.2% and Guledivici 36.6%. Suppuration was encountered in 57% of our cases.

Infection is naturally followed by fissure or rupture of the bile ducts due to development of bacteria in the bile. Infection, especially in the fissure syndrome, is not strikingly manifest. Postoperative analysis of case reports showed that a cyst fissured into the bile ducts and whose presence was not reflected by clinical symptoms produced notwithstanding moderate pains in the hypochondrium and a subfebrile state. In another case, infection consecutive to fissure, with a turbid fluid, had no clinical correspondent, not even high leukocytosis values.

Evident suppuration is, however, always accompanied by marked pain at the base of the thorax, with high oscillating temperature, subclinical icterus in most cases, alteration of the general condition and increased leukocytosis. All these signs are not obligatory and one or the other may be absent.

Suppuration of the cyst is followed by rupture, i.e. by a stable communication between the cyst and intrahepatic bile ducts, a biliocystic fistula through which the fluid courses to-and-fro, in terms of pressure on one and the other side of the fissure and of the site of the fistula. Thus, a fistula in the declive part of the cyst ensures good drainage of the cavity and seldom results in suppuration. Fistulas situated in the upper part of the cyst only permit partial evacuation. The contractions of Oddi's sphincter, its prolonged spasm result in stagnation of the bile in the main bile ducts and retrograde penetration of the bile into the cyst, which actually causes suppuration of the latter, since the bile contains pathogenic microbes, especially bacillus coli.

After attacks of cholangitis whose origin cannot always be identified, new cystobiliary fistulas may develop, draining the cystic cavity. In such cases suppuration may be attenuated, the cystic pouch shrivel and the content turn into a bilious magma that encompasses the daughter cysts.

Young, unisaccular cysts with declive fistulas have, in general, an aseptic evolution, whereas most older, multisaccular cysts have a septic evolution.

Suppuration may also be caused by anaerobic microorganisms and the evolution suddenly takes on dramatic aspects. In this instance, the cyst contains gases that can be detected at the radiologic examination (air-fluid level), i.e. a pyopneumohydatid.

However, the diagnosis is not readily established, because an air-fluid level with horizontal subdiaphragmatic fluid and slightly undulated membrane may also be encountered in simple suppuration.

b) **Rupture of the cyst.** Suppuration of a cyst leads to its rupture, but this may also occur after injury or effort. In one of our cases, rupture was caused by a fall from on high and, in another case, following a surgical manipulation. In such cases, rupture is followed by shock with its characteristic signs: pallor, cold perspiration, collapse of blood pressure, weak tachycardic pulse and loss of consciousness. To these are added anaphylactic phenomena: coughing, cyanosis, and peritoneal signs (nausea, vomiting, hiccoughing, peritoneal facies). Apart from rupture into the bile ducts, this may also occur into the free peritoneal cavity (Fig. 130), pleura, lungs and bronchi, gastrointestinal tract, pericardium, inferior vena cava.

Some authors consider that ruptures predominantly occur into the peritoneal cavity. However, our experience pleads for predominant rupture into the large bile ducts, but we also met with ruptures into the gastroduodenal tract and even the kidney.

Kourias, in a statistics of 1037 cases of hydatid cyst of the liver, gives the following proportion of ruptures into:

the bile ducts	43 cases — 4.15%
pleural cavity	8 cases — 0.77%
lung and bronchi	19 cases — 1.83%
gastrointestinal tract	3 cases — 0.29%

At the Congress of Oran, Devé communicated statistics of 1743 cases with data very close to those of Kourias as regards the proportion of ruptures.

In general, ruptures of the cyst are announced by severe pain in the right hypochondrium accompanied by shock, which may cause grave forms or cause death of the patient due to anaphylactic phenomena. Rupture of a cyst into the free peritoneal cavity may result in generalized hydatid peritonitis if surgery is not immediately performed. In four cases of rupture of the cyst into the free cavity we operated after 24 hours (one case), 10 hours (one case) and at a short interval in two cases, observing gradual attenuation of the severe signs; it remained only to treat the cyst itself and its dissemination. However, hydatoperitoneum followed

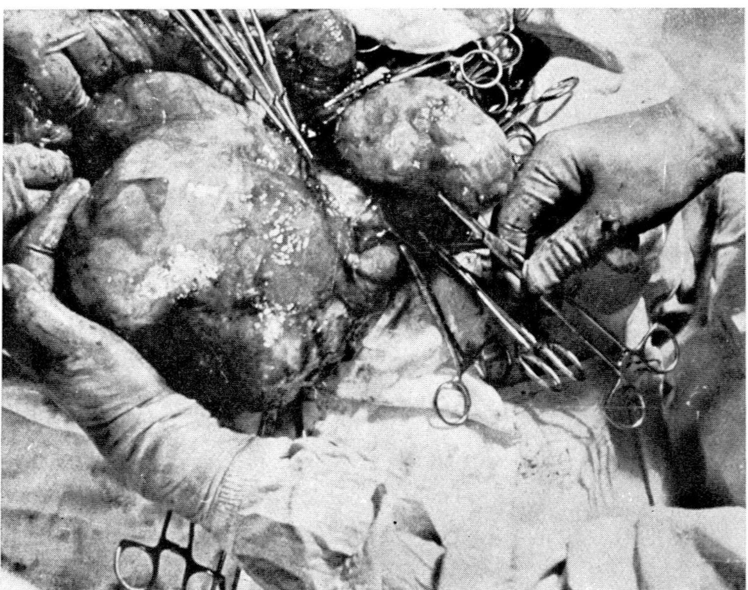

Fig. 130. — Rupture into the peritoneal cavity. Secondary peritoneal echinococcosis (patient *O.M.*, case 76).

in each case with multiple cysts (secondary echinococcosis), but both the choleperitoneum and the septicemic state were comparatively easy to control.

The differential diagnosis of rupture of the cyst into the free peritoneum must be established with perforated gastroduodenal ulcer, acute perforated appendicitis and ruptured extrauterine pregnancy. In case of ruptured cyst, peritoneal puncture will give a greenish, bilious fluid in which scolices may be found on microscopic examination.

In the attenuated forms, secondary echinococcosis of the peritoneum occurs with multiple seeding of hydatid cysts. The history of the case clearly showed rupture of the cyst, shock, gradual attenuation of the latter, and after some time evidence of secondary hydatidosis. Numerous round tumors of variable size, either elastic or fluctuating, can be palpated. Not all the cysts can be extirpated by repeated interventions and gradually a state of hydatid cachexia develops, followed by death.

One of our patients, *O.M.* (case 76), probably infested at the age of 17—18, when he exhibited allergic phenomena (pruritus, palpebral edema, etc.). At the age of 35, evidence was found of a tumor in the right hypochondrium, that was then neglected for 8 years. Rupture of the cyst into the peritoneal cavity, with severe shock, occurred, followed by apparent recovery. Surgery was performed two years later, extirpating 30 hydatid cysts of different size.

Another case of generalized hydatidosis was admitted to our department with a severe state of cachexia; marsupialization of some giant cysts was performed, but the complications led to death of the patient, as may be seen in the chapter on operative techniques.

Opening of the hepatic hydatid cyst in the pleural cavity is exceptional, because of the pleurodiaphragmatic adhesions that develop in suppurated hepatic cysts extending towards the thorax.

Case 111. S.C., male, aged 33, was admitted for a relatively hard cyst in the right hypochondrium. The liver and tumor could be palpated four finger breadths below the costal margin. Roentgenogram of the abdomen showed a typical "brioche" image in the right diaphragm. Calcium impregnation revealed the site of the tumor. Daughter cysts were eliminated in the feces. Surgery revealed multiple hydatid cysts in the left and right hepatic lobes and a cyst adherent to the mesocolon and perforated into it. Most of the cysts were suppurated and contained bilious magma. Cystotomy or pericystotomy was performed according to the access to the cysts. Suture of the colon at the level of the perforation. Drainage. Recovery after 50 days.

In the literature some cases of hydatid pyopneumothorax are reported, manifested by a tearing pain in the chest, followed by syncope and sometimes death. In case of survival, a bile-stained fluid is extracted by puncture (hydatid cholethorax). The fluid is as a rule infected, or secondary infection develops giving rise to pleural empyema. The treatment is that of purulent pleurisy, with removal of the hepatic hydatid and suture of the diaphragm.

One of our cases had a hepatic and a pulmonary hydatid cyst. After removal of the pulmonary cyst, the hepatic cyst extended towards the thorax, ruptured transdiaphragmatically, but in a symphized area. At operation, the diaphragm was sutured, the residual hepatic cavity was treated and pleural drainage instituted.

Opening into the bronchi with biliobronchic fistula is likewise a rare complication. Up to 1952, Kaplun only found 88 cases published in the literature. In Romania, N. Hortolomei (1954) discussed the treatment of this complication for the first time, and I. Juvara et al. (1958) published 7 cases studied over a 5-year period. We only encountered one case in our practice.

Opening of the hepatic hydatid cyst into the bronchi is the result of a longer or shorter evolution and is clinically manifested by characteristic massive vomiting of hydatid fluid or daughter cysts and bile in most cases.

Bronchopulmonary lesions almost always appear in the middle lobe of the lung and are caused both by the irritating action of the lung and by infection, finally resulting in irreversible pyosclerosis lesions. Once the pulmonary lesion is produced, it evolves on its own even after the hepatobronchial communication is suppressed.

The evolution of a biliobronchial fistula takes place in three consecutive stages: the hepatodiaphragmatic, the pneumobronchial and hepatobronchial stage, each one with different, characteristic symptomatic aspects. The most evident symptomatology is met with in the third stage when the cystic content is expectorated. The presence of daughter cells, membrane débris and especially bile pigments point to the diagnosis. Radiologic examination of the lungs reveals a circumscribed or diffuse opacity. The upper aspect of the liver appears to adhere intimately to the diaphragm, which loses its mobility on respiration.

Surgery is indicated in all cases and is urgent if we bear in mind the evolution of pulmonary lesions and rapid deterioration of the patient's general condition, due to the constant discharge of bile.

A complex treatment of the pleuropulmonary lesions is evidently necessary; this implies a thoracic approach that will permit removal of the hepatic hydatid cyst, exeresis of the irrecoverable right pulmonary lobe and suture of the diaphragmatic gap.

When the pulmonary lesions are mild, the abdominal approach is sufficient to remove the hydatid cyst and close the diaphragmatic gap. Recovery of the pulmonary lesions will then follow.

A rare event reported in the literature is rupture of a hydatid cyst into the gastrointestinal tract (stomach, more seldom the duodenum, jejunum or colon). The evolution is generally favorable, the cystic content being eliminated in the feces, as in one of our cases.

Patient *R.I.* operated in our clinic had two cysts, one on top of the other, in the right lobe and a central cyst perforated into the transverse colon. True spontaneous recovery took place with resolution of the remaining cavity of the perforated cyst and elimination through the feces even of pericystic sphacelae.

Rupture into the inferior vena cava has likewise been reported. In these cases death is caused by echinococcal embolism of the pulmonary artery and acute hydatid intoxication. Itorz and Angeles of Buenos Aires reported on a case of metastatic hydatidosis due to rupture of a hepatic hydatid cyst into the inferior vena cava. The patient, a 17-year girl, died following syncope. The postmortem examination revealed multiple abdominal cysts and a hepatic hydatid cyst with two perforations into the cava.

Very voluminous, suppurated hydatid cysts may also open on the skin. Ruptures into that pericardium and renal pelvis (one of our cases) have also been reported.

c) **Cirrhosis and hepatic hydatid cysts.** Among the complications that may occur in a patient with hepatic hydatid cyst is cirrhosis.

The presence of a hydatid cyst in the liver brings about anatomic changes, i.e. destruction of the parenchyma in the lobe involved and hyperplasia of the intact lobe. These compensatory hyperplasias that appear in the healthy lobe compensate in general the functions of the liver.

According to Bacques, destruction of the parenchyma is produced by embolism of the portal circulation, with reactive thrombosis and consecutive acute cellular degeneration. In addition to destruction of the parenchyma produced by grafting and growth of the cyst, lesions also appear in the immediate vicinity of the cyst, which may progressively extend to other more distant hepatic areas. The sclerogenic character of these lesions may lead to the onset of hepatic cirrhosis. The foci of necrosis caused by local circulatory disturbances, biliary stasis produced by different mechanisms, edema and infiltration in Dissé's spaces brought about by vasomotor allergic disorders are so many cirrhogenic factors added to one another in the course of hepatic hydatidosis.

This phenomenon was followed up in patient *M.I.* (case 75) with multiple cysts of the right and left hepatic lobes, on the fragments collected during the second intervention, when net evidence of cirrhosis was found.

The hydatid cyst may cause venous stasis by the compression it exercises upon the suprahepatic vein or the portal vein. In a posterosuperior location, the cyst may compress the veins on the posterior wall of the thorax or spinal column, producing accentuated venous stasis with hepatomegaly, portal hypertension and ascites. In this eventuality, histologic examination of the liver shows a fibrous tissue invasion with a starting point in the centre of the lobe and not at the margin as in cholestatic cirrhosis. The anatomopathologic picture produced closely resembles that described in the Budd-Chiari syndrome. Although this syndrome is seldom observed in the course of hepatic hydatidosis, Bourjeon and Pietri remark that hydatidosis should always be kept in mind in cirrhotics from regions with a high echinococcosis incidence.

The hydatid cyst may cause cholestatic cirrhosis by several mechanisms. Fissure of the cyst may cause discharge of the fluid into the bile ducts, causing edema of the mucosa and consecutive spasms of Oddi's sphincter, that accentuates biliary stasis and favors infection.

The problem of biliary dyskinesia in hepatic hydatidosis was also studied by P. Teodorescu et al. according to whom the mechanism of production of dyskinesia is a hyperergic reaction caused by discharge of the hydatid fluid into a sensitized organism, exercising its effect first of all upon the bile ducts. Cendan and Chiffert (cited by P. Teodorescu) consider that hydatid cyst developing in the hepatic parenchyma represents a foci of pathologic stimulation of the vascular receptors in Glisson's capsule, modifying the higher nervous activity and bringing about functional disturbances in the bile ducts.

Local reactions in the course of allergic manifestations may also cause cirrhotic modifications during the development of a hydatid cyst.

Deschiens and Poinier produced hepatic lesions by intramuscular injections of hydatid fluid.

Peretz-Fontana included fragments of hydatid membrane into the rabbit liver and observed their lysis in some instances, and in others a process of sclerosis propagating from the zone of the implant towards the periphery. According to this author, the sensitizing substance is pericystic chitin, although most investigators consider the polysaccharides and globulins in the hydatid fluid to be the true allergens. Therefore, polysaccharides and globulins are assumed to play the role of hydatid toxins, inducing anatomic lesions that may range from mild vascular permeability disturbances with edema and infiltration of Disse's space up to the histologic picture of hepatic cirrhosis.

Sometimes daughter cells or brood capsule fragments pass through the cystobiliary fistulas into the biliary system, producing obstruction of the main bile ducts, with all its consequences for the hepatic cell.

Inflammatory hilar adenopathy that accompanies some suppurated cysts may likewise compress the hepatic pedicle. In one of the patients operated by us, accentuated dilatation of the bile tree was observed following upon the marked hilar adenopathy which accompanied an infected cyst of the right hepatic lobe.

Thiodet reports on a similar case in which the pericystic inflammatory magma compressed the hepatic pedicle, resulting in obstructive jaundice, an important collateral circulation and hematemesis.

d) **Biliary lithiasis and hydatid cysts of liver.** In this connection, it is difficult to define whether the calculi developed prior to grafting of the hydatid cyst or as a consequence of the latter. At any rate, the concomitant existence of the two diseases may result in errors of diagnosis and mistaken therapeutic indications.

Case 21. Patient *L.M.*, aged 60, was admitted for pain in the right hypochondrium, transitory subclinical icterus, hepatic colic. Preoperative cholecystography: excluded gallbladder. Roentgenogram: image of a hydatid cyst in the right lobe. The operation revealed a hydatid cyst lying almost in the vesicular bed and microlithiasis of the gallbladder. Cystectomy and cholecystectomy (cystectomy through the gallbladder bed). Subhepatic drainage. Recovery in 15 days.

The local and general alterations produced by the hydatid cyst might have favored biliary lithiasis. In our statistics there were 5 patients with hepatic echinococcosis and calculi, in whom a causal relationship could be established between the evolution of the cyst and the presence of gallstones. However, we did not find evidence of gallstones due to hydatid cysts, i.e. lithiasis secondary to the presence of hydatid fluid in the bile ducts, where they might form nuclei around which the gallstones develop. This stands true even in the cases in which rupture of the cyst into the bile ducts took place.

In 1907, Devé coined the term "cholelithiasis of hydatid origin" and in his book on echinococcosis there is a special chapter dealing with "the hydatid cyst and lithiasis".

In 1948, this problem was taken up again by Alphonso Cendan who classified lithiasis in hydatid, parahydatid and common biliary lithiasis.

Parahydatid lithiasis may be the result of bile retention consecutive to biliary dyskinesia caused by the presence of the cyst or an endocanalicular obstruction, as recently observed in one of our cases (Fig. 115).

At any rate, parahydatid lithiasis is very rare and Cendan himself reports 1 case in 500 operated hydatid cysts of the liver.

Some authors admit a clinical form of posthydatid lithiasis, in which persistence of a residual cavity communicating with the bile ducts is assumed to be a source of formation of calculi.

From the foregoing passages it may be asserted that hydatid cysts actually represent a hepatobiliary disease in the course of which severe complications may develop, endangering the patients's life.

POSITIVE DIAGNOSIS

Biologic diagnosis. The presence of a hydatid cyst of the liver produces important toxic and allergic reactions in the human organism both at the site of development of the cyst (due to compression and to the reactivity of the affected organ) and in the rest of the body, caused by the biologic activity of the larva.

Therefore, on the one hand, there is a local defense reaction manifested at the level of the liver by the presence of the adventitial membrane and of an atelectatic zone with marked eosinophil infiltration, and, on the other, a hydatid anaphylactic and allergic reaction. Some of the local aspects have already been dealt with. We shall now discuss the general phenomena.

From the moment of infestation, owing to slow impregnation with hydatid fluid that has penetrated by dialysis into the general economy of the organism, biologic alterations with a specific and unspecific character take place. These may be made evident by a series of laboratory tests which may likewise be specific or unspecific. We are often faced with a marked increase in leukocytes and in the erythrocyte sedimentation rate. In other cases, more or less specific, urticarial anaphylactic phenomena develop.

The hydatid membrane appears to play the role of a filter and both the albumin remaining in the membrane and the ultrafiltrable products containing glucidic fractions — allergens (Peretz Fontana) or protein fractions — are readily revealed, as for instance by Casoni's intradermoreaction.

The protein fraction that cannot be dialysed through the intact membrane gives a delayed Casoni reaction. Therefore, the Casoni intradermoreaction should be read 10—15 minutes and up to 1 hour for the glucidic fraction, and after 24 hours for the protein fraction. The early reaction is encountered in all cases of hydatidosis, whereas the delayed reaction is the result of a rupture or fissure.

The test is considered positive when at the site of the antigen injection a yellowish-pink pruriginous papule appears, or a macule with an extensive zone of edema. When no reaction appears up to 1 hour, the test is considered negative.

In our statistics, the early Casoni reaction was present in 92.3% of the cases and the 24-hour test in 45.7%. This differentiation is not kept account of in other statistics. The results were in agreement with the intraoperative findings in 98% of the cases. However, in 8 cases the test was negative or slightly positive, although fairly large cysts were found at the operation.

Similarly, in 5 patients suspect of hepatic hydatid cysts on the basis of the clinical data, the Casoni test was positive or slightly positive and the operation revealed diaphragmatic hernia, penetrating ulcer of the liver and malignant tumors, suspected at the radiologic examination. Some of the mistaken results may be caused by repetition of the test, since it is known that Casoni's intradermoreaction repeated at a few weeks interval may give false positive reactions. In two patients with a positive Casoni test, but in whom the diagnosis of hepatic hydatid cyst was not confirmed intraoperatively, evidence was found of another parasite. Hence, the test cannot be considered as highly specific.

The late reaction was followed up at 24 hours and confronted with the intraoperative discovery of fissures of the cyst. In 59% of the cases a late positive reaction tallied with net abrasions, readily reflected in biliary disturbance of the fluid. Although not always trustworthy, it is certain that in all cases of fissure caused by infection of the cyst the Casoni test at 24 hours was positive. Other statistics mention the proportion of positive Casoni tests without making a difference between the early and late reaction: Cărpinişan (1952) 85—90%; Nana 78.4%; Juvara (1958) 77%.

During the last five years, in order to obtain repeated and correctly interpreted Casoni tests, we used, according to the indications of Dan Panaitescu, an antigen with slight pH variations, prepared with human hydatid fluid from pulmonary or hepatic cysts by the Dr. I. Cantacuzino Institute. The antigen was injected slowly in moderate amounts of 0.1—0.2 ml.

The reaction remains positive even after surgical extirpation of the cyst, up to 1—2 years, sign of persistence of the general biologic alterations. In addition, in some patients with a negative reaction, operated without any incidents, the test remained positive for about 6 months after the operation.

Eosinophilia. In the past, eosinophilia was considered particularly important for the biologic diagnosis of hepatic hydatid cyst. Later on it was discredited, but today it is believed that medullary eosinophilia has a high diagnostic value in the absence of peripheral eosinophilia.

Peripheral hypereosinophilia is of short duration and decreases with development of the cyst, so that its appearance may be considered to be linked to the onset of the disease. This has been called parasitic eosinophilia. When it appears late, it points to fissuring of the cyst and is, therefore, an anaphylactic hypereosinophilia (Devé). Boteri was the first to report on increased eosinophilia after injection of the antigen and discussed the possible stimulation of a latent eosinophilia.

In all our cases we found peripheral eosinophilia, the values ranging between 5 and 15%. In only 6 cases it attained 20% and in 18 cases it was only 2 to 4%.

It is not generally considered a specific test in the hydatid disease, but as in our cases we constantly found increased peripheral eosinophilia values, we should like to join those who sustain that, in the absence of other evident elements, an increase in eosinophilia within the limits shown should warn us of a possible undetected hydatidosis.

Patient *Z.I.*, with a four-year history of diffuse abdominal pain and hepatic colic accompanied by dyspepsia and nausea, was treated for a long time for chronic hepatitis. Eosinophilia ranged between 9 and 15%. The Casoni test repeated at long intervals was negative. Laparotomy revealed the presence of a hydatid cyst of the liver.

Increasing reference has been made to the so-called induced eosinophilia test, based upon Boteri's observation that a constant increase in eosinophilia takes place within the first days after injection of a certain amount of hydatid fluid to a patient with echinococcosis, whereas in healthy individuals eosinophilia is not modified.

In all cases suspect of hydatid cyst, we applied the induced eosinophilia test, and determined eosinophilia before and 3—4 days after the Casoni intradermoreaction. In 65% of the positive Casoni cases, an increase in eosinophilia was found.

In 15 cases, eosinophilia decreased by 5—7%, 30 minutes after the intradermoreaction (investigations carried out with the Dr. I. Cantacuzino Institute). In these cases, it probably was a question of hydatid allergy, and hypereosinophilia met with in the same interval probably reflects hydatid anaphylaxia. Application of these methods might lower the proportion of errors of diagnosis in hydatidosis. When eosinophilia appears within the first 30 minutes after the Casoni test, the allergic reaction may sometimes give a microshock that can be followed up even when the test is negative. When eosinophilia values fall or are not modified, one should check whether the test is not falsely negative. In case of hydatidosis, the modification is constant, either in the sense of an increase or decrease, and prof. Lupaşcu et al., applying the variation test of the proportion of eosinophilia, consider that eosinophilia determined before and 30 minutes after intradermoreaction increases the value of the Casoni test for the diagnosis of hydatidosis from 87 to 94%.

Another test, fairly widely used of late in Romania is the Weinberg-Pîrvu test based upon complement deviation, and considered positive in 90% of the cases. However, Thiodet sustains that the test is negative in intact cysts and positive in fissured, infected cysts. The test is not specific and the proportion of errors much higher than with the Casoni test.

Similarly, the value of the precipitation tests of the Fleig-Lisbonne, Walle-Confosto, Peretz-Fontana-Diodet and Prausnitz-Kustner type is questionable, and even in positive cases the results can only be interpreted in comparison to other tests and, evidently, to the clinical and radiologic examination.

Radiologic diagnosis. One of the most important means of investigations is the roentgenogram upon which the diagnosis of simple or multiple hydatid cyst is based in the first place.

Plain radiography. Ramond showed that the hepatic hydatid cyst opposes an identical absorption to passage of X-rays as the liver, giving a similar opacity. Calcified cysts give typical radiographic images, sometimes revealing the complete contour of the cyst walls, at other times outlining a simple curve against the hepatic shadow. In 87% of our cases the cyst was made evident by a plain X-ray, which may therefore be considered as furnishing serious arguments in favor of a positive or negative diagnosis. Multiple, layered calcifications can sometimes be seen continuing or not the shadow given by calcification of the cystic wall (Fig. 131). Such an image may be considered pathognomonic. Intracystic calcifications have likewise been noted and sometimes taken for vesicular gallstones. These images necessitate a differential diagnosis with biliary lithiasis, tuberculoma, syphilitic gumma, amebic abscess and hepatic infarct.

If the hydatid cyst is located in the center of the liver, the radiologic view will help to assess the volume of the liver, combining this method with the orthodiagram.

A cyst developing towards the upper surface of the liver will distort the diaphragmatic cupola and liver (image "en brioche", Figs 132 *a* and *b*). The values of these images are relative since the deformities are also observed in other diseases: voluminous, secondary cancer nodule, embossed syphilitic liver, interhepatophrenic adherential peritonitis, and epiplocele wedged into Larrey's gap. Most erroneous images are given by constitutional deformity of the diaphragm. Studies on the pathologic physiology of the diaphragm, especially when thoracic surgery began to progress, resulted in the identification of congenital or acquired anomalies and also of the role played by this muscle in the pathologic processes of the phrenic nerve or neighboring organs mediated by the two serous membranes that line it: the pleura and peritoneum. Starting from the concept of the motor and trophic action of the phrenic nerve upon the diaphragm, we postulated that the phrenic nerve is primarily involved in most deformities of the diaphragmatic cupola (see Chapter 6).

Based upon our clinical findings and experimental work, we showed that the phrenic nerve is, as a rule, involved in the pathologic process of spondylodiskarthrosis of the cervical vertebra, readily observed on the radiographies revealing the conjugate foramina.

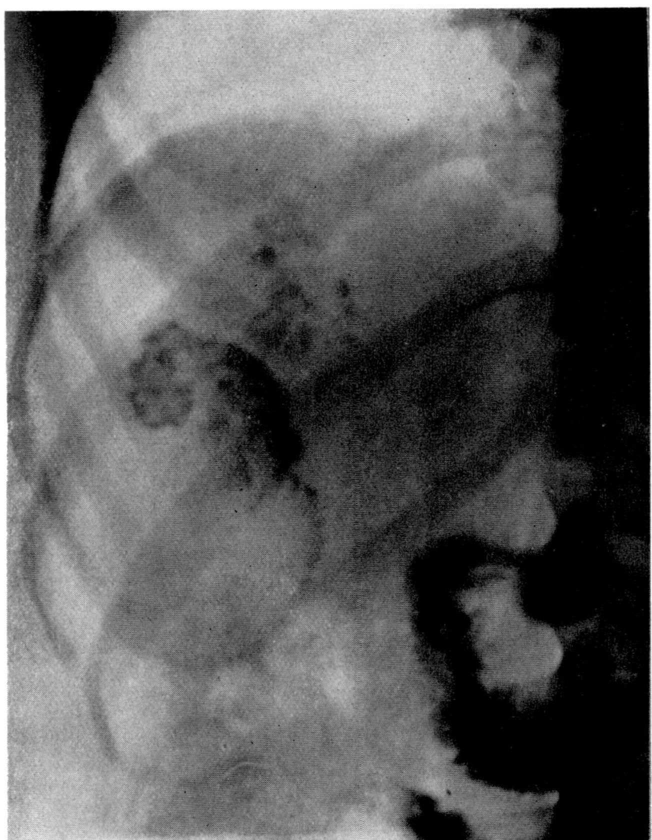

Fig. 131. — Calcified hydatid cysts of the right hepatic lobe (patient *I.C.*, case 111).

Clinical findings showed compression of the phrenic nerve at the level mentioned, with partial strangulation of the roots or even of the trunk, representing a center of chronic irritation that gives rise to differences in the tone of the diaphragmatic muscle. The diaphragmatic areas with a reduced or abolished tone take on a pseudocystic aspect, the liver being soft and readily moulded upon the deformities of the diaphragm in terms of the muscular tone. This assumption and the clinical findings were verified by experimental works. In this instance, as well as in all cases of assumed hydatid cyst of the upper aspect of the liver with deform-

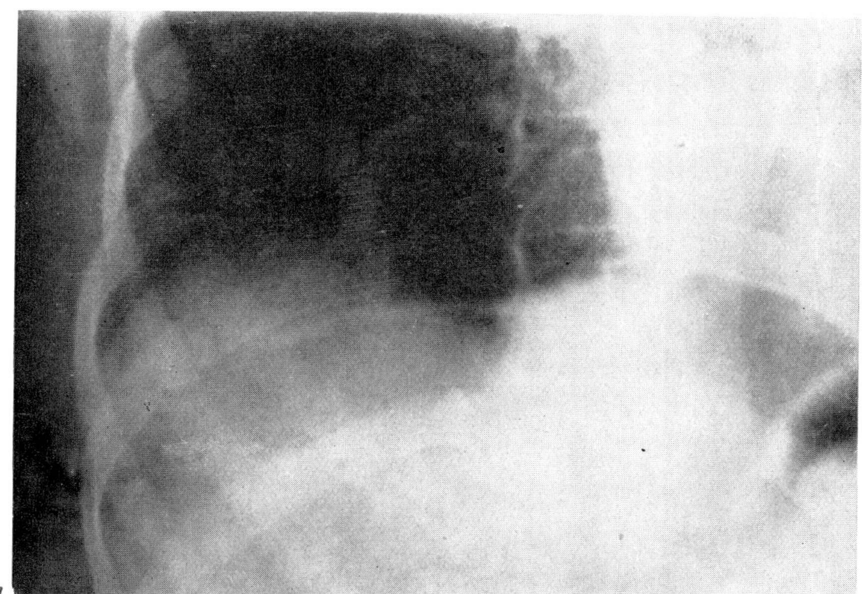

a

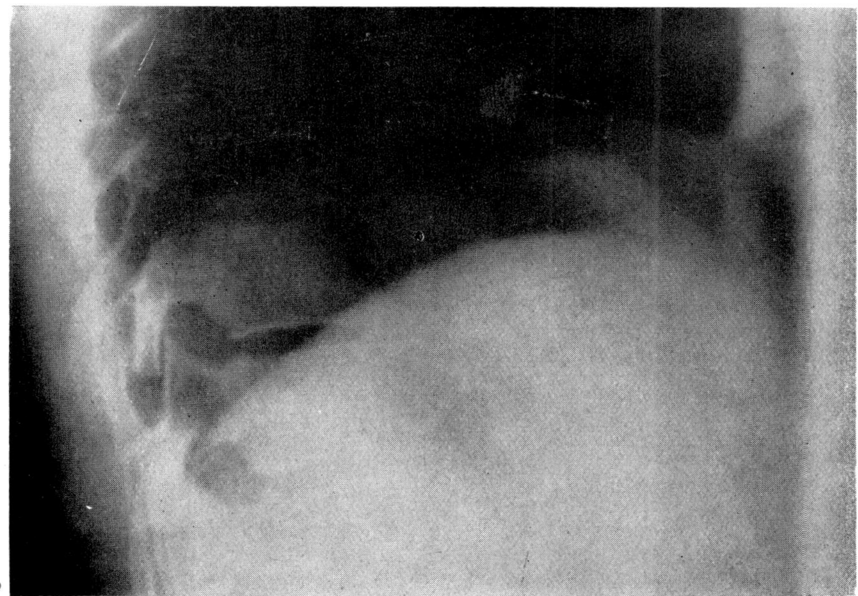

b

Fig. 132. — Plain abdominal roentgenogram. Cyst on the upper surface of the liver deformity of the diaphragm: *a)* front and *b)* side view (case 213).

ity of the diaphragmatic cupola, a radiologic side view of the spinal column in the cervical region is obligatory for detecting a possible pathologic process at this level which would give a correct interpretation of the deformity, and avoid a false diagnosis of hepatic hydatid cyst.

Deformity of the liver dome must be made evident both in front and side

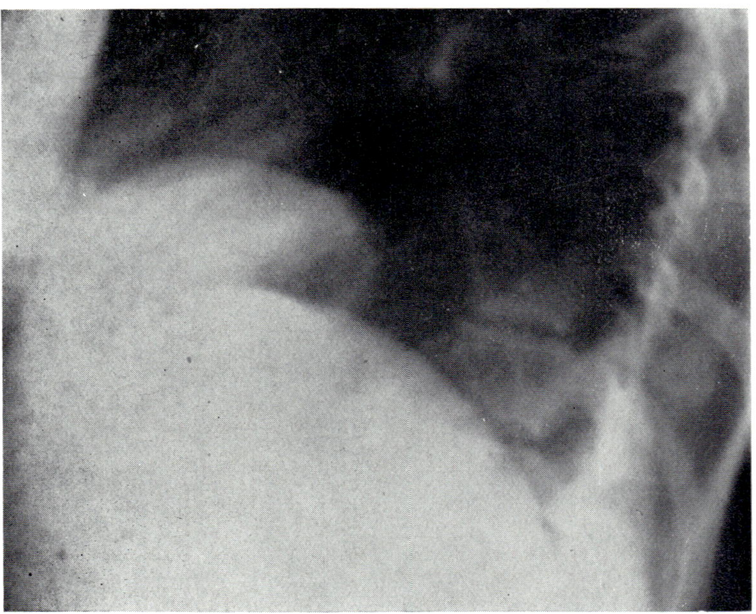

Fig. 133. — Plain abdominal roentgenogram, side view revealing distortion of the diaphragm.

views (Fig. 133), the latter being of particular importance since it can reveal certain swellings that may be characteristic of multiple hepatic hydatid cysts, whereas the front view only shows, in the same cases, simple raising of the right diaphragm. Suppurated cysts may give air-fluid level aspects (Fig. 134).

When the clinical examination indicates the existence of one or several pulmonary cysts, the image of a deformity on the side view is a certain sign of multiple hepatic cysts.

Although plain X-rays give very good results, it is not certain, and other complementary radiologic procedures have been used.

Pneumoperitoneum. Only superficial cysts are revealed by Alexandrini's method, and it should be resorted to only in pathologic states of the diaphragm with a radiologic aspect pointing to the presence of a tumor on the upper aspect of the liver. Air (carbon dioxide or oxygen 300—800 cm^3) is injected, detaching the diaphragm from the convexity of the liver and permitting examination of the upper aspect of the liver and interpretation of the abnormal shadow of the diaphragmatic region, the smallest swelllings often being visible. In this case too, both front and side views must be taken, preferably in a standing position.

In many cases, the patient must lie in a supine position or right or left lateral decubitus. This was necessary in 15 of our cases and in 3 of them the presumptive diagnosis was invalidated, demonstrating affection of the diaphragm

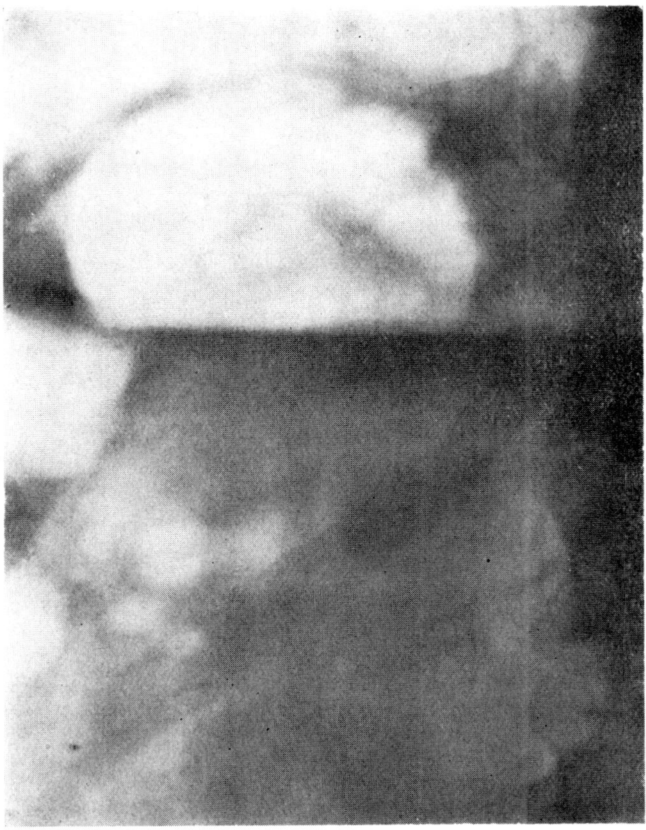

Fig. 134. — Plain roentgenogram showing subdiaphragmatic air-fluid image. Suppurated hydatid cyst of the upper surface of the liver (patient *N.C.*, case 115).

In 3 cases, pneumoperitoneum revealed distortions of the inner surfaces of the liver. This procedure was never applied in subjects with encapsulated and fibroadhesive peritonitis, considering it inefficient and even dangerous in such cases. It should be practiced only when the indications are very precise.

Retropneumoperitoneum may likewise be useful for discovering cysts of the posterior area. In general, it is not of great interest for the diagnosis of hepatic hydatid cyst.

It should be noted that pneumoperitoneum, retroperitoneum and gastroduodenal or colic insufflation cannot furnish elements of diagnosis in cases of central cysts or cysts of the posterosuperior zone, which are the more dangerous the closer they develop to Devé's so-called silent zone, burdened by a high mortality rate. Lagoss and Garcia mention 31 such cases in their statistics with 9 deaths.

Gastric X-ray with contrast medium is an indirect method that may reveal the contour of a cyst developing towards the midline (Fig. 135).

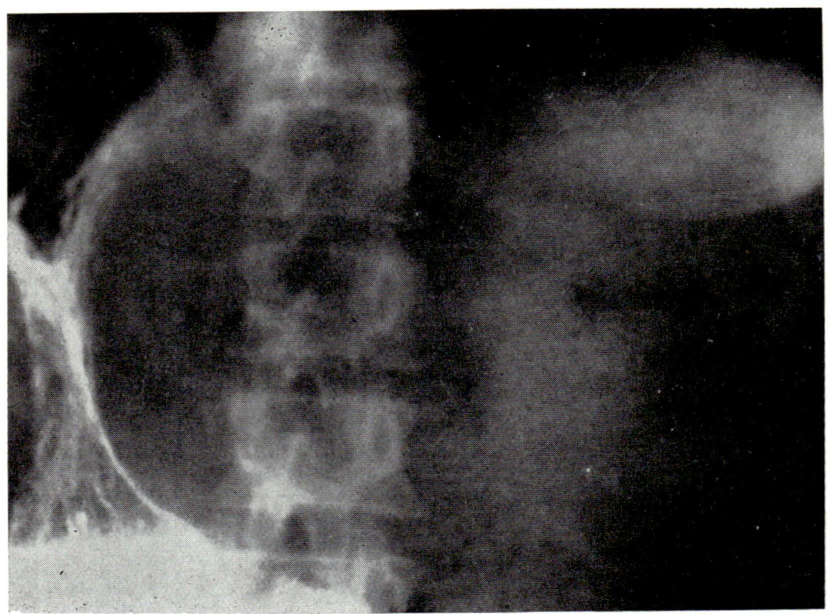

Fig. 135. — Gastric roentgenogram revealing a hepatic hydatid cyst with median growth (patient *P.E.*, case 120) (patient in ventral position).

Hepatography, recommended by Graham, does not give conclusive results. Various contrast substances have been used, but the disproportion between the volume of the gland and the comparatively small amount of biliary secretion makes it impossible to obtain a pertinent image. As the method is not always harmless and the results poor we have not used it.

Aortography may be considered, in principle, an ideal method, since vizualization of the capillaries ought to give in the hepatic zone circular images of lesser vascularity, but actually it only vizualizes correctly the trunk of the hepatic artery and the right and left terminal branches are only visible over a short distance. The parenchymatous capillary endings are never sufficiently injected. This method likewise presents certain hazards. Complications such as retroperitoneal hematomas, injuries of the kidneys, thrombosis of the mesenteric arteries have been reported; lethal cases have also been reported (Stanley Crawford). We only applied this method experimentally on dogs.

Modern methods of exploration. During the last 10 years, splenal and portal venography, and more recently stereoportography, have been successfully applied for the detection of central and posterosuperior hydatid cysts of the liver. These methods may confirm with certainty a diagnosis of hepatic hydatid liver and also furnish value details on the volume and eventually the number of cysts (single or multiple). Since 1954, we have performed pre-, intra- and postoperative cholangiography systematically. Bourgeon et al., on the basis of experience in almost 100 splenal and portal venographies for hepatic echinococcosis, assert that the study and treatment of this disease cannot be conceived today without these methods of exploration.

Splenal and portal venography. According to some authors, it is easy to perform and innocuous and gives a precise image of the hydatid cyst. We do not fully agree with this statement. Splenal and portal venography may also reveal deeper and posterior cysts, that cannot be detected by X-rays or any other method; they will show the relationship between the biliary tree and the eventual multiplicity of the cysts, their topography and size. The images obtained by this method are based upon the action of the cyst on the intrahepatic venous ramifications, amputation of one of the main branches of the portal vein, or an avascular area contrasting with good injection of the neighboring areas. Atrophy (cirrhosis of the infested lobe) and compensatory hypertrophy of the remaining healthy part may likewise be observed. False images are only given when the cysts are very small. Transparietal splenal and portal venography demands perfect technical conditions. Léger and others showed, however, that there are certain risks, as shown by the initiators of the method. Several lethal cases have been published. There are, certainly, indications for transparietal splenal and portal venography, but in view of the hazard involved we have given it up; a simple laparotomy may be considered less risky. Notwithstanding, splenal and portal venography remains an excellent value for locating smaller, central hydatid cysts, evidence of which was not found even on examination. For instance:

Case 120. Patient *P.E.*, aged 32, was admitted for a renitent tumor in the right hypochondrium. Plain X-ray of the abdomen showed a raised right diaphragm, and stomach displaced towards the left. Xyphoumbilical laparotomy: revealed a hard, enlarged liver. Direct examination and palpation did not detect any cystic formation. Splenal and portal venography outline the regular contour of a central tumor in the left hepatic lobe. The tumor was approached from the superior aspect of the left lobe, after previous puncture for extracting the hydatid fluid Cystostomy with ablation of the membrane and flattening of the remaining cavity. Drainage. Moderate postoperative cholerrhagy, which gradually diminished. Recovery was almost complete on discharge.

Preoperative cholangiography. The progress of hepatobiliary surgery during the latter years is unquestionably linked to the advance made in X-ray examination of the bile ducts. It is generally admitted today that the most conclusive data in hepatobiliary pathology are supplied by cholangiography. Preoperative knowledge of the morphologic and functional state of the intra- and extrahepatic bile ducts is of the utmost importance for the surgeon who must interpret and treat diseases of the liver.

Intravenous cholangiography with biligraphin was communicated for the first time in 1953 at the German Congress of Gastroenterology, held in Stuttgart, and represents an obvious progress in the preoperative diagnosis of organofunctional lesions of the bile tree (Fig. 136). However, in hepatic tumors it does not furnish sufficient data for the diagnosis.

Laparoscopic cholangiography recommended by Marcelo consists in initial pneumoperitoneum of 1—3 litres of air, followed by an incision two-finger breadth to the right of the umbilicus, through which the laparoscope is introduced. The gallbladder is punctured under laparoscopic control, introducing the contrast solu-

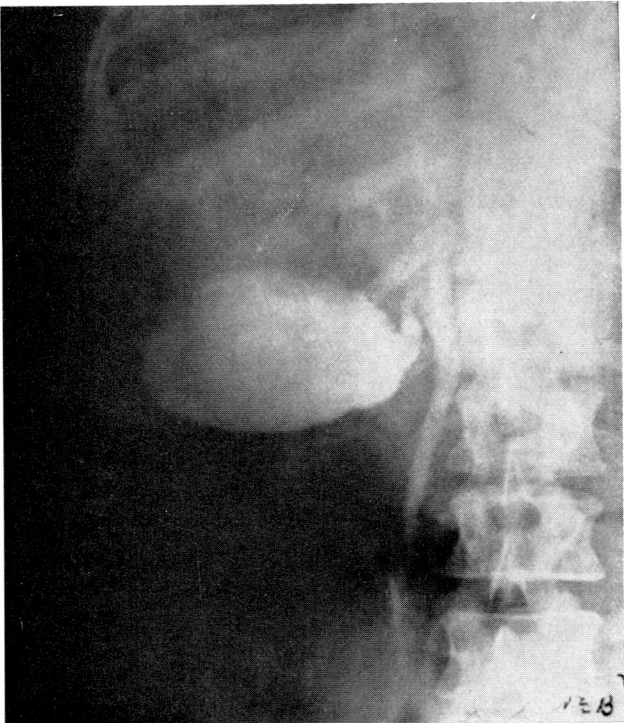

Fig. 136. — Cholangiography revealing the cyst and deformed extrahepatic bile ducts (case 193).

tion through a fine needle in order to avoid choleperitoneum. This may, however, prevent the obtaining of a sufficiently clear image.

Radiomanometry by preoperative transhepatovesicular puncture was recommended by Kapandji. After initial cholecystography, the gallbladder is punctured with a fine needle under radiologic control and radiomanometry performed. The drawbacks are the same as with the preceding method.

Cholangiography by hepatic puncture, advised by Carter and Saypol, was further developed by Léger. The left hepatic lobe is punctured through the epigastric region in the angle formed by the right costal margin and xyphoid. At this level, the left lobe is in the immediate vicinity of the costal margin, therefore there is no danger of injuring the cavity organs. However, there is a risk of puncturing a hydatid cyst with all its consequences. In one case, after attempting such a cholangiography we were faced with an emergency intervention.

The methods described give satisfactory and conclusive results, but they are not easy to apply and neither can they be considered without risk. They are not currently applied in practice.

Among all the methods mentioned, we consider preoperative cholangiography as obligatory, in view of the influence of hydatid cysts upon the biliary system. In two of our cases, preoperative cholangiography pointed to a diagnosis of hydatid cysts herniating in the main bile ducts.

Peroperative cholangiography. Peroperative exploration under manometric and cholangiographic control represents until now the best method of exploration, that cannot as yet be replaced.

Varied and extremely valuable data are obtained, and we consider that the method should be applied on principle for voluminous, multilobate or central hydatid cysts. Before attempting to carry out a cystectomy or planned hepatectomy, cholangiography will delineate the tumor and its relationship with the hepatic hilus.

At the French Congress of Surgery, in 1956, we read a paper showing, on the basis of demonstrative illustrations, the value of cholangiography in delimiting the margins of intrahepatic tumoral formations and revealing the connection of the tumor with the hepatic hilus (Figs 137 and 138).

Intraoperative radiomanometric control may reveal accentuated dyskinesia of the biliary tree that sometimes accompanies hepatic echinococcosis, owing to the interference of complex factors. Foremost among these are cystobiliary fissures which trigger oddian spasms and produce local irritation of the bile ducts (choledochitis), that becomes more accentuated as hydatid sand, membranes etc. are eliminated through these ducts.

Case 115. Patient *I.M.*, aged 45, admitted for jaundice and palpable subhepatic tumor. Cholangitis process three years after the subhepatic tumor was detected. Surgery revealed a hydatid cyst on the lower aspect of the right hepatic lobe, measuring 5 cm in diameter and with diminished pressure. Intraoperative cholangiography revealed a common bile duct packed full of daughter cysts. Cystectomy, choledochotomy, T-tube, external drainage. Cholangiography on the 12th day showed normal passage of the bile. Recovery.

The very presence of the cyst may constantly irritate the vascular receptors or those of Glisson's capsule; to this is also added sensitization of the organism following penetration into the blood flow of polysaccharides and albumins, with an allergic role. Evidence is supplied by radiocinematographic recordings of disturbances in the kinetics of the bile ducts in the course of hepatic echinococcosis.

Today, cholangiography is systematically practiced, when possible both before and after evacuation of the cyst. Peroperative cholangiography may furnish important data in multiple hydatid cysts of the liver.

The cyst also appears in the form of clear images (Fig. 138) precisely delineated by two or more opacified ducts that mould the parasitic pouch. To this is added compression of the vessels by the cyst. Particularly good results were obtained by peroperative retrograde cholangiography, introducing the contrast medium directly into the biliary tree after clamping the common hepatic duct above the cystic duct; on removing the clamp, a clear image of the function of the extra-hepatic ducts will be obtained.

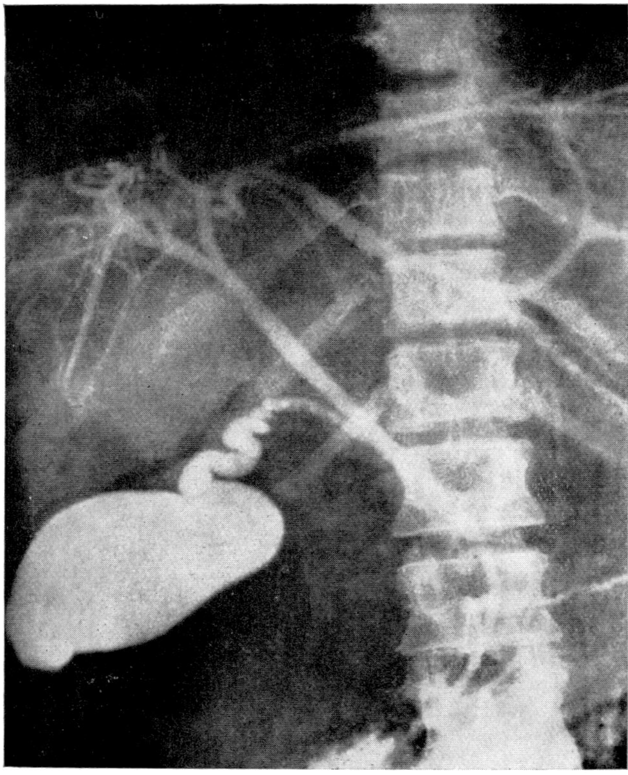

Fig. 137. — Intraoperative cholangiography shows the cyst and its relationship to the bile ducts.

One of our cases confirmed the necessity of performing intraoperative cholangiography.

Patient *M.N.*, with a voluminous cyst of the left lobe of the liver. The right lobe appeared intact on examination. Retrograde cholangiography, performed on principle, unexpectedly revealed the presence of a cystic formation in the right lobe; puncture confirmed the cholangiographic diagnosis.

Bourgeon, who likewise performed a great number of intraoperative cholangiographies showed that, by this means, he detected with the greatest accuracy a number of cysts that could not be detected by surgical exploration. Peroperative cholangiography may also supply data on the presence of daughter cysts in the common bile duct, pointing to the necessity of looking for the initial cyst in the liver, which was not found on surgical exploration. Such cases have also been published by G. Vergoz, Pol et al.

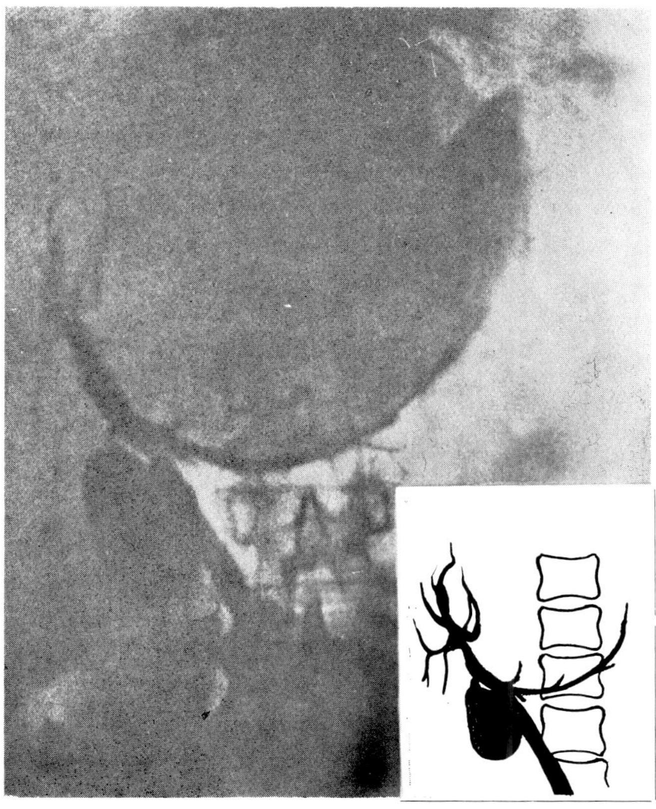

Fig. 138. — Intraoperative cholangiography. The cyst appears clearly delineated by one or several ducts which mould the circle of the parasitic pouch (patient *C.E.*, case 8).

Of still greater importance for correct surgical tactics is cholangiography after evacuation of the cyst, when it permits appraisal of the integrity and morphology of the intra- and extrahepatic bile duct system and, eventually, the existence of cystobiliary fissures.

Bourgeon shows that small, multiple cysts may pass undetected at the cholangiographic examination and recommends double cystography and cholangiography.

Postoperative cholangiography must be carried out in complicated cases, with persistent discharge of bile, and especially in residual cavities that are late in healing (Fig. 139). In these cases fistulography with contrast medium draws attention to the causes of delayed healing.

The radiologic methods of investigation in the diagnosis of single or multiple hepatic hydatid cysts, therefore, appear as fairly complicated and their interpre-

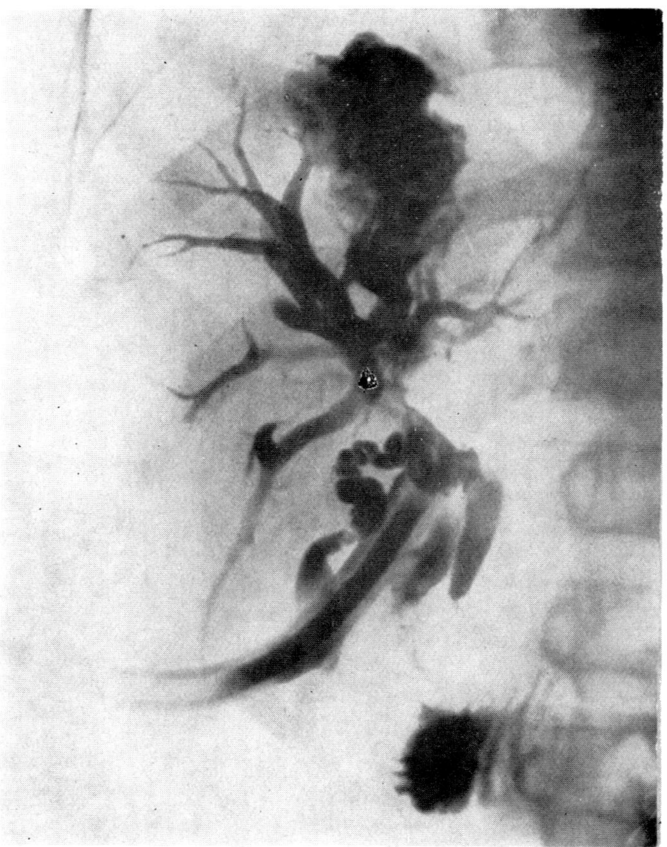

Fig. 139. — Postoperative cholangiography. Note communication of the cystic cavity with the common bile duct (patient *I.N.*, case 197).

tation and application requires basic competence. Application of these methods may be summed up schematically as follows:

Preoperative investigations: plain radiography, tomography of the liver, cholangiography with biligraphin and, rarely, splenal and portal venography.

Peroperative investigations: cholangiography and retrograde cholangiography before and after evacuation of the cyst, cystography and in some cases splenal and portal venography.

Postoperative investigations in case of complications: fistulography.

Hepatic scintigram (hepatogram). Increasing importance is attributed to hepatic scintigrams performed after the injection of rose bengal labeled with radioactive iodine. Rose bengal is eliminated through the blood only by the hepatic cells and, therefore, gives fairly complete indications concerning the activity of these cells, hepatic vascularity and transit of the blood through the liver. As a rule, radioactivity is uniform over the liver, reproducing the shape of the liver exactly. Hence, the scintigram may outline the contour of a compensatory enlargement or supply evidence of circumscribed lesions of the liver. In hydatid cysts, more or less voluminous, well delineated lacunae appear which help location of the cyst or cysts and facilitate the problem of the route of approach; the surgeon is also spared the ignominy of having "overlooked" a cyst (Figs 140, 141, 142 and 143).

TREATMENT OF THE HEPATIC HYDATID CYST

During the last few years a wide range of surgical procedures have been recommended in the treatment of hepatic hydatid cysts. The number of the methods proposed reflect their insufficiency; however, neither have the different means of medical treatment been abandoned, confirming the assertion of Tiodet that "the medical treatment of hydatidosis has and will always be attempted".

Biologic treatment. Problems linked to hydatid allergy and anaphylaxis have been amply studied and are fairly well known, but the questions of immunity in this disease are hardly understood. Although the patients with hydatidosis have specific antibodies, they are not immune and rupture of the cyst constantly results in secondary echinococcosis. It cannot be a question of acquired immunity, yet some mammal species exhibit natural immunity. Starting from this observation and from the facts that spontaneous recovery has been reported following calcification of the cyst and that the hydatid cystic fluid is a good antigen to which the organism responds by forming specific antibodies, some authors have tried different methods of vaccination or passive immunization in view of a biologic therapy of the hydatid cyst.

As far back as 1903, Devé attempted to create in the rabbit a refractory state to hydatid infection using an echinococcal antiserum. He was not, however, able to prevent the experimental infection.

In 1923 Petrov, and in 1939 Plotnikov likewise applied vaccinotherapy to patients with hydatidosis on a wide scale, but without results.

The problem was taken up again by Bartolome, Calcagno (1939), Rivas, Gobica, Mantilla (1944), Peretz-Fontana and Scaltritti, who did not obtain results with vaccinotherapy but, notwithstanding, reported certain changes in the host organism: a general sensitization that prevented severe accidents, and improvement of the patient's general state of health. As vaccinotherapy exercised no direct influence upon the parasite, they recommend its use as an adjuvant to the surgical treatment.

At the IVth International Congress of Hydatology (1952) held in Santiago de Chile various biologic therapeutic methods were proposed, using the complete

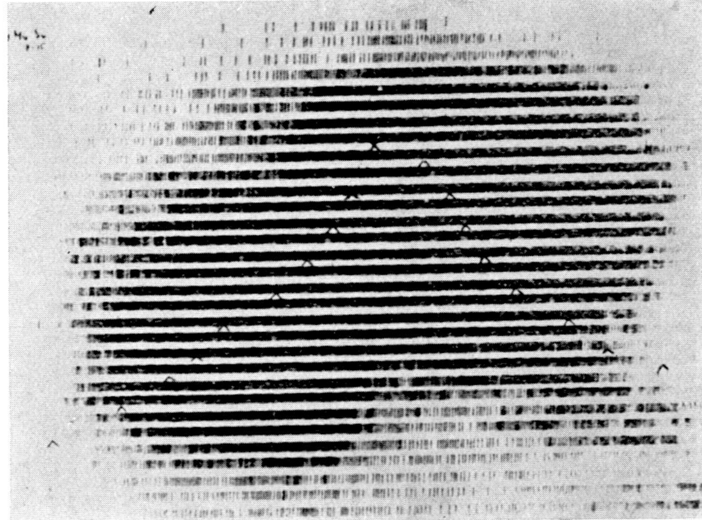

Fig. 140. — Hepatic scintigram with I^{131} rose bengal. Below the diaphragmatic cupola, note the absence of activity in the right upper half. The left lobe exhibits compensatory hypertrophy (patient *V.S.*).

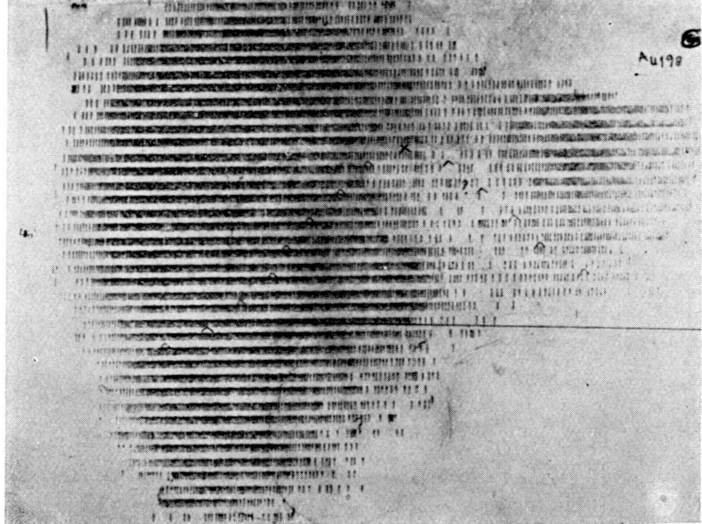

Fig. 141. — Hepatic scintigram with colloidal Au 198. Between the left and right lobe, a zone of poor uptake, of tumoral aspect. The hydatid cyst occupies segment II (patient *S.M.*).

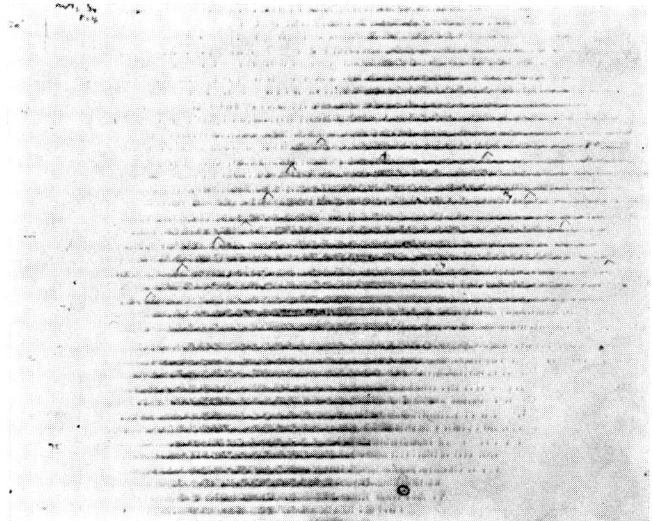

Fig. 142. — Hepatic scintigram. Right hepatic lobe replaced by a tumor mass with a fairly clear contour (patient *R.A.*).

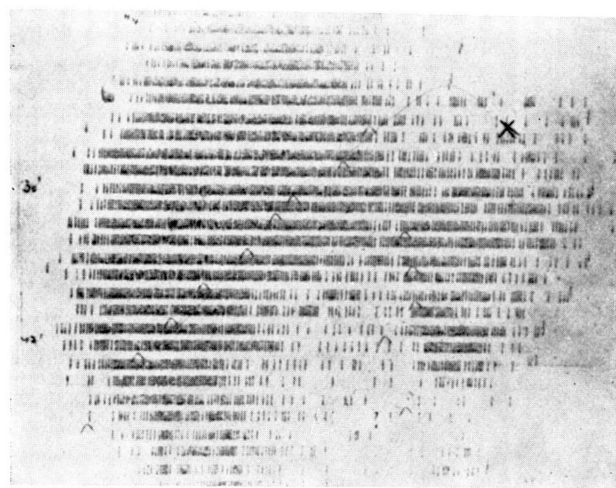

Fig. 143. — Scintigram supplying evidence of a cyst of the left and middle hepatic lobe, confirmed intraoperatively (patient *H.G.*, hase 395).

hydatid fluid or that previously treated with formaldehyde and heated, or combined with hydatid membrane and scolex extracts, with protein fractions from the hydatid fluid, etc. The results obtained showed the biologic treatment to be of interest in that it facilitates calcification of the cyst and produces desensitization manifested by disappearance of the skin reactions. However, as asserted by Rouques (1957), these treatments do not kill the parasite.

Chemical treatment. Numerous attempts have been made in the treatment of hydatidosis at killing the parasite *in situ* by chemical means. No satisfactory results were obtained. A few years ago, Cuervo introduced thymol in the treatment since he considered it to be little toxic and readily dialyzed, its antiparasitic activity being manifested by suppression of the activity of the germinative membrane. Thymol was dissolved in an iodate oily solution, iodine having the twofold advantage of being a parasiticide and of facilitating diffusion of the drug, the lipids and proteins serving as vectors. The 50% thymol solution in 2—3 cm iodate oil was administered in intramuscular injections. According to Cuervo, the treatment results in retraction of the germinative membrane, destruction of the parasite and resorption of the cystic content.

In a follow-up study of many cases treated by the Cuervo method, Peretz-Fontana reached the conclusion that it can only be applied in complicated, ruptured cysts.

We applied this treatment in several cases in our clinic in different forms of hydatid cyst, particularly in secondary generalized echinococcosis. Twenty cases were followed up for 2 years, interval during which 5 complete series of thymol iodate were administered; no changes were found, either in the biologic reactions or in the clinical course. During six operations after this treatment live parasites were found.

During the last four years, particularly in secondary echinococcosis, we combined the surgical treatment with paludrin; the patients were followed up for almost 4 years by the Division of Helminthology of the Cantacuzino Institute. This method is still in the experimental stage and conclusions cannot be drawn, but it may be mentioned that recovery was obtained in 6 of the cases and in two cases the results were not satisfactory.

Surgical treatment. The hepatic hydatid cyst is a disease with a complicated evolution, both as regards the development of the parasite and the effect upon the liver, and especially the biliary system. There can be no question of a generally accepted, readily applicable surgical procedures.

Modern concepts on the surgical treatment of hydatid cysts are based upon a closer understanding of the pathologic physiology of the liver and biliary system, the operation having in view not only to save the patient's life, but also to deal with the important hepatobiliary sequelae of surgery in the past.

The biliary affinity of the hydatid cyst, the direct and distal action upon the intrahepatic and even extrahepatic bile ducts, oblige the surgeon to pay constant attention to the functional integrity of the biliary system.

Puncture of the cyst with modifying injections is absolutely contraindicated, since the proligerous membrane is not influenced and the injection is inefficient and even dangerous.

Bearing in mind the great advantages of modern anesthesia and resuscitation, we must definitely give up, on choosing the therapeutic approach, all conservative treatments which are insufficient and certain conservative operations which only put off the complications.

From the foregoing paragraphs it results that surgery is the only radical method of obtaining recovery, irrespective of the site of the cyst.

Because of the varied forms in which the hydatid cyst appears, as regards its topography, number, size, evolutive phase, complications, the surgical methods must be individualized in each separate case. In choice of the surgical procedure, we must first of all keep account of the patient's general state of health.

It is not possible to establish strict rules of behavior in such cases, but, based upon the progress of surgery today, the surgical treatment can be discussed along general lines.

Following rupture of the cyst and hydatid intoxication, the patient may present hepatic insufficiency, a bad general condition, and the surgical intervention must be simple even with the risk of interfering several times, letting the organism and the liver recover in the meantime. But, as in pulmonary hydatid cysts, the surgeon should start with the idea of a possible exeresis and must be master both of non-anatomic and of controlled hepatectomies.

Our experience shows that multiple cysts often face the surgeon with situations in which combined procedures must be used, in terms of different factors.

Preoperative preparation. We have always paid particular attention to the preoperative preparation of the patient suffering from hepatic hydatid cyst. From the start, the patient should be put on a diet rich in carbohydrates and poor in fats. Hepatic extracts protecting the liver cell are administered, together with complex vitaminotherapy. In order to prevent anaphylactic shock, some authors and especially Devé recommend preoperative injection of progressive hydatid fluid antigen doses by subcutaneous route: 0.25 ml on the first day, 0.50 ml the second, 1 ml the third and fourth day. There were no hydatid toxic accidents in our clinic, irrespective of the anesthesia used.

Of late, having noted certain allergic reactions to formalin, the sensitivity of the patients to different drugs has been tested and the operation started under the protection of synthetic antihistaminics.

Route of access. At the Ist World Congress on Hydatid Cysts, in 1951, Peretz-Fontana recommended the median supraumbilical approach, which has the following advantages:

1. It facilitates manual exploration of the whole liver, except in rare cases of supra- or subhepatic adherences, by palpation of any swelling or part of modified consistence.

The left lobe can readily be explored with the right hand and, through a slit cut in the lesser omentum, the hilar region and Spiegel's lobe, then, even if a cyst has not been found, the convexity of the gland must be examined with the left hand introduced through the interhepatophrenic space, palpating it carefully up to the coronary ligament, on the upper aspect of the liver.

When one or several cysts are discovered on the convex aspect of the liver, the transpleurodiaphragmatic approach must be used in the same or a second stage.

2. The median supraumbilical approach has the advantage of permitting easy, rapid closure of the wound and does not predispose to eventration.

Already in 1952, Constantini proposed *thoracophrenolaparotomy* which broadly exposes to view both the convex and concave aspects of the liver, allowing for complete exploration; it is, however, too traumatizing to be used for a simple exploration. We have used this route of access only when the multiplicity of the cysts, or their site which is difficult to approach, has been established by prior abdominal explorative laparotomy.

In 40% of our cases a *broadened Sprengel incision* was applied since it exposes the entire gland, does not section the nerves of the abdominal wall and offers a good approach to the extrahepatic bile ducts.

Experience has shown that there is no ideal route of access and its choice must be guided by preoperative clinical and radiologic investigations and depends upon the number of the cysts, topography, direction of maximum development, possibility of transforming a laparotomy into a thoracophrenolaparotomy, when right hepatectomy becomes necessary.

The two main objects of the operation are: evacuation of the parasite and healing of the remaining cavity in the liver after removal of the parasite.

Treatment of the parasite. Although the most important surgical problems are linked to the treatment of the remaining cavity and function of the biliary system, particular attention must also be paid to the parasite. The immediate risk, and this should be emphasized as much as possible, is contamination of the operative field, which should be guarded against by packs moistened by a weak formalin solution, especially the peritoneal cavity closer to the cyst, in order to inactivate *in situ* the infestation potential of the parasite. Only after perfect isolation can puncture and aspiration of the cyst be performed.

In all cases, except calcified cysts, puncture was resorted to since we considered it useless to attempt enucleation of a live hydatid cyst from the liver parenchyma.

Puncture and aspiration is done with a thick needle (Fig. 144) in order to avoid discharge of the fluid into the peritoneal cavity, i.e. the risk of secondary echinococcosis. The puncture should be performed as close as possible to the center of the exposed surface of the adventitia. In our experience, it was necessary to puncture the hepatic parenchyma in only 20 cases. With multiple cysts, hidden from sight, the cyst is palpated and only after it is emptied is a second cyst punctured through the residual cavity of the first. Evacuation of the cyst should be done by suction, since daughter cysts or brood capsules may obstruct the needle.

In general, after aspiration of about a quarter or even half the content of the cyst, when the adventitia becomes flaccid and the pressure is lowered, the cyst is sterilized by injecting 2—4% formalin, which gives the best results according to all authors. The amount of formalin introduced is proportional to the volume of the cyst and the amount of hydatid fluid withdrawn (Fig. 145).

Although the experiments carried out in animals demonstrated the absence of any nocuous effect of formalin, either in the peritoneal cavity or bile ducts, certain drawbacks have been reported, such as the allergic reactions mentioned and a case of prolonged reflex spasm of the common bile duct. To this may be added the case of the Argentine surgeon Calleri: total stenosis of the common bile duct after cystectomy, which he attributed to formalin. Hence, we consider that it should be used with certain precautions. In the patients tested who showed a high sensitivity to formalin we resorted to alcoholization of the cyst, as in pulmonary hydatid cysts. No incident was noted.

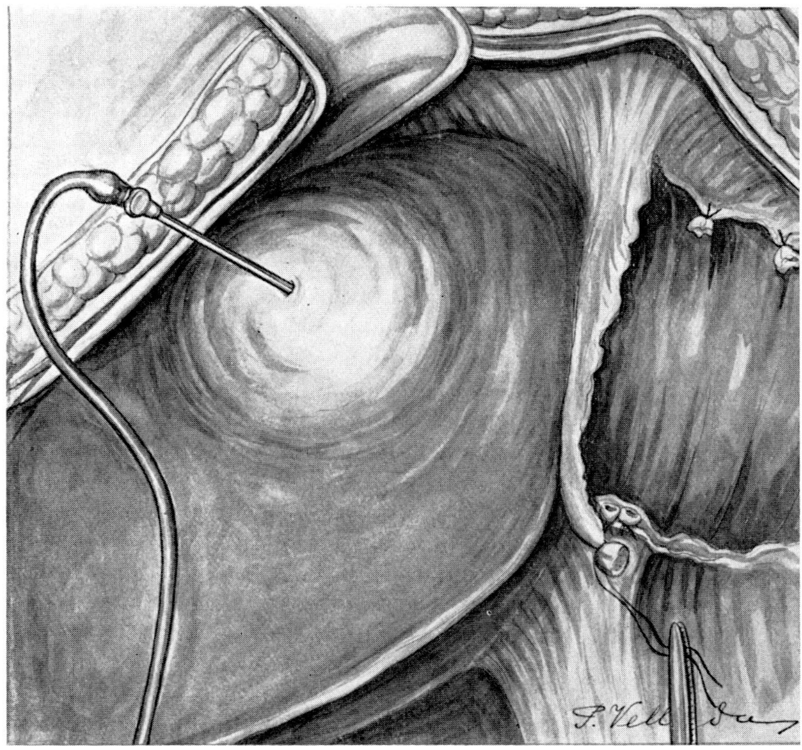

Fig. 144. — Puncture with a thick needle and tube, avoiding diffusion of the fluid in the peritoneal cavity (the same patient as in Fig. 157 *a* and *b*, with anatomic left lobectomy for multiple cysts).

Emptying of the cyst. After sterilization, the whole content of the cyst is emptied by a broad opening starting from the orifice of the puncture (Fig. 146). Once the cyst is empty, the entire brood capsule is carefully drawn out (Figs 147 and 148). All daughter cysts should be previously removed. Only after removing the capsule is the surgeon faced with the problem of choosing the surgical procedure. The cysts situated over the cupola of the liver are approached by thoracophrenolaparotomy (Fig. 149).

Different surgical procedures in the treatment of hydatid cysts. The various techniques used will now be discussed from the standpoint of our experience, emphasizing their advantages and drawbacks, indications and contraindications.

Once the parasitic content has been removed, the most adequate procedure for treating the remaining cavity (a very delicate surgical problem) must be chosen, bearing in mind the thickness of the adventitia, bile duct injuries and size of the

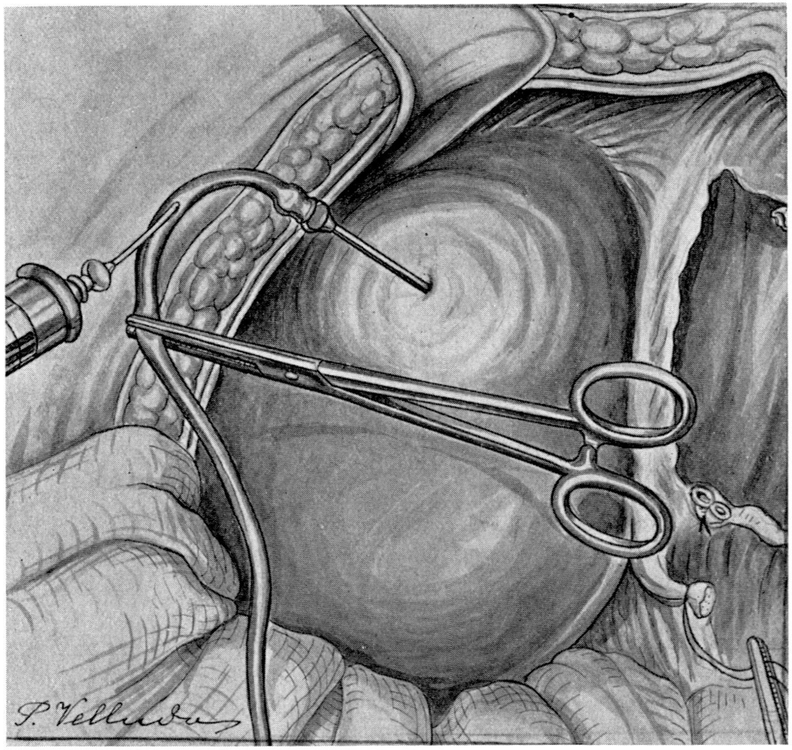

Fig. 145. — Injection of formalin after partial emptying of the cyst.

remaining cavity. Intrahepatic lesions of the biliary tree are of the greatest importance in choice of the procedure. Exeresis is not always possible, nor is it necessary.

Cystotomy. We shall first analyze the surgical techniques and procedures that leave the adventitia *in situ*. Cystotomy consists in puncture of the cyst followed by formalin treatment or alcoholization and evacuation of the brood capsule (Figs 144—149). Simple cystotomy can only be applied in small, young cysts.

Simple cystotomy should not be taken for primary closure, which implies operative reduction of the pericyst planes. The disadvantages of the method consist among others in the serohemorrhagic or even biliary exudate that cannot be resorbed and forms a new, non-parasitic cyst.

Some authors, of whom Yovanovitsch, show that by this procedure only half of the patients recover *per primam*. Referring to 79 cases, Yovanovitsch showed that the non-parasitic cyst persisted in half the cases, the operation having transformed a parasitic into a non-parasitic cyst, exposed to suppuration. Suppuration occurred in 23 cases, a reoperation being necessary, and in one of five cases a biliary fistula developed.

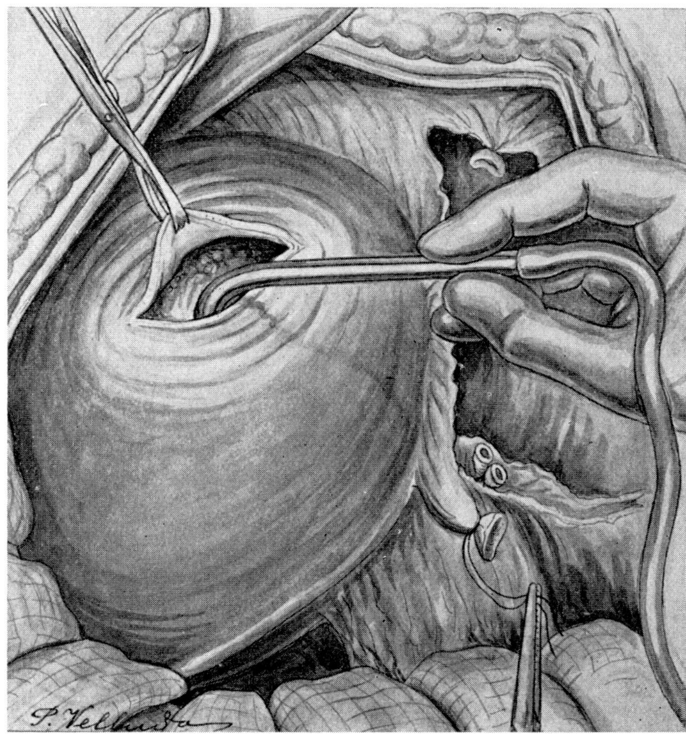

Fig. 146. — Emptying of the cyst with the electric suction pump.

Demirlau, however, warmly recommends simple cystotomy and reports 201 cures in 217 cases. Our experience has shown that the procedure is ideal provided the indications are correct (young, non-infected cyst, therefore without fissures into the bile ducts), the liver and intraabdominal pressure closing the cavity within a very short interval. Many of our cases confirmed this, as for instance:

Case 264. Patient *M.I.*, aged 25, admitted with hepatomegaly. Clinical and laboratory diagnosis: hepatic hydatid cyst. At the operation, a hydatid cyst measuring 6 cm in diameter was found in the left lobe. The anatomical situation and adhesions of the omentum prevent *de visu* approach of the cyst. After treatment of the cavity, cystotomy was performed. The brood capsule was extracted and the cystic cavity was abandoned without drainage. Normal postoperative course. The patient was discharged after 10 days. There was no febrile period and the radiographic control a year later revealed no sign of residual cavity. Two years later, the patient was operated for umbilical hernia. The zone of the cyst was examined during the operation and was found to have a normal hepatic consistence; biopsy at this level likewise showed normal hepatic tissue.

Simple cystotomy was performed by us in 67 cases. In some cases, it was applied only in some of many cysts, other procedures being used for the other cysts.

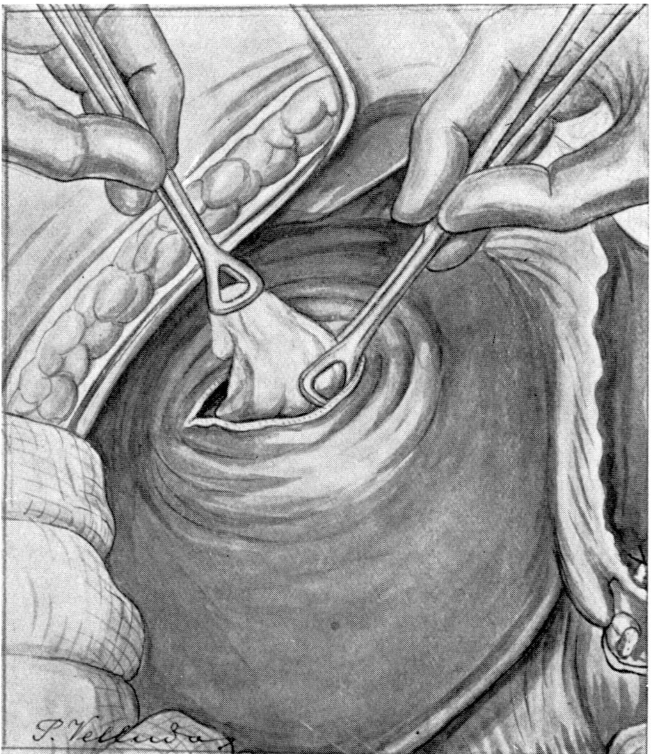

Fig. 147. — Extraction of the brood capsule.

Only 2 patients had fever for a longer period and in one of the cases a reintervention was necessary for draining the cavity. As the procedure was often practiced without correct indications, it has been very much discredited and is less recommended in the literature.

The indication of cystotomy is restricted to cysts in the prefissure stage, i.e. a young, small, clear cyst with intact parasitic vesicle, negative at cholangiography or the methylene blue test, with a poorly organized pericystic membrane, that readily contracts when the cystic content is evacuated.

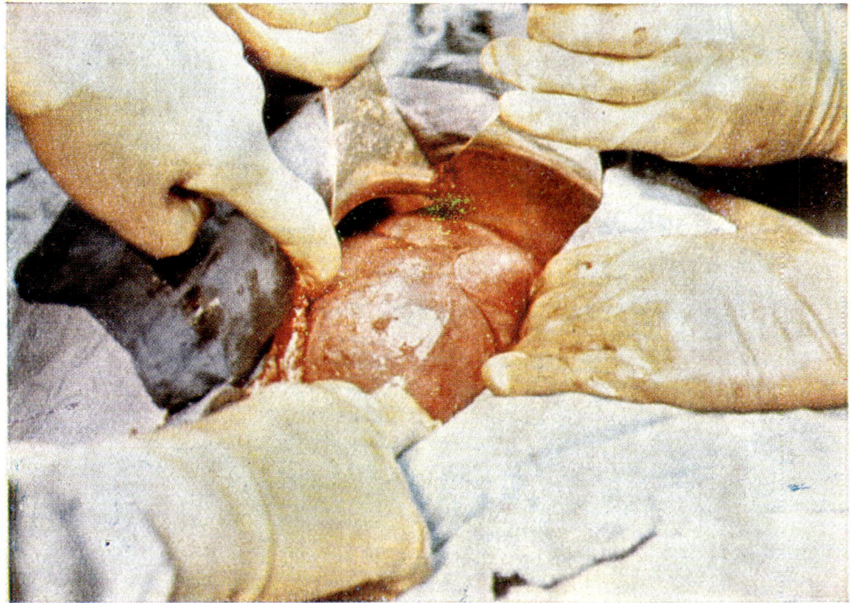

Fig. 148. — Cyst elow the cupola of the liver approached by thoracophreno-laparotomy.

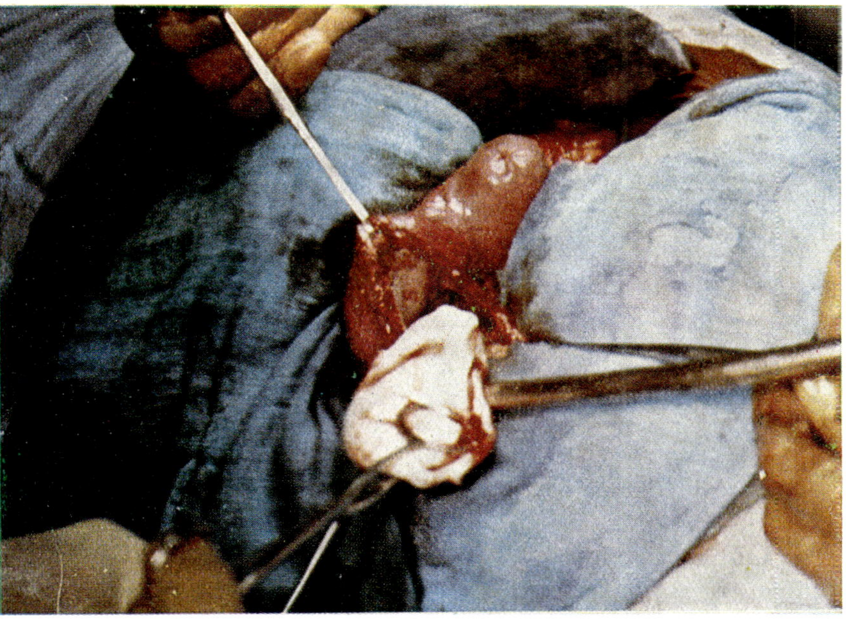

Fig. 149. — After perfect isolation of the operative field and formalinization. extraction of the brood capsule.

Authors such as Cronwell and Vegas, Delbet, Olivier and Llobet-Varsi, Ivanisievici, Oulié and Toole observed the frequency and gravity of serous biliary, air-fluid or hematic pouches, that are often suppurated after applying simple cystotomy. They consider the incidence rate of complications to be of 30 to 40%. The possibility of a late hydatid reinfectation *in situ* also exists.

The cause of the complications resides in the fact that almost all the cysts are fissured, which can be easily demonstrated by injecting methylene blue into the gallbladder. The appearance of the dye in the cystic cavity shows that the cyst was fissured and that serious chances existed, after cystotomy and primary suture, of suppuration starting from infection of the bile ducts. Devé also showed that any reduced pouch is under the influence of the bacteriologic state of the bile.

According to the authors mentioned, a great number of hepatic hydatid cysts are fissured and, still more important, in the period immediately after the fissure is formed, the parasitic vesicle remains for a comparatively long interval clear and unchanged, the infection being latent and only revealed by cultures.

This was confirmed in our experience, and in 10 cases in which a clear fluid was cultured infection was found.

Cystotomy and reduction of the residual cavity without drainage. This technique includes a series of procedures used in terms of the evolutive phase, complications, size and topography of the cyst.

The remaining cavity is left free and safety drainage is instituted close by. Pexy of the sutured pouch to the peritoneal aspect of the abdominal wall is then performed (Llobet-Varsi).

Reduction of the cavity without drainage is known as *Posadas'procedure* and consists in lining the cavity after extraction of the parasite. The similar Bobrov procedure consists in suturing the remaining pouch to the parietal peritoneum.

Most authors, based upon a fairly large number of cases, consider these procedures as simple and benign. The pericystic membrane that has not been removed is gradually resorbed. Using this technique, Constantini reports 115 recoveries, Gerolanos 128, and Carlos Rivas 160 recoveries, without complications.

The technique of cystotomy with sectioning of the pericystic membrane over a fairly large surface, and especially plombage of the remaining cavity with omentum, has been broadly used by us without any drawbacks. We used this technique in 87 cases, even in the presence of moderate fissures made evident by cholangiography or visible with the naked eye; before plombage with omentum, the fissures were closed with X-sutures. The omentum is fixed to the margin of the cavity, and sometimes the Guedj tunnelling method is used. In most cases a drain tube was introduced at a distance.

There were no complications among our cases operated by this procedure, neither did intrahepatic abscesses or important cholerrhagia develop. We recommend this procedure in the cases in which exeresis raises difficult technical problems or problems linked to the patient's general state of health.

Although *plombage with omentum* has been criticized by some authors, we applied the procedure whenever possible, that is when a sufficient viable flap could be obtained for plombage. There are several advantages: a moderate discharge of bile is rapidly arrested. When the pericyst is not too thick, the cavity diminishes and the secreted fluid is absorbed. In the course of several reoperations, we had the occasion to observe a true revascularization of the inner aspect, that favors progressive resorption.

Good results were also obtained by leaving the cavity open into the peritoneum. After emptying the cyst, we sometimes sectioned the extrahepatic part of the cyst and fixed the margins of the liver with continuous suture and eventual suture of the visible ducts. The procedure is similar to that recommended by

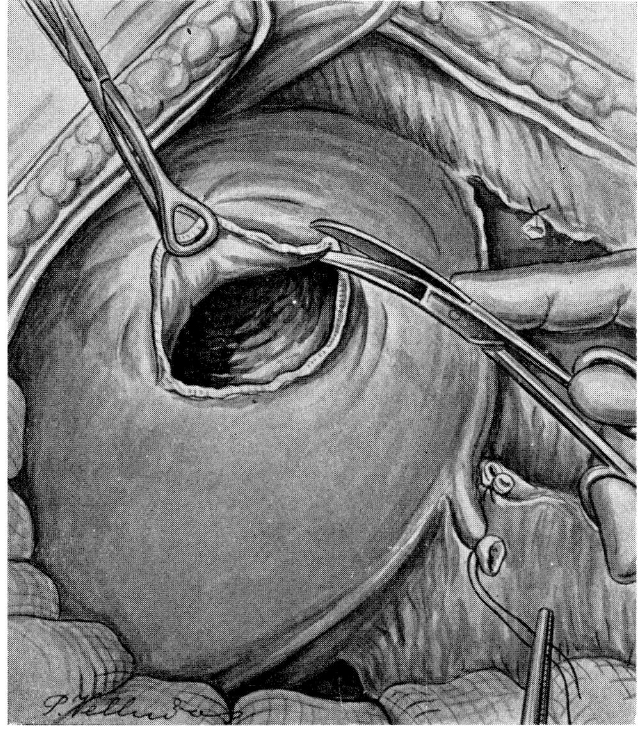

Fig. 150. — Cystectomy and removal of the operculum (Lagrot).

Lagrot and Coriat: sectioning "en collerette" of the extrahepatic portion of the cyst, therefore "flattening" of the cyst, with contingent drainage of the peritoneal cavity, especially with a view to introducing antibiotics (Figs 150, 151 *a* and *b*). However, the danger of choleperitoneum cannot be overlooked.

The Lagrot and Coriat procedure is applied to cysts developing on the surface of the liver, producing a mere swelling up to giant tumors that descend in the pelvis. The technique starts with packing off of the peritoneal cavity, as with the other techniques, puncture, formalin treatment, evacuation of the fluid and extraction of the brood capsule, after which the protruding part of the cyst, where white hyaline patches can be seen and no hepatic tissue is found, is broadly

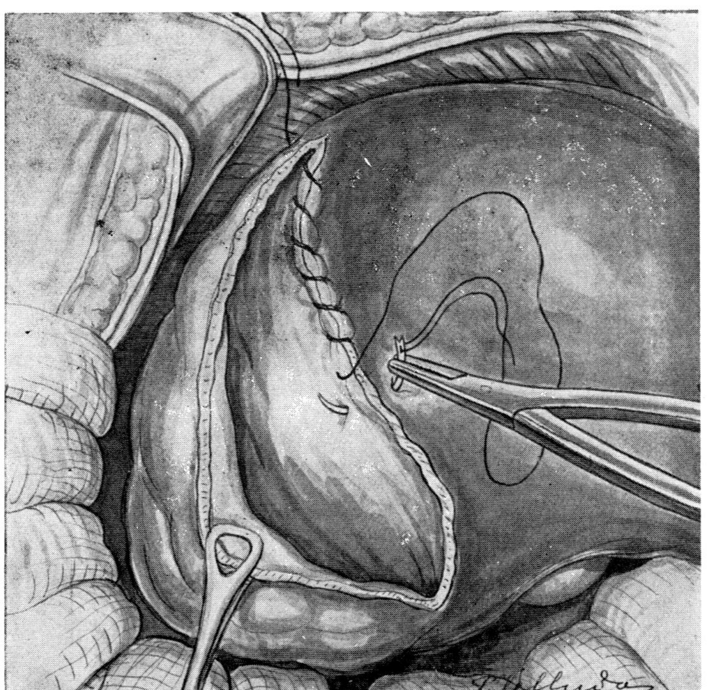

a

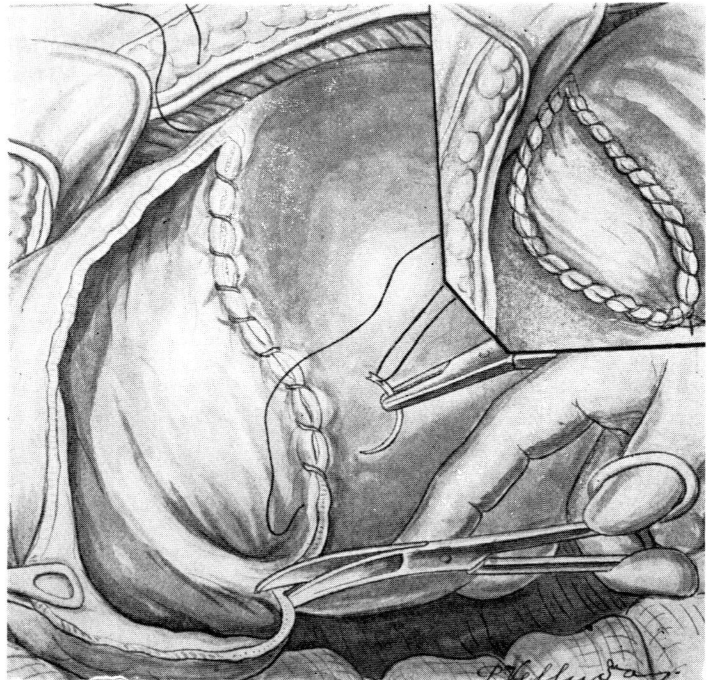

b

Fig. 151 . — Broad resection of the pericyst (*a*), followed by suture of the section edges (*b*).

excised. The part to be excised is split in four and each flap is cut off with the electric cautery from the margin of the normal hepatic parenchyma, without sacrificing any portion of the recoverable tissue. Section of this sclerosed tissue is not followed by bleeding or only slight bleeding and hemostasis can be done by X-sutures or by interrupted suture along the edge of the parenchyma.

In this way, the prominent part of the pericyst and the outer sclerosed, irrecoverable portion of the hepatic parenchyma are removed. The cyst is flattened and only a small portion of the fundus remains, that disappears fairly quickly as no kind of retention is possible.

The fundus of the cyst is not extirpated as in total cystectomies or pericystectomies, the hepatic tissue in this area being readily recoverable when it is no longer compressed by the parasitic tumor. This also avoids the hazard of accidents, since the fundus is intimately connected with the blood vessels and bile ducts.

Omentoplasty is considered useless and difficult to carry out (especially in cysts of the upper surface of the liver or in multiple cysts) and sometimes dangerous (traction of the large curvature of the stomach, adhesions, etc.).

The operation usually ends by closing the abdominal wall anatomically, leaving a narrow tube for introducing the antibiotics. A small amount of bile sometimes drains through the tube for 2—3 days. The tube is removed on the 4th or 5th day.

In infected or suppurated hydatid cysts, it is absolutely necessary to instil antibiotics.

In the cases of calcified hydatid cysts, resection of the prominent part of the cyst should be completed, when possible, by detaching the calcified plaques from the fundus with the greatest care.

In hydatid cysts adherent to important formations (hepatic pedicle, diaphragm, kidney, duodenum, small intestine, colon), the operation generally consists in removing the operculum of the cyst, without touching the parts of the adventitia intimately adhering to any of the formation mentioned; flattening of the cyst will be sufficient to ensure recovery.

This procedure was applied by us in 14 cases of large cysts of the undersurface of the liver or multiple cysts, in some of which plombage with omentum could not be done.

Case 19. Patient *M.D.*, aged 36, was admitted to our clinic for the presence of a large subhepatic tumor, jaundice, accentuated eosinophilia and intensely positive Casoni test. Laparotomy revealed a hydatid cyst on the undersurface of the liver, developing posteriorly. The cyst pressed upon the hepatic pedicle and extrahepatic bile ducts. After formalin treatment, the brood capsule was extracted and the operculum removed, the adventitial zone adherent to the hilus remaining intact. Drainage. Rapid recovery within 15 days.

The residual cavity after resection of the adventitia may be left wide open to allow the peritoneum to absorb the exudate at the level of the remaining pericyst.

In multiple cysts of the liver operated in a single stage, each cyst is treated successively as if it were a single cyst.

The anatomic results of such an operation are satisfactory. In two cases, reoperated for other locations, only slight retraction of the parenchyma was noted and even that was identified with the help of the adhesions that had developed — a sign of the former intervention.

Surgery is not possible in case of important biliary fistulas, either because of the risk of a choleperitoneum or because of an encysted bilious collection.

Drainage of the remaining cavity into the bile ducts (sphincteroplasty, choledochoduodenostomy).

Among the cystotomy procedures with reduction of the pouch without external drainage is *drainage of the remaining cavities into the bile ducts.* In two cases we were faced with specific situations: after evacuation of the cyst, fissure of the remaining cavity into a fairly large bile duct was found, the slit measuring more than 10 mm. As there was no other chance of solving the bile discharge but by facilitating drainage of the intra-and extrahepatic bile ducts, we resorted to sphincteroplasty. In one case, ascending cholangiography was performed after clamping the common bile duct; the operation obviously helped drainage of the bile and disapearance of the bile discharge. In the second case, the problem was solved only at the reoperation, by choledochoduodenostomy, ensuring broad drainage of the extrahepatic bile ducts. In most of our cases, we performed choledochotomy with external drainage, since it decompresses the damaged common bile duct, favoring drainage of the cavity, and permits postoperative control cholangiography, which will supply data on healing of the residual cavity and allow for an efficient local treatment.

Case 219. Patient *G.M.*, aged 63. The disease dated back 14 years. Presenting signs: jaundice, cholangitis phenomena, large tumor of the right hypochondrium. Intraoperative cholangiography revealed rupture of the cyst into the bile ducts. Cystotomy in one stage was not a solution as the cholerrhagia persisted. At the reoperation, a very dilated common bile duct, containing daughter cysts, was found. Choledochoduodenostomy was performed. Favorable postoperative course; discharge of bile ceased on the third day. Recovery after 25 days.

Internal drainage in the bile ducts was recommended by Goinard already in 1959.

Cystotomy followed by marsupialization. Marsupialization (Lindemann and Landau) is one of the oldest procedures applied in the surgical treatment of hepatic hydatid cysts. The procedure consists in stitching the edges of the adventitia to the margins of the parietal incision, which is only partly sutured in order to drain the cyst, following exclusion of the peritoneal cavity. The method appears simple but has many drawbacks and serious precautions must be taken. According to Curutchet, "the intervention lasts half an hour and the postoperative consequences half a year".

Indeed, marsupialization has the great disadvantage of delaying recovery by creating a fistula which may close very slowly. Cholerrhagia in itself — as shown by Mallet-Guy — not only leads to protein and hydromineral imbalance after some time, but results in the infectious process that is generally associated with the loss of bile, with aggravation of the late prognosis due to the persistence of suppuration from the cystic pouch. Recovery is delayed the more, the larger and the older the cyst, i.e. when the pericystic membrane is more calcified. Calcification of the membrane renders the cyst wall rigid and prevents their collapse. Control of the marsupialized cavity with the aid of retractors and frontal mirror show that the suppurative process results in sloughing at the level of the pericystic membrane, the sloughs separating and producing a profuse discharge of massive lymph and serum infiltrate that forms between the hepatic parenchyma and the slough. This inevitably exposes to infection and a still greater loss of salts and proteins. At first, calcification raises a barrier between the hepatic parenchyma and the marsupialized pouch, but detachment of the calcified area will increase hydromineral and protein losses, as well as the absorption of toxins from the infected pouch. This aggravates the local and general postoperative course. Separation of the sloughs sometimes results in injury of the bile ducts in the vicinity of the pouch and, consequently, in accentuated discharge of bile, propagation of the infection and attacks of cholangitis. The treatment with antibiotics does not give the expected results because they penetrate difficultly into the sclerosed, poorly vascularized area. Apart from trailing biliary fistulas that end in cachexia and death (in 10 of 92 cases in the statistics of Yovanovitsch and 4 of 18 in that of Rivas), cases of severe secondary hemorrhage and even relapses *in situ* have been reported.

Even if sloughing does not take place, the pericystic parenchyma is replaced, as shown by Danicico, by sclerous tissue that favors persistence of the cavity. At times, alteration of the parenchyma is very accentuated and results in fibrous transformation of certain large areas, involving more than half the liver. Fibrosis strangles the bile ducts, obliterates the vessels, with stasis and thrombosis, which favor further suppuration of the residual cavity and bile ducts.

Bearing these drawbacks in mind, we avoided marsupialization as much as possible.

However, in one case it became obligatory: there were multiple localizations of the cysts, one being particularly large, then the patient's general condition and the behavior of the pericystic membrane towards the hepatic parenchyma also influenced us.

The postoperative course was particularly difficult and the necessity of continuously correcting the biochemical constants confirmed the general disadvantages of the procedure. Any other procedure in this patient, aged 73, would have been impossible because of the large site of the cyst, the location and difficult approach in the peritoneal cavity. The patient died three months after the operation.

The only advantage of marsupialization appears to be its simplicity and rapidity, but today it is considered obsolete. If the cyst is not open towards the bile ducts, the cavity becomes infected, and if it is open discharge of bile will develop.

Today, it can only be conceived as a first stage, as an attempt to save extremely severe cases, or to gain time up to reoperation and exeresis.

Statistics show a high mortality rate not only when marsupialization is applied in extreme cases, but also when it is currently used: 30—40% deaths and unresolved situations in 50—60% of the cases.

Drainage of the cavity, by a thick Pezzer tube. According to some authors, it is but a hidden marsupialization and the same hazards of infection and cholerrhagia are involved.

Although this is true along general lines, in 5 cases in which we applied this procedure removal of the drain after 10—12 days was followed, in case of patent intra- and extrahepatic bile ducts, by closure of the wall and arrest of the discharge, bile always running along the routes of lesser resistance. As long as drainage exists, the lesser resistance is towards the exterior, Oddi's sphincter representing all the same an obstacle; the moment in which the drain is removed and the cavity walls are closed, the internal route becomes more accessible. This procedure was resorted to in the cases in which technical difficulties prevented plombage or closure and in which there was no possibility of postural drainage of the extrahepatic bile ducts. When drainage was suppressed, the gauze strips saturated with bile showed gradual diminution of discharge, followed by recovery (Fig. 152 *a* and *b*).

Cystojejunostomy, recommended by Goinard and Pellisier, was practiced by us in two cases. The sectioned cysts left a cavity which was sutured by a Y-shaped anastomosis to a jejunal loop. This shunt was necessary because of the persistence of accentuated discharge of bile after emptying the cyst. The advantage of the procedure stands in efficient drainage not only of the declive parts, but also of those that show a tendency to retention. The drawback — of lesser importance — is the persistence of the excluded loop after retraction of the cavity. At any rate, the loop must be sufficiently long not to produce reflux. In the second case, this procedure was applied in the second stage because of persistence of a biliary fistula with massive discharge.

Exeresis procedures. The methods of total or partial resection of the adventitia include total or partial cystectomy, cystoresection and planned hepatic resections.

Cystectomy or pericystectomy has in view partial or total removal of the adventitia of the pericyst. This is the most rational and physiologic operation, if we bear in mind the danger of leaving the adventitia *in situ*. The adventitial membrane is a sclerous and often calcified tissue that is the main obstacle preventing closure of the cavity; it is at the same time an infected tissue that communicates with the bile ducts and maintains their infection. The pericyst may often be a source of local relapses. R. Bourgeon, who showed the necessity of removing the adventitia, calls this procedure a pericystectomy. The term cystectomy might be maintained only for mass removal of the cyst and adventitia, as recommended by Pozzi in 1889, and applied by Napalkov in 1904; Melnikov subsequently studied the operation in detail.

These authors insist that any complicated or infected hydatid cyst should be removed together with the brood capsule, without opening the cyst; this, according to Napalkov, guarantees against peroperative dissemination and avoids postoperative complications, relapses included.

The procedure has proved useful, especially in infected cysts with thickened walls, and small calcified cysts (Fig. 153).

Yovanovitsch considers that an ideal cystectomy (Fig. 154), as conceived by Napalkov, is difficult and dangerous for the hepatic parenchyma, since a bile duct or blood vessels may be readily injured, resulting in severe intraoperative complications that cannot be always controlled.

Hence, Yovanovitsch recommends cystectomy with an open pouch. This operation is comparable to the techniques of Hugon and Dubau applied in pulmonary hydatid cyst.

Pericystectomy (Fig. 155 *a* and *b*) will be described according to the technique of Yovanovitsch, although he actually calls it cystectomy. It includes formalin treatment or alcoholization in order to avoid the danger of dissemination, after which the brood capsule is extracted; the forefinger of the left hand is introduced

a

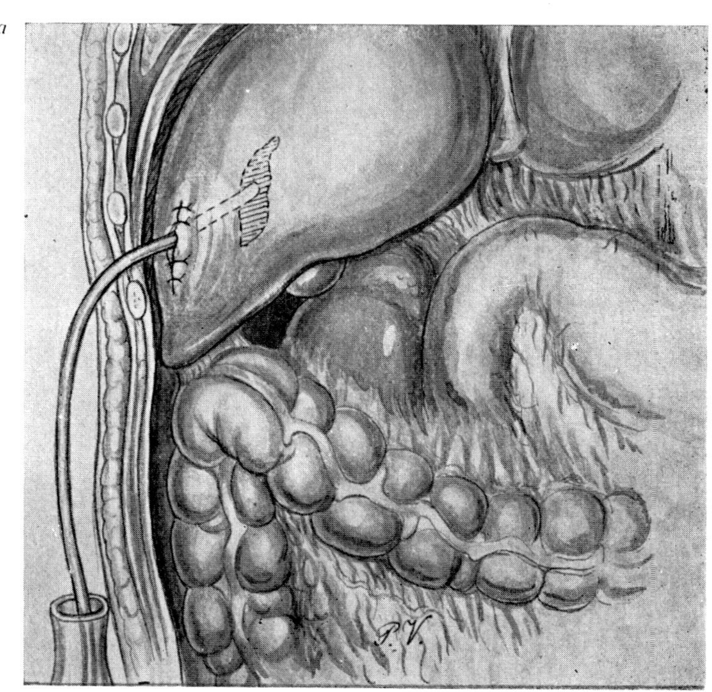

b

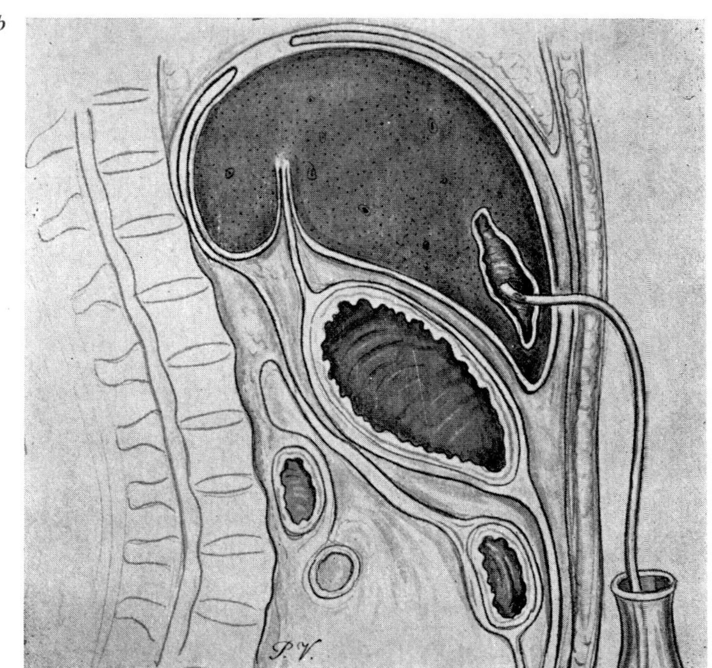

Fig. 152 *a* and *b*. — Drainage of the cavity of a central cyst.

into the cavity in order to stretch the cyst wall between it and the thumb, facilitating separation of the membrane from the hepatic parenchyma by slow attentive dissection; according to Yovanovitsch, the "cautery should caress the surface of the cyst" (a technique similar to dissection of a hernial sac).

A scraper can be used in case of calcified cysts. It is generally possible to remove the whole membrane, but sometimes it can only be excised in fragments.

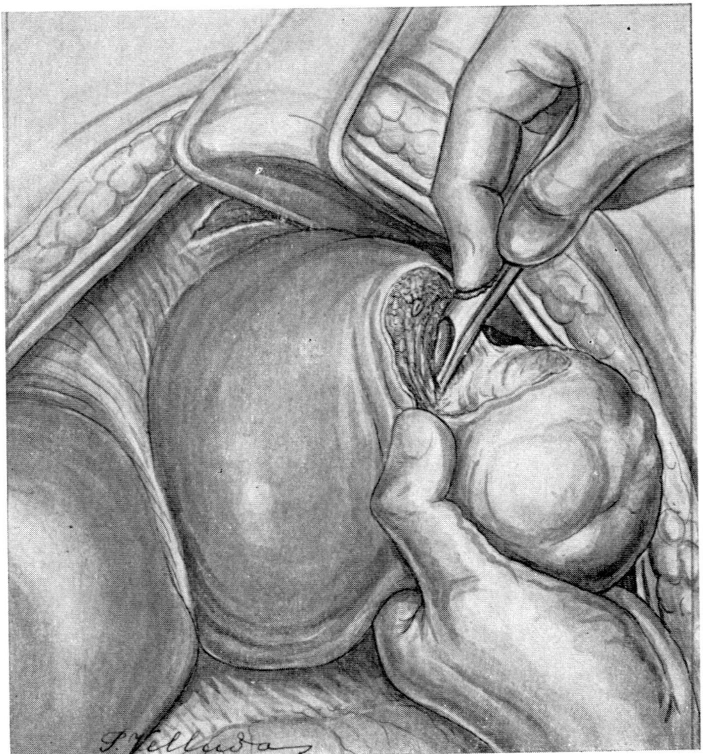

Fig. 153. — Cystectomy for calcified cyst.

After removal of the membrane, a healthy bleeding surface remains that can be sutured immediately, as for instance in the uterus after myomectomy.

When the remaining pouch is suppurated, suture is replaced by hemostatic tamponade and antibiotics. The cavity is then packed with an omentum flap.

In order to avoid intraoperative discharge of bile and hemorrhage the largest bridles are clamped and ligated. The vessels and bile ducts are not severed from the beginning, but previously clamped and ligated, and even attached, in order to avoid their retraction into the depth of the hepatic parenchyma.

When the fundus of the pouch is situated in areas that may be considered dangerous or inaccessible (hepatic hilus, vena cava, etc.), it is advisable not to remove the pericyst. A subhepatic drain should be introduced in all cases.

Partial cystectomy or pericystectomy implies leaving of the pericyst *in situ* in the vicinity of the larger vessels and bile ducts, as in Mabot's procedure. Extirpation of a good part of the pericyst makes it easier to approach the walls and

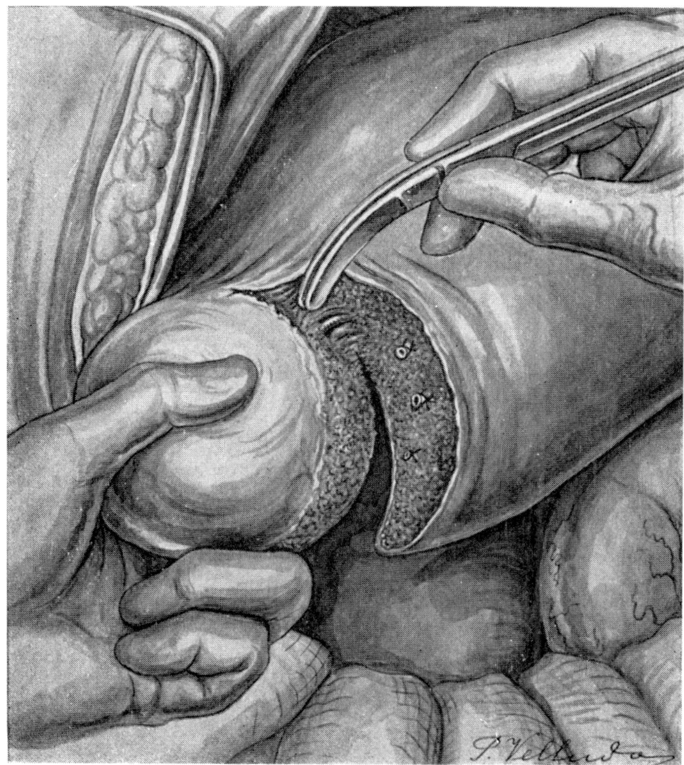

Fig. 154. — Ideal cystectomy.

in some cases the parenchyma may be completely sutured onto the remaining pericyst, with or without omentoplasty. Contact drainage should be performed in these cases, too.

Cystectomy, applied in 60 of our cases, has the great advantage of being radical, removal of the pericystic adventitia factually solving the problem of the remaining cavity.

Leaving of the membrane *in situ*, as with the other procedures, exposes the patient to two great risks: local hydatid recurrence and intrahepatic septic foreign body.

Indeed, the microscopic examinations revealed the presence of inclusions with scolices within the pericystic membrane, which at any moment may result

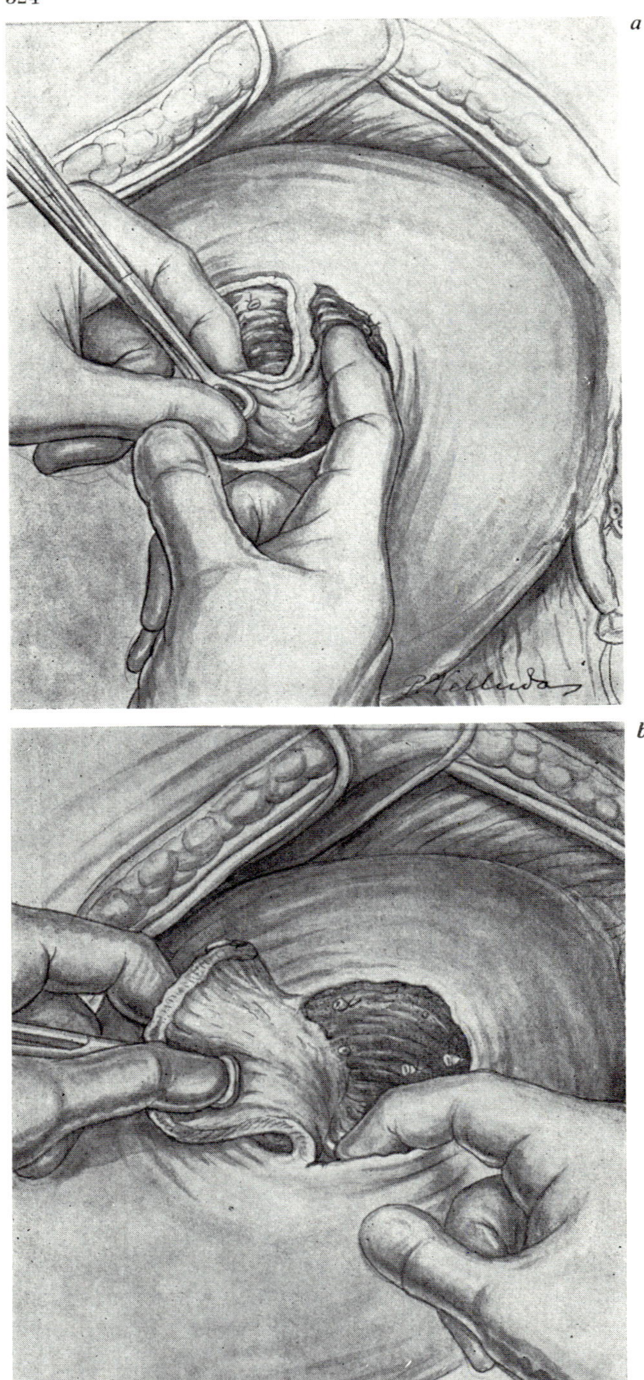

Fig. 155 *a* and *b*. — Pericystectomy with open pouch.

in relapse. Melnikov and other authors, in their studies on the anatomy and physiology of the pericystic membrane, showed that it is formed of fibrous, fasciculate, nonvascularized connective tissue deriving from the viscera but with an anatomophysiologic behavior of its own, depending both upon the parasite and upon the liver.

The young evolutive cysts have a thin membrane, difficult to detach from the liver and through which hydromineral exchanges take place. At the level of this membrane a continuous calcification process develops, increasing and individualizing the pericyst.

The amount of calcium contained in the pericystic membrane may attain impressive figures in comparison to the calcium content of the liver parenchyma. This calcification has proved to be directly proportional to the vitality of the parasite and the intensity of the hepatic reactions.

The calcification process is more accentuated on the internal aspect of the pericystic membrane, the external aspect remaining lax.

In general it is considered that the pericystic membrane is a means of defense of the organism against the parasite. From the above it may be concluded that cystectomy or pericystectomy is more readily performed in cases of older calcified cysts than in younger evolutive cysts, through the membrane of which intense nutritive exchanges take place.

A young, uncalcified membrane will oppose less resistance to healing of the remaining cavity after extirpation of the parasite, than a calcified membrane.

A thick, more or less calcified membrane is almost always infected. In this connection we have already described the role of fissures into the bile ducts, in the triggering and maintenance of infections of the pericyst.

Consequently, the pericystic membrane should be considered as a septic foreign body situated within the hepatic parenchyma.

Another question which has given rise to many discussions is that of the presence or absence of inclusions with scolices in the pericystic membrane and of whether the adventitia by a mechanism of exogenous proliferation can become infiltrated with daughter cysts.

According to Yovanovitsch, parasitic formations, included in or neighboring the pericystic membrane, are found in one of seven cystectomies. These are exogenous vesicles deriving from the germinative sand produced by the brood capsule and which are included in the pericystic membrane and sometimes even in the adjacent hepatic parenchyma in the form of more or less separate diverticuli. The existence of these formations had already been described by Devé. Others, among whom Constantini, deny the existence of such formations. Although in our cases we never met with such proliferations, we always pleaded for pericystectomy in long-standing cysts, based upon the data in the literature concerning numerous recurrences occurring *in situ*, which lend support to the possible existence of parasitic formations able to develop in the pericystic membrane. Therefore, removal of the pericystic membrane is strongly to be advised, provided it is technically possible without endangering the patient's life or producing severe complications.

Partial cystectomy has also certain drawbacks, which may, however, also be due to technical mistakes, such as scraping of the endocyst or its gradual thinning, which do not permit a controlled technique, a minute progressive and methodical maneuver separating the pericyst from the healthy tissue with detection and ligation of the blood vessels and ducts before severing. The healthy tissue can be sutured or lined.

The hazard of intra- or postoperative hemorrhage must also be kept in mind especially with cysts situated close to the vascular hilus. In such cases, it is recommended to leave *in situ* the fundus of the fibrous sac that is in contact with the large vessels of the hili. The fact that the pericyst is surrounded by a vascular and biliary crown encrusted in the hepatic parenchyma, consequently with the risk of severing a blood vessel or bile duct, should never be overlooked.

On establishing the indication or contraindication for a cystectomy or pericystectomy, the following elements should be had in view: fissuring of the cyst into the bile ducts, the site and volume of the cyst, the patient's general condition. Before cystectomy, some of the means of investigation mentioned must be applied, of which cholangiography before and after evacuation of the contents of the cyst is the most important. Cystectomy will be indicated in:

— young, recently fissured cysts, i.e. exposed to secondary suppuration if not treated by cystectomy. The adventitia should be raised, the vessels and fissured bile ducts ligated in the pericystic pouch and the hepatic wound sutured;

— calcified cysts, that can be raised *en masse* when situated on the cleavage plane between the adventitia and liver; as a rule it is free of blood vessels;

— suppurated cysts;

— cysts opening into the bile ducts, since choledochotomy with drainage is not sufficient to obtain recovery.

Bearing these facts in mind, we agreed with other authors on the contraindications of the operation and do not apply it in cases of:

— very young, non-suppurated cysts, where cystotomy without drainage and with simple reduction is the most indicated operation as already mentioned;

— central cysts of small size that should not be operated until they exteriorize;

— cysts with a difficult location in the hilus of the liver or very close to the inferior vena cava. Less radical measures are indicated in such cases;

— giant cysts that demand resection of the fibrous coat and sometimes partial hepatectomy or even lobectomy;

— multiple cysts of the left lobe, when it is preferable to carry out left hepatectomy. This is fully justified since in order to remove multiple cysts the surgeon is obliged to resect the altered pericystic parenchyma, severing a number of regional and segmentary pedicles, and therefore putting out of action an important part of the hepatic gland. Actually, in such cases cystectomy or pericystectomy is a blind hepatectomy.

Very good results were obtained by us in 50 cases of partial cystectomy or pericystectomy on an open, evacuated cyst. In relatively young and often non-fissured cysts we used simpler methods. Bourgeon considered partial or total pericystectomy as the procedure of choice in case of complicated cysts and a thick adventitia with biliary fistulas.

In multiple cysts operated in a single stage, each cyst is treated successively as if it were a separate cyst.

In case of multiple cysts of the liver and peritoneal echinococcosis, some authors recommend treating the liver cysts in a first stage and the peritoneal cysts in a second stage. Although the importance of this tactics has been emphasized, we have successfully operated all the cysts in the same operative stage, since we considered it illogical to temporize.

Hepatectomy for hydatid cyst: *Non-anatomic resection or cystoresection.* In agreement with the modern tendencies in the treatment of hydatid cysts of the

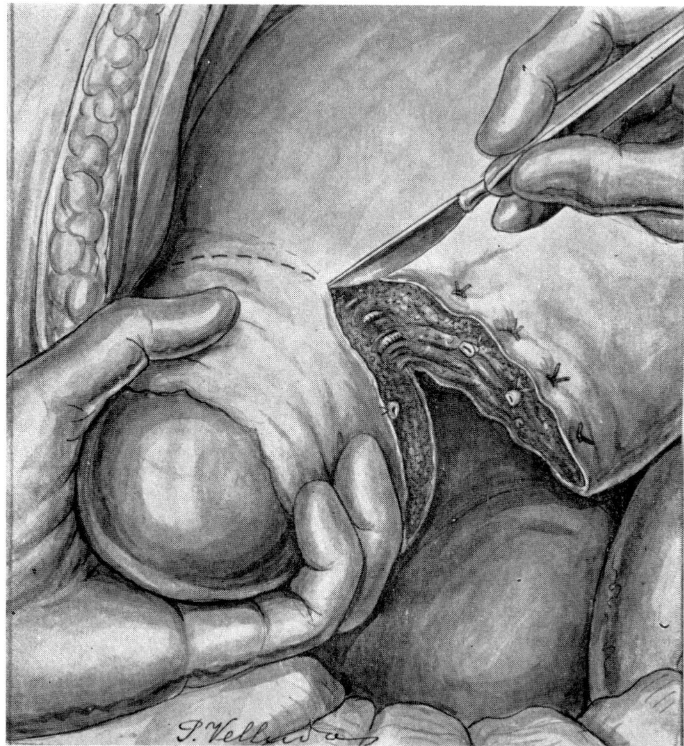

Fig. 156. — Cystoresection. Part of the neighboring parenchyma is also removed.

liver, and firstly with Bourgeon who defended radical surgery of the hydatid cyst during the latter years, we applied non-anatomic resections or cystoresection in 22 cases. In these cases this procedure appeared to be the most radical and sure and with the lowest sacrifice of the organ.

In general, the cysts have thickened, suppurated walls and are favorably located towards the outer margin of the liver, with a thin surrounding hepatic tissue, definitely jeopardized as a rule.

The operation (Fig. 156) consists in removing the cyst with the adventitia and part of the involved parenchyma. Actually, a resection limited to the level of the cyst. This implies either resection of some pedicles *de visu*, or prior stay U-sutures along the whole length of the part to be excised and its sectioning. The cut part is sometimes sutured with continuous catgut stitches, controlling the tightness of the ducts by retrograde cholangiography through the gallbladder or common bile duct, after clamping the latter.

The residual recess is rapidly occupied by the neighboring organs without any drawbacks. In all the 22 cases operated in this way, recovery *per primam* was obtained without complications.

Controlled hepatectomy implies resection of part of the liver (segment, region, half the liver or even more) containing the cyst, after prior ligation of the pedicles of this portion. Our practice amounts to 14 controlled hepatectomies for hydatid cyst of the liver. The indications depend upon the size of the cyst or number of the cysts and irreversible alteration of the hepatic tissue.

Controlled or anatomic hepatectomy (Fig. 157 *a* and *b*) is indicated only in cysts including a whole lobe, or in diffuse, racemose cysts.

Normally, hypertrophy of the residual liver preexists, and its absence points to circulatory disturbances in the parasite-free liver and is, therefore, a contraindication for hepatectomy. The technique shall not be described, as it has already been dealt with in detail in the chapter concerning controlled hepatectomies.

The treatment of calcified hepatic hydatid cyst implies understanding of the fact that calcification does not mean spontaneous recovery of an old cyst. Calcification may also be encountered in young cysts, although more seldom than in older cysts in which the pericystic adventitia is formed by successive layers of calcium. As a rule, these calcified cysts have a biliary core with a magma that visibly bears the imprint of infection. This lends support to the point of view of Devé who asserted that calcification does not implicitly mean death of the parasite. Calcification is a complication that may have severe consequences. The presence of a calcified cyst in the hepatic parenchyma is followed by fissures of the bile system, opening into the pericyst, upsetting the entire vascular architecture and contributing to the onset of cirrhosis by cholostasis. To this is added the danger of an "exogenous vesiculation" owing to the presence of the parasite in the pericyst.

The concentric calcium lamellae in the adventitia fit into one another like "tiles on a rooftop", forming a rigid, resistant shell that can no longer be pared off. In the past, attempts were made to empty these cysts, followed by marsupialization, but the results were most unfortunate because of the irreversible rigidity of the cyst wall, which favors an endless discharge of bile, suppuration or hemorrhage.

We have frequently encountered calcified hydatid cysts, either single or next to uncalcified cysts of the liver. The 28 calcified cysts treated by us represent 8% of our statistics; 18 were men and 10 women. In 27 cases recovery was obtained, and in one case of giant calcified cyst, that occupied almost all the right hepatic lobe, an attempt at right hepatectomy was followed by death.

Case 51. Patient *P.M.*, aged 31, was admitted for a large tumor in the right hypochondrium. Eosinophilia 23%. Positive Casoni test. Phenomena of anaphylaxis. The first symptoms of the disease dated back 16 years. A diagnosis of hydatid cyst was made and confirmed intraoperatively. The cyst was partly calcified. Cholangiography revealed multiple large openings towards the intrahepatic bile ducts. Anatomic right hepatectomy was performed, under difficult

a

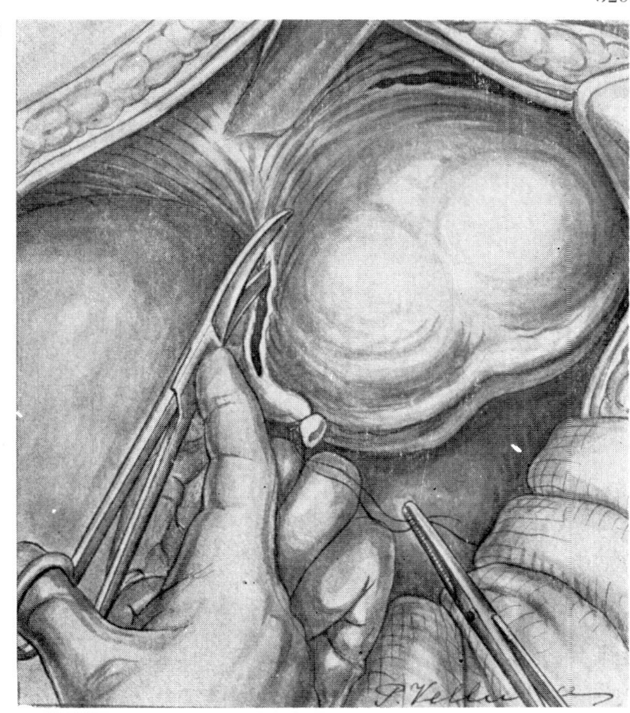

b

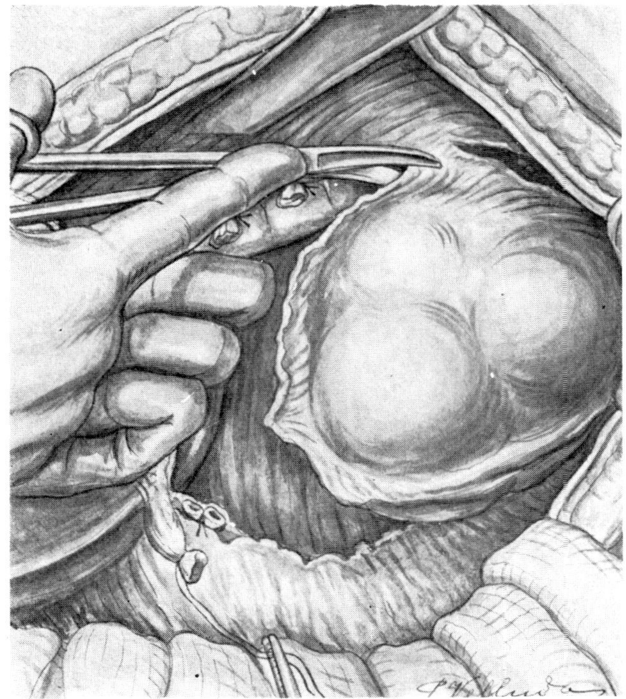

Fig. 157 *a* and *b*. — Left lobectomy for multiple cysts of the liver.

conditions. Excessive peroperative hemorrhage, ending in collapse and death in spite of intensive therapy.

Choice of the operative approach was dictated by our way of conceiving the presence of the calcified cyst in the liver, resorting in principle to exeresis procedures. In our statistics there are 8 cystectomies (Napalkov), 10 cystoresections and 10 controlled hepatectomies. The procedures were chosen in terms of the site of the cysts, their number and size. Extraadventitial cystectomies were always carried out on closed cysts and finished by suture of the hepatic parenchyma. The thick resistant membrane, the relatively easy cleavage, the ligatures performed one after the other, avoided complications (cholerrhagia or hemorrhage); hospitalization averaged 8 to 14 days.

Cholangiography was useful because it demonstrated rupture of the pericyst and in two cases the presence of dead daughter cysts in the extrahepatic bile ducts; choledochotomy was combined either with external drainage or with choledochoduodenotomy. In two cases — one with colic fistula and the other with choledochoduodenotomy — fragments of calcified hydatid membrane were eliminated in the feces.

Most cystoresections were performed for marginal cysts, at times very voluminous, occupying the whole lobe and having calcified walls, over two thirds or all the surface.

The intimate adhesions that develop between the calcified cyst and the neighboring organs, or mesocolon and hilus, give rise to particular problems. We preferred in all these cases, after surgery of the liver, to leave upon these formations a pericystic crust, at the same time ensuring efficient drainage.

Although we performed 10 anatomic hepatectomies for calcified hepatic cysts, we consider cystoresections preferable and only the extent of the lesion and the location of the cysts obliged us to resort to hepatectomies.

The treatment of concomitant cysts of the liver and lung. Concomitant cysts of the liver and lung were encountered in 16 cases and of the liver and mediastinum in one case.

Ideal in the treatment of such localizations would be a single operation. This, however, is only possible when the pulmonary cyst is located at the base of the right lung or even middle right lobe and the hepatic cyst on the upper surface of the liver. This combination was met with in 5 cases.

Case 213. Patient *C.T.*, aged 37, was admitted for thoracic pain, coughing, tumor in the right hypochondrium. Plain X-ray of the abdomen revealed a round opacity measuring 3 cm in diameter in the right middle lobe. Preoperative diagnosis: right pulmonary hydatid cyst and hepatic hydatid cyst. Both foci were treated concomitantly by right thoracotomy and Sprengel laparotomy. Recovery without complications.

We considered that thoracophrenolaparotomy is to be preferred in such cases. In half of the cases mentioned we resorted to this procedure.

In cases of multiple cysts of the liver we preferred to perform thoracotomy in a second stage. We proceeded in this way in a case of marked abdominal development of a cyst, with compression of the bile ducts which obliged us to approach the hepatic cyst first. In such cases jaundice must be dealt with in the first instance. In another three cases in which jaundice was recent, laparotomy was carried out at the same time as thoracotomy.

In one patient both a mediastinal and a hepatic hydatid cyst were found.

Case 4. The patient *M.N.*, 29 years old, operated 3 years previously for hydatid cyst of the right hepatic lobe, was admitted for vomiting, coughing, loss of body weight, dull cardiac sounds, pain in the epigastrium, fever. Tomography and teleradiography revealed a formation, probably cystic, at the level of the mediastinum, which continued with a hepatic opacity in the left lobe. The clinical and radiologic diagnosis was confirmed by transparietal splenoportography. Thoracotomy. Pericardotomy. After evacuation of the cyst which was suppurated, rupture of the diaphragm was detected with the presence of a second cyst in the left lobe of the liver. Hepatic pericystectomy, drainage of the thoracic and abdominal cavities. Recovery after 25 days, without complications.

Problems of surgical methods. The surgeon, faced with the extraordinary variety of the forms taken on by the hydatid disease of the liver, actually has at his disposal only a small number of techniques. Careful choice of the procedure in each case is the only way to obtain good results.

One cannot start on an operation for hepatic hydatid cyst with preconceived ideas. The surgeon must, therefore, be closely acquainted with all the procedures, so as to be able to meet any situation according to the factors that have to be taken into consideration: the content of the cyst, site, involvement of the bile ducts, number of cysts, etc. Of particular importance is the existence of biliary fistulas.

When there is no biliary fistula, a simple operation — cystotomy for instance with or without resection — must result in recovery very rapidly. In our statistics, 75% of the cases recovered rapidly, and 60% *per primam* after 10—15 days. Exeresis was only applied when the cysts were situated marginally, were very large and surrounded by a wide area of definitely involved hepatic tissue.

In case of biliary fistulas one of the radical methods must be used: pericystectomy or internal drainage of the pericystic pouch.

The same problem may also be considered from the viewpoint of the cystic content. A clear content and a thin, supple pericyst can be treated by simple methods, postoperative discharge of the bile not being important. A radical operation can only be justified by considerations of a topographic order.

Whenever the fluid is turbid, purulent, biliary, therefore with evident fissures into the bile ducts, and the pericyst is thickened, the surgeon should have in view removal of the pericyst and drainage of the extrahepatic bile ducts.

Calcified cysts represent a special problem; in general, their treatment implies total cystectomy or pericystectomy.

Similarly, the *location* in the liver influences the attitude of the surgeon to a great extent (Fig. 158 *a, b, c, d, e, f*). The most difficult situation is that of the deep, central hydatid cysts, communicating with the bile ducts and vessels.

Choice of the operative procedure in terms of the site of the lesion. According to F. Lagrot and P. Coriat, it is very seldom that a diagnosis can be made in true central locations of the cyst. In general, a smaller or larger swelling appears on the surface of the liver. These authors recommend surgery nevertheless, because even if it is not possible to flatten the cyst it will be possible to open the cavity and obtain recovery. When the cyst is indeed central, then this method cannot be used. After puncture and formalinization, the cavity could no longer be found and was abandoned. Two years later, at another operation, there were no longer any signs of hydatid cyst and the hepatic tissue was of normal consistency.

Polar cysts, on the external margin of the liver are generally treated by radical operations of the cystoresection type or by the flattening procedure of Lagrot and Coriat, with contact drainage.

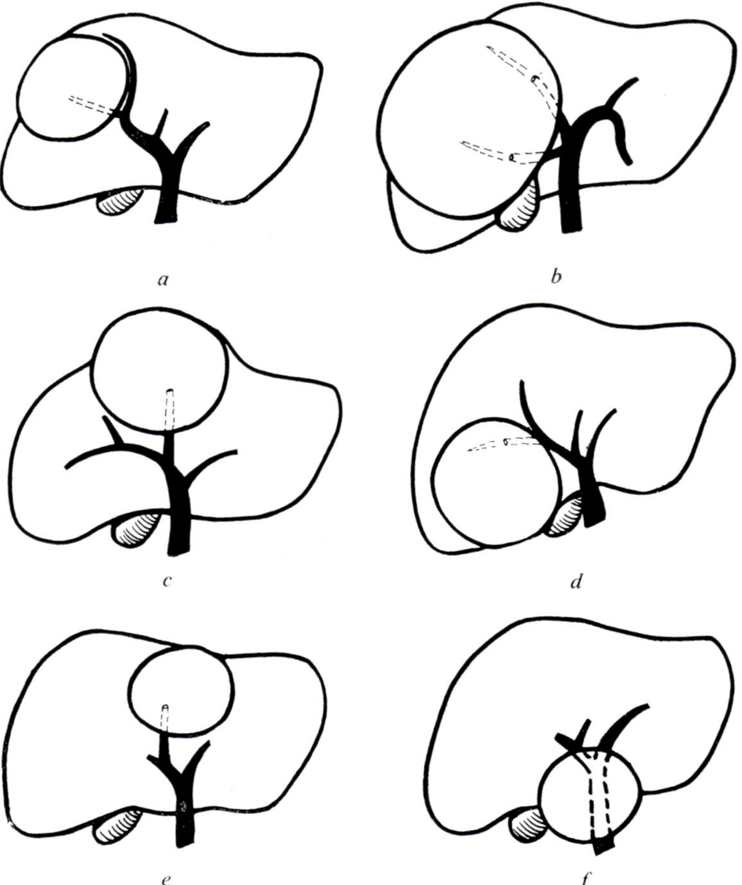

Fig. 158. — Different, more frequent locations of the hydatid cyst. *a)* right polar cyst; *b)* dextromedian; *c)* of the cupola; *d)* of the under surface; *e)* central superior; *f)* central inferior.

The cysts localized on the cupola of the liver and the posterior cysts may be approached by thoracophrenolaparotomy (see Fig. 149), performing a pericystectomy after severing the triangular ligament.

The cysts of the undersurface permit a more varied treatment, it being possible to apply almost any of the procedures listed. The incidence of multiple cysts with this localization is very high (36% in our statistics). In general, it may be asserted that one of two patients has multiple cysts.

Hydatid cysts opening into the bile ducts. The best approach in such cases of rupture into the bile ducts and obstruction of the common bile duct appears to be that of establishing the procedure from case to case, the patient's general condition being one of the most important arguments.

In all cases a good preoperative preparation is obligatory, in an attempt to correct the biological constants and hepatic functions. Intraoperatively, the liver should be explored with the greatest attention in order to detect the cysts both by current means and by cholangiography. The gallbladder and bile ducts must likewise be explored by the same means, since they may also contain daughter cysts.

The procedure is chosen according to the location of the cyst and of the obstruction, and the patient's general state of health.

In central cysts that are not exteriorized, we have used simple drainage of the common bile duct.

When the obstruction is in the bile ducts, choledochotomy is not sufficient; both the right and left hepatic ducts will have to be catheterized, washed and aspirated until opening and drainage of the conduit is obtained.

When the patient's condition permits, an attempt should be made to operate the hepatic cyst and open the bile ducts in the same stage.

When the volume and location of the cyst demands hepatectomy, this must be performed be it either anatomic or controlled, and we have not hesitated to do so even after biliary drainage if it was necessary.

When the patient's state of health was very poor, the simplest procedures were applied together with choledochotomy for deobstruction, and followed or not by sphincteroplasty or choledochoduodenostomy, according to the cholangiographic indications.

On summing up our attitude, we again insist upon the inadvisability of large operations with the sacrifice of normal tissue and great hazard, especially as the simple and even the conservative methods have given good results. The choice of the procedure must depend upon a series of factors, among which:

— the site and volume of the cyst, its relationship with the liver pedicles;
— pathoanatomic alterations of the cyst, parenchyma and pericyst;
— the patient's state of health.

On the basis of our experience, choice of the procedures may be schematically represented as follows:

Cystectomy or pericystectomy :

— pediculate cysts;
— young, recently fissured cysts;
— multivesicular cysts, with a thick wall and infected, biliary content;
— calcified cysts;
— cysts opening into the bile ducts.

Cystotomy followed or not by drainage :

— small recent cysts with a clear fluid without pathologic alterations of the parenchyma and pedicles.

Cystotomy with flattening of the cavity :

— in all cases in which the pericyst can be resected.

Cystoresection and controlled hepatectomy:

— voluminous cysts occupying half the liver or an extensive area;

— multiple cysts within an area limited to half the liver;

— alveolar echinococcosis in a single lobe or segment, in half or even more than half the liver.

Surgery of the hepatic hydatid cyst is a complex problem that raises questions of intraoperative diagnosis, methods and technique.

After a careful summing up of all the elements mentioned, the surgeon must choose the method presenting the lowest hazard and at the same time that which will result in complete and rapid recovery, avoiding postoperative complications.

REFERENCES

1. Aucev N., Atanasov A., Khirurghiya, 1964, *3*, 26.
2. Andreoiu C., Andriu V., Chirurgia, 1956, *2*, 231.
3. * * * *Archives internationales de la Hidatidose*, vol. 16, Paris, 1957.
4. Atucha I., Rev. Chir., 1955, **58**, *4*, 225 .
5. Bacques P., Sem. Hôp. Paris, 1956, **32**, *62*, 3210.
6. Bakaloudis P., Mém. Acad. Chir., 1968, **94**, *12—13*, 424.
7. Bejan I., Covaci P., Timişoara med., 1958, *1—2*, 179.
8. Bernandini P., *Congrès International de Gastroentérologie*, Bruxelles, June 1—6, 1964.
9. Bidulescu A., Popescu S., Mocanu V., Chirurgia, 1962, *2*, 223.
10. Boulvin R., Acta chir. belg., 1957, **49**, *3*, 890.
11. Bourgeon R., Marseille chir., 1957, **9**, *2*, 272.
12. Bourgeon R., Pietri H., Sem. Hôp. Paris, 1957, **33**, *14*, 910.
13. Bourgeon R., Pietri H., Sem. Hôp., 1952, *61—52*, 2460.
14. Bourgeon R., Pietri H. et al., Afrique franç. Chir. (Alger), 1956, **14**, *3*, 202.
15. Bourgeon R. et al., Rev. int. Hépatol. 1956, **6**, *8*, 997.
16. Bourgeon R. et al., Afrique franç. Chir., 1957, **15**, *2*, 135.
17. Bourgeon R. et al., Arch. Mal. Appar. digest., 1954, **43**, *2*, 168.
18. Bourgeon R. et al., Presse méd. 1953, *74*, 1515.
19. Bourgeon R. et al., Maroc méd., 1954, **347**, 316.
20. Bourgeon R. et al., *Traitement chirurgical actuel de kyste hidatique du foie*, Congr. Franç. Chirurgie, 1961.
21. Bourgeon R., Moniel J., Mém. Acad. Chir., 1964, **90**, *11—12*, 355.
22. Burghele Th., Bora A., Chirurgia, 1935.
23. Burghele Th., Bora A., Niţescu, Chirurgia, 1938, *11—12*, 905.
24. Burlui D., Raţiu O., Condiescu M., Chirurgia, 1967, *5*, 403.
25. Burlui D., Condiesco M., Manesco G., Lyon chir., 1968, **64**, *2*, 220.
26. Buţureanu Vl., Rev. med. Chir. (Iaşi), 1958, *2*, 299.
27. Carcasonne M., Marseille chir., 1958, **10**, *4*, 510.
28. Chereseto P. L., Surgeons, 1959, **31**, *4*, 375.
29. Chevnier L. E., France méd., 1958, **21**, *2*, 83.
30. Chiricuţă I., Manoliu C., Rosner O., Chirurgia, 1956, *3*, 431.
31. Ciobanu St., Butnaru M., Petrila P., Chirurgia, 1960, *1*, 67.
32. Ciobanu St., Butnaru M., Rev. med. Chir. (Iaşi), 1962, *2*, 273.
33. * * * Presse méd., 1951, *70*, 1401.
34. Costescu N., Viaţa med., 1960, *8*, 633.
35. Covali N., Chirurgia, 1960, *1*, 55.
36. Dante T., Chirurgia (Uruguay), 1964, *3*, 335.
37. Demirieau J., Mém. Acad. Chir. Paris, 1956, **82**, *14—15*, 470.
38. Devé F., *L'echinococcose primitive*, Masson, Paris, 1949.
39. Devé F., *L'echinococcose secondaire*, Masson, Paris, 1949.
40. Enev K., Khir. (Sofia), 1964, **16**, *60*, 497.

41. Făgărăşanu I., Burlui D., Albu E.,Microbiol. Parazitol. Epidemiol., 1965, **10**, *3*, 203.
42. Făgărăşanu I., Albu E., Cohn A., *Aspectele chirurgicale şi medico-sociale ale chistului hidatic hepatic. Consideraţiuni pe marginea experienţei noastre în tratamentul chistului hidatic*. In *Omagiu lui St. G. Nicolau*, 1965, Ed. Acad., Bucharest, p. 405.
43. Făgărăşanu I., Aloman D., Probleme de terapeutică, 1965, **9**, *1*, 9.
44. Făgărăşanu I., Aloman D., Chirurgia, **9**, *4*, 495.
45. Făgărăşanu I., Dobrovici N., Med. int., 1957, *1—4*, 36.
46. Fraissee I. H., Arch. Mal. Appar. digest., 1958, **47**, *5*, 620.
47. Gheorghescu B., Brasia I., Med. int., 1964, **16**, *4*, 453.
48. Gherasim M., Pascu Paszter, Chirurgia, 1959, *1*, 67.
49. Gherman I., Debau M., Med. int., 1965, *10*, 1149.
50. Goinard P., Pégulbo V., Pélissier V., *Le kyste hidatique. Thérapeutique chirurgicale*, Masson, Paris, 1960.
51. Goinard P., Pégulbo, Afrique franç. Chir. Alger, 1958, **16**, *4*, 350.
52. Goinard P., Toulouse méd., 1956, **57**, *1*, 29.
53. Guedj P., J. Chir. (Paris) 1967, **93**, *2*, 191.
54. Haratular St., *Tratamentul chirurgical al chistului hidatic de ficat* in *Conferinţa chirurgicală interregională privind problemele chistului hidatic*, Constanţa, 1957.
55. Juvara I., Manescu G., Vasilescu D., Lyon chir., 1958, **54**, *3*, 405.
56. Juvara I., Rădulescu D., Prişcu A., *Probleme medico-chirurgicale de patologie hepato-biliară*, Ed. Medicală, Bucharest, 1969.
57. Kourias B., Presse Méd., 1961, *4*, 105.
58. Kourias B., J. Chir., 1957, **74**, *2*, 138.
59. Kourias B., Mantonakis S., J. Chir., 1968, **96**, *1—2*, 21.
60. Lagrot F., Coriat P., Sem. Hôp. Ann. Chir., 1957, *7—8*, 475.
61. Lagrot F., Coriat P., Ann. Chir., 1961, **15**, *13—14*, 877.
62. Lagrot F., Coriat P., Lyon Chir., 1959, *55*, 826.
63. Lougs O. F., Sociedad Montevideo, 1958, **42**, *6*, 179.
64. Lupaşcu Gh., Panaitescu D., *Hidatidoza*, Ed. Acad., Bucharest, 1968.
65. Mandache Fl., Ghergut A., Popescu M., Chirurgia, 1965, *12*, 1097.
66. Miniconi P., Algérie méd., 1956, **60**, *12*, 1023.
67. Olivier Cl., *Chirurgie des voies biliaires extra — et intrahépatiques*, Masson, Paris, 1961.
68. Palma R., G. ital. Chir., 1958, **14**, *2*, 163.
69. Panaitescu D., Microbiol., Parazitol., Epidemiol., 1964, **9**, *3*, 235.
70. Panaitescu D., *Contribuţiuni la studiul diagnosticului imunologic al hidatidozei umane*, Doctoral thesis, Bucharest, 1962.
71. Panaitescu D., Microbiol., Parazitol., Epidemiol., 1960, *3*, 217.
72. Papahagi E., Chirurgia, 1959, *2*, 281.
73. Peretz-Fontana V., Arch. int. hidatid., 1956, **16**, 509.
74. Pongrátz E., Gyöngyösi G., Orvosi hetilap, 1961, *41*, 1937.
75. Popescu C., Chirurgia, 1958, *2*, 263.
76. Popescu V., Chirurgia, 1959, *1*, 91.
77. Purastu F., Rev. Med. Sarda, 1958, **60**, *5*, 501.
78. Rassi L., Ass. Med. Brasil, 1955, **2**, *1*, 69.
79. Setlacek D., Niculiu Gh., Stănescu M., Popa Gh., Chirurgia (Buc.), 1967, *2*, 105.
80. Simitsch T., Epizoot., 1961, **1**, *3—4*, 738.
81. Slurian S., Titescu V., Chirurgia, 1963, **12**, *5*, 767.
82. Ştefănescu N., Rev. Med. Chir., 1964, *4*, 1013.
83. Teodorescu D., Viaţa med., 1958, *2*, 1211.
84. Teodorescu D., *Anchetă privind boala hidatică în România* in *Conferinţa interregională privind problema chistului hidatic hepatic*, Constanţa, 1957.
85. Teodorescu P., Bercovici S., Med. int., 1957, *8*, 1246.
86. Thiodet I., Maroc méd., 1956, **378**, 1080.
87. Tordjman G., Bandale S., Bendabati R., Lyon chir., 1966, *3*, 370—376.
88. Ţurai I., Chirurgia, 1959, *4*, 489.
89. Vergoz G., Mém. Acad. Chir., 1958, **84**, *1—3*, 57.
90. Vernejoul E., De Courbier, Marseille chir., 1956, **8**, *3*, 338.
91. Wechsler L., Antohe E., Rev. Med. Chir. Iaşi, 1964. *4*, 931.
92. Yovanovitsch B., Sem. Hôp. Paris, 1959, 13.

CHAPTER 8

BENIGN TUMORS OF THE LIVER

Benign tumors of the liver present a very varied structure according to the different tissues from which they arise.

However, only certain types of benign tumors are more frequently encountered, which we shall deal with in the following pages.

Although studied by many authors, these tumors have been differently interpreted, as results from the various terms used; the very attitude of these authors towards one treatment or another and towards the mode of appraising the prognosis greatly varies. The problem has been rendered more difficult by the close resemblance between some aspects observed in hepatic postaggressive processes (alteration, regeneration, reaction) and certain morphologic aspects of the benign tumor processes, or even those on the borderline of malignancy.

This is also reflected in many cases by the inability of the histopathologist to draw a line between benign and malignant only on the basis of cytologic peculiarities (E. Gall, in Schiff). Moreover, in establishing the variety of the tumor the histologic examination is not always sufficient and must be completed by the macroscopic data supplied by the surgeon (polycystic disease or solitary parasitic cyst, etc.).

Bearing in mind that, as a rule, the incidence of benign hepatic tumors is fairly low, we shall not study the cases of unusual interest (for instance the single case of leiomyoma published by Rios-Daienz in 1965), but shall insist especially upon those which are comparatively more frequent and whose diagnosis and uncertain evolution raise problems and impose an active therapy.

The numerous present classifications of hepatic tumors, based upon morphologic and pathogenic criteria are known to present several drawbacks, so that we propose to use a morphologic-clinical classification, in which the practitioner may more readily list a given case and establish its prognosis and therapy.

A. HEPATIC ADENOMA

Adenomas are tumors formed of adult, well differentiated cells, developing in glandular organs; they are often encapsulated. In the liver the epithelial cells take on two aspects — the liver cell and the cells of the intrahepatic bile ducts — and adenomas of the liver also present two varieties:

— benign hepatomas, with cells sometimes closely resembling the cells of the hepatic trabeculae;

— benign cholangiomas, recalling in various ways the cells of the intrahepatic bile ducts from which they derive.

PATHOLOGIC ANATOMY

Macroscopically, hepatic adenomas appear as round or oval formations of variable size (1.5 mm in diameter up to the size of a child's head — Alain Mouchet), the color of the hepatic parenchyma, or somewhat lighter (Bockus). The tumor may be single or multiple, without manifesting any special predilection for certain areas in the liver. They gradually tend to become subcapsular, protruding upon the surface of the liver (sessile form) and more seldom have a large pedicle.

Adenomas may be encapsulated or without a well defined capsule.

Microscopic aspects. *Liver-cell adenoma* (benign hepatoma) is formed of polygonal cells sometimes identical to those of the hepatic cords. These cells tend to form cords grouped at times into lobules or separated by bands of fibrosis. The bile ducts show a lesser tendency to proliferation (numeric disproportion between the two kinds of epithelial cells). Vascular ectasia and lymphocytic infiltrates are likewise noted. The tumors themselves may exhibit zones of more accentuated cellular proliferation, with cells of varied size and tinctorial affinity, whose nuclei likewise vary in number and size (Henson).

The tumor may appear either in the form of a simple hepatic dysembryoma (solitary adenoma — Lecène), well encapsulated and with a well defined lobulation, or as a trabecular adenoma in which the full cellular cords do not have a lobular arrangement and the tumor is not encapsulated (Alain Mouchet).

Adenomas of intrahepatic bile ducts (benign cholangioma) are sometimes small and more seldom encountered according to some authors (Sherlock).

Their structure recalls that of the cystadenoma because the cells, arising from the intrahepatic bile ducts, are cuboid or prismatic and more homogeneous than the liver cells. These cells, displaying a canalicular arrangement, delimit a lumen that is sometimes larger and contains the secretion of the cells which become gradually smaller and flatter. At times it is difficult to differentiate between a cholangioma with the evolution of a cystadenoma and the polycystic disease or the structure of the solitary cyst (Sherlock).

There also exists a form in which the two elements (liver-cell and duct elements) are to be found in equal proportions: mixed adenomas (Sherlock) or cholangiohepatoadenomas (Henson) that correspond to a form described at the beginning of the century by Albrecht under the name of hamartoma. The tumor, with its clearly differentiated elements but with a disorganized arrangement, is more often met in children (they might be congenital) and show a rapid growth necessitating an early intervention.

CLINICAL STUDY

Incidence. Adenomas are relatively seldom identified in the clinic because of their association to other affections of the liver that draw the clinician's attention (cirrhosis); however, they appear more often on necropsy protocols methodically drawn up.

In the course of 47 years, in the Mayo Clinic there were 13 hepatic adenomas, of which 5 clinically manifest liver-cell adenomas, 7 small asymptomatic cholangioadenomas discovered incidentally, and 2 hamartomas with rapid growth and voluminous tumor.

Age. Liver-cell adenoma appears to be the tumor of young adults, cholangioadenoma is more often encountered in patients with a longer hepatic past history (38—60 years, according to Henson), and mixed adenoma (hamartoma) in childhood.

Sex does not appear to be of importance.

The present study includes the most common aspects: liver-cell adenoma or adenoma of intrahepatic bile ducts.

Symptoms. The initial phases are always masked by the accompanying hepatic disease; ascites, hematemesis and dysproteinemia are present in 20% of the adenoma cases (Bockus). However, when the neoformation reaches a certain volume it gives signs of clinical and functional disturbances.

In most cases the tumor is palpable, painless or tender on palpation; it may be firm, with a smooth surface or else several nodules may be felt on the upper explorable surface of the liver (multiple adenomas).

The patient seldom complains of pain, he only feels a vague discomfort, especially after meals (mutual compression — Agaev). The pain is seldom sharp, with the clinical picture of acute abdomen, when rupture of the adenoma with intraperitoneal hemorrhage has occurred (Smirnov).

The *biologic tests* are not pathognomonic and are not characteristic of the disease.

The *radiologic examination* may supply useful information; the standard roentgenogram (bases of the thorax and lower half of the abdomen) may show an enlarged liver or a tumor forming a common body with the liver. Pneumoperitoneum may help to identify certain tumors that do not appear on the standard front view.

Barium meals may reveal the presence of esophageal varices, the stigmata of cirrhosis, that often accompany hepatic adenoma; the lesser gastric curvature may be displaced or lengthened, moulding the tumor, and the colic angle descended.

Splenal and portal venography may reveal a hepatic lacuna with a more precise contour than that of an abscess (Bockus). However, neither venography nor the scintigram present distinct signs of hepatic cyst or tumor.

✦

It may, therefore, be concluded that, apart from the misleading signs (of the accompanying disease) or uncharacteristic signs (of compression), only when the tumor itself becomes accessible to palpation or is made evident radiologically is the question of a diagnosis of hepatic adenoma raised.

This shows how difficult it is to establish a diagnosis preoperatively. In the following pages several of the pre- and intraoperative diagnostic aspects will be discussed, mentioning only those aspects which reflect the difficulties encountered in establishing the diagnosis or the limitations of our present possibilities. It should be emphasized that the scintigram shows the contour of hepatic cysts of any kind, including metastatic tumors or primary cancer (zones of lower uptake), but does not clearly differentiate a liver-cell adenoma (with a metabolism analogous to that of the normal liver) from the remaining parenchyma. The cholangioadenoma can be detected, but is often overlooked because of its small size.

DIAGNOSIS

The following problems will be discussed: the diagnosis of tumor, of benign tumor, and its variations — a final stage seldom reached preoperatively, but at any rate obligatory intraoperatively (in cooperation with the anatomopathologist).

Is there a hepatic tumor ? The following aspects should be eliminated:

— supernumerary hepatic lobe;
— *hepar lobatum ;*
— hydatid cyst;
— hepatic syphilis;
— hypertrophic cirrhosis;
— colic, gastric or pancreatic tumors;
— vesicular hydrops.

Is the tumor benign ? A very slow growth (almost stationary), a good general condition, the absence of local symptoms (or attenuated subjective signs), the absence of fever, point to a benign tumor.

Hepatic adenoma ? When the preoperative diagnosis has reached this stage, it should be differentiated from hemangioma (with a variable volume in terms of effort) and from a solitary cyst (renitent, whereas the adenoma is firm).

In most cases the question arises of a tumor that is visible and palpable intraoperatively; all forms of parasitic or nonparasitic cysts are readily eliminated by their characteristic aspect and consistency.

Hemangioma is very different in aspect, as it is purplish and reducible.

Regeneration nodules that appear in a visible cirrhotic liver are small and very numerous.

Even if the foci represent multiple adenomas, this is no longer of interest, as they are not operable. The histologic examination alone may elucidate the question.

These stages in establishing the diagnosis are not always regularly gone through and a tumor may be discovered intraoperatively, whose probable benign character was not established preoperatively.

The differential diagnosis should be established with:

— Secondary adenocarcinoma (as a rule metastases of tumors of the gastrointestinal tract): multiple whitish yellow tumors in an otherwise unmodified liver.

— Primary carcinoma of the liver (tumor, often but not obligatorily single): due to its rapid growth, the tumor is often large when the patient decides to accept the operation and fever develops. Actually, the attitude is the same in case of carcinoma or an assumed benign tumor: resection in healthy tissue whenever possible.

Needle biopsy is not a useful means of diagnosis because an encapsulated hemangioma or a hydatid cyst cannot always be excluded, and the puncture in such cases may be fatal or have severe side effects.

Even if it is possible to exclude formations with a fluid content, biopsy puncture is not indicated, as the small amount of material collected cannot ascertain the benign character of the tumor and may lead to grave errors of diagnosis and indication.

Laparoscopy does not imply great hazard, but offers very little information in a problem in which diagnostic difficulties exist even in the course of explorative laparotomy. Completion with a biopsy does not increase its efficiency to the same extent as it involves risk and disadvantages.

Laparoscopy is performed under aseptic conditions, the same as any surgical intervention, with previous pneumoperitoneum.

Under local anesthesia, a small incision is cut in the right hypochondrium and the laparoscope is introduced. This permits examination of most of the undersurface of the liver and a small part of the upper surface (under favorable conditions and in the absence of perihepatitis) and of the gallbladder. Other parts of the gastrointestinal tract may also come within the range of the laparoscope.

A small fragment is collected from the apparently modified area and from the intact area, for comparison. Hemostasis is accomplished by diathermo- or electrocoagulation, hemorrhage being minimal.

Therefore, there is a clinical preoperative and an intraoperative stage of the diagnosis, completed by extemporaneous histologic examination. The latter is based upon study of the tumor, but also keeps account of the aspect of the peritumoral tissue.

It is worthy of note that liver-cell adenoma and cholangioadenoma develop as a rule in a liver that has undergone prior structural changes, especially cirrhosis, the coexistence of which has been frequently noted (I. Kaufman).

It is known that in cirrhosis destructive and cicatricial lesions alternate with regenerative islets of both epithelial elements. The small, regenerative nodules are not encapsulated; they tend to compress the portal network, thus autoregulating the intensity of regenerative proliferation by reducing the portal blood flow (Mann). The transition from regenerative to adenomatous proliferation is only possible when certain undetermined factors would prevent this autoregulation. This implies that the adenoma is an exaggeration of the lobular, cellular recovery process (i.e. regeneration). Cholangioma recalls the hyperplastic nodules that develop in the intrahepatic bile ducts in the rabbit in the course of certain parasitic diseases; the fact that small cholangiomas frequently appear in geographical regions infested by intestinal parasites (Gall) should not be overlooked.

This accounts for the difficulties that sometimes arise in determining the regenerative or neoplastic character of adenomas of the liver (Abrikosov). However, it should be borne in mind that the regenerative islets are disseminated throughout the whole liver (not only within a few centers as the adenoma), that they are not enclosed in a capsule (as the adenoma frequently is) and, moreover, are very small.

An opposite aspect of the problem is the definition of the benign character of adenomas. Some authors (Hanot, Gilbert, Letulle) attribute a malignant character to all adenomas of the liver. Others have found it very difficult to delimit the fundamental benign character of an adenoma (Kaufman), and still others (Sherlock) even deny the possible malignization of a hepatic adenoma (although they admit invasion of the blood vessels and metastases). Faced with the difficulties of drawing a line between a benign or a malignant adenoma, some authors have proposed a gross appraisal in terms of the diameter of the tumor: any adenoma with a diameter of 2.5 cm is probably malignant (Gall). This appears to be a very arbitrary classification.

Neither does the number of adenomas categorically indicate a tendency to malignization, since there may be cases of long-standing multiple adenomas.

The lack of homogeneity of the cellular aspects appears to be of greater importance (especially the presence of mitosis), as well as the absence of the capsule, certain clinical features (rapid growth, sensitivity or pain at the site of the tumor, low fever), and alkaline phosphatase alterations when normal values were recorded in the near past.

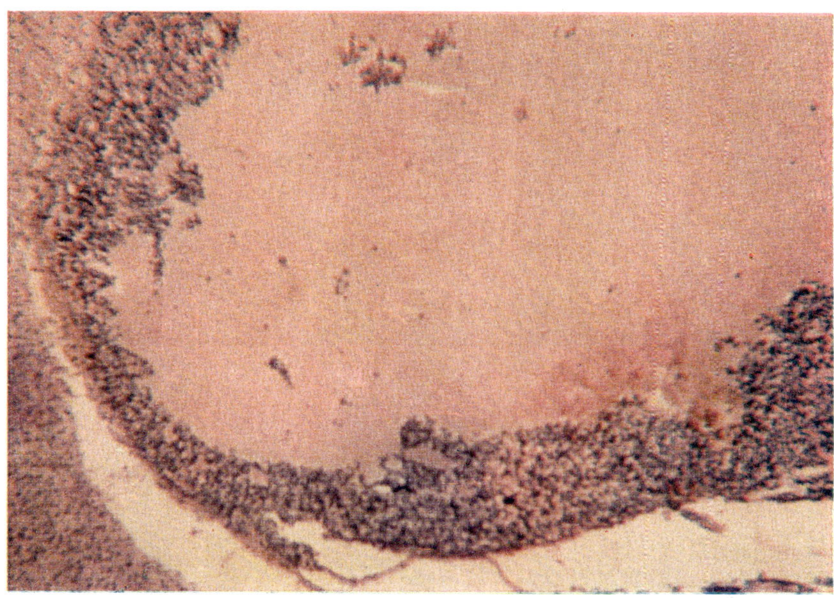

Fig. 159. — Liver cell adenoma. Adenomatous proliferation with cellular necrosis.

The relationships between the regenerative phenomena, hepatic adenomas and malignant hepatoma may be followed up in Figs 159, 160 *a*, *b*, 161 *a*, *b*, 162 *a*, *b* and 163.

PROGNOSIS

Although the lesion is histologically benign, it has a powerful malignant potential. It does not seem correct to adopt either an unfounded optimism (Sherlock) or the pessimism of other authors (Letulle), but to consider hepatic adenoma as a lesion whose benign character is not always demonstrable.

The tumor, by its constant growth, will induce with time phenomena of compression; its removal may be difficult and involve sacrifice of large hepatic areas. The prognosis is good in encapsulated liver-cell adenoma and more reserved in the non-encapsulated trabecular adenoma.

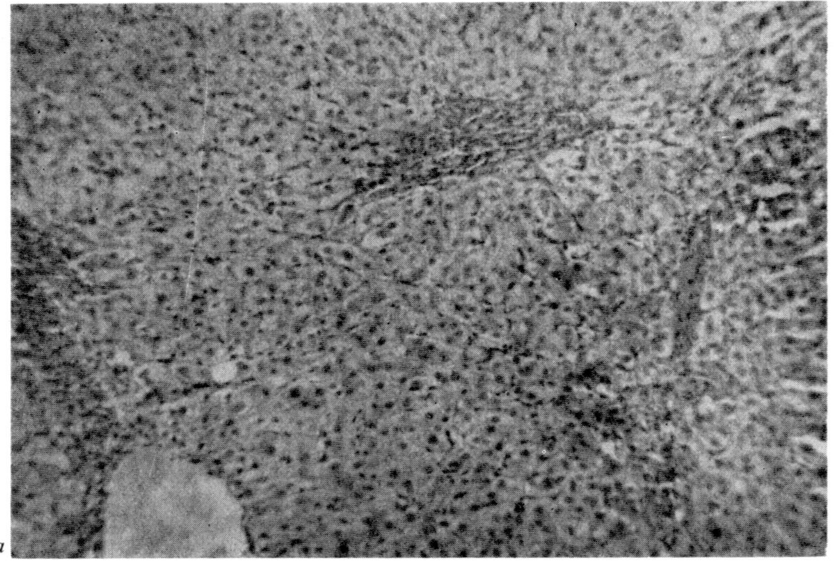

a

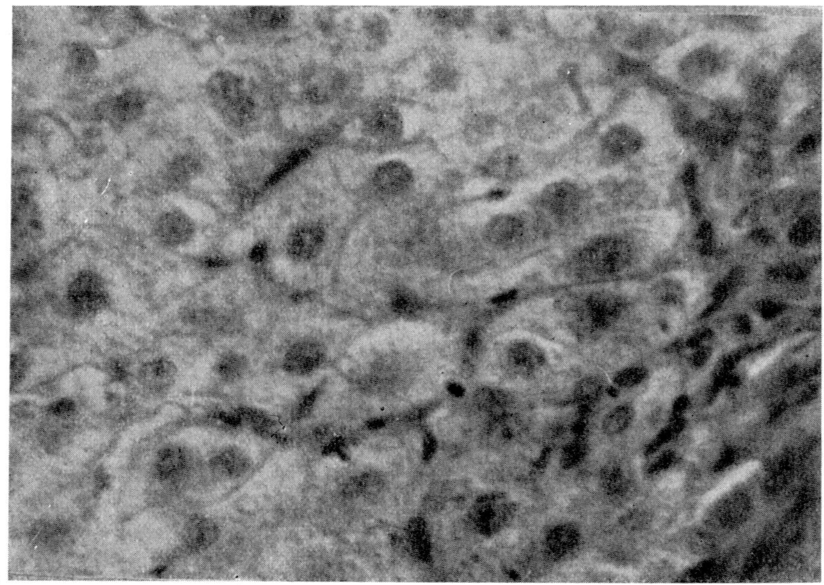

b

Fig. 160 *a* and *b* — Cellular regeneration in the course of chronic hepatitis.

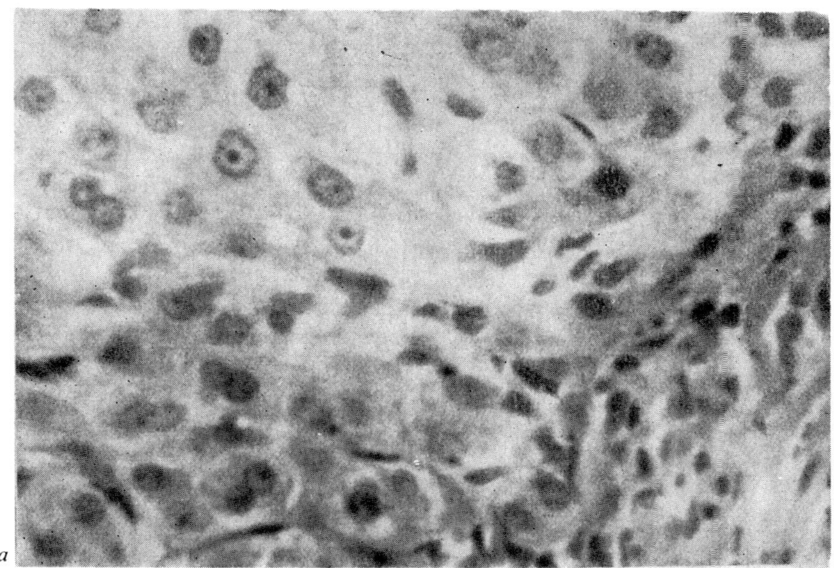

a

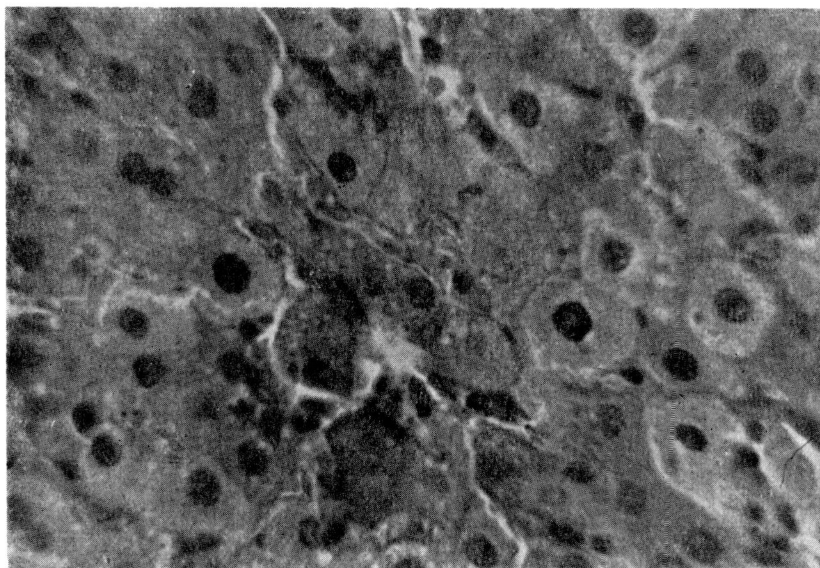

b

Fig. 161 *a* and *b* — Intense cellular regeneration in the course of chronic hepatitis.

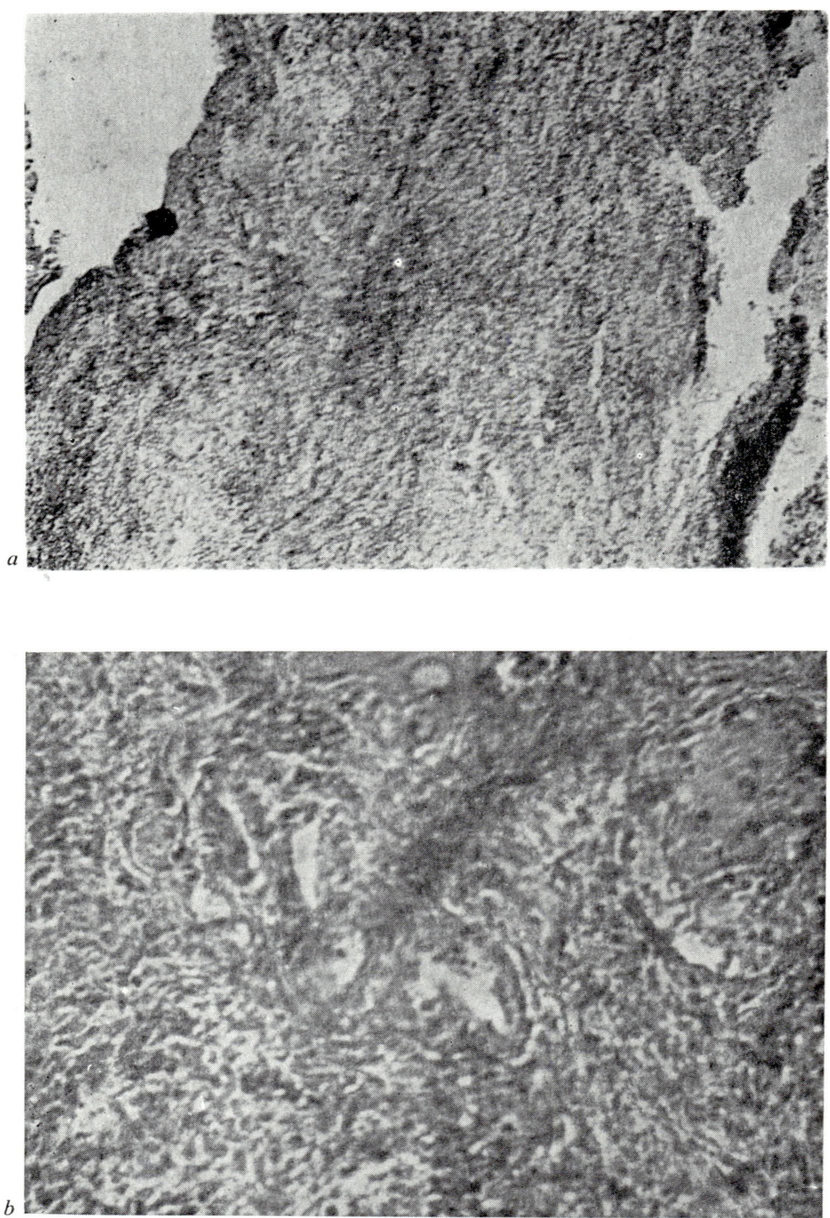

Fig. 162 *a* and *b* — Accentuated proliferation of biliary neocanaliculi in annular cirrhosis.

Surgery often gives good results (Aurousseau, 9 resections and 9 recoveries), but relapses occur in up to 30% of the cases (Wallace, 1941).

TREATMENT

In view of the uncertain prognosis, the general indication will be excision of the tumor with section of healthy tissue, whenever this can be done without too great hazard. The indications must be individualized in each case.

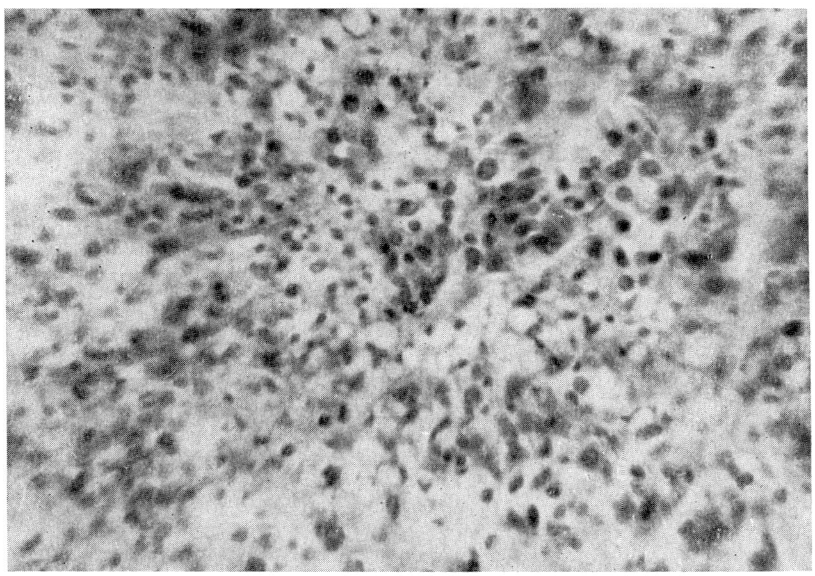

Fig. 163. — Liver carcinoma. Dark cells in the center of the image.

Pedunculate adenoma is essentially a surgical form, even when discovered casually during an operation.

Multiple adenomas cannot be considered surgical lesions when disseminated throughout the whole liver; but there must be no error of diagnosis with the hyperplastic regenerative nodules of cirrhosis. A characteristic fragment should be collected for the histologic examination.

When the nodules are disseminated in a single lobe, then planned lobectomy can be performed, under conditions of team work, with the corresponding resuscitation — anesthesia.

In solitary adenoma occupying the left lobe, or almost the whole lobe, planned or non-anatomic lobectomy may give good results.

For solitary adenoma of the right liver, enucleation is preferred whenever possible, ending with omentoplasty for packing the residual cavity. Right hepatectomy implies high operative hazard, that outweighs the lesser hazard of the adenoma.

Therefore, on establishing the operative indication the operative risk should be weighed against the potential risk of the adenoma when left to evolve, also taking into account the patient's age, physiologic moment, pathologic sequelae, etc., before making a decision as to a radical or conservative approach.

REFERENCES

1. ACHAVAL A., TAUWE W. N., GAMBILL E. E., Proceedings of Mayo Clinics, 1965, **40**, *3*, 206.
2. BOCKUS L. H., *Gastroenterology*, vol. III. W. S. Saunders, Philadelphia, 1953, p. 278.
3. BRZHOZOVSKIY A. G., *Chastnaya khirurghiya*, Medghiz, Moscow, 1954, p. 390.
4. CRĂCIUN E., *Introducere în morfologia patologică*, Ed. medicală, Bucharest, 1958, p. 261.
5. DAIENZ-RIOS J. L., Arch. Pathol., 1965, **79**, *1*, 54.
6. FEY B., MOCQUOT P., OBERLIN S., QUÉNU H., TRUFFERT P., *Traité de technique chirurgicale*, Masson, Paris, 1942, p. 35—50.
7. LETULLE M., *Anatomie pathologique*, vol. III, Masson, Paris, 1931, p. 1946.
8. MOUCHET A., *Nouveau précis de pathologie chirurgicale*, Masson, Paris, 1957, p. 210.
9. SCHIFF L., *Bolile ficatului*, Ed. medicală, Bucharest, 1964, p. 565—602.
10. SHERLOCK SHEILA, *Diseases of the liver and biliary system*, Blackwell, Oxford, 1955, p. 505.
11. *** *Klinicheskie ocherki operativnoy khirurghii*, Medghiz, Moscow, 1954, p. 314.
12. *** *Mnogotomnoe rukovdstvo po khirurghii*, vol. VIII, Medghiz, Moscow, 1962, pp. 260—272; 306—308.

B. NON-PARASITIC CYSTS OF THE LIVER

Cystic formations of the liver form a chapter in surgical pathology that has not yet reached a definite classification.

Up to the end of the 18th century, the most naive and fantastic interpretations were given to the collections of fluid in the liver.

In 1760, Pallas separated a group of cysts with detachable membrane, to which he attributed an animal origin, being the first to refer to the relationship between the hydatid cyst and echinococcus; thus he isolated the large group of *hydatid cysts* which we have studied in a separate chapter.

Non-parasitic cysts were described almost 100 years later.

In 1846, C. Benjamin Brodie evacuated by puncture a hepatic cyst in a young patient; several authors question whether it was a non parasitic cyst (Geist).

The visceral polycystic disease (hepatorenal) only drew the attention of pathoanatomists in 1856, when the first case of non-parasitic cyst of the liver, verified at necropsy, was described by Brisbane (cited by Wickle and Charache, 1956). Other authors attribute the first conclusive description either to Glotz in 1864 (Bulganov, Bregadze) or to Bristowe, in 1855 (Henson). Hufeland, Virchow, Lejars studied the visceral polycystic disease with frequent renal and more seldom hepatorenal localizations.

The polycystic disease of the liver was found by F. Ackman (up to 1931) in eleven of 6,141 necropsies.

In 1856, Michel published a case of solitary hepatic non-parasitic cyst found in a 60 year old man who died from diarrhea.

In literature, there are several cases of non-parasitic solitary (uni- or multilocular) cysts of the liver.

Up to 1937, S. Sherlock found 188 cases and a further 195 cases up to 1942, but did not show whether this was a mathematical total or if she had checked the documentary material to remove the insufficiently characteristic cases.

Up to 1956, Geist found 193 cases of solitary hepatic cysts, checked operatively and histologically (it is the most accurate statistics as regards discrimination of the doubtful cases).

Perreau found less than 250 published cases up to 1965.

The discussions on the unitary pathogeny or particular forms of the solitary cysts and of the polycystic liver have not yet been brought to a close, although many authors, starting with Lenormand and then Bockus, Rachet and Geist, studied the two anatomoclinical aspects separately (solitary cyst and polycystic liver).

The other forms of non parasitic cysts (Bockus, Bregadze, (Henson): *cystadenoma* (proliferative multilocular), *pseudocyst* (degenerative tumoral), *teratoma* (dermoid), *lymphangioma* and *ciliate endothelial cyst* have been individualized, but are seldom encountered.

In the present study we shall deal exclusively with the first two forms of non-parasitic cysts of the liver:

— polycystic disease of the liver (with or without association of polycystic kidney);

— solitary cyst of the liver (uni- or multilocular).

Irrespective of the pathogeny, account shall be taken of the practical aspects (diagnosis and therapy), concomitantly studying both forms and showing the difference between them. The familial character, the association with cystic lesions of other organs, are arguments in favor of a faulty development that takes place already in the intrauterine period (congenital disease) without being able as yet to define what conditions determine a polycystic liver or a solitary cyst.

PATHOLOGIC ANATOMY

The disease is comparatively rare. The most frequent association is that with cysts of the other organs, the kidneys especially, more seldom the pancreas, ovaries, lungs, brain, pituitary, breast, peritoneum, spleen; 56% of the cases are associated with renal polycysts according to Davis, and renal polycysts are associated to hepatic polycysts in 19—33% of the cases according to Comfort.

The size of the cysts varies very much: the smallest are microscopic and the largest the size of a pregnancy at term. They are located within the mass of the hepatic parenchyma or on the surface and are at times pedunculate. Most of them are to be found in the anteroinferior portion of the right lobe. The outer surface is smooth, greyish-blue and glossy, the inner surface is irregular and translucent. The thickness of the walls is as a rule small and there is no cleavage plane between the cyst and the surrounding hepatic tissue. The content is clear, serous, yellowish or brown, fluid or viscous, containing albumin, cholesterol, bile acids and pigments, and sometimes fatty acids, red blood cells and leukocytes. As a rule, the pressure of the fluid is lower than in the hydatid cyst.

Microscopically, the wall is composed of three layers: an internal epithelial layer formed of cuboid or cylindrical cells, which may often be absent; a dense, middle layer, poor in cells and vessels, and an external, lax layer with connective elastic and muscular fibers and many cells and blood vessels. In the external layer, dilated bile canaliculi can be observed, as well as inflammatory infiltrates; the neighboring hepatic parenchyma may be compressed and atrophied. Both the solitary and multiple cysts in the liver have the same origin: an anomaly of the intrahepatic bile ducts.

Several theories have been emitted to explain the genesis of these cysts:

1. The inflammatory theory (Virchow) — by intrafetal cholangitis with obliteration of the canaliculi and retrograde cystic dilation.

2. The neoplastic theory — cystadenomas developing from the bile ducts.

3. The dysembryoplastic theory (Albrecht) — by exaggerated proliferation of the intrahepatic bile ducts during the embryonic period.

4. The degenerative theory (Morris, Tyson). No general consensus has been reached concerning the pathogenic mechanism, but the neoplastic theory and the degenerative theory have been widely accepted among specialists, although both account for a number of cases, but not all of them.

ETIOLOGY

In spite of the relatively rare occurrence of non-parasitic cysts, a certain predominance of the female sex has been noted (90 women to 26 men according to Rizzo, cited by Bregadze). The age at which the disease is most frequently encountered are the third and fourth decades, but asymptomatic forms have been encountered at necropsy at all ages, from newborn children to old subjects.

Finally, an important feature is the aspect of a familial disease taken in the broadest meaning of the word, that is in the same family there are cases of hepatorenal polycystic disease, polycystic liver or solitary cyst of the liver; ovarian or pancreatic cysts are more seldom found in the same family.

CLINICAL STUDY

Non-parasitic cysts of the liver may develop for a long time without drawing the attention of the patient. The disease may therefore be said to present an initial clinical period of latency that may last for a long time and even a lifetime (rare cases discovered at necropsy).

After some time, between the ages of 40 and 60, the disease becomes manifest with symptoms that, although not fully characteristic, point to the visceral aspect of the disease and may raise a suspicion of the disease itself when the patient is carefully examined.

Subjective symptoms. The patient often has a feeling of *tension* in the supra-umbilical region, a symptom which may be the only one for several years (as in one of our cases).

Pain develops as a rule much later and has certain particular features: it is continuous, with a very slow but gradual tendency to become more accentuated.

It is felt especially in the epigastrium or the upper right quadrant of the abdomen, sometimes irradiating towards the shoulder or subscapularly.

Pain is more often felt in single cysts due to their rapid growth and to the large volume they sometimes attain, filling the whole abdomen (Ochsner, 1938, cited by Fani). On the other hand, the constant, discrete tension or weight felt above the umbilicus is more often encountered in the clinical picture of polycystic liver.

Sudden change in the pain of a patient with non-parasitic cyst, either solitary or polycystic, that suddenly becomes unbearable, means that one of the complications which we shall deal with lower down has occurred.

The *functional symptoms* are not characteristic.

1. During the period when the disease is well tolerated, moderate compression of the neighboring viscera takes place, as well as irritation of their interoceptors. The manifestations are especially digestive: anorexia, nausea, unpredictable vomiting, gaseous distension or constipation.

2. In the advanced stage of the disease, accentuated disturbances may occur in bile excretion with jaundice (a phenomenon seldom encountered).

3. Nervous functional disorders may likewise develop in the terminal phase of the polycystic liver associated to polycystic kidney; these disorders are produced by renal insufficiency rather than by hepatic deficit.

4. In the end period, hepatic insufficiency may develop, but only if it is not associated to a polycystic kidney that curtails the evolution and does not give time to the morphologic alterations to spread to the whole liver.

General symptoms. The patient's general condition is seldom altered, except in the end stage of the polycystic disease when a true "pseudoneoplastic cachexia" develops (Rachet). The disease may evolve without fever, except in the case of complications.

The *local examination* supplies information and sometimes reveals signs, although the patient does not yet feel ill.

1. *Local examination* shows a deformity of the abdominal wall, which will vary in terms of the size of the cyst. A solitary cyst may simulate a tumor producing a local deformity, whereas in the polycystic liver several comparatively large cysts (containing up to 1000 ml — S. Sherlock), next to less voluminous cysts, are observed.

2. *Palpation* will inform us upon the variety of the cyst. The polycystic liver, dotted with formations of a renitent consistency, is often very large and we may encounter what Fiessinger calls "an enormous, silent liver" in which pain is hardly felt and is far from corresponding to the impressive total deformity of the liver. Therefore, a characteristic of the polycystic liver on palpation is the size of the organ and the round formation disseminated in both lobes (case 3, *W.R.*).

Both kidneys may be likewise enlarged. Luzzato (cited by Rachet) showed that 17% of the patients with a polycystic liver had multiple cysts in the kidneys. According to other authors, more than half (56%) of the patients with a polycystic liver suffered from multiple visceral cysts, affecting the kidneys as well.

With a solitary cyst, the liver is only partly deformed, the small cyst protruding slightly on the under surface of the right lobe (by preference) or the left (case 1, *S.I.*), and may range up to a large cyst occupying the whole abdomen

(Parry) and beside which the liver appears to be an annex of the cyst to which it has given rise (case 2, *P.E.*).

3. *Percussion.* The cyst gives a dull sound if intestinal loops do not come in between, and auscultation gives no relevant information.

Complementary examinations:

1) A *plain radiologic examination* in a standard position is of capital importance, as the partly deformed liver or that covered by formations with a circular contour can be detected and will guide the surgeon towards one or other of the two anatomoclinical forms. Pneumoperitoneum may create optimal conditions for this examination.

2) A *barium meal* will give relevant information. The stomach may be displaced, descended, and may adhere to the neighboring deformed liver. Sometimes, a false aspect of "lacunar image" may be observed, as in the case of Andina. Barium enema shows an aspect that the surgeon must be acquainted with: the colon displaced to the left and downward shows that the subhepatic formation belongs to the liver (S. Munroe Jr., 1942).

3) *Angiography and cholangiography* (intravenous) furnish data on the vasculo-biliary elements surrounding the cysts (Bennet, 1964). This may help us to appraise preoperatively the number of the more voluminous formations and their size, but does not help us to appraise the nature of the disease.

4) The *scintigram* (with radioactive rose bengal) outlines the exact location and size of the cyst, which are represented by zones of inactivity against the homogeneous background of the liver that has taken up the radioactive substance. The smaller cysts can not be detected, especially those of less than 10 mm in diameter.

5) *Laparoscopy* may elucidate the nature of the cyst, but fails to show whether the cyst is parasitic or not.

6) It is considered characteristic of non-parasitic cysts that the liver tests are not altered even when the liver is very deformed (Henson, etc.). This is worthy of note, but it should not be forgotten that in the final stages of the polycystic disease with a hepatic localization hepatic insufficiency may be reflected by the dysproteinemia tests.

7) Among the other laboratory tests are:

— Blood urea which increases in the hepatorenal polycystic disease due to renal failure.

— Bilirubinemia may increase in certain clinical forms of the disease.

— Leukocytosis accompanies rupture of a non-parasitic cyst; discrete leukocytosis may also be observed in periods of quiescence.

The period of clinical latency that may sometimes last a lifetime may also be very short. In the case of Clatworthy, hepatomegaly became evident at the age of 5 months, when the patient had to be operated; however, as a rule the liver is normal at birth even in case of polycystic disease. The known cases of dystocia of fetal origin in hepatorenal polycystic disease are due to the exaggerated enlargement of the kidneys and not of the liver (Sherlock).

The first signs of the disease appear as a rule between the ages of 30 and 40. In the pure hepatic polycystic disease or solitary cyst, this period is tolerated up to the age of 60, whereas in the hepatorenal polycystic disease renal insufficiency curtails the evolution and the patient dies around the age of 45.

Spontaneous evolution increases the number and size of the cysts. Due to predominance in the clinical picture of a single symptom, several *clinical forms* may appear:

1. *Associated* in the renal-polycystic disease; this phenomenon belongs to the clinical picture of the polycystic liver in 56% of the cases, but only 19 to 33% of the patients with a polycystic kidney also have a polycystic liver (Sherlock).
2. *Pseudoascitic forms.* It is especially the solitary giant cyst that may be misleading at a more superficial examination (Constantini).
3. *Polycystic liver associated with the presence of pleural fluid.* As already mentioned, the disease occurs more often in women, and such cases are difficult to differentiate from the Demond-Meigs syndrome (ascites, hydrops of the chest, ovarian fibroma).
4. *Painful forms.*
5. *Forms with a digestive symptomatology.*
6. A latent, blatant or rapid *evolution.*
7. *Complicated forms.*

COMPLICATIONS

1) *Rupture of the cyst,* with a clinical picture of perforation ("stabbing pain") and peritoneal reaction accompanied by alteration of the patient's general condition and fever.

2) *Torsion of a pedunculate cyst* seldom occurs, since the cyst itself is very rare; torsion may simulate peritonitis or visceral torsion (Geist).

3) *Intracystic hemorrhage* causes a sudden increase in volume and tension, with accentuation of spontaneous pain.

4) *Infection of the cyst* may be more frequent than expected, since moderate leukocytosis may be encountered in the course of the disease: however, suppuration of the cyst, reported by some authors, is actually very rare. A. Bell found 7 cases up to 1966.

5) *Rare complications:* ascites due to compression of the portal vein; jaundice caused by compression of the liver pedicle; obstruction caused by compression of the intestine.

DIAGNOSIS

a. *Positive diagnosis.* The difficulties encountered in establishing the diagnosis vary from case to case.

1. Detection at a routine clinical examination in a patient over the age of 30, of a wholly or partially enlarged liver, without signs of hepatic insufficiency, a good general condition and normal biologic tests.

Repeated examinations show no local changes and the patient's state of health remains good.

It is probably a solitary non-parasitic cyst, or a polycystic disease. A correct diagnosis can only be made if the existence of this condition is not overlooked.

2. A patient between the ages of 30 and 40, complaining of right subcostal pains and with an enlarged liver and kidneys, is probably suffering from the hepato-renal polycystic disease. Determination of the Van-Slyke urea clearance coefficient, together with urography showing enlargement of the kidneys, will confirm a diagnosis of plurivisceral polycystic disease.

3. A patient comes to consultation with a slightly altered general state of health, pain in the right hypochondrium and shoulder; a renitent formation is felt on the undersurface of the right lobe. Moderate leukocytosis, normal liver tests, normal functional tests of the kidneys. This clinical picture may correspond to the clinical phase of "non-parasitic solitary cyst", but, in order to ascertain the diagnosis, a differential diagnosis must first be made.

b. *Differential diagnosis:* 1) *Solitary non-parasitic cyst* of the undersurface of the right lobe:

— when the size of the cyst is small or medium, it may be considered as hydrops of the gallbladder. If there is no contraindication (fever, intense pain), duodenal intubation and the Meltzer-Lyon test will produce B bile of normal color and amount; this excludes *cholecystic involvement;*

— when the liver is very voluminous it may simulate ascites, but the dullness can only be detected over the liver irrespective of the patient's position; the hepatic tests will exclude a *cirrhosis;*

— irrespective of the volume, it may be taken for a *hydatid cyst*. In such cases, Casoni's intradermoreaction and induced eosinophilia should be performed, but other elements may also be helpful: the hydatid cyst is as a rule firmer to the touch than the solitary cyst.

A subcapsular hydatid cyst may present fremitus (an inconstant but pathognomonic sign) and an older cyst may be calcified (X-ray examination). Even if doubts still exist, which often happens, an error is not grave since both diseases are surgical. In most cases the diagnosis is rectified only intraoperatively.

A non-parasitic cyst may also be confounded with *hepatic hemangioma:* in this case the tumor presents a systolic murmur and its size may vary from one examination to another.

The differential diagnosis should also be done with *solitary hepatic adenoma*, which is however firmer; an uncertain diagnosis can only be elucidated intraoperatively at gross examination.

Voluminous cyst associated with pleural exudate in a female might suggest *Demond-Meigs syndrome;* a vaginal touch will detect the ovarian fibroma.

Cyst of the undersurface of the liver may be confounded with a *retroperitoneal tumor*, which likewise develops slowly and does not alter the patient's health. In this case, barium enema will reveal a colon that is raised and pushed forward, and not descended and displaced to the left as in a cyst of the liver. As a matter of fact, the enema only indicates the intrahepatic and not the retroperitoneal site of a palpable formation.

Barium enema may invalidate a diagnosis of tumor of the *transverse colon* and also that of the transverse mesocolon.

Preoperatively, it is very difficult, if not impossible, to differentiate clinically a solitary cyst from an *accessory lobe-Riedel*, but a ^{131} y rose bengal scintigram is helpful.

A solitary cyst in the left lobe (a less frequent site) may be taken for *hypertrophy of the lobe* or *enlarged kidney (hydronephrosis)*, in which case urography or ureteropyelography will elucidate the case. In rare cases it may be confounded with the *spleen*. Careful examination will detect the spleen in its recess.

2) *Polycystic liver* (without polycystic kidney).

The liver is deformed and enlarged, and may be confounded with:

— *Hypertrophic cirrhosis*, which is accompanied by splenomegaly and alteration of the hepatic tests.

— *Metastatic cancer of the liver :* the patient's general condition is severely altered, and large hard nodules can be felt; the alkaline phosphatase test is modified. The original tumor must be found.

— *Lobate syphilitic liver* is a difficult diagnosis, because the biologic tests must be repeated after reactivation and the local examination confronted with the history of the case and laboratory tests. At any rate, the syphilitic liver behaves like a cirrhosis, with functional deficit and positive dysproteinemia tests, seldom encountered in the course of the hepatic polycystic disease.

Alveolar echinococcosis distorts the liver and may simulate a portion of polycystic liver with clustered cysts. The Casoni test is as a rule negative in the alveolar parasitic cyst. The diagnosis can be established at biopsy.

3) Among the *complications* are ruptures of the cyst, manifested by fever, leukocytosis and locally as peritonitis (rigidity), which may be misleading, especially when preceded by functional gastrointestinal disturbances. When in doubt, explorative laparotomy should not be temporized, being infinitely preferable to a fatal delay in the event of an undetected perforated duodenal ulcer.

c. *Operative diagnosis.* As a rule, direct examination of the liver at laparotomy will exclude other conditions and help to establish the diagnosis. Peroperative puncture will exclude a hydatid cyst.

A localized or disseminated distribution throughout the whole organ differentiates the *solitary unilocular cyst* (or even multilocular cyst) from the polykystic liver.

Competent histologic examination of the specimen will differentiate it from:

— *pseudocyst* (cavity in the tumor with cystic degeneration). Lorrimer performed an anatomic right lobectomy for cystic tumor of the right lobe of the liver; the histologic examination showed a pseudocyst developing in a mesenchymoma;

— *hepatic alveolar echinococcosis* (Rachet): a central zone of necrosis surrounded by flat vesicles. No scolices were found in the fluid and the puncture was therefore useless;

— the *so-called epithelial cyst* (with ciliate epithelium — Bockus);

— *cystadenoma*, proliferative histologic aspect;

— *lymphangioma :* histologic aspect characterized by the existence of an inner endothelial lamellar coat;

— *teratoma :* complex tumor;

— *traumatic pseudocyst*, covered with fibrous lamella and not with epithelium; a severe injury is found in the past history of the case.

This shows the importance of biopsy in surgery of the liver, as emphasized by some surgeons (Schottenfeld).

To conclude this chapter on diagnosis: *puncture must be avoided* in preoperative exploration of a patient suspect of cystic formation of the liver: biopsy puncture rarely collects characteristic fragments from the wall of the non-parasitic cyst, because of its structure; in case of hydatid cyst, it exposes the patient to untoward anaphylactic accidents, notwithstanding the synthetic antihistaminics of today which have reduced their gravity. Moreover, when the renitent formation is not a non-parasitic cyst but a hemangioma, the hazard of an internal hemorrhage is very serious and involves the surgeon's responsibility.

PROGNOSIS

Cysts grow progressively and increase in number. This spontaneous evolution can only end in two ways:

— substitution of the functional tissue by cystic formations;

— the appearance of accidents and complications.

Hence the disease, benign histologically, should not be viewed with too much optimism.

Actually, the period of latency and tolerance lets the patient lead an almost normal life for a fairly long time; however, on establishing the prognosis (immediate or late), account must be kept of the general features of the disease, the clinical form and evolutive moment.

The following situations may be met with:

a) *Hepatorenal polycystic disease in the latent phase:*

— immediate prognosis: good;

— late prognosis: very poor (death at the age of 40—45).

b) *Hepatic polycystic disease:*

— immediate prognosis: good;

— late prognosis: fairly good *quo ad vitam;* functionally, reserved.

c) Solitary non-parasitic uni- or multilocular hepatic cyst:

— immediate prognosis: good;

— late prognosis: reserved because of the complications, and progressive growth of the cyst and adhesions to neighboring viscera, the operation itself becoming more difficult and risky in the late phases of the disease.

SURGICAL TREATMENT

Therapeutic methods. The therapeutic methods may be separated into *palliative* and *curative*.

Palliative methods: 1) *Transparietal puncture of the cyst* is only permitted when the diagnosis is certain (after previous laparotomy). The contents of large cysts, which cause pain and complications due to compression of the neighboring viscera, may be evacuated at regular intervals.

2) *External surgical drainage* and *marsupialization* are readily performed surgical methods, but which have serious drawbacks:

— the postoperative treatment lasts very long;

— the hazards of a residual long-standing fistula are very high (F. Jones, 1923).

3) *Internal drainage. Anastomoses of deep, voluminous cysts* to the gastro-intestinal tract exposes the patient to enterocystic infection and cannot be recommended. It is not a solution but rather a means of masking the disease.

Curative methods (radical). As even in solitary cysts small cysts may exist around the large central cyst (multilocular aspect), a non-parasitic cyst can seldom be cured by non-anatomic hepatectomy (wedge-shaped, enucleoresection) and still more rarely by cystectomy (Făgărăşanu, Gologorskiy, Mesleaninov, etc.). It is often necessary to resect larger areas. Therefore, in the surgical treatment of non-parasitic cysts of the liver (when operable), anatomic resection (right or left hepatectomy), lobectomy and more seldom segmentectomy should be performed.

Indications. 1) Hepatorenal polycystic disease cannot be treated surgically, and only certain accidents or complications will oblige us to resort to surgery, i.e. to drainage or puncture of the more voluminous cysts. In general, any intervention should be avoided (case 3).

2) The *purely hepatic polycystic disease* presents a similar problem from the surgical point of view, but the favorable anatomic acini-like arrangement (Rachet) of the localized forms (that form the transition towards the multilocular solitary cyst) and the localization in a single lobe may justify hepatic resection (case 2).

3) The *solitary non-parasitic cyst* (uni- or multilocular), irrespective of the size, should be operated in view of the growth of these formations (case 1).

Both the etiopathogenic (Prete: congenital malformation of a hepatic segment) and the technical arguments plead in favor of an anatomic resection, since the safety of large resections is based upon compliance with the vasculobiliary topography.

Problems of anesthesia-resuscitation and operative techniques.

1) *Anatomic hepatectomies* are broad operations performed in most cases by thoraco-abdominal approach (thoracophrenolaparotomy).

The anesthesiologist specialist in resuscitation should examine the patient carefully (respiratory function, circulation, electrolyte balance), including the liver functions as a matter of routine, although there are no deficits as a rule.

Modern criteria are best met by closed-circuit endotracheal anesthesia; by using ganglioplegics and antihistaminics in potentiating doses, good protection is obtained against operative shock and smaller amounts of anesthetic are used, of particular importance in operations on the liver.

Loss of blood from the large vessels must be avoided by a correct surgical technique; however, capillary hemorrhage from the remaining hepatic surface has only partly been solved.

Anesthesia under controlled hypotension has been recommended by some authors, but this obliges the specialist in resuscitation to return "volume for volume" the blood lost in case of hemorrhage of the large vessels.

Controlled hypotension reduces very much or even avoids capillary hemorrhage. Our experimental investigations also confirmed this fact in resections of the liver.

In order to reduce intraoperative hemorrhage, some authors recommend compression of the liver pedicle. On studying the "liver depleted of blood" (ischemic), Bernhardt et al. (1955) reached the conclusion that the best results are obtained under hypothermia, since the period of temporary ischemia may be prolonged. They assert that hepatic resection under hypothermia with temporary ischemia is more advantageous than under controlled hypotension.

Apart from the different means employed for suturing the sectioned hepatic surface, an attempt was made to prevent hemorrhage by fluid nitrogen. Serra devised a special cautery from the tip of which fluid nitrogen dropped; congealing thus obtained over the incised surface avoids hemorrhage for a few minutes, after which the larger vessels appear and can be ligated separately. Brunschwig obtained good results in anatomic hepatectomy with this cautery.

2) *Anatomic hepatectomies* are described in the respective chapter.

For non-parasitic cysts, left lobectomies (Claget, 1944, cited by Sherlock) and total right hepatectomies have been carried out (Clatworthy, 1956) successfully.

In Romania, the first anatomic left hepatectomies were reported by I. Făgărășanu (1956) for non-parasitic cyst.

In these operations the route of acess must be very broad:

— thoracophrenolaparotomy along the right 8th rib (Lortat-Jacob — for right hepatectomy);

— transverse laparotomy combined with left thoracophrenotomy, as used by Clatworthy in children and Brunschwig in the adult;

— median laparotomy combined with right thoracophrenotomy, joining above the umbilical region (Ciobanu);

— median xyphoumbilical laparotomy, giving full satisfaction in total left hepatectomy, performed under spinal anesthesia.

Right hepatectomy consists in severing the right hepatic glissonian pedicle between two ligatures, the right suprahepatic vein between ligatures and the 2—4 accessory right suprahepatic veins, exposing the sagittal vein that must not be resected and dividing the parenchyma to the right of the main fissure.

Clatworthy, for a non-parasitic cyst of the right liver, performed a similar operation using certain artifacts.

In order to identify the bile ducts more readily on the sectioned surface, he injected a dye into the common bile duct, clamping it; the dye came out through the sectioned ducts, which were easily detected and clamped (technique adopted by Bourgeon-Perreau).

In order to avoid the discharge of bile, as well as bile stasis within the first few days after the operation, the common bile duct was drained.

Total left hepatectomy is more readily performed by hilar approach, when the hilus is accessible; this implies severing between two ligatures of the left hepatic artery, left portal vein, left hepatic duct (if it can be individualized) and then, mobilization of the liver, exposure and ligation of the left suprahepatic vein above its confluence with the sagittal vein, which must not be severed. The gallbladder remains adherent to the right liver.

In a case operated by us, the hilus could not be approached and we resorted to the scissural approach which reversed the operative stages, since it began with the suprahepatic pedicle, opening posteriorly the large scissura in order to reveal the hilar plate where the mass of the glissonian pedicle was ligated.

The left liver also received from the coronary artery of the stomach another important arterial branch, which had to be ligated and severed.

Peroperative cholecystocholangiography may be necessary in order to detect the site at which the two hepatic ducts join in Glisson's plate (I. Făgărăşanu).

The surface of the resected liver should be peritonealized with the large omentum (in the case described we used, however, the falciform ligament).

Postoperative cholangiography with biligraphin permits good anatomofunctional control (I. Făgărăşanu).

RESULTS

Broad hepatectomies are well tolerated. A particular problem is that of right hepatectomy when two thirds of the liver parenchyma are removed. It is known that up to 70% of the liver can be resected without causing severe or lasting functional disturbances. However, it cannot be sustained that such broad resections do not produce disturbances even in the experimental study. Lokhatiuk (1957) demonstrated in the dog that resection of 30—70% of the liver lowers bile secretion up to the 26th day, followed by recovery only on the 90th — 93rd day after the operation (however, somewhat reduced when 70% of the liver is resected).

In humans, Tumer (1923) and Velikoretzkiy (1934) showed that in broad resections of the liver the only test modified is the BSP test; according to Pickrell and Cay, there is a delay in 30% of the cases.

Abdol Islami and G.T. Pack (1956) showed that after total right hepatectomy for malignant tumors (70—80% of the liver) serum bilirubin increased with obstructive jaundice; this is accounted for by compression of the hepatic trabeculae and therefore of the bile ducts by the blood vessels, dilated by the increased portal flow in the remaining parenchyma.

The prothrombin time increases slightly without showing a tendency to hemorrhage.

Proteinemia (serine + globulins) collapses postoperatively and cannot be normalized by plasma perfusions or protein lysates.

Plasma electrolytes: serum Na and phosphates are slightly reduced, the remaining mineral components not being modified.

Amoniemia is not modified even after the postoperative administration of amigen; experimentally, in dogs, ammonium chloride tolerance after resection of 70% of the liver remained the same as in the normal animals.

These changes do not involve the general status, which remains normal. Therefore, in certain cases, total right hepatic resection can be performed.

Excision, according to the older statistics of Davis (1937) mentioned in Sherlock's book, gives a mortality rate of 22% after operations for solitary nonparasitic cysts of the liver; however, Geist reports a mortality rate of 5.1% in 193 operated cases up to 1955: 6 died after aspiration or drainage (palliative treatment), 1 died after marsupialization, and 3 after total or partial excision. Of the 122 cases operated between 1924 and 1955 only 3 patients died, so that the mortality rate can actually be considered to be of about 2.4%, which fully justifies operation of the non-parasitic cyst of the liver. The two cases operated by us gave excellent early and late results.

In order to illustrate the diagnostic and operative difficulties, here are three clinical cases:

Case 1. Patient *S.I.*, aged 32. Diagnosis: solitary non-parasitic subcapsular cyst of the liver. The onset dated back 8 years, with mild localized pain below the left costal margin. During the last 6 months, the pain became unbearable and forced the patient to come to hospital.

Palpation showed a renitent formation, the size of an orange, situated below the left costal margin.

Surgery (January 14, 1957) revealed a superficial cystic formation, measuring 12 cm in diameter, in the left lobe of the liver. "Closed sac" cystectomy was performed. The histologic specimen is represented in Fig. 164. Recovery within 12 days.

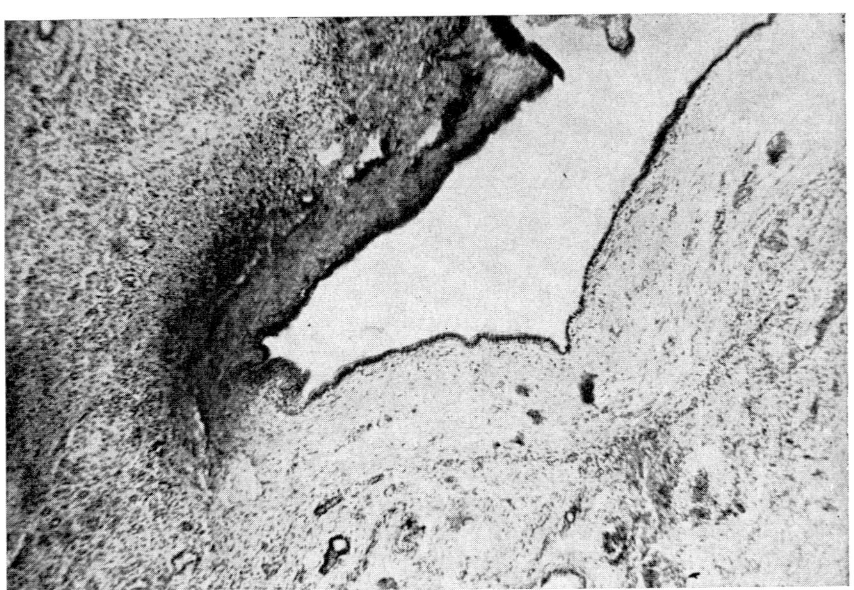

Fig. 164. — Solitary, non-parasitic cyst of the liver. Microscopic aspect: cystic cavity, lined by a single epithelial layer and surrounded by dense sclerosis tissue.

Case 2. Patient *P.E.*, aged 58 was admitted on April 4, 1956, with a sensation of epigastric plenitude and epigastric tumor.

The first signs dated back one year: uncharacteristic gastrointestinal disorders, gases, constipation, sensation of gastric plenitude. The patient was not alarmed.

Two months prior to admission, the patient noted a painless formation that gradually increased in size.

Presenting signs: good general condition; nothing relevant on examination of the different organs and systems.

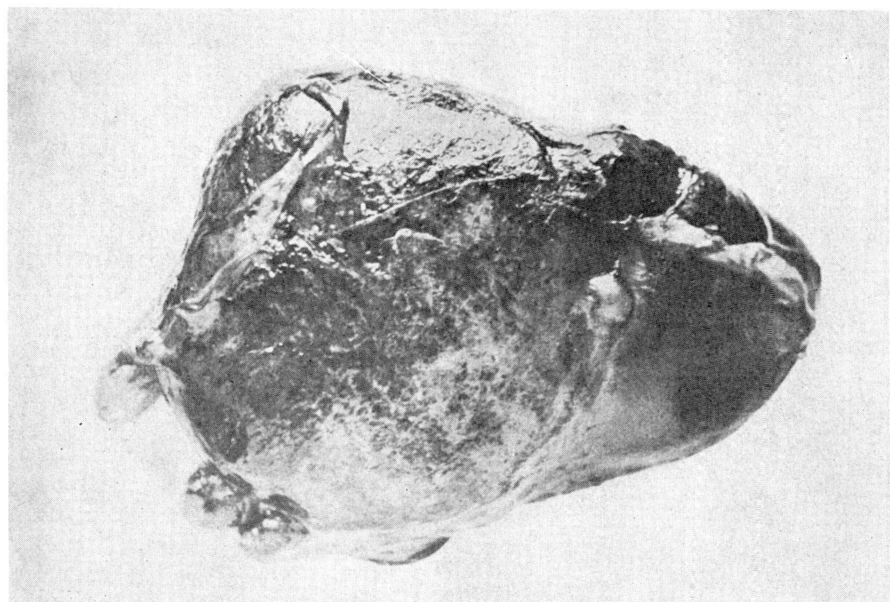

Fig. 165. — Polycystic liver: operation specimen (controlled left hepatectomy). Cranial aspect.

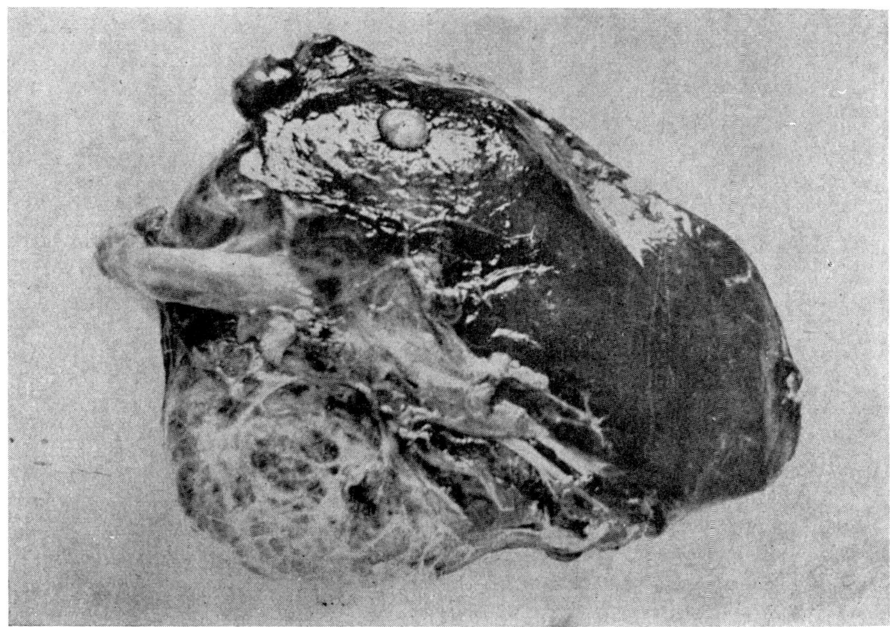

Fig. 166. — Polycystic liver: operation specimen (controlled left hepatectomy). Caudal aspect.

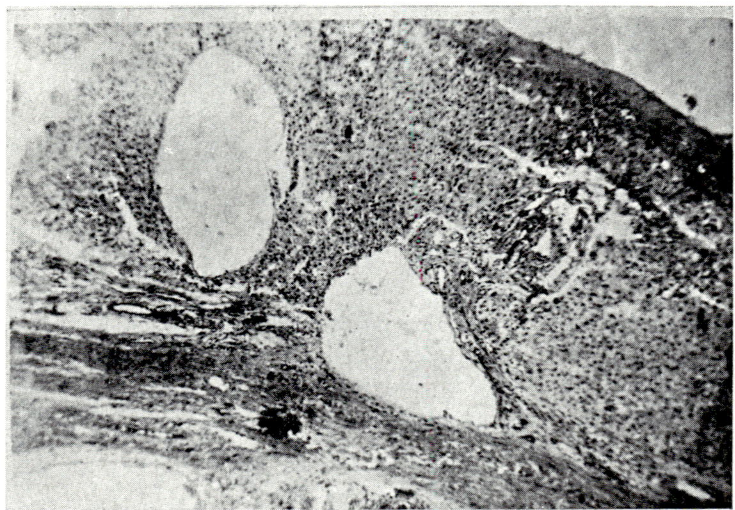

Fig. 167. — Polycystic liver. Note cystic formations separated by the hepatic trabeculae.

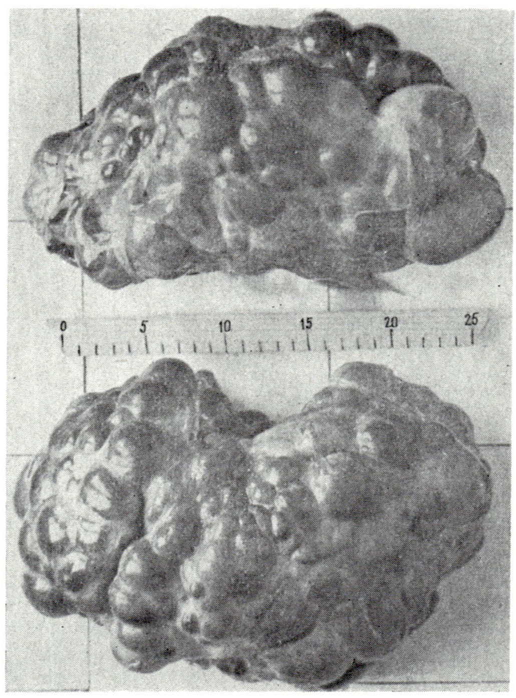

Fig. 168. — Polycystic kidney (necropsy specimen). The same case as in Fig. 169. Predominant renal involvement (hepatorenal polycystic disease).

Local examination revealed deformity of the abdomen in the epigastrium and right hypochondrium. A renitent formation, the size of an adult fist, could be felt in the epigastrium, painless, with a rough irregular surface, moving with the respiratory motions. The spleen could not be palpated.

X-ray examination : gastrointestinal tract normal. Laboratory test: no significant changes Casoni test negative, eosinophilia 3%. Presumptive diagnosis: hydatid cyst of the liver Explorative laparotomy was indicated.

Operation (April 20, 1956): xyphoumbilical laparotomy under spinal anesthesia showed that the left lobe and quadrate lobe were transformed into a polycystic mass, except for a smal zone on the posterior part of the left lobe. Diagnosis: polycystic liver.

Intraoperative cholangiography: amputated left hepatic duct.

Anatomic total left hepatectomy (Figs 165 and 166); the operative difficulties encountered decided us to choose the scissural approach in order to reach Glisson's pedicle. After isolation and ligation of the left suprahepatic vein in the posterior part of the main fissure, exposed by section of the falciform and left triangular ligaments, the whole of Glisson's pedicle was ligated. The most important arterial branch of the coronary artery was ligated and severed. Total resection of the left liver. Peritonealization with the falciform ligament that was sutured to the lower aspect of the liver. Subhepatic drainage.

Postoperative course: after 3 days the drainage tube was removed; recovery of the operative wound within 10 days.

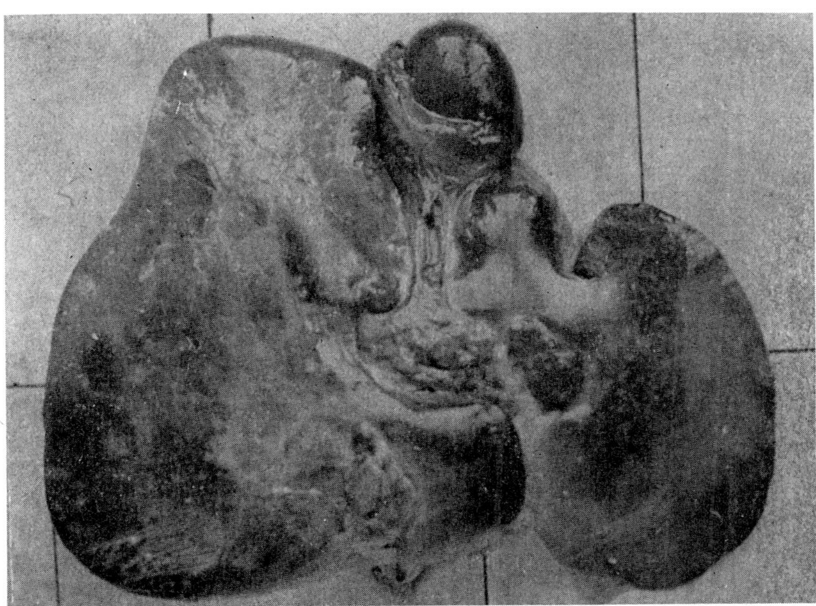

Fig. 169. — Polycystic liver, caudal aspect. Surface deformed by cystic formations (necropsy specimen).

Histologic findings: Glisson's capsule slightly thickened, subcapsular hepatic islets with modified trabecular structure, surrounded by connective tissue with numerous thick collagen fibers and accentuated diffuse lymphopolyblastic inflammatory infiltrate.

Numerous bile canaliculi, some of normal size, others slightly dilated with a monolayered epithelium. Rare cysts with a cuboid cell epithelium. Some cysts visible with the naked eye have a flat endotheliform epithelium, surrounded by a thick connective lamellar capsule. The cyst had a low protein content and stained with eosin (Fig. 167).

Postoperative cholangiographic control showed the presence of the gallbladder at the edge of the right liver and normal intra- and extrahepatic bile ducts.

At reexamination 2 months after the operation, the patient was in excellent health and the liver tests were within normal limits. After 18 months the situation was the same. Urography revealed a left renal cyst close to the pelvis, about the size of a cherry.

Case 3. Patient *W.R.*, aged 45. Diagnosis: hepatorenal polycystic disease; uremia.

The disease, that had lasted 3 years, presented marked aggravation during the last two months. On December 14, 1956, the patient was admitted to the hospital for the third time, with azotemia, nausea, headache, disorientation. The clinical examination showed enlarged, nodular kidneys. Three weeks after admission, the patient died from uremia.

Necropsy: enlarged kidneys (40 cm long) with a macro- micropolycystic aspect (Fig. 168). On the surface of the liver (of normal size), numerous irregularly disseminated, unequal cysts. Uni- and multilocular cysts in all the hepatic lobes (Fig. 169 and 170).

The patient's sister also suffered from polycystic kidney and uremia.

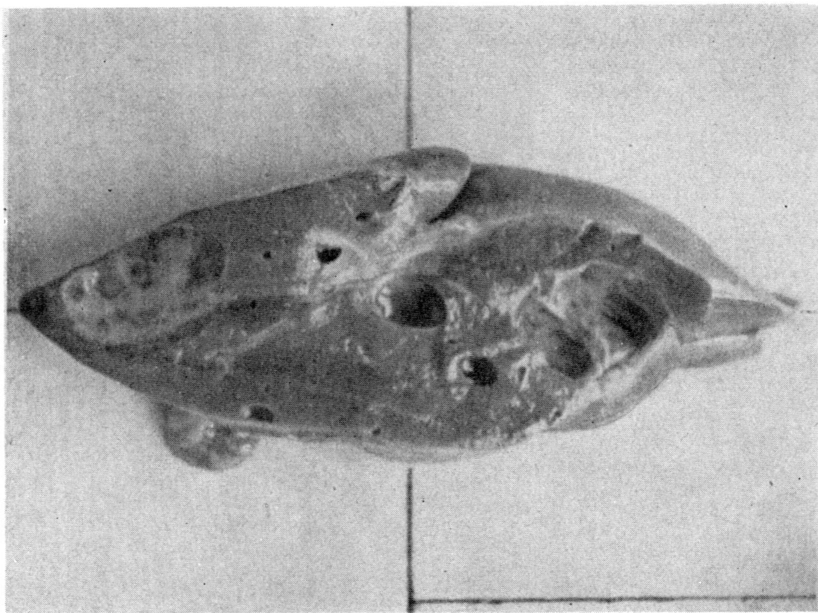

Fig. 170 — Polycystic liver. Cross section. Cystic cavities, isolated or confluent, often central, surrounded in places by sclerosis (white bands) (necropsy specimen).

REFERENCES

1. Abdol I. G., Pack G. T., Miller Th., Surgery, 1956, **39**, *4*, 551.
2. Andina M. I., Khirurghiya, 1959, *9*, 126.
3. Bel A., Tete R., Hartemann E., Chapuy P., Girard M., Arch. Mal. App. digest., 1966, **55**, *3*, 235.
4. Bennet J., Chalut J., Parat A., Prot D., Presse méd., 1964, **72**, *15*, 877.
5. Bernhard W. F., Mc Murrey J. D., Curtis C. H., New Engl. J. Med., 1955, **253**, *5*, 159.
6. Bockus H. L., *Gastroenterology*, vol. III, W. B. Saunders, Philadelphia, 1953, p. 375.
7. Boyd W., *Pathology for the surgeon*, 7th ed., W. B. Saunders, Philadelphia, 1956, p. 264.
8. Brunshwig A., Bull. Soc. Int. Chir., 1955, **14**, *3*, 370.
9. Brunshwig A., Cancer, 1955, **8**, *6*, 1226.
10. Bulgakov P. P., Vestn. Khir., 1960, **84**, *4*, 114.
11. Cavallini A., Francolini C, Minerva chir., 1955, **10**, *12*, 608.
12. Chipail Gh., Diaconescu M., Wexler L., Chirurgia, 1953, **3**, *4*, 72.
13. Ciobanu St., Chirurgia, 1956, **5**, *2*, 163.
14. Ciobanu St., Chirurgia, 1957, **5**, *4*, 495.
15. Ciobanu St., Chirurgia, 1957, **5**, *3*, 434.
16. Clatworthy W., Boles G., Surgery, 1956, **39**, *5*, 850.
17. Făgărăşanu I., Popescu Gh., Aloman D., Chitlaru L., *Hepatectomii tipice şi atipice* in *Ses. ştiinţ. Acad. R.P.R.*, 1956, vol. 6.
18. Făgărăşanu I., Chitlaru L., Rozemberg A., Chirurgia, 1956, **5**, *4*, 507.
19. Făgărăşanu I., Ionescu-Bujor C., Constantinescu C., Probl. Ter., 1958, **9**, *2*, 82.
20. Fani L. E., Finkel I. I., Sov Med., 1958, *7*, 118.
21. Geist D. C., Surgery, 1955, **71**, 867.
22. Gologorskiy V. A., Sov. Med., 1958, *7*, 134.
23. Gugusvili L. L., Khirurghiya, 1957, *5*, 138.
24. Henson W. St. Jr., Gray H., Dockerty B. M., Surg. Gynec. Obstet., 1957, **104**, *1*, 63.
25. Henson W. St. Jr., Hallenbeck A. G., Gray K. H., Dockerty B. M., Surg. Gynec. Obstet., **104**, *2*, 302.
26. Henson W. St. Jr., Gray K. H., Dockerty B. M., Surg. Gynec. Obstet., 1957, **104**, *3*, 551.
27. Lokhatiuk A. S., Vestn. Khir., 1957, *1*, 61.
28. Lorrimer S., Ann. Surg., 1955, **141**, *2*, 246.
29. Lortat-Jacob J. L., Robert H., Bull. Soc. Int. Chir., 1955, **4**, *3*, 357.
30. Mancuso M., Natalini E, Del Grande, Policlinico, 1955, **62**, *5*, 259.
31. Meschyaninov A. I., Vestn. Khir., 1958, *12*, 80.
32. Perreau P., Guntz M., Renier J. C., Arch. Mal. App. digest., 1965, **54**, *9*, 882.
33. Prete A., Gaz. ital. Chir., 1955, **11**, *11*, 1241.
34. Rachet J., Busson A., Duhamel J., Sem. Hôp., 1963, **29**, *15*, 73.
35. Schottenfeld L. E., Amer. J. Digest. Dis., 1955, **22**, *5*, 129.
36. Serra P. A., Brunshwig A., Cancer, 1955, **8**, *6*, 1234.
37. Sherlock Sheila, *Diseases of the liver and biliary system*, Blackwell, Oxford, 1955, p. 554.
38. Velikoretskiy A. A., Kasankina T. N., Khirurghiya, 1955, *5*, 11.
39. * * * *Monogotomnoe rukovostvo po khirurghii*, vol. 8, Medghiz, Moscow, 1962, p. 309.

C. HEPATIC HEMANGIOMA

HISTORY

Hemangioma is "a tumor formed of exuberant and disproportionate formations of ectatic blood capillaries or blood pools" (Letulle).

As these vascular tumors frequently occupy a superficial location on uncovered sites (face, limbs), they drew the attention of older observers, such as Ambroise Paré (1517—1590), who called them *signe* (Pierre Delbet).

With time, the terms used to describe these tumors became more numerous and reflected the evolution that took place in the mental attitude of the physicians and anatomists towards the significance and structure of these formations.

Starting with De Graefe's "angiectasis", the terms used come closer to our present concept and include a larger sphere, reflecting the etymologic significance of the word.

Boyer (1757—1833) called them "cavernous tumors". Then, Philippe van Walther coined the name of "telangiectasis", which has, however, today a more precise significance.

Follin finally called it "angionoma", and Virchow simplified it to "angioma", term used at present. This is, briefly stated, the history of hemangiomas.

The history of angiomas of the liver is simpler; owing to their deep location, they have only been investigated since the second half of the 19th century.

Steffen (1882) published anatomical findings concerning extensive hemangiomas occupying large areas in the liver. Surgeons and physicians attempted to establish a preoperative clinical diagnosis.

Schroetter showed that a systolic murmur heard over the epigastric region and hypochondrium indicates the vascular origin of the hepatic tumor. Although J. L. Faure (in Delbet) doubted this (Schroetter's patient was not operated), today we find in literature 2 of 6 operated hemangiomas of the liver, diagnosed preoperatively, with this sign (Velikoretzkiy: the two cases of Lomovitzkiy).

In an attempt to establish the diagnosis, puncture has also been used; it is, we believe, superfluous to recall the cases of Broca and Terrier who died following hemorrhage caused by puncture of hepatic hemangiomas (J. L. Faure).

Several surgeons indicated laparotomy because the condition could not be diagnosed preoperatively. The most daring attempted to extirpate the vascular tumor, as appeared logical. In this way, many observations were gathered concerning hemangiomas of the liver.

In Romania, I. Iacobovici encountered several cases of hemangiomas of the liver (*Chirurgie*, vols. I and II, 1944).

Stout, in the statistics of the Presbyterian Hospital, found, up to 1932, 17 benign tumors of the liver, of which 13 hemangiomas (Bockus).

In 1939, Ghenzburg gathered from world literature 49 cases of operated hemangioma (Murlaga); and 66 were found up to 1942 (Schermaker in Bockus).

Murlaga added to the international statistics of Combé, with 71 hepatic resections (up to 1946), the cases of Ansimov, Nicolski and his own, raising the number to 74 in 1951.

In some countries, hepatic hemangiomas are systematically operated; thus, in the U.S.S.R., Velikoretzkiy recorded 29 resections up to 1954, and Gorbinova 30 up to 1957.

Until August 1963, Berman found 80 resections for hemangiomas, to which may be added one of our cases, one of Stoian's and one of Alexandriyski's, that is 83. L. Schiff considers angioma as the most frequent benign tumor of the liver.

PATHOLOGIC ANATOMY AND ETIOPATHOGENY

Hemangioma is a comparatively rare, single or multiple tumor, sessile, seldom pedunculate (Greville Young, 1964), predominantly situated on the upper surface of the liver, of various sizes, from that of a pin head up to that of a walnut, or even of an entire lobe. The color is reddish-violet or bluish, according to the degree of blood stasis. It may be surrounded by a capsule or, when the latter is missing, it seems to be confluent with the surrounding tissues.

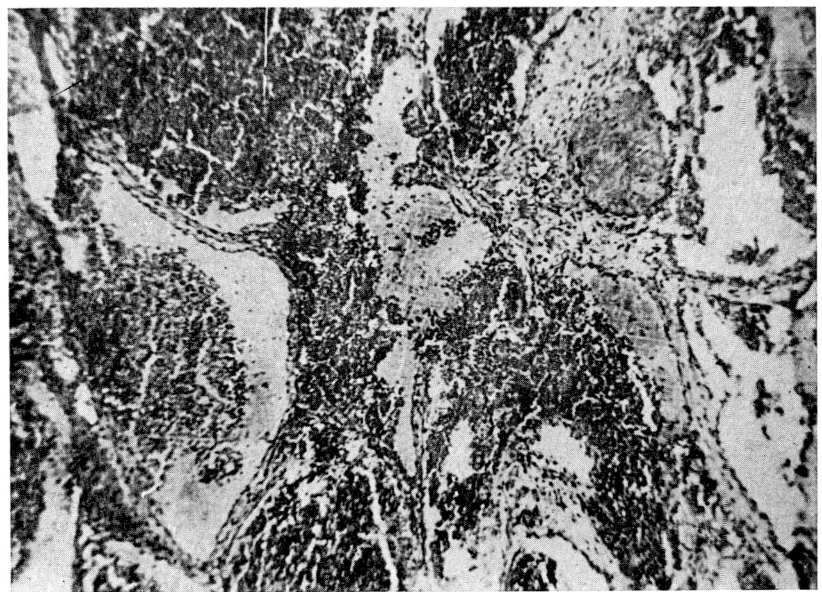

Fig. 171. — Hepatic hemangiocavernoma. Note large vascular lacunae, full of red blood cells, separated by thin septa.

Microscopically, it appears as a clustering of vascular lumina of various size, lined by endothelium and surrounded by connective stroma. Several types are differentiated according to the histologic structure:

a) *Cavernous hemangioma*, or hemangiocavernoma, is the most frequently encountered in the liver and is characterized by large vascular lacunae and stroma reduced to fine connective septa (Figs 171 and 172).

b) *Capillary hemangioma*, rarely found in the liver, with narrow vascular lumina and more abundant stroma.

c) *Scirrhous hemangioma*, with collapsed or closed vascular cavities, rich fibrogenetic stroma, considered as a form of involution of angiomas.

d) *Hemangioendothelioma*, that presents signs of active endothelial proliferation and may be related to malignant hemangioblastic tumors.

Signs of inflammation, thrombosis and organization are often observed, with hyalinization and calcification of the stroma.

Several etiopathogenic theories exist concerning the morphogenesis of hemangioma:

1. Inflammatory (Virchow), due to transformation of a granulation tele-angiectatic tissue.

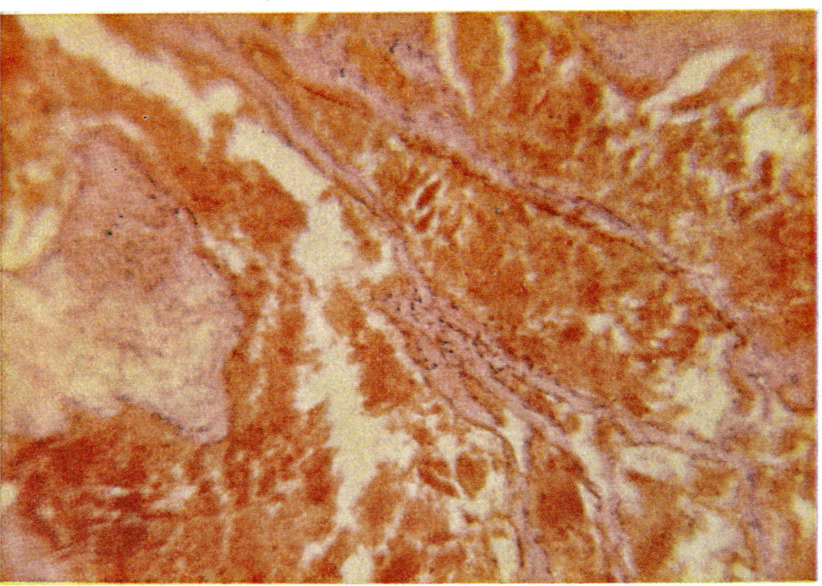

Fig. 172. — Liver hemangioma. Dilated, anastomosed sinusoid capillaries, full of red blood cells.

2. Postnecrotic vasodilatation *a vacuo*, consequent to a limited necrosis o the liver (Ziegler).

3. Vasodilatation due to circumscribed stasis (Schmieden), with consecutive cavernous ectasis.

4. Posthemorrhagic organization and transformation of a voluminous hematoma.

5. Dysgenetic (Albrecht, Ribbert, Sabin, Schafer), due to a developmental anomaly in the course of embryogenesis of the vascular system, with persistence of the decidual vessels. The frequent appearance in childhood (50%), the high familial incidence, the multiplicity of the localizations, the stationary or slow evolution and organoid structure lend support to the latter assumption. However, there are no morphologic criteria on the basis of which the neoplastic or dysembryoplastic origin of these tumors can be asserted apart from the clinical criteria of evolution. It is also admitted that certain cases of angiomas represent true angioplastic tumors.

CLINICAL STUDY

Hemangioma of the liver forms part of the congenital tumors that usually draw the attention of the bearer only after the age of 30 to 40, before which a long period of latency may be assumed to exist.

Subjective symptoms. 1. The earliest symptom is as a rule a vague sensation of weight, of continuous pressure in the epigastrium or right hypochondrium; the patient is not alarmed at first and one or two years may pass before he is fully aware of the local symptoms.

2. The patient then begins to have undefined pain, at times subcostal, which occasionally radiate towards the shoulder or subscapularly.

The pain may be continuous and exasperating because it never ceases day or night, probably due to distension of Glisson's capsule by the vascular tumor under tension due to its growth. The size of the tumor depends upon the hemodynamics of the return circulation to the right heart; hence, sudden changes may occur in the volume of the tumor, producing sharp, interrupted pain, taking on the aspect of *right subcostal painful seizures.*

3. Not characteristic and misleading are the persisting headaches and resistance to current treatments.

Functional symptoms are not as a rule typical: nausea and vomiting, and sometimes only anorexia.

General symptoms. Although the mechanism is difficult to explain, the patients often complain of fatigue and loss of weight.

Local examination will show:

1. The size of the tumor, whether it is large or small, whether it occupies a posterior site (rare) without deformity of the subcostal region; in larger, anterosuperior hemangiomas, asymmetrical deformity of the anterior abdominal wall may be observed in the right upper quadrant — a swelling that moves when the patient breathes (downward on inspiration, upward on expiration).

2. The patient himself often palpates the region at the first subjective symptoms. An enlarged lobe may be found, apparently smooth (rare cases of centrolobular hemangiocavernomas), or one or several tumors may be individualized on the liver surface, exhibiting several particular features: they are less firm than the surrounding parenchyma, not actually painful, yet the patient complains that the discomfort is increased on pressure. The size of the tumor may vary very much, in terms of the circulation — Caroli.

In general, the hemangioma located subcapsularly forms part of a hepatic lobe whose tissue surrounds it. However, it may sometimes be pedunculate (Sheila Sherlock) and in this case it is palpable the same as a tumor neighboring the liver and moving with it in the course of respiration movements.

3. Percussion will show nothing relevant besides the dull sound of the tumor formation.

4. Auscultation is a simple method of exploration, unfortunately used very little in examination of the abdominal viscera. Schroetter was the first who based the diagnosis of hepatic hemangioma on auscultation of the systolic murmur over

the tumor. Surgery subsequently confirmed the preoperative diagnosis. The same phenomenon was also observed by Beck (A.V. Smirnov).

The clinical examination must be completed by several supplementary examinations that are particularly useful when correctly performed.

1. *X-ray examination* of the liver has taken on an increasing importance with technical progress.

— Plain radiography in standard postures (front and side views) may show an increase in the volume of the liver or distortion.

— Pneumoperitoneum is necessary when the tumor is located on the convexity of the lobe and is projected upon the clear field of the pulmonary base: the air penetrates between the diaphragm and the liver, and the hepatic site of the tumor is more readily detected.

— Barium meal (Bockus) completes the X-ray examination and will show any displacement of the stomach, duodenum, transverse colon or hepatic angle, with a normal configuration and moderate functional disorders.

2. *Angiography* is not a widespread method, although already in 1954 R. Bourgeon and H. Pietri concluded that splenal and portal venography may give useful indications on the site of intrahepatic tumors.

3. *Scintigram* may be used to outline the contour and location of a hemangioma in the liver, the same as for other benign tumors without a specific metabolic activity of the liver cell. Voluminous tumors are more evident.

4. *Laparoscopy*, practiced as far back as 1901 by Kelling, is today greatly facilitated by the set of Marcelo Royer and Sclari, permitting optical exploration after pneumoperitoneum.

Technique: pneumoperitoneum is performed under local anesthesia in the right hypochondrium, then through an incision in the anterior abdominal wall made with a trocar, the laparoscope is introduced. Caroli showed the use of laparoscopy for establishing the exact preoperative diagnosis of hemangioma. It is notwithstanding seldom used by surgeons.

5. *Cholangiography* may be carried out either pre- or peroperatively for diagnostic purposes.

— Preoperative: intravenous cholangiography with biligraphın (the most innocuous); transparietovesicular cholangiography (Kapandji); transparietohepatic cholangiography (Carter-Saypol, 1952).

— Peroperative cholangiography gives very precise indications (I. Făgărășanu: *Anatomic and Non-anatomic Hepatectomies, 1956*). In 1935, Velikoretskiy reports on a case of hemangioma of the left hepatic lobe in which cholangiography revealed the contour of the tumor by the way and place in which the intrahepatic bile ducts were compressed.

6. The functional liver tests show no alterations. However, in one case of voluminous hemangioma of the right lobe, intolerance to novocaine developed with the accentuation of hepatomegaly. As novocaine is inactivated in the liver, it may be deduced that over a certain limit growth of the vascular tumor will impair the functional capacity of the liver.

7. Among the other tests, mention can be made of Gorbinov's case in which he found an ESR of 50 mm/hour, although the tumor measuring 13/10/8 cm was a hemangioma.

EVOLUTION

The evolution of hepatic hemangioma is progressive.

The first signs appear between the ages of 30 and 40 after a long preclinical period and, after that, become gradually more accentuated.

The small initial size of the vascular tumor accounts for the latent preclinical phase; as it grows in size, signs specific to the tumor develop, or symptoms caused by displacement or compression of the neighboring viscera.

In the preclinical period, hemangioma may be incidentally discovered in the course of laparotomy for another disease; it may be sharply curtailed by the onset of complications, either under the influence of a physiologic (pregnancy, the case of Caroli-Ricordeau) or a pathologic state, modifying the circulatory regimen and bringing about an increase in the rate of growth of the vascular tumor.

Complications may develop at any moment.

COMPLICATIONS

We are far from sharing the optimism of some authors who let themselves be deceived by the apparent inactivity of this histologically benign formation.

The following are the complications of a hemangioma (J. K. Berman):

a) necrosis / malignization;

b) development beyond the limits of easy operability;

c) rupture.

a. *Necrosis* is very rare (Berman observed it in a newborn infant); *malignization* or fibrous cicatricial transformation is likewise very rare (Corman-Murlaga).

b. *Development beyond the limits of easy operability* may occur at any moment, especially in young patients in whom the rate of growth of these tumors is more rapid.

In women, pregnancy represents a critical period that may bring about an increase in the size of the tumor, necessitating the sacrifice of large areas of the liver (Caroli — right hepatolobectomy for postpartum hemangioma).

In the first phases of development, a hemangioma may sometimes be extirpated relatively sparingly (non-anatomic hepatectomy), but once it has increased in size anatomic resection of a segment, or more frequently of a lobe, must be performed; in the latter case, we may be faced with a large scale operation because of the volume and topography of the tumor.

This is the true risk of temporization, justified by the apparent benign character of hemangioma of the liver.

c. *Rupture* is a dramatic, and as a rule fatal accident; it cannot be foreseen and may occur whatever the patient's age or the duration of the disease.

By its structure and subcapsular location, a hemangioma does not offer favorable conditions for spontaneous hemostasis and death occurs by intraperitoneal hemorrhage.

In one of Pozzi's cases, this much dreaded complication was produced in the mother following the efforts of birth.

There is also the case of Hendricks who observed fatal rupture of a hepatic hemangioma in a 2-day-old child (cited by J.K. Berman).

DIAGNOSIS

a) A *positive diagnosis* is presumptive in most cases It is based upon:

— Slow evolution, especially in women aged 30 to 40, is not reflected as a rule upon the patient's general condition.

— Asymmetrically enlarged liver (tumor of one lobe, or isolated growth of one lobe).

— Tumor varying in size at the different examinations, renitent, painless or only slightly painful.

— Auscultation of a systolic murmur over the tumor, the *only sign that can be considered pathognomonic*, should be carefully carried out on the course of a local examination for a hepatic tumor of undetermined origin.

In general, the auxiliary examinations determine the site of the tumor and its topography with respect to the hepatic structure (X-ray examination, chol-angiography); laparoscopy will establish a correct preoperative diagnosis if the location of the tumor makes it accessible to this examination.

We should also like to mention that puncture *must be rigorously contra-indicated* whenever the origin of the tumor is not determined and the suspicion exists that it may be a hemangioma.

Biopsy puncture of the liver is a method that must be reserved prevalently to non-surgical cases (hepatitis, precirrhotic states, biopsy control of the regene-rative potential of the liver) and not in surgical diseases with a chronic evolution. In hemangioma, as well as in hydatid cyst and non-parasitic cyst, it is formally contraindicated, the very structure of the tumor not permitting the removal of fragments suitable for conclusive examination.

Only in cases of acute evolution with signs of inflammation (abscess) can needle biopsy be used without any inconvenience.

Differential diagnosis. 1) The differential diagnosis must first be made with primary or secondary malignant tumors that have a rapid local development, and early alteration of the patient's general condition, which is not observed in the evolution of an uncomplicated hepatic hemangioma.

Special attention should be paid to hemangioendothelioma, likewise a vas-cular tumor, but with a marked character of malignancy (actually a structural form of hepatic sarcoma, according to Titu Vasiliu).

2) The differential diagnosis must then be made with diseases with a chronic evolution, that are as a rule accompanied by characteristic biologic reactions:

— hepatic syphilis (positive Bordet-Wasserman and dysproteinemia tests);

— hydatid cyst of the liver, in which the Casoni test and eosinophilia are generally positive; it is considered a firm, renitent or even hard tumor.

3) There is a further category of diseases with which the differential diag-nosis is difficult:

— Hepatic adenoma *(well encapsulated tumor)* "is a firmer tumor than hemangioma, of a volume that is not variable but steadily, slowly and progres-sively increasses" (Boyd). It is difficult to establish this diagnosis clinically be-cause puncture which would facilitate the answer is contraindicated.

— Non-parasitic cyst of the liver.

In polycystic liver, the diagnosis is more readily made because it is altogether exceptional that a hepatic hemangioma should involve so many vascular islets; moreover, the polycystic liver often coexists with bilateral polycystic kidneys, revealed at urography. On the other hand, with the solitary non-parasitic cyst of the liver the differential diagnosis is very difficult; we may discern a lesser consistency than that of the hemangioma and the characteristic vascular fremitus of angioma (when the latter is perceptible). Similarly, the non-parasitic cyst is as a rule clearly delimited. It results, therefore, that the clinical diagnosis is often difficult and must be completed by laparoscopy or rather by explorative laparotomy. The diagnosis is readily established intraoperatively, as the tumor is subcapsular and has a characteristic macroscopic aspect. Microscopic examination of the resected part confirms the diagnosis invalidating that of hemangioendothelioma, the only tumor that resembles it macroscopically.

PROGNOSIS

We have given an outline of the spontaneous evolution of untreated hemangioma of the liver.

Bearing in mind the progressive character of this formation, as well as the existence of a period of slow evolution, it is difficult to formulate a comprehensive prognosis.

The prognosis should be individualized as follows:

— It may be generally accepted that small superficial hemangiocavernomas of the liver, casually discovered, with the aspect of a vascular spot, not of surgical interest, have a *good prognosis.*

— The bulging hemangiomas, even in the preclinical period, have an *immediate good prognosis*, but the *late prognosis is reserved.*

The immediate prognosis is reserved in young athletes or pregnant women when the hemangioma is in the clinical phase.

TREATMENT

Indications. Therapeutic indications will be discussed in the following cases:

1. Small hemangioma (vascular spot), latent, incidentally discovered.
2. Small latent bulging hemangioma, incidentally discovered.
3. Palpable hemangioma.
4. Hemangioma causing pain and discomfort.

1) *Small hemagioma*, discovered on the occasion of another operation, is not of particular interest, except in newborn children; in such cases, when a small hemangioma is discovered in the course of a pylorotomy, the child should be kept under observation and the family warned of the possibility of a subsequent operation at the first signs of growth of the tumor.

2) *Latent bulging hemangioma* may be discovered during a laparotomy for another disease, and in principle should be removed. If the operation is not too complicated (cholecystitis, gastric resection for chronic duodenal ulcer, epigastric hernia,

etc.) and if the location of the hemangioma permits an easy extirpation (marginal anterior site, etc.), then the tumor should be operated. On the other hand, if the disease for which the operation is performed is severe (perforated ulcer, acute pancreatitis) or necessitates a complex intervention (duodenopancreatectomy), or when excision appears to be very difficult, the operation for hemangioma should be put off for a later date.

3) *Palpable hemangioma* does not always cause discomfort or pain and is difficult to diagnose clinically.

Therefore, we should start with an explorative laparotomy or, when a previous laparoscopy has been carried out, extirpation of the vascular tumor should be indicated.

4) *Hemangioma that causes pain and discomfort* must categorically be operated, and the operation should not be put off, especially in young athletes and pregnant women.

Although Schumaker (cited by Bockus) reports on two cases of liver hemangiomas that recovered following irradiation (hard Roentgen rays), we believe that the efficiency of this treatment is doubtful and necessitates the application of large doses over a small area. Roentgentherapy or the sclerosing treatment should only be resorted to when the vascular tumor by its extent and site has rendered the operation impossible. A conservative treatment will only result in renewal of the evolution after some time; we have had to perform left lobectomy for hemangioma after a sclerosing treatment applied in another department.

Bearing in mind the aggravation of the evolution of a hemangioma during pregnancy, we consider that:

— it is indicated to terminate pregnancy in the first trimester and operate the hemangioma:

— if the patient is already in the eighth month, Cesarean section should be recommended in order to avoid the effort of birth, treating the hemangioma subsequently.

Operative methods. Hepatic surgery raises numerous difficult problems; the liver is friable, richly vascularized and exposed to the hazard of choleperitoneum when injured.

Several operative techniques with minimal risk have been devised (see chapter on hepatectomy).

When comparatively restricted areas are to be resected in hemangiomas of medium size, then the technical difficulties are smaller.

The key of success is to remove the vascular tumor by cutting into the healthy parenchyma. Certain precautions must be taken to avoid hemorrhage and the discharge of bile. This type of limited resection in the vicinity of the pathological process, in the healthy parenchyma *(non-anatomic resection)* must be reserved for hemangiomas of small size, therefore diagnosed in due time.

In contrast, for over ten years so-called controlled hepatectomies have been performed, in which account was kept of the anatomic landmarks, resecting a clearly individualized vasculobiliary area (segment, lobe) in which the pathologic process developed. Characteristic of this type of intervention is identification of the lobar or segmentary pedicle, which must be ligated in order to reduce to a minimum the hemorrhage and discharge of bile from the sectioned parenchyma.

This type of resection must be reserved for voluminous hemangiocavernomas, in which a blind non-anatomic resection would expose the patient to the risk of having to ligate essential elements of the remaining parenchyma. Anatomic resections have been performed for large, hepatic hemangiomas, with good results (Caroli, left lobe, 1955; Heitz, right hepatectomy, 1956; Stoian, left lateral lobe, 1959).

Non-anatomic resection for hemangioma.

The types of non-anatomic resection which are used in the treatment of hepatic hemangioma are: superficial resection, wedge-shaped resection and marginal resection.

These limited surgical procedures demand, however, that particular attention should be paid to the anesthesia and an adequate route of access.

Anesthesia should be perfect, permitting at any moment extending of the surgical field, since nothing guarantees preoperatively that we shall not be obliged to perform an anatomic lobectomy, due to the size of the tumor and its depth. This is not easy with local anesthesia. Therefore, spinal anesthesia should be applied or, still better, closed endotracheal anesthesia, the only method that permits at any moment extending of the surgical field by thoracophrenotomy, when this is found necessary.

The route of approach to small or medium size hemangiomas (the only ones that permit non-anatomic resection) will be laparotomy that can be readily modified. The most advantageous from this point of view is xyphoumbilical laparotomy that can eventually be combined with thoracophrenolaparotomy (along the eighth rib), the two incisions joining together above the umbilicus; actually, the abdominal incision is a Rio-Branco incision.

Resuscitation consists of oxygen and replacement of blood loss, volume by volume, with a small addition of isotonic glucose solution in slow continuous, uninterrupted perfusion. When anesthesia of the pedicles is well done, (or disconnection with ganglioplegics), operative shock should be non existent.

In all these types of hepatectomy, hemostasis of the resected surface must be very carefully attended to.

The technical problem of hemostatic suture has preoccupied many surgeons.

In Romania this technique was studied as far back as 1894—1896 by Bălăcescu and then by Amza Jianu, (Iacobovici, Făgărăşanu, Chipail, Plătăreanu, C. Popescu have also performed non-anatomic hepatectomies).

There are still many surgeons who have tried to improve hemostatic sutures. Thus, in 1956, Robinson and Butcher proposed the use of a metallic loop (instead of a needle) in order to avoid perforation of the intrahepatic vessels.

Along general lines, there are two modes of performing a non-anatomic resection, with hemostasis of the remaining surface:

a) Around the tumor to be resected one or two rows of stay-sutures are applied and the parenchyma is then incised under protection of *previous hemostasis*, completed by omentoplasty over the resected surface.

b) Temporary hemostasis (temporary clamping of the hepatic pedicle, as performed by Berman in children; compression of the resected part between the hands of the surgeon's aid, as performed by Gorbinov) is followed by resection and hemostasis with ligation of the large vessels on the resected part, completed by omentoplasty (with sutures) along the whole resected surface for hemostasis of the small vessels, or suture of the whole resected surface with two ivalon bands (Krippaene and Herr, 1963).

In one patient *(M.St.*, 40 years), we performed a wedge-shaped resection of the left hepatic lobe under protection of hemostatic sutures with stay-sutures. A vascular tumor (hemangioma), the size of an orange, occupied the anterior margin of the left lobe. After covering the section surface with omentum the abdominal wall was closed without drainage. The patient recovered and was discharged after 10 days.

Alexandriyski, with the same indication, performed a right anterior marginal non-anatomic resection (1958).

We performed an anatomic hepatic lobectomy in a 62 year-old patient, 20 years after a sclerosing treatment, with favorable results (April 1966) (Fig. 173 *a* and *b*).

Results. Murlaga found in world literature 74 operated cases of hepatic hemangioma (in 1951); in 63 cases, non-anatomic or anatomic resections were performed, and in 11 cases a palliative treatment (cauterisation, tamponade).

It results, therefore, that in 86% of the cases hemangioma could be operated by hepatic resection.

Bockus (1953), analyzing an international statistics, mentioned that of 56 resected hemangiomas only one patient died postoperatively, the remaining patients being considered as surgically recovered and cured.

Velikoretskii (1955) showed that in 11 of 29 hemangiomas operated in the USSR anatomic resections were performed, and in 18 cases non-anatomic resections; none of the patients died postoperatively.

In 1956, Melnikov reported three deaths in 32 cases of hepatic hemangioma operated in the USSR.

In order to illustrate this chapter, the report of a clinical case follows.

Patient *M.St.*, aged 40, was admitted with attacks of epigastric pain and pain in the left hypochondrium. Headache and constipation.

The patient began to suffer five years previously. At first the epigastric pain was mild, but then increased in intensity and spread to the left hypochondrium, occurring in painful attacks that lasted several hours.

During the last year, the patient suffered from chronic constipation and headache.

Clinical findings. The general condition of the patient was comparatively good.

Respiratory and circulatory system: nothing relevant.

Local examination: in the epigastrium and left hypochondrium a renitent tumor formation could be palpated, the size of an orange, with a rough surface; the formation followed together with the liver the respiratory movements and was vaguely tender on palpation.

Hemogram: leukocytes: 16,000. Normal formula; red blood cells 4,414,000; Hb = 79%. BW negative; ESR = normal; hepatic tests = normal.

Gastrointestinal radioscopy: normal aspect and dynamics.

Preoperative diagnosis: hydatid cyst (?), explorative laparotomy is recommended. Operated (April 3, 1954) under spinal anesthesia: xyphoumbilical laparotomy.

On the anterior margin of the left lobe of the liver a tumor formation the size of an orange, purplish, slightly embossed, elastic and partly reducible by compression. Wedge-shaped resection

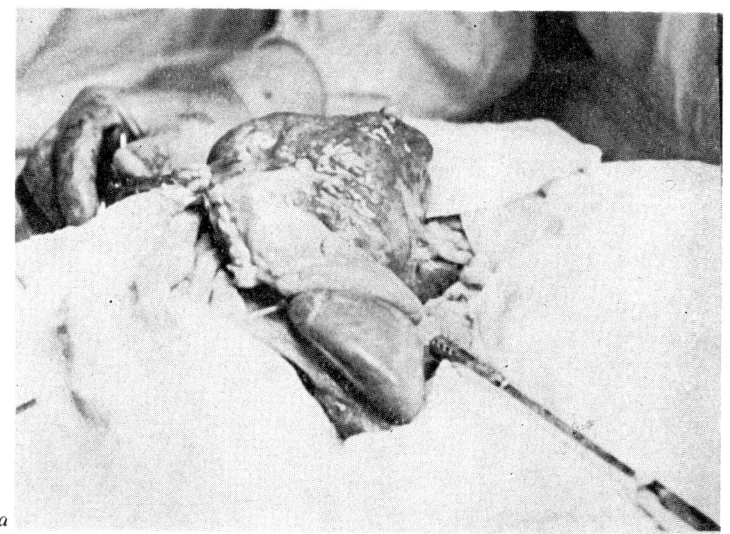

a

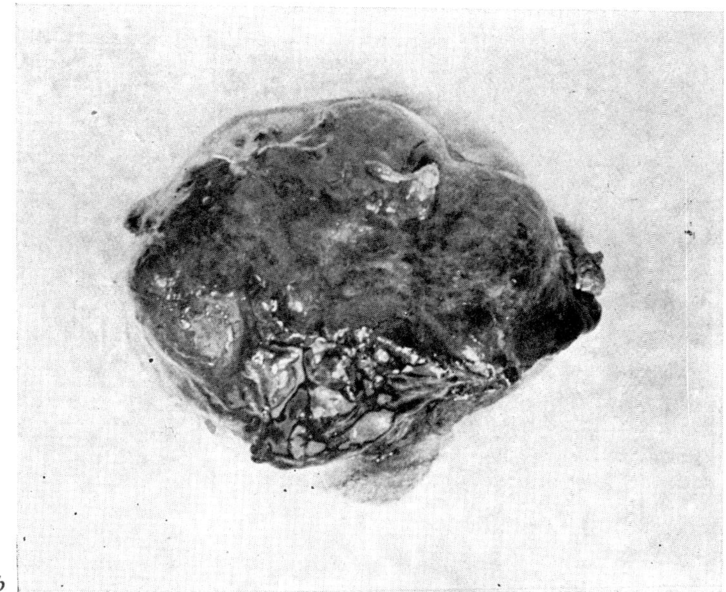

b

Fig. 173. — Relapsing hemangioma of the liver 20 years after sclerosing treatment.

a. Intraoperative aspect; *b.* operative specimen (anatomic left lobectomy).

in the healthy parenchyma up to the limit of the tumor, under the protection of hemostasis with stay-sutures, ligated to the under surface of the liver.

Peritonealization of the sectioned surface with omentum. Hemostasis and cholestasis being perfect, the wound was closed without drainage. Uneventful postoperative course. Sutures were removed on the seventh day. Surgical recovery and discharge on the tenth day.

Histological examination: hepatic hemangiocavernoma (Fig. 174).

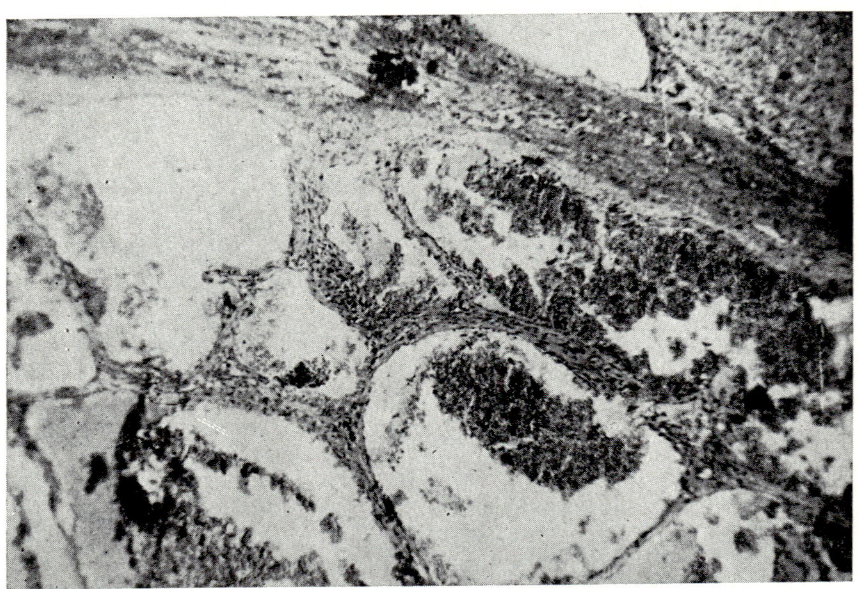

Fig. 174. — Hemangiocavernoma of the liver (patient *M.St.*). Non-anatomic resection of the left hepatic lobe. Microscopic aspect.

In conclusion, hepatic hemangioma (hemangiocavernoma) is a benign histologic formation which, however, exposes the patient to particularly severe complications.

The diagnosis is difficult, but may be established preoperatively. An uncertain diagnosis in the common cases, a reserved prognosis in the cases in which a positive diagnosis has been made, imposes a radical surgical treatment.

Hemangioma should be removed by non-anatomic or anatomic hepatectomy, according to the extension and connection of the tumor with the intrahepatic vasculobiliary elements.

Hepatectomy (non-anatomic or anatomic), performed correctly and as early as possible, will result in recovery, the patient fully regaining his working ability.

REFERENCES

1. ALEXANDRIISKI M. V., Nov. khir. Arkhiv, 1958, *3/213*, 100.
2. BERMAN J. K., KIRKOFF P., LEVENE N., Surgery, 1955, **71**, *2*, 249.
3. BOCKUS H. L., *Gastroenterology*, vol. III, W. B. Saunders, Philadelphia, 1953, p. 353.

4. BOYD W., *Pathology for the surgeon*, 7th ed., W.B. Saunders, Philadelphia, 1956, p. 263.
5. CAROLI I., ETEVE-RICORDEAU, Rev. méd. Chir., Foie, Rate et Pancréas, 1955, *3*, 39.
6. DELBET P., *Hémangiomes. Traité de chirurgie clinique et opératoire*, vol. I, Baillière, Paris, 1896, p. 439.
7. FAURE J. L., *Tumeurs du foie* in *Traité de chirurgie clinique et opératoire*, vol. VIII, Baillière, Paris, 1899, p. 239.
8. GORBINOV E. I., Vestn. Khir., 1967, *6*, 130.
9. GREVILLE Y., Brit. J. Surg., 1964, **51**, *7*, 505.
10. HEITZ I., Lyon chir., 1956, **51**, *1*, 107.
11. IACOBOVICI I., *Chirurgie*, vol. I, fasc. II, ed. Socec, Bucharest, 1944, p. 774.
12. LETULLE M., *Anatomie pathologique*, vol. 1, Masson, Paris, 1931, p. 130.
13. * * * *Medicina internă*, vol. III, Ed. medicală, Bucharest, 1956, p. 211.
14. MELNIKOV A. V., Khirurghiya, 1956, *1*, 38.
15. MURLAGA S. H., Khirurghiya, 1951, *3*, 55.
16. ROBINSON J., GARVEY R., BUTCHER, Surgery, 1956, **40**, *2*, 391.
17. SCHERLOCK SHEILA, *Diseases of the liver and biliary system*, Blackwell, Oxford, 1955, p. 575.
18. STOIAN M., STOIAN E., NEDELCOV P., Chirurgia, 1959, **8**, *5*, 779.
19. ȚURAI I., GEROTA D., *Chirurgia căilor biliare extrahepatice*, Ed. medicală, Bucharest, 1957, p. 66.
20. VASILIU TITU, *Manual de anatomie patologică clinică*, 2nd. ed., Ed. Universitară, Sibiu, 1957, p. 693.
21. VELIKORETSKII A. N., KASAKNINA R. N., Khirurghiya, 1955, *5*, 44.
22. * * * *Mnogotomnoe rukovodstvo po khirurghii*, vol. VIII, Medghiz, Moscow, 1962, p. 313.

CHAPTER 9

MALIGNANT TUMORS

A. PRIMARY MALIGNANT TUMORS
CARCINOMA
PATHOLOGIC ANATOMY
CLINICAL STUDY
LABORATORY TESTS
RADIOLOGIC EXAMINATION
BIOPSY PUNCTURE
LAPAROSCOPY
RADIOISOTOPE SCANNING
DETECTION WITH ULTRASOUNDS
DIAGNOSIS
TREATMENT
PRIMARY SARCOMA AND MALIGNANT HEMANGIO-ENDOTHELIOMA

B. SECONDARY MALIGNANT TUMORS
ETIOLOGY
PATHOGENY
PATHOLOGIC ANATOMY
CLINICAL STUDY
LABORATORY TESTS
DIAGNOSIS
TREATMENT

A. PRIMARY MALIGNANT TUMORS

CARCINOMA

In Romania as in the rest of Europe, primary malignant tumors of the liver are relatively rare in the clinic in comparison to other tumors, but can no longer be considered exceptional as shown in the statistics at the beginning of the century. The real increase in the incidence of these tumors implies a closer understanding of the possibilities of establishing a precise and early diagnosis, in order to increase the chances of the surgical treatment. Unfortunately, due to the limited possibility of discovering the tumor in an early stage and its extremely severe course, surgery usually fails. In most of the successful operations, the tumor was small and discovered incidentally in an initial phase of development, in the course of an operation on the upper abdomen for various diseases of the organs situated in this region.

Carcinoma of the liver is more frequent than sarcoma, and in this chapter the latter will not be separately dealt with as its symptomatology, clinical course and treatment closely resemble that of carcinoma.

PATHOLOGIC ANATOMY

Hepatic tumors are classified by S. Sherlock and by other authors according to their origin (table 3).

According to their gross appearance, Egger divides primary hepatic tumors into:

1. The *nodular form*, the most frequent, encountered in 62 to 83% of the cases in various statistics, and almost always accompanied by cirrhosis; the liver is enlarged, including within its mass numerous nodules of different size, ranging from a pinpoint to several centimeters in diameter. A unicentric theory on the origin of these nodules assumed the existence of a single, initial malignant tumor from which numerous metastatic tumors arise in the rest of the liver. According to the *multicentric theory* the tumors arise simultaneously from numerous adenomatous formations produced by nodular cirrhotic hyperplasia.

Table 3

Origin		Tumor	
		Benign	Malignant
Epithelial tumors	Liver cells	Hepatoma (adenoma)	Hepatoma (liver-cell carcinoma)
	Intrahepatic bile duct	Cholangioma	Cholangiocarcinoma
Connective tissue		Fibroma	Sarcoma
Blood vessels		Hemangioma	Hemangioendothelioma

2. The *massive single tumor* is met with in almost a quarter of the cases; it occupies a major portion of a hepatic lobe, as a rule the right one. The association with cirrhosis seldom occurs in the massive form of carcinoma. Some tumors may be surrounded by small cancerous nodules but, characteristically, the liver is not invaded for sometime by the tumoral process. Necropsy or operations on the upper abdomen may sometimes reveal small single, hard tumors of a whitish, grey or yellowish color. These do not represent an anatomopathologic form proper, but the incipient stage of development of a massive tumor. The fact that single malignant tumors of the liver are classified from the pathoanatomic point of view as massive shows that single tumors of small size are seldom found and have not been classified. Surgically, the single, massive tumor, especially in the incipient stage of development is the only pathoanatomic form in which a radical treatment can be attempted.

3. The *diffuse form* is more seldom encountered than the preceding ones, representing in Egger's classification about 12% of the cases in Europe (almost twice the proportion in certain African statistics). The liver is not enlarged, sometimes having a subnormal weight (650 g in the case of F.C. Roulet). Miliary hepatic carcinomatosis, involving the whole organ, develops against a background of atrophic cirrhosis. In such cases the surgical treatment is no longer possible.

From the *microscopic* point of view (Figs 175, 176 and 177), hepatic carcinomas may be separated, as already shown, into two main forms: *malignant hepatoma*, developing from the liver cells and *malignant cholangioma* deriving from the epithelium of the intrahepatic bile ducts. Most anatomopathologists agree with this classification, a certain disaccord still persisting with regard to the mixed forms. At any rate, these mixed hepatobiliary carcinomas, also called *malignant hepatocholangiomas* are frequent although their exact statistical proportion has not been established. Among the pure forms of carcinoma, malignant hepatoma is more frequent than cholangioma: 70—85% as against 15—30%; malignant hepatoma is almost always associated with cirrhosis in contrast to the cholangioma which only appears to be associated with cirrhosis in about 25% of the cases in Europe and more seldom in Africa.

In carcinoma, intrahepatic dissemination is very common (Figs 178, 179 and 180), distal metastases are surprisingly rare, although the tumoral cells have the property of invading the intrahepatic branches of the vena porta and hepatic veins, penetrating into their lumen. The metastases that appear at a distance are usually found in the lungs. Sometimes the tumoral cells pass beyond the pulmonary barrier, penetrating into the circulation and fixing themselves upon different organs supplied by the branches of the aorta, as a rule on the bones. Metastases of the liver cell carcinoma maintain the peculiarities of the liver cells from which they arose, for instance the capacity of secreting bile; in other cases they are completely anaplastic, modify their histologic structure and lose their functional properties.

Invasion of the regional lymph nodes is common in carcinomas of the liver. As a rule the lymph nodes of the hilus and hepatic pedicle are at first invaded. Lymphatic dissemination at a distance is seldom observed, the same as with dissemination through the blood circulation. Neoplastic invasion of the mediastinal lymph nodes is seldom noted. It is very likely that the low proportion of

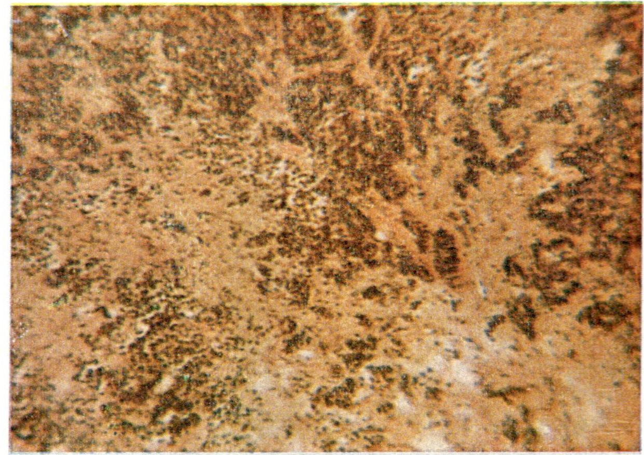

Fig. 175. — Hepatocellular carcinoma (Van Gieson; obj. 3). Intense lobular necrosis and perilobular inflammation.

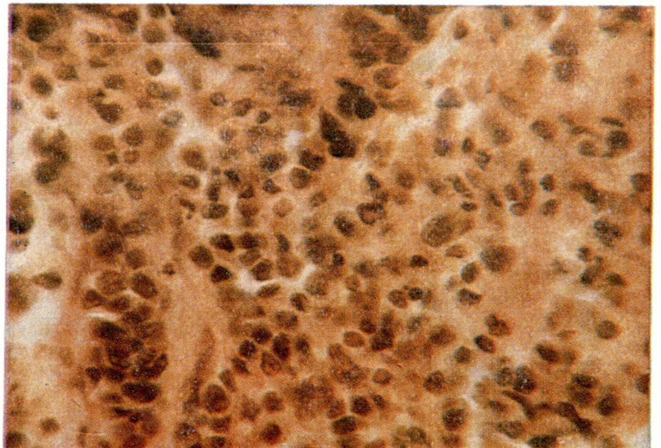

Fig. 176. — Detail of Fig. 175 (obj. 7). Neoplastic cells of various size, some giant with nuclear anomalies.

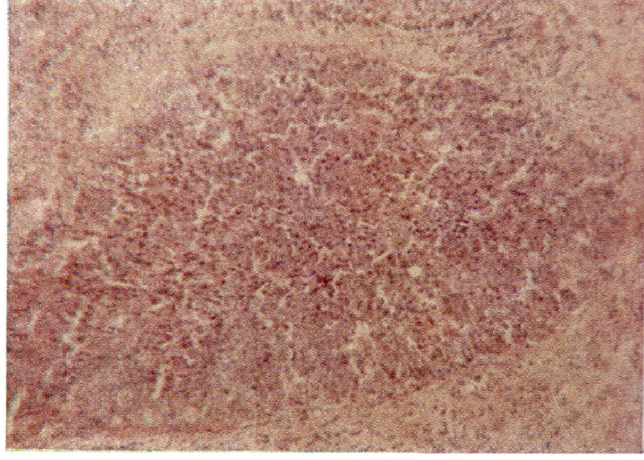

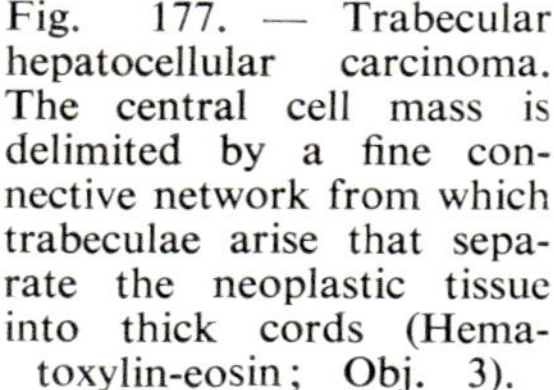

Fig. 177. — Trabecular hepatocellular carcinoma. The central cell mass is delimited by a fine connective network from which trabeculae arise that separate the neoplastic tissue into thick cords (Hematoxylin-eosin; Obj. 3).

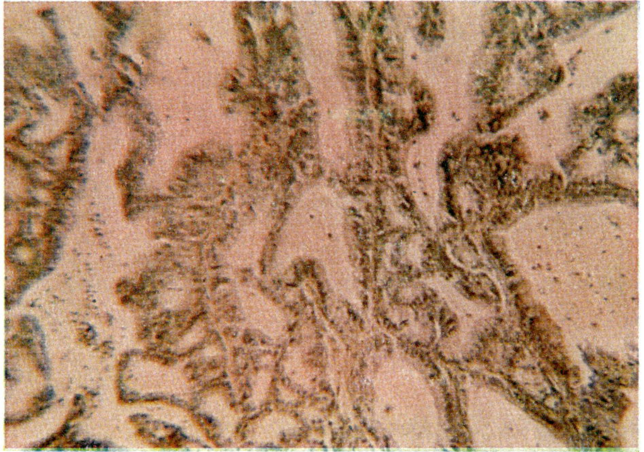

Fig. 178. — Massive metastasis of a polypous carcinoma in the liver (Van Gieson; obj. 3).

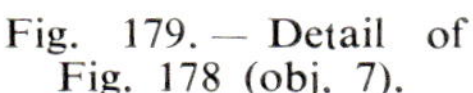

Fig. 179. — Detail of Fig. 178 (obj. 7).

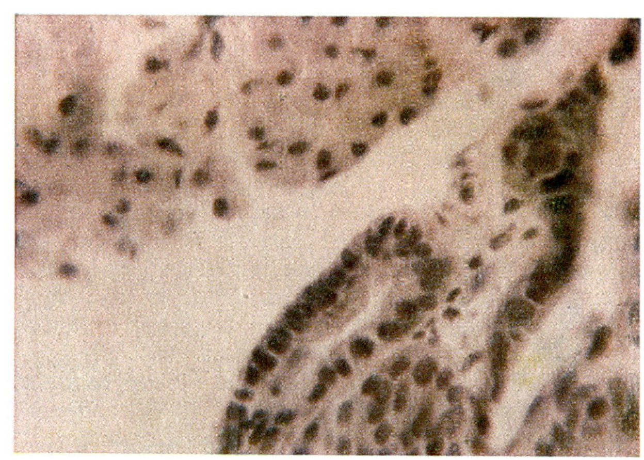

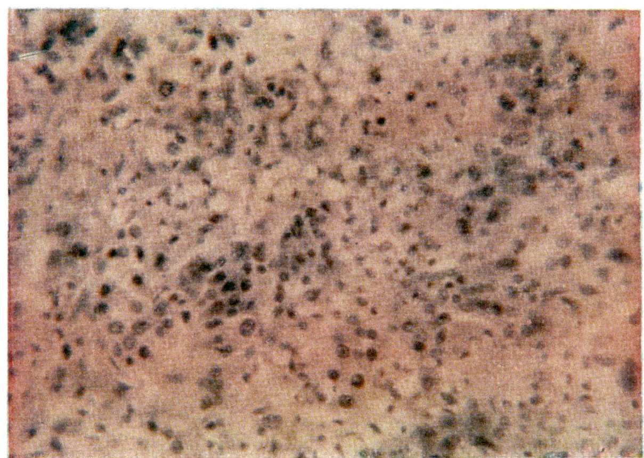

Fig. 180. — Metastasis of malignant melanoma of the liver in a patient with a primary tumor in the region of the buttocks (Hematoxylin-eosin).

distal dissemination of a hepatic carcinoma by lymphatic or circulatory route is not due to any biologic properties of these tumors but to the rapid evolution of the disease that puts an end to dissemination of the tumor at an early date.

CLINICAL STUDY

Hepatic cancer has three clinical peculiarities that make discovery of the disease possible only in a very advanced stage of development:

1. insidious onset;
2. the lack of specific subjective symptoms;
3. rapid course of the disease.

At first, little distress is felt, and the patient does not consider it necessary to go to the doctor's. About three fourths of the patients consult the doctor after about three months' evolution. The initial symptoms gradually become more accentuated and in the meantime other symptoms are added, reflecting a particularly severe state. Approximately three fourths of the patients come for loss of body weight, anorexia or abdominal pains. About two thirds discover by themselves the presence of a tumor in the region of the liver. In decreasing order, the patients complain of: marked asthenia, abdominal distension, jaundice, fever, diarrhea, nausea, vomiting, edema, cutaneomucous bleeding, hematemesis, etc.

Clinical findings. *Hepatomegaly* is a major objective element encountered in approximately 80% of the patients with hepatic cancer. Hepatic dullness over the right medioclavicular line increases by 5—10 cm and much more in many cases. The liver is palpable, as a rule hard and may have a smooth surface and a hard, sharp anterior border, intersected by deep incisurae. In more than half the patients, the surface of the liver and anterior margin are mammilated, with numerous nodules of variable size, mostly hard, sometimes soft. The abdominal wall may be thin in some cases, when hard or even fluctuant tumors can be felt. In rare cases, the whole liver is not enlarged but a tumoral swelling can be felt as a rule on the right half of the liver. This clinical aspect of tumoral liver corresponds to the pathoanatomic form of massive carcinoma with solitary tumor.

Pain in the right hypochondrium, epigastrium or lumbar region is a frequent symptom encountered in about 70% of the patients. In general it is caused by rapid distension of the liver capsule. At first the pain is not continuous and appears when walking or during muscular work. Later the pain becomes continuous and as a rule not too accentuated, rather like a feeling of pressure in the epigastrium. Pain is felt, or becomes more acute, when the patient lies on his left side, due to mechanical causes, explained by traction upon the ligaments of a liver that has greatly increased in weight.

Dyspeptic disturbances are frequently encountered in these patients but are not specific. Anorexia, ballooning, nausea, vomiting, diarrhea appear either separately or together and are of variable intensity. The patient loses weight and cachexia develops in the end stage.

Jaundice is not constant, generally mild, and appears in about 50% of the cases. It is caused by the compression exercised by the tumor upon the intrahepatic bile ducts, or by massive destruction of neoplastic tissue. The intensity of the jaundice does not always run parallel to the degree of spread of the tumor.

Ascites is to be found in 40–50% of the hospitalized patients and corresponds to portal hypertension due to intrahepatic block caused by concomitant cirrhosis, or by extrahepatic block due to recurrent thrombosis of the vena porta. Tumoral invasion of the intrahepatic branches of the vena porta takes place against the blood flow, up to obstruction of the main trunk. Due to stasis, blood thrombi are added to the tumoral thrombi. Thrombosis of the vena porta explains why the portal hypertension syndrome becomes suddenly more accentuated or has a sharp onset, in some patients in which ascites, splenomegaly and hematemesis develop rapidly. In many cases, the ascites fluid is hemorrhagic because of the fragility of the capillary vessels or rupture of a tumor on the surface of the liver due to necrosis of the neoplastic tumor. After paracenthesis the ascites fluid rapidly forms again, but in most cases does not contain neoplastic cells.

Fever. Many patients have a subfebrile state; in other cases fever may be due to the resorption of toxins from the neoplastic tissue or to dysfunction of the liver cell, reflected upon the thermoregulating centers. Fever may also be of septic origin, due to infection of necrotic foci or to cholangitis caused by pressure of the tumor upon the bile ducts.

Dyspnea, a late symptom, is brought about by very voluminous tumors that push the right diaphragm upwards, or in the more advanced stages by pulmonary metastases.

Cirrhosis is frequently encountered in liver cancer. Apart from splenomegaly and a collateral venous circulation, vascular stars, palmar erythema, gynecomasty, etc. can also be observed.

Clinical forms. According to the predominance of one symptom or group of symptoms, various clinical forms of liver cancer have been described. Thus, Lin Chao-ch'i et al. individualized 10 clinical forms to which he added two rarer ones:

1. hepatomegalic — the most frequent form;
2. simulating an abscess of the liver;
3. cirrhotic;
4. with obstructive jaundice;
5. with intraperitoneal hemorrhage;
6. hypoglycemic;
7. lithiasic (simulating lithiasis);
8. chronic hepatitic (simulating hepatitis);
9. intraabdominal cystic;
10. diffuse carcinomatous;
11. leukemoid;
12. paraplegic (with vertebral metastases).

According to the authors this separation into 12 clinical forms facilitates the diagnosis, but they are not fixed forms and may undergo frequent changes in terms of the evolution.

M. Payet et al. describe 4 clinical forms, with an unequal incidence.

1. *Tumoral form* in about 70% of the cases corresponding to the hepatomegalic form of the foregoing classification.

2. *Febrile form*, simulating the tropical amebic liver abscess, is encountered especially in the warmer regions of the globe. This category does not include numerous subfebrile cases, representing about 50% of the cases. In forms simulating a liver abscess, the temperature may rise to 39°—40°C/102.2°—104° F and remain in a plateau or oscillate intermittently the same as malaria fever. The patient's general condition rapidly alters, the liver progressively becomes larger, leukocytosis rises to 20,000—50,000, with predominant neutrophil polynuclears. The presence of jaundice or ascites plead for cancer. In many cases the diagnosis is established following explorative puncture.

3. *Malignant cirrhosis.* The disease appears with signs of decompensated cirrhosis and evolves very rapidly because of massive cancerous invasion of the liver. The patients are usually admitted 1—2 months after the first symptoms, which are vague at first. After admission the average survival is of 15—20 days, whatever the treatment. Death is brought about by acute hepatorenal insufficiency, uremia and severe jaundice.

4. *Atypical forms.* M. Payet et al. describe numerous atypical forms, the most important appearing to be those which are classed according to the mode of expansion of the tumor.

a) Forms with *endothoracic development* include the fairly rare cases in which the tumoral liver presses the diaphragm and right lung upwards, producing atelectasis: the lower edge of the liver does not exceed the costal margin and half the xyphoumbilical distance. The clinical manifestations are especially of the respiratory type. The diagnosis can only be established by puncture. The radiologic images closely resemble those given by pachypleuritis.

b) The *pseudorenal form* likewise includes rare forms in which the tumor develops posteriorly and downwards, simulating a renal tumor with lumbar contact and ballotement. Urography gives images that are difficult to interpret and biopsy puncture alone can establish the diagnosis.

Evolution. The interval between the onset of the clinical disease and death is on the average 6 months. In decreasing order of frequency, the causes of death are: hepatic coma, hemorrhage from the tumor or esophageal varices and cachexia. G. Macchioro found in the literature some very rare cases, with a clinical course of 2—4 years. One patient in the series of Lin Chao-ch'i lived 3 years and 11 months with a malignant hepatoma initially verified by biopsy and after death at necropsy. The incipient malignant lesions preceded the clinical onset of the disease by several months.

In certain clinical forms, the duration of the disease is much shorter. In the febrile form, simulating a liver abscess, the course of the disease is about 3 months. In malignant cirrhosis the evolution is supraacute, death occurring within 15 to 20 days after the onset of the first major symptoms. Fever, jaundice and early ascites, a marked collateral circulation are the signs of a rapid evolution.

In some cases, the course of the disease may be silent or even asymptomatic. Death may occur suddenly, after a short clinical course, with sharp pains, vomiting, diarrhea, simulating an acute abdominal syndrome. In most cases death is caused by thrombosis of the vena porta in patients with an undeveloped collateral circulation. In other cases, a massive intraperitoneal hemorrhage may develop in the course of an effort or abdominal injury, by rupture of the tumor on the surface of the liver. The tumor must be of very low consistency to rupture tumors necrosed in the center, with richly vascularized, friable walls. This intraperitoneal hemorrhage may be very massive, ending in shock and death.

LABORATORY TESTS

Patients with carcinoma of the liver may suffer from various degrees of anemia and leukocytosis.

Anemia is the more accentuated, the more frequent and massive the hemorrhage. In most cases the red blood cell count is of 2,500,000 to 3,500,000/mm^3.

Leukocytosis is as a rule of about 10,000 with 80% neutrophils. The leukocyte count is higher in the form simulating a liver abscess. In the pseudoleukemic form, Lin Chao-ch'i et al. found leukocyte counts up to 123,000, with 95—99% neutrophils. In any cirrhotic with leukopenia, the appearance of leukocytosis that cannot be explained by an intercurrent disease, suggests the possibility of a liver carcinoma.

Plasma proteins show normal or low values; the albumin/globulin ratio is low and sometimes inversed. Plasma protein electrophoresis reveals in most cases hypergammaglobulinemia, reversing the A/G ratio; α_2 globulin is the most increased fraction.

The *liver tests* (thymol turbidity and zinc sulfate test) are normal in half the patients, especially at the beginning of the disease, then become positive and more intense towards the end. The BSP test is more sensitive and positive in almost all the patients.

Serum transaminase and aldolase show higher values in about 50% of the patients.

Prothombin index falls below 75% in at least one third of the patients.

Serum bilirubin is slightly increased in anicteric patients.

Two tests are considered more important for establishing a diagnosis of carcinoma of the liver: blood glucose and serum alkaline phosphatase. In general, hypoglycemia is more or less accentuated and alkaline phosphatase increases. When the other laboratory tests are negative and these two tests intensely positive in the direction shown, they may be considered to give a diagnostic orientation, without being specific of liver carcinoma.

Recently, Lin Chao-ch'i et al. published the preliminary results of a laboratory study concerning the reaction of the urine to deoxyribonucleic acid. They considered this test to be highly specific, since it was positive in all the patients with hepatic carcinoma and negative in 96% of the cases of uncomplicated cirrhosis and 100% of normal subjects. The authors do not discuss the principles of the test.

The fact that most of the laboratory tests are slightly positive or normal is accounted for by the high capacity of the liver cell to supplement the functional deficiencies of a large part of the liver deeply altered from the pathoanatomic point of view. It is sufficient for a quarter of the hepatic tissue to remain intact for the functional necessities of the organism to be met with. Therefore in patients with carcinoma, without cirrhosis, neoplastic invasion must be extremely advanced for the hepatic test to be strongly modified. In patients with concomitant cirrhosis, the initial alteration of the tests is determined by the degree of cirrhosis. To the end period are added the changes brought about by the degree of cancerous invasion of the liver.

RADIOLOGIC EXAMINATION

Of all the radiologic examinations, *plain X-ray* of the liver gives the best results comparable to those of more complex methods; it is readily performed and the least harmful. Small tumors, especially those located in the center of the hepatic parenchyma or those protruding on the undersurface of the liver cannot be detected by a plain X-ray. Moreover, even when the image of a tumor is detected, its nature cannot be established at the radiographic examination.

In some cases, in which the tumor or tumors come in contact with the right diaphragm, giving radiographic images show a circumscribed swelling, or irregular swellings on the diaphragm. Corroborated with the clinical examination, this irregular aspect of the diaphragm is very important in the diagnosis of liver carcinoma. Therefore, plain X-rays are recommended in all suspect cases. The image must be taken in different projections, in front, side and oblique positions.

Pneumoperitoneum increases the value of a roentgenogram, separating the liver from the diaphragm; the tumor formations can be more clearly discerned as belonging to the liver. Pneumoperitoneum is contraindicated in weak patients or those without ascites. At the end of a paracentesis, after evacuation of the ascites fluid, a moderate amount of air can be injected in order to establish a more precise diagnosis.

In suspects of liver carcinoma, a pulmonary radiologic examination is necessary so as not to overlook possible metastases. Barium meal is also recommended as it may reveal displacement of the stomach down and leftwards, or of the hepatic angle of the colon in tumors of the right lobe, compressed by the liver tumor. Esophageal varices depending upon the associated cirrhosis, without being of great diagnostic interest in carcinoma of the liver, complete the patient's general status.

No simple and efficient method has yet been found to visualize the liver, comparable to urography and cholangiography by intravenous route. Hepatography with thorotrast, the best method proposed to date has been given up as it was discovered that this substance produced liver sarcoma in the patients to which it was administered.

Splenal and portal venography, performed for the first time in liver carcinoma by F. Lagrot et al. in 1954, gives well visualized hepatographic images, provided the contrast medium is allowed to fill the liver. The radiographs must be taken at least 15 seconds after the end of the injection since in the first seconds only the large branches of the vena porta are visualized. On the positive radiographs, the tumor or tumors appear as one or several filling defects. Splenal and portal venography has not been adopted as a current diagnostic method in liver tumors since it involves certain risk, especially in patients with a weak general condition or clotting disturbances. Moreover, it has a high index of error. Falsely negative results are frequent because of the impaired intrahepatic portal circulation which opacifies badly in the, as a rule, cirrhotic liver of patients with liver carcinoma. In many cases with venous shunts the opaque substance is lost in the general circulation before reaching the liver.

Selective hepatic arteriography by transaortic route is a method frequently used today: it avoids dilution of the contrast substance in the aorta and gives a very clear hepatographic image in experimented hands. This method is inefficient only when the contrast substance of the arterial blood dilutes 1:5 in the portal blood, giving a poor hepatographic image.

Hepatic phlebography has the same defects and advantages as arteriography. It is difficult to guide the catheter from the cava into the hepatic veins, even by a skilled hand. The results are often poor and disproportionate to the amplitude of the method.

BIOPSY PUNCTURE

An essential examination for the diagnosis of carcinoma of the liver is biopsy puncture, at first used by Iversen and Roholm in 1940 and now widely applied in many countries. In patients with enlargement of the liver the transparieto-abdominal route should be chosen for the puncture. When the tumor is palpable, the needle is introduced directly into the tumor. When the liver does not exceed the costal margin, the intercostal route of approach is preferable. The product collected varies: normal or cirrhotic liver tissue, neoplastic tissue, eventually purulent magma or magma resulting from the residual necrosed tumoral tissue. Sometimes only blood or bile is extracted or the gross aspect shows a non-homogeneous aspect and consistency, which points to the presence of a malignant growth.

Biopsy puncture of the liver is *contraindicated* in coagulation disturbances, especially when the prothrombin index falls below 60%. Even when the coagulation tests are normal clotting substances should be administered before the puncture and ascites fluid extracted in order to reveal eventual hemorrhage and to palpate the liver for the puncture more readily. Cytologic examination of the sediment may in some cases reveal cancerous cells. Puncture is likewise contraindicated when the patient's general condition is altered since even a slight hemorrhage may represent a particularly severe incident, and in hepatobiliary suppurations, because of the risk of peritonitis. In the latter case the contraindication may be questioned since it is difficult to differentiate the febrile or subfebrile forms of carcinoma from hepatobiliary suppurations. In the tropical regions where biopsy punctures were done in a large series of patients in order to differentiate liver abscess from cancer, there were extremely rare cases of peritonitis.

The results of a blind puncture have a casual character as long as the needle has not been introduced directly into a tumor, palpable below the costal margin. If the result is negative, the puncture may be repeated. In the regions in which carcinomas of the liver are more frequent, surprisingly few mistakes are made. In China, H.L. Chung found positive biopsy puncture results in 76.1% of the cases of carcinoma. W.S. Ch'ien gives a percentage of 92.3%, therefore only 7.7%

falsely negative results. In Europe, where we probably have a more restricted experience in biopsy puncture, positive results are obtained in only about half the cases checked anatomically.

Biopsy puncture is not of great interest for the *early* diagnosis of liver carcinoma. After more than 3000 punctures in cases of cirrhosis, J. Delarue and L. Frühling observe that no incipient carcinoma was detected. The only cases of incipient hepatoma were found at necropsy among the patients with cirrhosis who died from hemorrhage caused by portal hypertension. Even if in such cases an incipient carcinoma were suspected, it would have been almost impossible to detect with the tip of the needle in the course of 2—3 punctures, a small tumor located within such a large organ as the liver.

Several severe and even fatal accidents have been recorded after biopsy puncture. A. Singh et al. report 3 severe hemorrhages and a biliary peritonitis after 410 punctures performed in a hospital of Punjab, India; all three patients recovered. M. Payet after more than 1000 punctures had a fatal case of hemorrhage.

LAPAROSCOPY

The idea of observing intraperitoneal lesions with an optical instrument introduced through the abdominal wall has tempted many investigators. Some of them have a vast experience in this direction. However, the value of laparoscopy has been contested, not so much the method itself as by comparison with explorative laparotomy, which is preferred by most surgeons.

The following laparoscopic images correspond most probably to cancerous lesions of the liver:

— candle-like patches over the liver surface;

— hard whitish or pseudocystic nodules; by laparoscopic "palpation", the consistency of the nodules can be tested in comparison to the surrounding liver tissue;

— an enormous, single tumoral mass, with a polylobate surface, sometimes pseudocystic.

According to F. Pergola et al., the laparoscopic diagnosis is limited by the following factors:

1. The diagnosis is not possible when the cancer nodules are located centrally or posteriorly;

2. Multinodular carcinoma may be confounded with certain forms of posthepatitis cirrhosis;

3. Primary carcinoma cannot be differentiated from metastatic cases, as the primary tumors are sometimes umbilicated the same as the secondary ones. When associated cirrhosis is found, it is very likely a primary tumor as metastases seldom appear on a cirrhotic liver.

Laparophotography has not substantially improved the method. On the other hand, biopsy puncture under laparoscopic control certainly gives better results. Several authors, among whom Righi Riva et al., F. Pergola et al., prefer this method to blind puncture which they avoid. The tumor is more readily detected and hemorrhage is avoided; pseudocystic nodules should not be punctured, especially when blackish in color since they may correspond to blood pools that will flood the peritoneal cavity when the needle is withdrawn. Tumors of vascular origin, which are generally pulsatile should likewise be avoided.

RADIOISOTOPE SCANNING

During the last ten years, both the function and the morphology of the liver have been successfully studied with the help of radioactive isotopes. In some medical centers, the method is now currently used for the diagnosis of malignant tumors of the liver, as well as in other diseases of this organ. In 1953, L. A. Stirrett et al. described for the first time a method for detecting hepatic metastases with radioactive isotopes. The method was soon extended to primary malignant tumors.

At the beginning, serum albumin labeled with radioactive iodine — ^{131}I — was used, but the results were not very good as the capacity of the tumoral tissue to take up radioactive albumin does not differ sufficiently from that of the surrounding tissue, to give contrast detectable on the records. In 1955, G. V. Taplin et al. used rose bengal combined with radioactive iodine. Rose bengal being a tetrafluorescein tetraiodate, one of the common iodine atoms may readily be substituted by a ^{131}I-labeled atom. In addition, sodium, carbon and especially radioactive gold are also rapidly taken up by Kupffer cells; in about 20 minutes 80% of the substance is concentrated in the liver.

At present two products are currently used in the diagnosis of malignant tumors of the liver: ^{131}I rose bengal and radioactive colloidal gold — ^{198}Au. Most investigators, among whom W. Schumacher, J. Caroli, etc. prefer rose bengal although it is more expensive, to ^{198}Au.

— With the aid of rose bengal both the morphologic and the functional aspect of the liver can be studied. After injection of the substance, radioactivity is determined over the cephalic region and the liver. The more rapid the accumulation in the liver, the greater its functional capacity. In a healthy individual the curve reaches a peak after 5—6 minutes. Rapid decrease of radioactivity in the cephalic region to half the maximum values shows a good functional capacity of the liver. In the normal individual, radioactivity half life should not exceed 12 minutes in the cephalic region. In certain injuries of the liver cell, it may last up to 50 minutes. According to J. Caroli, ^{131}I rose bengal is superior to the non-radioactive functional tests.

— As it is more rapidly eliminated than ^{198}Au, ^{131}I rose bengal produces milder irradiation, even less dangerous than that of the current roentgen diagnostic examinations. The substance is to be found after an hour and a half in the jejunum and is eliminated with the feces within 24 hours; in cirrhotics about 25% is eliminated through the urine.

For morphologic determinations, 50—100 μc ^{131}I rose bengal or an equal amount of ^{198}Au are injected by intravenous route. Lately, ^{131}I biligraphin, in 200—300 μc amounts has also been used. The amounts of the substance used are directly proportional to the subject's body and volume of the liver. Recordings are taken after 15 minutes when ^{131}I rose bengal is used, after 20 minutes with ^{198}Au and after one hour with ^{131}I biligraphin.

The cost of a scintiscanner for recording radioactivity is approximately equal to that of a roentgen apparatus. W. Schumacher who has dealt in detail with this problem finds the Szintophot Sp. 31, made in Germany, very satisfactory. In our clinic we are using a Scinticart apparatus. The apparatuses have a scintillation counter, a multiplier tube, focussing collimator, a linear amplifier and an electromagnetic complex for recording the pulses transformed into horizontal rows of short vertical lines which in the aggregate show the distribution of a radioactive tracer substance; the denser the lines, the higher the radioactivity in the region corresponding to the liver. Absence of the tracing or a gap in the tracing shows that the radioisotope has not been taken up and corresponds to a pathologic process.

Various terms have been used for the graphical representation: gammagram, or scintillography by the French, isotopographic image by the Italians and radioisotope scanning by the English and Americans. In Romania, scintillogram or scintigram is used. The qualities of the image are expressed in terms of contrast, opacity, resolution power, clear or diffuse aspect. When the detector is driven back and forth across the organ, from the diaphragmatic aspect of the liver towards the undersurface, there is time for the gallbladder to fill with ^{131}I rose bengal or ^{131}I biligraphin. A hepatocholecystogram is obtained, since the scintigram also exhibits an opacity that outlines the gallbladder.

The value of the scintigram increases when recorded on a film upon which a roentgenogram of the liver is taken; this facilitates interpretation of the results, the anatomic reference points helping to locate the lesions more precisely.

Hepatic scintigram of malignant tumors shows a single or multiple defects (Figs 181, 182 and 183). However, by this method only tumors of a given size and depth can be detected. Friedell, Intyre and Rejali, who attempted to establish a definite relationship between the diameter of the tumor, its depth and the possibility of detecting it by radioactive isotopes, built a liver-like container, which they filled with a weak ^{131}I solution and air-filled plastic balloons of various size, simulating hepatic tumors, and found that the latter should measure at least 2.5 cm in diameter in the right lobe and 1.5 cm in the left lobe to appear on the scintigram. W.Y. Chao found that tumors at 10 cm depth should measure at least 10 cm in diameter to be detected and those at 5 cm depth at least 5 cm diameter.

In contrast to metastatic tumors, primary tumors of the liver have been comparatively little studied by scintigraphy, although the method has proved highly efficient for the diagnosis. In Caroli's opinion, it is superior to other diagnostic methods, such as laparoscopy, hepatic arteriography, splenal and portal venography. He considers scintigraphy comparable to a good laparophotography in several colors, combined with multiple hepatic punctures.

Friedell et al. uphold that a hepatic scintigram with radioactive isotopes may help to establish a differential diagnosis between a primary malignant tumor of the liver and a cystic tumor, for instance hydatid, although both appear as defects on examination with ^{131}I rose bengal, ^{198}Au and ^{131}I biligraphin. On repeating the hepatic scintigram with ^{131}I albumin the hydatid cyst continues to be impermeable to the radioactive substance, i.e. a solitary defect as at the first examination, whereas

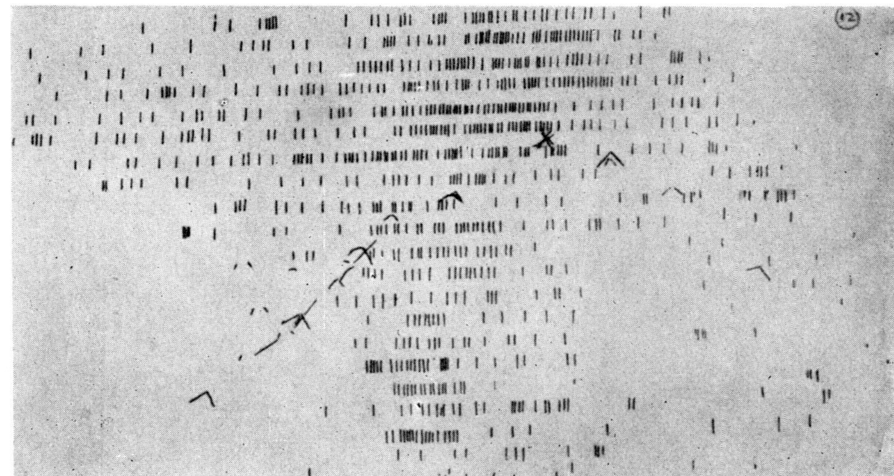

Fig. 181. — Hepatic scintigram of patient *C.N.* suffering from primary carcinoma of the liver. Right lobe almost entirely occupied by the tumor (^{131}I rose Bengal). The reference points mark the costal margin.

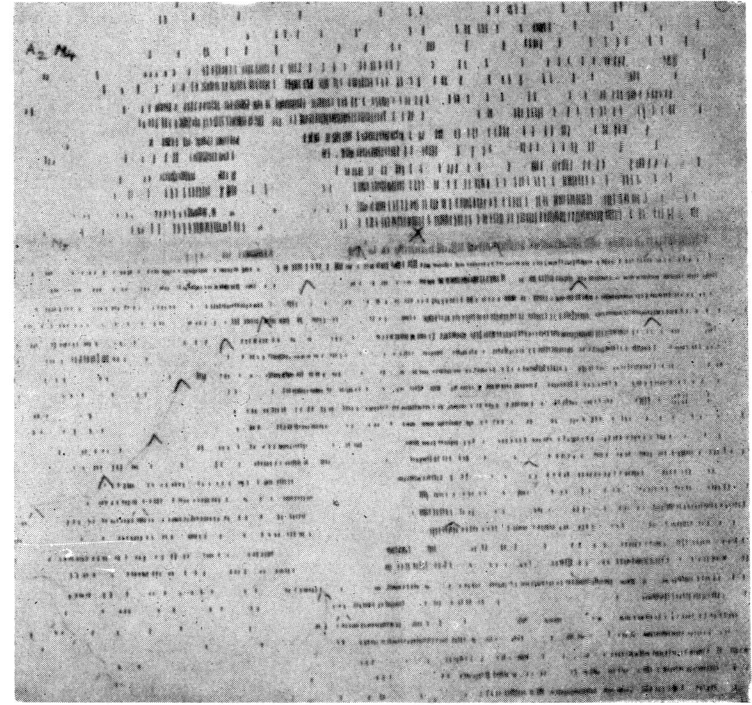

Fig. 182. — Hepatic scintigram of patient *B.G.* suffering from malignant tumor of the sigmoid colon with multiple hepatic metastases. Enlarged liver, with many "gap" images.

the malignant tumor takes up ^{131}I albumin, and becomes as opaque as the rest of the liver. We obtained conclusive results with scintigraphy when the metastatic or the primary tumors were large, and the diagnosis had not raised any special problems. In incipient primary tumors, the only ones in which an early diagnosis would be very useful, this method can only furnish information when the tumor has a diameter of more than 2—3 cm.

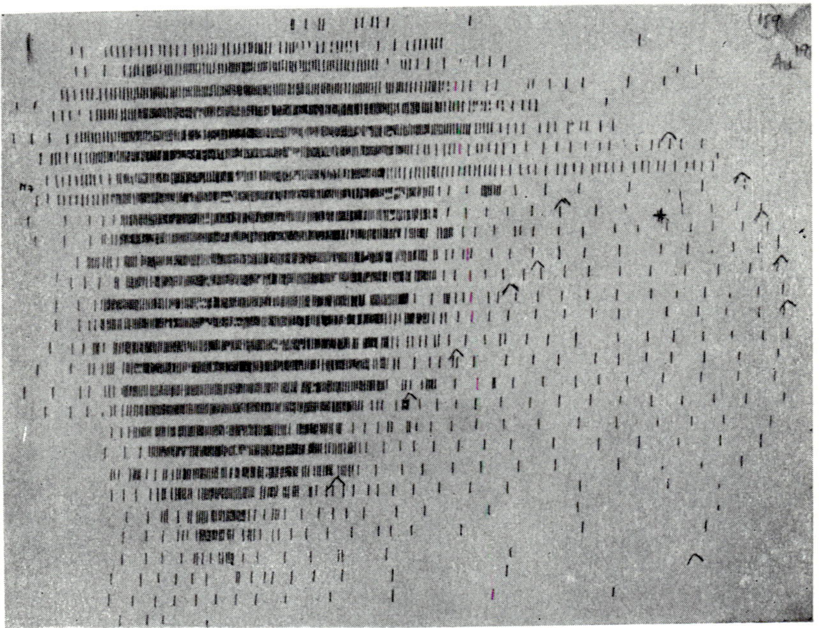

Fig. 183. — Hepatic scintigram of patient *B.E.* suffering from malignant gastric tumor with massive invasion of the left lobe of the liver.

DETECTION WITH ULTRASOUNDS

For several years a new method has been tested, in a clinic in Shanghai, for detecting malignant tumors of the liver, i.e. ultrasound detection. With a special apparatus for emitting ultrasound waves, at a given frequency, certain differences may be detected in the way in which the tumor and the surrounding liver parenchyma reflect the waves, due to the different physical properties of these tissues.

In a series of 40 cases, checked by anatomic examination, the diagnosis by ultrasounds was correct in 33 cases. In 3 cases the results were falsely positive and in 4 cases falsely negative. Lin Chao-ch'i published the results obtained and stated that the method can be improved upon. Preliminary studies show it to be a valuable aid in the diagnosis of primary malignant tumors of the liver.

DIAGNOSIS

Great difficulties are encountered in the diagnosis of cancer of the liver during the acute stage of the disease, and in the incipient period it is almost impossible to establish. In the regions with a low incidence, carcinoma of the liver is discovered in most cases in the course of an explorative laparotomy or at necropsy. When the incidence is higher, the diagnosis is more readily established, at any rate in the end period, due to the greater clinical experience of the doctors. Ascites, jaundice and cachexia are considered the terminal signs of liver carcinoma.

In the course of diagnostic investigations, the clinical examination represents the first and probably most important stage since it will give a valuable orientation as regards selection of the cases for study by other methods of investigations. From the clinical point of view, the most important signs of probability are the following:

1. Progressive enlargement of the liver especially when it has a hard, irregular surface because of multiple nodules.
2. A solitary, voluminous nodule in a patient with cirrhosis.
3. A solitary nodule in a non-cirrhotic patient is highly suspect of malignancy when it grows very rapidly.
4. Cirrhosis with a malignant onset or cirrhosis that suddenly deteriorates.
5. Internal spontaneous hemorrhage especially at menopause in women, and in men.
6. Hepatomegaly with ascites shows a high probability of the presence of a carcinoma in a very advanced stage. In most cases, cirrhosis is not accompanied by ascites as long as the liver is hypertrophic.

The approximate value of the different methods of investigation that complete the clinical examination was shown in the previous chapter. The diagnosis can be established with certainty only following the pathohistologic examination, the other methods indicating in the best of cases a diagnosis of probability. In the statistics of 330 cases of Wang Ch'eng-en and Li-Kuo-ts'ai, the anatomic diagnosis was checked in a certain number of cases. In 83.7% of these cases the diagnosis was established on the basis of the clinical, radiologic and laboratory examinations. In 16.3% of the cases, special procedures were necessary: biopsy, puncture, ultrasound, pneumoperitoneum, peritoneoscopy, hepatoarteriography and laparotomy. In the first group of patients there were 23.5% falsely-positive results, invalidated by laparotomy or necropsy.

Differential diagnosis. In the geographical regions with a low incidence of liver carcinoma most cases are wrongly diagnosed before laparotomy or necropsy. Here are some of the main diagnostic mistakes:

Metastatic cancer. In many cases of metastatic cancer the primary tumor may be found, as a rule, on one of the intraabdominal segments of the gastrointestinal tract. Moreover, the hepatic scintigram may reveal secondary tumors since the way in which radioactive albumin iodine is taken up differs in primary tumors.

Cirrhosis may simulate cancer or may be associated to cancer in the course of its evolution. Sometimes it is necessary to resort to many methods, including exploratory laparotomy in order to be able to establish the diagnosis.

Abscess of the liver may be taken for the febrile form of carcinoma. On puncture, a characteristic viscous pus will be withdrawn. The diagnosis is very difficult even in the course of laparotomy. W. Schumacher had in his care four patients in whom the abscess was only discovered after the second or third successive laparotomy and only due to location of the purulent collection by scintigraphy. According to M. Payet when in doubt, the patient should be treated as having an amebic abscess, thus offering a chance of recovery to the patients in which the suspicion of cancer was not confirmed.

Cancer of the gallbladder is very difficult to differentiate from carcinoma of the liver. However, in most cases the patients with vesicular cancer are old lithiasic patients whereas hepatic carcinoma generally develops in cirrhotics.

Other malignant tumors of the neighboring organs as a rule of the pancreas, require special methods of diagnosis.

Intraperitoneal hemorrhage due to rupture of the hepatic tumor may simulate an acute hemorrhagic pancreatitis, rupture of the spleen, perforated ulcer and other acute abdominal diseases. The diagnosis is established in the course of the explorative laparotomy.

Pseudocystic malignant tumors may be taken for a cyst of the liver or pancreas especially in patients with a satisfactory general state of health.

Early diagnosis. As already mentioned, liver carcinoma can only be discovered in the incipient phase of development in very rare cases. Even if the methods of investigation whould be more accurate, the efficiency of an early diagnosis would not be greatly improved since as long as a suspicion of cancer does not exist, the patient is not examined in detail. The evolution is at first oligo- or asymptomatic, then unspecific disturbances develop and carcinoma is only suspected or confirmed when the tumor or tumors take on a high degree of development so that the stage of curability has already been exceeded. By early diagnosis we do not mean only detection of the cases in which the volume of the tumor is very small. Rare cases have been reported in which large tumors had been removed with success which at first appeared to be inoperable both from the technical and the prognostic points of view. Starting from the idea, accepted in general, that the tumor has been diagnosed early when it could be resected, such voluminous tumors may be considered as in an early stage of development not so much by their size but by the favorable site of their location in the parenchyma and in a single hepatic area. There are, therefore, different degrees of an early diagnosis.

As regards small, incipient tumors, there appear to be only two possibilities of diagnosing them: (1) a tumoral nodule may sometimes be discovered by palpation when it develops on the surface of the liver, on the anterior edge or below the chondrocostal margin and when the abdominal wall of the patient is not too thick. The patient does not come to the doctor because of the symptomatology brought about by the presence of the small tumor, which is actually asymptomatic, but because of disturbances produced by different diseases of the upper abdominal organs. Once detected, such a tumor should be punctured for a histological examination. It is preferable even when the result is negative, to carry out an explorative laparotomy. Followed up, the tumor may increase raising to a clinical suspicion of carcinoma but then the most favorable therapeutic moment has probably already passed. (2) In other extremely rare cases, a small malignant tumor may be discovered incidentally, in the course of an operation in the upper abdomen, that has no direct connection with the hepatic tumor.

TREATMENT

To-date, the only method of treatment of primary carcinoma of the liver that has given good results, even if fairly restricted, is surgery. The other methods applied can only be considered as palliative.

General chemotherapy has been abandoned in favor of regional chemotherapy. By the general route of administration, however large is the dose of the active substance, it is impossible to obtain a tumoricide concentration in the cancerous focus. In regional chemotherapy, a 10-to 20-fold concentration can been obtained in the focus capable of destroying the tumoral tissue partly or of arresting its development for some time. Among the substances used, thiotepa has given the best results with the lowest intolerance. Several routes of administration have been used: the right gastroepiplooic vein, hepatic artery, right gastric epiploic artery, which appears to be the most convenient. The polythene catheter introduced in the artery may be left for 20 to 30 days without producing vascular thrombosis. Small repeated doses of the active product are introduced through the catheter. Lin Chao-ch'i who used this method in 12 cases of primary liver carcinoma, obtained, in his opinion, very good results. The pain disappeared and the volume of the liver was reduced. However, there is no case published in which complete sterilization of the tumor has been obtained by chemotherapy.

Radiotherapy with radioactive cobalt, ^{60}Co, has not given satisfactory results. Although the volume of the liver decreases in most of the cases treated, the state of health deteriorates. Cobaltotherapy should not be applied to patients in poor condition with deficient hepatic function, ascites, jaundice, metastases.

Other radioactive isotopes have also been tried, especially ^{198}Au with inconstant results.

Regional chemotherapy is superior to radiotherapy in patients with hepatic carcinoma but cannot be substituted for the surgical treatment. It can only be applied to inoperable patients with a general satisfactory state of health, i.e. in diffuse or multinodular carcinoma and in some cases of massive, inoperable carcinoma.

Surgical treatment. The first successful resection of the liver for primary carcinoma was performed by Schrader in 1890. At the last control, seven years after the operation, the patient showed no sign of relapse.

Until 1940—1950 several sporadic cases of hepatectomy for primary carcinoma were published, the technique used being that of non-anatomic resections. Since then the number of cases sharply increased due to the general progress of surgery and to improvement of the technique of resections which made extirpation by controlled hepatectomy possible even of a voluminous tumor. Notwithstanding hepatectomies in general, and especially those applied in liver carcinoma, cannot be considered as current operations because of the extremely restricted possibilities of discovering a single primary malignant tumor in an initial state of development and because of the high risk implied by the operation.

The principle of an early and radical operation should stand at the basis of the surgical treatment of malignant tumors of the liver and of any other organ. We have already shown the causes that prevent an early diagnosis. If we reduce the problem to a minimum, that is to the number of cases in which a single, small hepatic tumor was incidentally discovered in the course of an operation on the upper abdomen, it may be asserted that any such tumor should be extirpated. Therefore, the surgeon must be acquainted with the technique of resection of the liver in order not to regret having left *in situ* a perfectly resectable tumor. Extirpation of voluminous tumors demands, however, a far greater experience in hepatobiliary surgery.

In operations with very high operative hazard such as broad hepatectomy, the only justification is the radical aspect. Therefore palliative operations are questionable if not directly contraindicated. Such operations have sometimes been performed in cases of very large tumors that pressed upon the neighboring organs and the abdominal wall. In this way, at the expense of a high mortality rate, it was possible to prolong the life of some patients by several weeks or months.

In order to comply with the rules of a radical operation, it is necessary for the resection plane to be at a distance from the tumor in the apparently normal hepatic tissue. Analysis of the cases published showed that the survival mean is the longer, the more removed is the resection plane from the tumor. The minimal accepted distance is of 2 cm but within the limits of the possibilities offered, the surgeon should try to extend it to 5 cm. In most cases published in which the operation is described in detail, the limit of safety is of less than 2 cm, the resection plane passing tangent to the tumor. When no tumor tissue visible with the naked eye has been left *in situ*, such a resection may be considered as a radical operation but with smaller chances of survival for longer periods.

The indications for hepatectomy in malignant tumors of the liver result from the foregoing paragraphs. In general, the operation is indicated when the patient's condition is satisfactory, when resection is technically possible and offers a sufficient guarantee of being radical, without untoward operative hazard, in comparison to the expected results.

For resection to be technically possible, the hepatic hili must not be invaded by the tumor. The resection must be thus conceived so that at the end of the operation the residual liver, perfectly vascularized, should not contain any visible tumor tissue. The tumor must be single or in the case of multiple tumors, they should be grouped within the portion of resected liver.

Contraindications. The operation is contraindicated in patients in a poor condition, with a tendency to cachexia, jaundice, edema and marked ascites, as well as in the clinical forms with a severe, febrile onset, or those simulating an abscess of the liver.

In a large number of patients, Chinese surgeons report a high mortality rate after simple explorative laparotomy in patients with liver carcinoma (over 29% of the cases). Similarly, alteration of the liver function was more accentuated in the patients that died than in the survivors. Hence they contraindicate surgery when several of the hepatic tests are even moderately altered (albumin/globulin ratio, bilirubin, serum transaminase and alkaline phosphatase).

Volume, extent and site of the tumor. The volume of the tumor is not a contraindication for resection when there are no metastases and when its location is favorable to hepatectomy. Wang Ch'eng-en, in a series of 21 patients in which resection was possible, observed that before the operation the tumor only appeared resectable in 6 cases. As regards the extent of the tumor process, we have already shown that palliative resections are not worth while. The operative hazards are very high and it appears useless to accept them in order to extirpate a tumoral formation only partly, when we know how often the results are fatal even when the tumor has been resected in its totality. The deeper the tumor is located towards the posterior border of the liver or the hili (portal hilus and posterior hilus of the hepatic veins), the more unfavorable the conditions for resection. When the tumor has developed close to the hili, or has invaded them, resection is contraindicated both because of the extreme risk of the operation and because dissection will not be possible up to the limits of oncologic safety. In such conditions, the large vessels of the liver ought to be sacrificed, which is not possible and only reduces the operation to a palliative intervention with terribly high risks.

Finally, the contraindication may be implied by the surgeon's lack of experience in hepatobiliary surgery or an inadequate equipment.

Preoperative preparation. In the preoperative period, the functions of the different organs and especially of the liver should be determined. An attempt should be made to correct certain deficiencies in order to avoid per- and post-operative complications. A diet rich in carbohydrates, proteins and vitamins is recommended. Three to four days before the operation, wide-spectrum antibiotics are administered, to lower the resorption of intestinal toxins and let the liver relax to a certain extent. In view of the rapid evolution of carcinoma, the preoperative treatment should be as short as possible.

Anesthesia. Endotracheal anesthesia with ether or fluothane is indicated. Hypothermia has also been envisaged. Intraabdominal hypothermia with cold normal saline, applied by the Chinese surgeons, allowed them to prolong clamping of the hepatic pedicle beyond the usual limits.

Operation. Longitudinal, transverse or oblique laparotomy is carried out, according to the size and site of the tumor. The incision may be enlarged, the new incision branching off over the abdomen or thorax. The risks are greater in broad hepatectomies when the abdominal approach alone is used.

Choice of the type of operation. After determining the lesions, it will be established whether the tumor is resectable from the technical and prognostic points of view, then the type of hepatectomy which involves the lesser risks and offers the highest possibilities of a radical intervention will be chosen. Wedge-shaped hepatectomy is indicated in small tumors on the anterior aspect of the liver; for large tumors left lobectomy, left hepatectomy, simple right or broad right hepatectomy will be performed according to the site and extent of the tumor. The techniques are described in detail in the chapter on resections of the liver. It should be decided how much of the hepatic parenchyma is to be left *in situ* to ensure a satisfactory function, compatible with life. Analysis of a large series of cases with advanced cirrhosis, generally associated with carcinoma, shows that less than half the liver parenchyma must be resected. Broader hepatectomies can be envisaged when the patient's condition is satisfactory and the liver function tests are good.

Results. The number of patients operated for primary carcinoma of the liver is relatively low in comparison to operations for other diseases of this organ, but has increased very much during the last few years. In 1956, K. Stucke found 94 cases published in the literature. 13 patients survived for less than 3 years and only 3 for 5 years. Somewhat later, Lichtman (cited by Plauchu in 1960) found 223 cases with a survival of 1—5 years.

In a statistics of 330 cases, in 10 Chinese clinics, published by Wang Ch'eng-en in 1963, resection was performed in 130 cases, i.e. 6.2% before 1957. There were 100 controlled and 30 non-anatomic hepatectomies. No relapses were found after 1 year in 6 patients, after 2 years in 2 cases, after 3—4 years in 3 cases, after 5 years in 1 case. Relapses occurred after 1—6 months in 9 cases, after 1 year in 3 cases, and in 1 case after 2 years and 1 case after 5 years; 33 patients died within the first 6 months, 7 after 1 year and 2 after 2 years.

Operative mortality has increased of late as resections are now attempted that were considered impossible before. After non-anatomic hepatectomies for carcinoma, the mortality rate is approximately 15% and after anatomic resections about 30%, due to the larger proportion of the resection and not to its nature. The highest proportion of deaths is reported after right hepatectomies: about 50%.

In general, the immediate and late results of surgery in liver carcinoma are considered very poor. Bearing in mind the short survival of unoperated patients, the operation is worth attempting in all incipient cases incidentally discovered in the course of an operation and even in more advanced cases when certain favorable conditions prevail: the patient is in good condition, the tumor is compatible with resection, the surgeon is skilled in hepatobiliary operations.

PRIMARY SARCOMA AND MALIGNANT HEMANGIOENDOTHELIOMA

Primary sarcoma of the liver (Figs 184 and 185), with its different histologic variants — sarcoma with round or giant cells, fibrosarcoma, hemangiosarcoma, melanosarcoma — is seldom encountered in the clinic. G. Willeford and V.A. Stembridge gathered almost 100 cases from the literature reviewed up to 1950, mostly discovered at necropsy. *Malignant hemangioendothelioma* (malignant hemangioma or hemangioblastoma) closely resembles sarcoma as regards the scarcity of the cases.

The diagnosis of these tumors is as difficult as that of carcinoma. Malignant hemangioma has a more rapid clinical course, it develops as a multiple cavernous tumor that readily ruptures, producing severe intraperitoneal hemorrhage. Clinically, this tumor is sometimes diagnosed with a certain probability when a fremitus can be perceived over the liver.

The following case is that of a child operated for hemangiosarcoma, a mixed tumor of connective and vascular origin.

B.I., aged 4 and half months was admitted to the Surgical Department of the State Hospital no. 12 on January 10, 1963 for an epigastric tumor observed two weeks previously. The child developed normally. The epigastric tumor was the size of an orange (about 8 cm in diameter), hard and sharply delimited. The X-ray examination revealed a tumor with a regular contour, developing ventrally rather than dorsally. The tumor pushed the diaphragm upwards and the stomach and transverse colon downwards. Apart from an increased erythrocyte sedimentation rate, the other laboratory tests showed nothing significant (hemogram, urine, serum transaminase, plasma protein electrophoresis). Explorative laparotomy under ether anesthesia revealed a well delineated tumor on the anterior aspect of the left lobe of the liver. The tumor was extirpated by controlled left hepatectomy, since left lobectomy would not have warranted

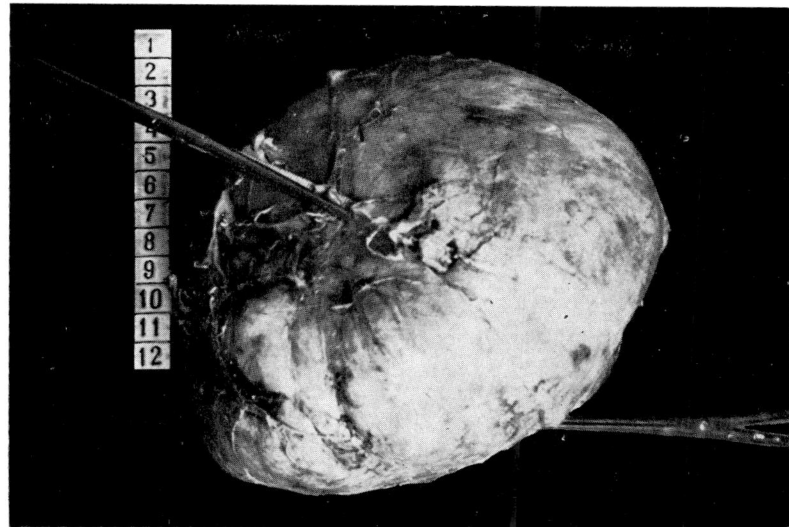

Fig. 184. — Voluminous hepatic tumor (primary sarcoma); operative specimen after right hepatectomy. Diaphragmatic aspect of the right lobe with swellings produced by the underlying tumor. The specimen weighed 1250 gm. The patient survived 2 years and 1 month after the operation.

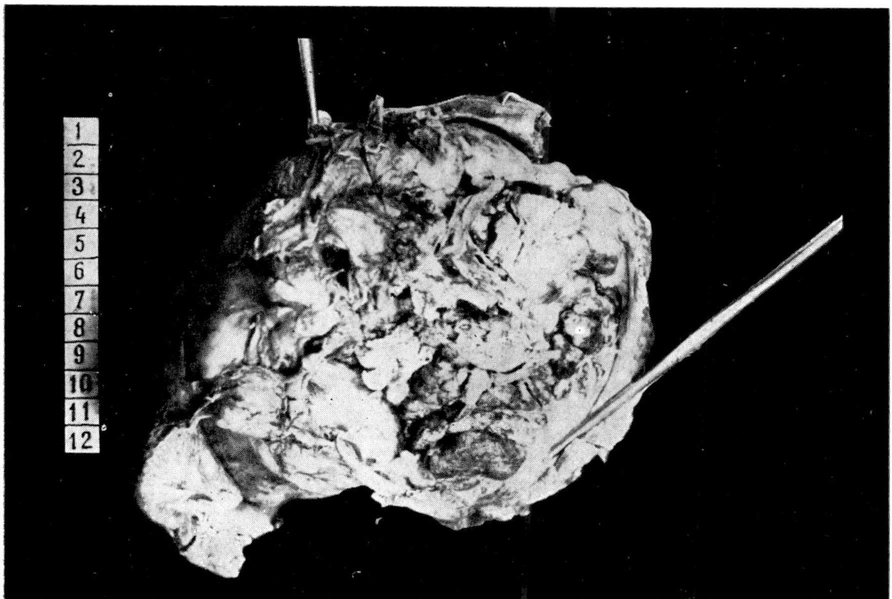

Fig. 185. — The same tumor as in Fig. 184 seen from another angle.

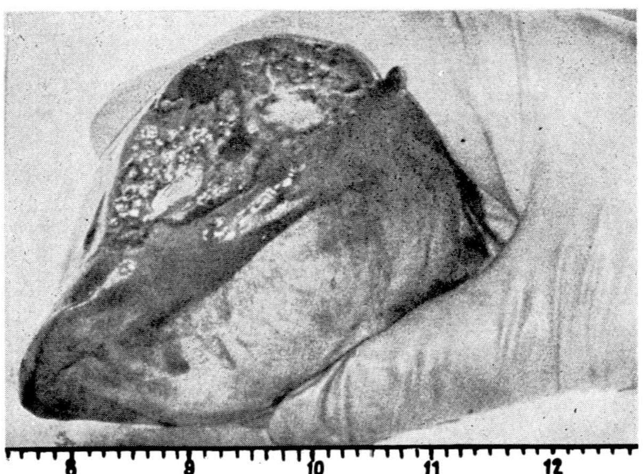

Fig. 186. — Left hepatectomy for hemangiosarcoma (child *B.I.*)

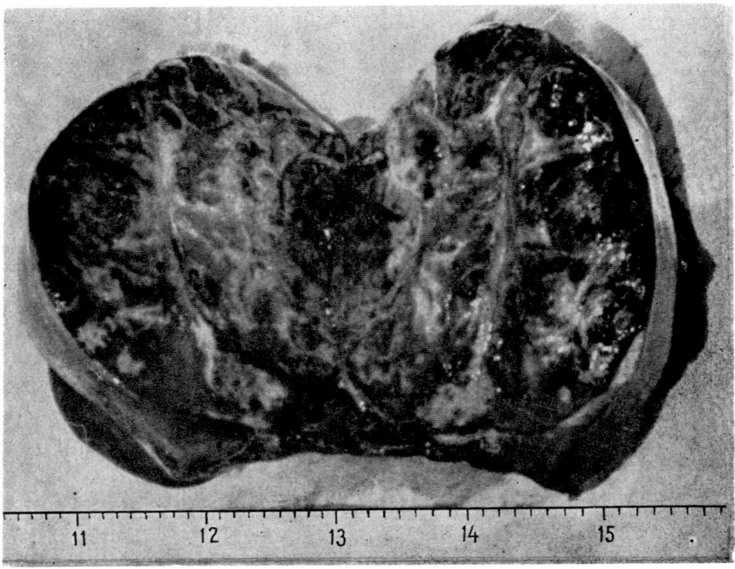

Fig. 187. — The same tumor, sectioned.

a radical operation. There were no complications. The tumor emptied of blood weighed 210 gm (Figs 186 and 187), and was enveloped by a thin capsule formed of nodules the size of a cherry, separated by fibrous septa starting from the capsule. The tumor tissue formed of round cells was invaded by numerous dilated blood vessels. One year and 3 months after the operation, the child had developed well and showed no signs of relapse.

B. SECONDARY MALIGNANT TUMORS

ETIOLOGY

Among the malignant tumors of the liver, secondary tumors represent about 96% of the cases, therefore are about 25 times more frequent than the primary tumors. In one of three patients with extrahepatic primary malignant tumors hepatic metastases will develop in the course of the disease. The proportion is still greater when the primary tumor is to be found in an organ supplied by the portal circulation: in almost 50% of the cases a secondary malignant tumor will develop in the liver. It is generally accepted that hepatic metastases are more frequent than the pulmonary ones, especially when the primary tumor belongs to the organs supplied by the portal circulation. H.E. Walther of Zurich is perhaps the only one who, on rich pathoanatomic material, found more pulmonary than hepatic metastases in primary carcinoma of the intraabdominal segments of the gastrointestinal tract.

In the clinic the proportion of metastases to the liver was lower than that found at the histologic examination. R.W. Raven, in a statistics on 818 cases of primary carcinoma of the stomach, colon and rectum, treated in the Marsden Hospital in London, found metastases in 21.5% of the cases. Kaufman (cited by K. Stucke) gives the following proportion of hepatic metastases: in carcinoma of the pancreas 50.5%, of the gallbladder 39.5%, of the stomach 33%, intestines 33%, breast 32%, esophagus 23.5%, thyroid 18%, uterus 12%. According to Kettler, 24.6% of the hepatic metastases derive from bronchopulmonary carcinomas.

PATHOGENY

Propagation to the liver of extrahepatic malignant tumors does not always take place by metastatic route proper, but often also by direct invasion of the surrounding organs. Tumors of the pancreas, kidneys, adrenals and especially of the stomach may invade the liver by contiguity, and tumors of the gallbladder may come in contact directly with the liver by continuity without interposition of the peritoneum. Other means of direct non-metastatic invasion also exist, by extension of the tumoral process along the afferent and efferent blood vessels of the liver and by retrograde lymphatic route towards the neighboring organs.

Embolic metastases are far more frequent than the secondary tumors produced by direct invasion. Isolated neoplastic cells, or groups of cells, detach themselves from the primary tumor, penetrate into the blood vessels and reach the liver by the vena porta or hepatic artery. The high incidence of metastases to the liver is brought about by two main factors:

1. The liver behaves as a filter that retains the neoplastic material brought by the vena porta. However, in primary malignant tumors in the portal area pulmonary metastases may be produced directly, without hepatic seeding, which shows that the neoplastic cells have not been retained by the hepatic filter or that they have reached the lung without passing through the liver, i.e. through the anastomoses between the portacaval system.

2. In comparison to other organs supplied by the branches of the aorta, metastases to the liver produced by arterial route are very frequent because of the favorable medium offered by the liver to the development of tumors, its extremely active metabolism and rich circulation.

PATHOLOGIC ANATOMY

Under the favorable conditions found in the liver, metastases grow rapidly and in their turn metastasize by portal and lymphatic route, invading the whole liver with tumor nodules. The liver, full of nodules, may sometimes increase very much in size. Sheila Sherlock cites a case reported by Weber, in which the liver weighed 21.5 kg.

Metastatic nodules, more consistent than the hepatic parenchyma, are as a rule the size of a walnut or cherry. In some cases miliary dissemination takes place throughout the whole organ or only within part of it. The color of the nodules is whitish-yellow or whitish-grey. At the gross examination, they appear as small swellings on the surface of the liver, each with a depression in the center giving it an umbilicated aspect. This feature is caused by necrosis of the central zone of the nodules.

In contrast to primary carcinoma, which is associated in most cases to cirrhosis, metastatic tumors are seldom encountered in cirrhotics, as noted by E.A. Gall, F. Pergola, etc. One of the causes of this pseudoimmunity is the development of portacaval shunts consecutive to intrahepatic block. The neoplastic cells in the portal territory penetrate more readily into the caval circulation than into the liver.

Microscopically, the metastatic tumor generally resembles the primary tumor from which it arose; however, an anaplastic process sometimes takes place, giving it a particular histologic structural aspect.

CLINICAL STUDY

The symptomatology is determined both by the primary and the secondary tumor process, or only by one of these components. In general, however, a state of accentuated fatigue, loss of body weight and a sensation of distension in the region of the liver are added to the clinical picture of the primary disease. The liver is enlarged and when the abdominal wall of the patient is very thin and atonic, one can sometimes palpate hard and eventually umbilicated nodules over the surface of the liver exceeding the chondrocostal margin.

In the course of the disease the clinical picture is aggravated by complications due especially to spread of the tumor process. Edema of the lower limbs may develop due to blocking of the inferior cava vein. Jaundice, which at first is absent or mild, rapidly becomes more accentuated, caused by invasion of the hepatic ducts. Ascites appears as a consequence of spread of the tumoral process to the peritoneum. Invasion of the branches of the hepatic veins and penetration into their lumina of the tumor process produces pulmonary microembolism with fragments of neoplastic tissue and pulmonary metastases. In some cases, intraperitoneal hemorrhage may occur spontaneously or following a slight abdominal injury, producing rupture of a tumor nodule on the surface of the liver. Cholangitis may be caused by obstruction of the hepatic ducts.

As a rule, death supervenes from hepatic or hepatorenal insufficiency. The liver functions remain satisfactory for a long time even when the tumoral process is very advanced. When the liver functions are severely involved, not even 20 per cent of the liver tissue has remained intact.

LABORATORY TESTS

Hemogram points to slight anemia and increased leukocytosis up to 30,000—50,000, with accentuated neutrophilia.

Liver functional tests: Bilirubinemia is normal or slightly increased (when both hepatic ducts are obstructed, bilirubin is excreted through the ducts that are still free); increased alkaline phosphatases, increased alpha or gamma globulins; increased BSP retention.

Biopsy puncture of the liver is only positive in half the cases, that is in the very advanced cases. In the incipient cases with a single tumor or a few nodules, the chance of extracting fragments of tumor tissue is very reduced even after repeated punctures.

Laparoscopy (peritoneoscopy) and laparophotography are methods of investigation whose utility has been challenged by many authors. Laparoscopy is considered by some surgeons as fairly accurate and less traumatizing than explorative laparotomy. When multiple metastases of a primary carcinoma are discovered at laparoscopy, the patient is saved from a useless laparotomy.

The laparoscopic diagnosis of liver metastases is more readily established than that of primary carcinoma. The metastatic origin of a hepatic tumor, when the existence of the primary tumor is unknown or uncertain, is based, as a rule, upon the absence of cirrhotic lesions and the umbilicated aspect of the tumors. However, not all nodular tumors are umbilicated and not all metastases take on a nodular shape; some are flat, others miliary, pseudocystic or infiltrative. In such cases a hepatic puncture should be performed under laparoscopic control.

Radiologic examinations have the same value in liver metastases as in primary carcinoma.

Investigations with radioactive substances. In 1953, L.A. Stirrett et al. described a new method for the detection and location of liver metastases with the aid of human serum albumin iodate with ^{131}I which is a radioactive isotope of this halogen. The radioactive albumin is injected by intravenous route and the liver scintigram recorded after 24 hours. According to these authors, the metabolic activity of metastases being at least 30% higher than that of the normal liver tissue as regards serum albumin, the tracer is prevalently taken up by the metastases. According to S. Sherlock, the increased capacity of metastases to take up ^{131}I albumin is due to the increased patency of the tumor capillaries for albumin. In contrast to the scintigrams obtained with rose bengal ^{131}I or ^{198}Au when liver metastases appear in the form of uptake defects, on the scintigram with ^{131}I-albumin these tumors correspond to aspects of increased irradiation.

In a group of 240 patients with different malignant tumors, studied by Stirrett et al., 53 had metastases of the liver verified at laparotomy. In 49 cases, the metastatic tumors were discovered by preoperative scintigrams. Therefore, there were only 4 falsely negative results (besides 6 falsely positive results, not confirmed at surgery). If we bear in mind that at the clinical examination only 11 of these series exhibited signs of metastases, the scintigraphic method appears to be particularly useful. Subsequent investigations confirmed the use of this method in the detection of liver metastases.

DIAGNOSIS

In the advanced stages of liver metastasis, the clinical diagnosis is as a rule easy to establish: a patient with a known primary malignant tumor, treated or not surgically, undergoes at a given moment evident aggravation of his general condition, accompanied by hepatomegaly, subclinical icterus or even accentuated jaundice.

When the abdominal wall is thin and of low tonicity, tumor nodules that are sometimes umbilicated can be palpated on the surface of the liver. The appearance of ascites and pulmonary metastases remove any doubts concerning the diagnosis.

Attentive follow-up of the clinical course of patients operated for malignant tumors may detect the onset of hepatic metastases in less advanced stages when the clinical signs are still discrete. In most cases, this clinical finding is superfluous since once the diagnosis is confirmed, the surgical treatment can no longer give results. An early diagnosis may be made in the following three events, very rarely encountered in practice:

1. At the preoperative control of the liver which is obligatory in the course of any resection of a primary malignant tumor of an intraabdominal organ, a single hepatic metastasis can be discovered which may be extirpated both from the technical and the prognostic point of view.

2. Solitary metastatic tumors of the liver can be discovered in the course of control surgical interventions (second-look), in patients in which the primary tumor was extirpated.

3. In these patients, repeated scintigrams after the operation appear to guarantee that evidence will be found of metastases, in a sufficiently early stage to be operated. However, it is known that only tumors larger than 2 cm in diameter can be detected by the scintigraphic method, at least until now.

TREATMENT

The prevention of metastases. 1. Radical extirpation of primary malignant tumors in an early stage.

2. The use of mild operative maneuvers in the course of this extirpation. Any strong pressure exercised upon the tumors may detach isolated neoplastic cells or

groups of cells from the tumor which will be carried to the liver or another organ by the blood flow. In order to prevent these intraoperative seedings, it is recommended to ligate the vascular pedicle of the tumor and to clamp the lumen of the segment involved close to the tumor.

Curative treatment. The indications, contraindications and technique of extirpation of liver metastases are very similar to those described in the treatment of primary malignant tumors. Solitary metastases alone are extirpated and only under conditions when radical resection is possible. A solitary metastasis will not be resected when radical extirpation of the primary tumor was not possible. In multiple metastases, even when grouped within a limited area, hepatectomy is contraindicated according to most authors.

To-date, few hepatectomies have been performed for hepatic metastases. Until 1956, K. Stucke found in the literature 136 hepatectomies for metastasis with an average survival of 5 years in almost 6 per cent of the cases. Complete statistics have not been published since then. Although the average survival is low, it confirms the hypothesis of Wangensteen on the possibility of single neoplastic emboli transported from the organs of the portal territory to the liver. In this case, hepatectomy appears to be justified when the patients are carefully selected.

Malignant tumors of the liver produced by direct spread from the surrounding organs may sometimes be extirpated *en bloc* with the primary tumor when the latter is located in the stomach or gallbladder. Wedge-shaped hepatocholecystectomy, a radical operation used in malignant tumors of the gallbladder, may be applied when involvement of the liver is still in an incipient stage. The late results obtained by us and other authors in such cases, were very poor. In 2 cases we obtained a survival of 7 and 6 years which shows that this operation can be consistently performed when the hepatic pedicle is not invaded.

Malignant gastroesophageal tumors sometimes spread directly to the left lobe of the liver which they partly invade. Extirpation of such tumors is very difficult and presents great hazard. In three cases in which esophagogastrohepatectomy was performed, there were three deaths. Death was not caused by hepatectomy but by the amplitude of the operation in general demanded by extension of the lesions. In a single case in which the left lobe presented a small metastasis easily removed by limited non-anatomic hepatectomy, esogastrectomy was followed by a survival of more than two years.

REFERENCES

1. Batzenschlager A., Réville P., Weill-Bousson M., Bull. Ass. franç. Cancer, 1961, **48**, *3*, 347.
2. Berman C., South Afr. med. J., 1955, **29**, *51*, 1195.
3. Bockus H. L., *Gastroenterology*, W. B. Saunders, Philadelphia, 1953.
4. Brunschwig A., Bull. Congr. Soc. int. Chir., 1957, 1123.
5. Bungeler W., Eder M., Dtsch. med. Wschr., 1960, **85**, *22*, 959.
6. Burghele T., Proca E., Chirurgia, 1958, *6*, 909.
7. Cachéra R., *Maladies du foie*, Flammarion, Paris, 1953.
8. Caroli J., Jammet H., Renault H., Sem. Hôp., 1958, **34**, *14*, 442.
9. Coleman J. A., Haines R. H., Philips C., Gastroenterology, 1954, **27**, *2*, 166.
10. Couinaud C., Presse méd., **63**, *21*, 417.
11. Couinaud C., J. Chir., 1954, **70**, *12*, 933.

12. * * * J. Amer. med. Ass., 1954, **154**, *9*, 767.
13. Evans J. A., Mujahed Z., J. Amer. med. Ass., 1959, **171**, *11*, 7.
14. Făgărășanu I., Aloman D., *Notre expérience concernant le cancer de la vésicule biliaire*, in *XVIIe Congr. Soc. Intern. Chir.*, Mexico City, 1957.
15. Făgărășanu I., Popescu C., Aloman D., Probl. Ter., 1958, **9**, *1*, 8.
16. Făgărășanu I., Aloman D., Chirurgia, 1960, **9**, *4*, 495.
17. Făgărășanu I., Aloman D., *Diagnosticul precoce al tumorilor maligne de ficat, căi biliare și pancreas*, Communicated at the Oncology Department, Bucharest, December, 1962.
18. Gall A. E., A.M.A. Arch. Pathol., 1960, **70**, *2*, 226.
19. Hepp J. et al., Acta chir. belg., 1961, **60**, *5*, 493.
20. Köhn K., *Das primäre Leberkrebs*, Springer, Berlin, 1955.
21. Lagrot F., Afr. franç. Chir., 1959, **17**, *3*, 153.
22. Lin Chao-Chi et al., Chin. med. J., 1962, **81**, *5*, 303.
23. * * * Lancet, 1956, **271**, *6946*, 782.
24. Macchioro G., Minerva med., 1962, **53**, *50*, 1960.
25. Melnikov V. A., Anal. rom. sov. (Chir.), 1956, **10**, *3 (11)*, 78.
26. Myasnikov A. L., *Bolezni pecheni i zhelchinych putei*, Medghiz, Moscow, 1961.
27. Ollino P. et al., Minerva med., 1958, **45**, *67—68*, 3199.
28. Otaki A., Read A. E., Stubbs J., Sculthorpe H., Brit. med. J., 1960, *5194*, 256.
29. Payet M., Camain R., Pene P., Rev. int. Hépatol., 1956, **6**, *1*, 1.
30. Pergola F., Ligneraux J., Cachin M., Sem. Hôp., 1961, **37**, *48—49*, 2433.
31. Plauchu M. et al., J. Méd. Lyon, 1960, **41**, *961*, 171.
32. Ponomareva E. D., Anal. rom. sov. (Med. gen.), 1956, *4*, 64.
33. Quattlebaum J. K., Surg. Clin. N. Amer., 1962, **42**, *2*, 507.
34. Reifferscheid M., *Chirurgie der Leber*, G. Thieme, Stuttgart, 1957.
35. Righi Riva G. C., Di Marco G., Manfredi G. C., Minerva med., 1961, **52**, *81*, 3482.
36. Roulet C. F. et al., *Cancer primitif du foie et des voies biliaires*, Masson, Paris, 1958.
37. Salzberg S., Georgescu I., Morf. norm. patol., 1957, *3*, 238.
38. Schumacher W., Dtsch. med. Wschr., 1962, **87**, *7*, 347.
39. Sherlock Sheila, *Diseases of the liver and biliary system*, Blackwell, Oxford, 1955.
40. Singh A., Jolly S. S., Singh S., A.M.A. Arch. int. Med., 1960, **105**, *3*, 424.
41. Stucke K., *Leberchirurgie*, Springer, Berlin, 1959.
42. Wang Ch'eng-en, Li Kuo-ts'ai, Chin. med. J., 1963, **82**, *2*, 65.
43. Ton That Tung, *Chirurgie d'exérèse du foie*, Ed. Langues Etrangères, Hanoi, 1962.

CHAPTER 10

RESECTIONS OF THE LIVER

During the last ten to fifteen years, marked progress has been made in surgery of the liver, due especially to the perfecting of anesthesia and resuscitation, to which were added a better knowledge of the anatomy and pathologic physiology of the liver and the pre- and peroperative use of portal phlebography and cholangiography. It is now possible to carry out broad resections of the liver, such as right hepatectomies, which were considered impossible some 20 years ago. Lesions considered inoperable can now be extirpated under satisfactory technical conditions. The clinical experience of the surgeons and anesthesiologists, under whose care the patient is, ensures the success of the operation, reducing operative hazard to a minimum. Anatomic or controlled hepatectomies, with separate ligation of the biliovascular pedicles of the resected portion, broaden the therapeutic possibilities of hepatic surgery. Non-anatomic resections maintain their value as a method of treatment affecting the more accessible parts of the liver.

THE HISTORY OF HEPATECTOMY

There are three periods in the history of hepatectomy:

— *the first period*, which lasted to about 1880, is characterized by experimental investigations, and a few emergency resections in the clinic when part of the hepatic parenchyma protruded through an abdominal wound. The first one to attempt resection of hepatic lobes in dogs appears to be Giuseppe Zambeccari, who showed in 1680, together with Ciaparglini, Neri and Bonucci that most of the experimental animals fully recovered about 15 days after operation. In 1716, Giovanni Berta resected a portion of the hepatic parenchyma that herniated through an abdominal wound. Berta was probably acquainted with the work of Cornelius Celsus "On Medicine", dating back to the first century A.D., which describes this operation.

— In *the second period*, experimental investigations became more numerous and clinical resections of the liver were performed for various chronic diseases. Priority for resection of the liver is attributed to Ohlshausen (1882), to Lins who extirpated a solid tumor in 1886 and to Loreta who performed a resection for hydatid cyst in the same year. In this period which lasted to 1940—1950, non-anatomic resections were performed, i.e. resections of the liver along a line that closely followed the contour of the tumor to be extirpated.

The technique of hepatectomy gradually progressed and the cases published increased in frequency, starting with 25 cases found in the literature by I. R. Penski and M. M. Kuznetzov in 1894 and ending with more than 1000 cases in 1955 (collected by A. Brunschwig).

Marked progress in the technique of non-anatomic hepatectomy was made in 1896 when Penski and Kuznetzov published their principles of hepatic hemostasis, whose value is still recognized. U-sutures are passed through the full thickness of the hepatic parenchyma and on tightening them the small vessels coursing through the liver are ruptured and the larger blood vessels and bile ducts are gathered together and bound closely. Use of a blunt needle, which pushes aside the hepatic vessels, likewise proved to be a technical improvement.

— In *the third period*, anatomic hepatectomies were currently instituted. In 1912, Wendel performed a right controlled hepatectomy with direct ligation, in the hilus, of the right branch of the portal vein and hepatic duct, removing a voluminous adenoma, weighing 940 gm. A year later, the patient remained in good health.

In 1939, Mayer-May and Ton That Tung performed a controlled left hepatectomy for a hepatic tumor; in 1940 V. Pettinari and 1949 R. W. Raven extirpated the whole left lobe of the liver. The number of hepatectomies increased and in 1952 J. L. Lortat-Jacob carried out the first broad, controlled right hepatectomy and in 1953 J. Sénèque published the first true left hepatectomy. The various considerations in regard to hepatic resection were discussed in detail at the XVIth Congress of the International Society of Surgery, held in Copenhagen in 1955.

In Romania, too, hepatectomy drew the attention of our surgeons, the promotors being I. Bălăcescu and Amza Jianu, whose contributions to the technique of hepatic hemostasis are well known. The first left hepatectomy was performed by one of us (Făgărăşanu, 1956). Th. Burghele and others carried out the first anatomic right hepatectomy in 1958.

The progress made in hepatic exeresis has been attributed to a more detailed understanding of the anatomy and pathologic physiology of the liver, but actually these were already well known at the end of the 19th century. If after some sixty years of non-anatomic resections the surgeons began to approach the liver at a level considered the most dangerous, i.e. the hilus, in order to ligate separately the pedicles of the portion of the liver to be resected, it is due to the advance of surgery and of medicine in general. J. L. Lortat-Jacob showed that the success of his first extended right hepatectomy was due to his experience in thoracophrenolaparotomy for portal decompression.

THE ANATOMIC BASES OF HEPATECTOMY *

The concept of Claudius Galenus on the anatomy and physiology of the liver was prevalent up to the end of the 16th century. Based upon speculation rather than anatomic study and experiments, Galenus believed that the liver was the center of hematopoiesis and distribution of the blood in the organism, the site of origin of the veins and the source of animal heat. The anatomic studies of Vesalius in the 16th century led later on to the discovery of the laws of blood circulation (Harvey, 1628).

The first scientific demonstration of the hepatic circulation was given by F. Glisson in the 17th century, who perfused the liver with a mixture of water and milk introduced from an ox bladder connected with the portal vein. The mixture passed through the liver to the portal vein and then to right atrium. As the liver gradually changed its color, Glisson concluded that the fluid did not only pass through the large vessels but also through the capillaries.

The liver was studied with the microscope by Malpighi in 1685, who considered it had a glandular role. Ferrein, in 1749, concentrated especially on the arterial circulation in the liver. F. Kiernan (1833) gave a detailed description of the intrahepatic distribution of the biliovascular branches.

---

* See Chapter 1.

The segmentary architecture of the liver, based upon the distribution of the intrahepatic biliovascular branches, was fundamentally studied by Hugo Rex in 1888, by Mall in 1906, by A. Melnikov in 1923—24 and by others. Inner segmentation of the liver was taken up again in 1948 and 1951 by C.H. Hjortsjö who compared stereoscopic cholangiographies with corrosion preparations of the bile ducts injected with colored plastic material. Further investigations confirmed the data of Hjortsjö and completed certain details.

It is known that the branches of the afferent portal pedicle are distributed throughout the hepatic parenchyma in zones that are almost independent of one another from the viewpoint of circulation, separated by planes lacking voluminous portal ramifications, i.e., the fissures, through which the branches of the hepatic veins pass. Each unit or subunit of the segmentary system of the liver is supplied and drained by two vascular pedicles, the same as the whole liver. These pedicles cross one another without coming in direct contact. The afferent pedicles emerge radially from a common center, from the portal hilus of the liver, and the efferent fan-like pedicles converge towards the inferior vena cava, at a certain distance from the portal hilus. This anatomic arrangement, specific of the liver, renders anatomic resection of certain segment units or subunits far more difficult than in other organs in which the efferent vessels follow in a retrograde direction the same pathway as the afferent vessels. Another difficulty arises from the location of the hepatic veins in the fissures that separate two portal territorial units. In the course of an anatomic resection performed along the fissure plane, the branch of the hepatic vein can be easily damaged if measures of precaution are not taken. As the hepatic veins drain both the resected portion and the neighboring areas, its injury would suppress the route of venous return of the remaining tributary hepatic tissue, resulting in more or less extensive necrosis according to the importance of the damaged vein. Therefore, in the course of an anatomic hepatectomy, the afferent and efferent vessels that correspond as exactly as possible to the resected portion of the liver should be ligated.

Yet, the danger of ischemic gangrene and hepatic infarct, consecutive to disproportionate ligation not corresponding to the portion of resected liver, must not be exaggerated. The hepatic segments, not separated by connective tissue septa, are partly dependent from the vascular point of view. Small vascular branches may pass beyond the fissures towards the neighboring units. As they are usually small, bleeding can be controlled after opening the fissure by current hemostasis procedures. Moreover, the cleavage planes are crossed throughout the liver by sinusoid pseudocapillaries which, within certain limits, supplant the arterioportal supply or the venous drainage, interrupted by ligation of the vessels within the areas next to the resected portions.

The anatomy of the portal vein, of the intra- and extrahepatic bile ducts and especially of the hepatic artery exhibits an infinite number of variations and anomalies. The pattern of the hepatic veins appears to be more constant. Intraoperative recognition, at any rate of the variants of the main trunks and branches of the first order, is obligatory if grave mistakes are to be avoided. Ignorance of the variants of the smaller branches may, in the last instance, lead to a supplementary sacrifice of hepatic tissue.

As already mentioned in the chapter 1, the liver is a segmental organ with delimited vascular and biliary cleavage planes, which form the anatomic basis for liver resections — hepatectomies (right or left), lobectomies and segmentectomies. In surgical practice, controlled resections in their order of frequency are left lobectomy, resection of the third segment, left and right hepatectomy. Right, left or bilateral paramedial segmentectomy, right lateral segmentectomy, planned resection of segments 4,5 and 6 are seldom reported in medical literature.

Right hepatectomy corresponds to planned resection of the right hepatic region along the main lobar fissure, maintaining the integrity of the sagittal vein, affluent of the left hepatic vein. The following are ligated and sectioned: 1) The biliovascular pedicle of the right liver containing the right hepatic artery, the right branch of the vena porta and right hepatic duct; 2) the right hepatic vein at its drainage site into the inferior cava, and 3) the right branches of the sagittal vein (Fig. 188).

Left hepatectomy or planned resection of the left liver necessitates ligation of the left branches of the afferent pedicle, left hepatic vein and left branches of the sagittal vein (Fig. 189).

Extended hepatectomy implies resection of a hepatic region together with the paramedial segment of the neighboring area.

Left lobectomy corresponds to resection of the classical left lobe, to the left of the left segmental fissure. It is also a segmentectomy, because the left lobe includes, according to most authors, all the lateral segment of the left hepatic region. Only C. Couinaud considers the lateral segment as a limited portion left of the segmental fissure that separates segment II from segment III, the classical left lobe corresponding to the left division according to the architecture of the liver based upon the distribution of the hepatic veins. Practically, in left lobectomy, the following must be ligated and resected:

— The branch or branches of the *recessus umbilicalis* that supply segment III together with the arterial and biliary ramifications;

— the left lateral vein (with the accompanying artery and bile duct);

— the left hepatic vein before it joins the sagittal vein (Fig. 190).

Planned resection of segment III necessitates ligation of the branch or branches from the left horn of the umbilical recess together with the arterial and biliary branches that accompany them and the hepatic vein of segment III, a branch of the left hepatic vein.

Planned resection of segments IV, V and VI is theoretically possible. Practically, it is difficult to ligate the pedicles of these segments according to the principles of planned resections because they are deeply buried within the liver parenchyma. Therefore, segmentectomy along an approximate cleavage plane is actually a non-anatomic hepatectomy. It is both useless and dangerous to look for the afferent vascular pedicles of these segments at their emergence from the large trunks.

The dorsal segments I, II, VI and VIII are not accessible to anatomic or non-anatomic resections because they are too deeply located. Moreover, any section along the cleavage planes that limit these segments will encounter the hepatic veins whose ligation would jeopardize venous drainage of the surrounding segments (right hepatic vein in case of segments VII and VIII and left hepatic vein in resections of segments I and II).

THE PHYSIOLOGIC BASES OF HEPATECTOMY

A detailed knowledge of the anatomy of the liver was necessary for perfecting the technique of hepatic resections but a close understanding of the pathophysiologic changes after resection was also obligatory. Numerous investigators tried

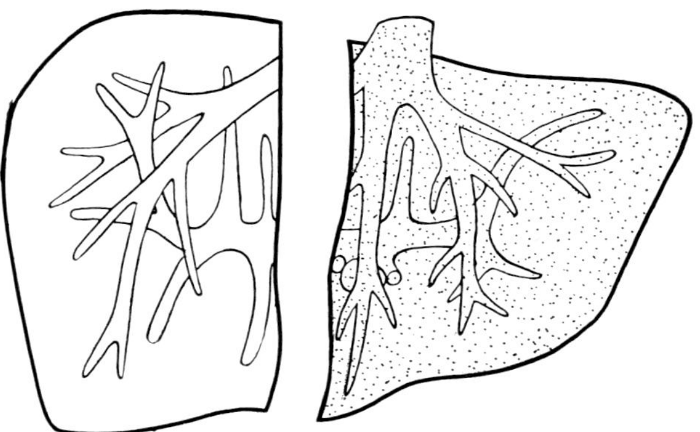

Fig. 188. — Right hepatectomy. The transection plane passes a little to the right of the main fissure, intercepting the right branch of the portal vein and the other components of the right Glisson pedicle, the right hepatic vein and the right branches of the sagittal vein.

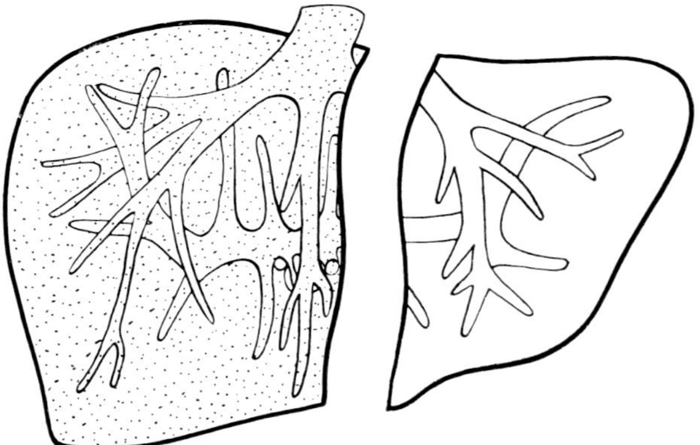

Fig. 189. — Left hepatectomy. Transection of the left Glisson pedicle, left hepatic vein and left branches of the sagittal vein. The section plane through the parenchyma passes a little to the left of the main fissure.

to elucidate the question of the tolerance of the organism to extended hepatic resections and determine the transformations that take place in the residual liver.

In 1890, Ponfick showed that resections including up to three fourths of the volume of the liver are compatible with survival of the experimental animals. These data were confirmed, in the course of the same year, by Podvysotzki, then by Meister, Glück and others. As it was clinically observed that hepatectomy within broader limits is well tolerated by the patients, it was admitted that tole-

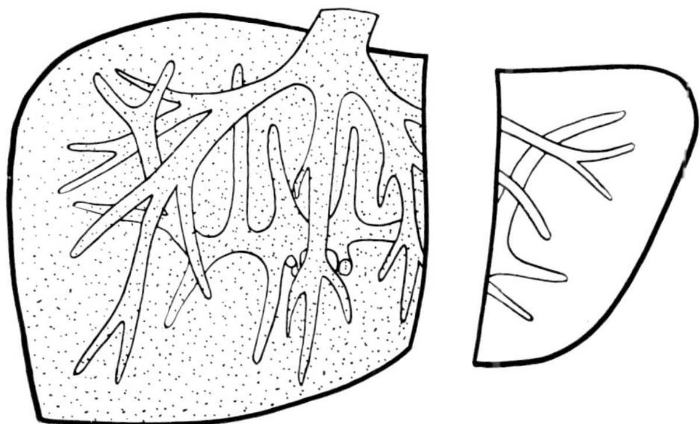

Fig. 190. — Left lobectomy.

rance in humans was comparable to that of the experimental animals, provided the residual portion of the liver has no lesions that might reduce its functional capacity. This was confirmed in 1952 by J.L. Lortat-Jacob who at his first extended right hepatectomy left only a residual portion of the liver the size of a fist. In the clinic, the exact ratio of the resected to the residual liver cannot be established, because the extirpated part generally contains a tumor mass that modifies the volume-weight relationships.

HEPATIC REGENERATION

The changes that take place in the residual liver represent one of the most interesting biologic phenomena. After partial hepatectomy, the liver rapidly regenerates, reaching the weight of the normal liver after 4 to 6 weeks. After repeated experimental resections in the same animal, the liver does not exhaust its regeneration capacity. If the animal survives, regeneration is more rapid and complete the more extended the resection and the more deeply injured the resected part. The fact that the whole amount of arterioportal blood passes through the residual liver accounts for the regeneration phenomenon. Some cases of jaundice with a benign evolution that appears after extended hepatectomy might be caused by the compression exercised by the blood-charged vessels upon the intrahepatic bile ducts.

The "regenerated" liver gains weight but not its initial form. If in the dog four of the seven lobes of the liver are resected, the remaining three lobes will be enlarged, but the resected lobes are not regenerated. Therefore, it actually is a compensatory hyperplasia and hypertrophy and not a regeneration. The next day after surgery, the liver cells divide, and mitosis is accelerated in the following days, then decreases and ceases completely after 4 to 6 weeks. At first the liver gains about 50 gm per day.

Apart from the volume of the resected portion, there are also other factors known to stimulate hepatic regeneration such as:

— *Humoral factors of regeneration* have been made evident in hepatectomized animals. In experiments with cross-circulation, a compensatory hypertrophy has been observed in the non-hepatectomized animal (G.T. Pack and A.H. Islami). Carnot noted that the normal liver becomes hypertrophic when the animal receives the serum of a hepatectomized animal.

— The hypothesis according to which the *venous portal output* in the residual liver is a factor stimulating regeneration, has been confirmed. Arterialization of the portal blood hastens regeneration, and an Eck fistula slows it down (G.T. Pack and A.H. Islami).

— The *postoperative diet* with a high caloric and protein value likewise hastens regeneration. More than after any other operation, hepatectomy necessitates the taking up of complete alimentation as soon as possible.

Among the *pharmacodynamic agents* to which a stimulating action is attributed are vitamins B and K, testosterone propionate, substances of the cortisone group and wide spectrum antibiotics, especially tetracycline.

Few direct observations on hepatic regeneration have been possible in man. Reoperations have shown that the liver regains its weight but takes on a new, more spherical shape.

BIOCHEMICAL CHANGES AFTER HEPATECTOMY

Both the experimental and the clinical data show that after extended hepatectomy alterations in hepatic function occur, revealed by laboratory tests. Maximum alterations occur 24 to 48 hours after operation and return to normal is observed during the following 4—5 weeks. The tests show: decrease of total proteins and increase of globulins (Lanutti and Parentela; Lewis et al.); positive Takata-Ara; decrease of the prothrombin time; decrease of glycemia; increase in serum alkaline phosphatase concentrations, increase in bilirubinemia, cholesterolemia and transaminases. These changes are not specific for hepatectomy, since they are also found in other operations involving other organs. Zucker et al. (1957) drew attention to certain humoral changes that increase the hazard of hemorrhage after hepatectomy. According to their experimental data, after resection of the liver, fibrinolytic activity increases very much and that of thrombocytes, prothrombine and factors V and VII decreases. These changes become more accentuated with hypothermia.

THE INDICATIONS AND CONTRAINDICATIONS FOR HEPATECTOMY

In order to establish the indications and contraindications for resection of the liver, the operative hazard must be balanced against the advantages of surgery. This principle should be applied to any operation, but especially to one involving such a high risk as hepatectomy. Wishing to apply the most up-to-date clinical techniques, the surgeon may be tempted to resect a whole hepatic lobe in order to extirpate a benign tumor, for instance, which could have been removed by another type of resection. In this way, a technically difficult operation could have been avoided, obtaining a better result without sacrificing a disproportionately large amount of hepatic tissue.

The patient, the disease, the surgeon who operates and the type of resection are the four elements that must be taken into account on appraising the operative risk in hepatectomy.

1. *The patient's general condition.* Advanced age, unsatisfactory general condition because of the liver disease or other coexisting disease, are factors that increase operative hazard. Severe hepatic, respiratory, circulatory or renal insufficiency are categorical contraindications as long as there is no favorable response to the preparatory treatment.

2. Another factor is the extent and site of *hepatic damage*, and its cause. Hepatectomy is more risky, the more extensive the lesion, the more malignant or the closer it is to the efferent and afferent hilus. On establishing the indications and contraindications for hepatectomy, account should also be taken of the intraoperative histologic examination, cholangiography, etc.

3. The *surgeon* should be acquainted with hepatobiliary operations, from the first stage of a simple operation on the liver to the most complex, because otherwise the operative hazard is considerably heightened.

4. The *type of resection*, imposed by the lesion likewise plays an important role in appraisal of the operative hazard. According to the increasing danger of technical difficulties that characterize them, hepatectomies may be classed as follows: minimal biopsy resection, marginal resection, wedge-shaped resection and elliptical resection, planned resection of segement III, planned left lobectomy, left hepatectomy and right hepatectomy. From this sequence, it might be inferred that planned hepatectomies are more difficult and risky than non-anatomic resections, although theoretically prior ligation of the vascular pedicles ought to diminish the operative risk. Actually, planned resections are more difficult because of the extension of exeresis. The same type of exeresis, for instance left lobectomy, practiced according to the rules of non-anatomic resections, is more risky.

Before starting a hepatic resection the surgeon should raise the following questions:

1. *Is the operation useful and are there sufficient guarantees that it will be radical?*

Resection of Riedel's abnormal lobe is useless as long as torsion has not occurred or the pedicle is not too long, threatening torsion.

Similarly, resection of a portion of the liver, when polycystic disease has extended to the whole liver, is useless.

Although technically possible, it is absolutely useless to extirpate a malignant hepatic tumor only partly, leaving tumor tissue *in situ*, or else to extirpate totally a malignant tumor in the presence of multiple metastases in other organs.

2. *Is the resection technically possible?* (bearing in mind the extent of the hepatic lesion). In order to appraise the technical possibilities, listing of the liver tissue affected will show whether its resection will leave the afferent and efferent circulation and biliary drainage intact. Technical possibilities should also be

appraised in terms of the extension of the lesion to the neighboring anatomic structures: vena cava, vena porta, etc.

3. *Which is the indicated type of resection?* A non-anatomic resection should always be given preference when the two foregoing conditions are met. However, if there are not sufficient guarantees that it will be radical, or if the non-anatomic resection would endanger the blood supply to the remaining liver, an anatomic hepatectomy must be performed.

Although indicated in many diseases of the liver, resections are seldom performed in hospital practice; indications are varied but not frequent. The small number of resections of the liver to date are due not only to technical difficulties, but also to the rarity of the cases in which they are indicated.

Congenital malformations. Resection of Riedel's *abnormal lobe* in case of torsion or long pedicle.

Congenital solitary cyst: anatomic or non-anatomic hepatectomy, according to the size of the tumor and degree of destruction of the hepatic tissue. As a rule, cystectomy alone is sufficient.

In *umbilical hernia of the embryonic type*, in the newborn, part of the liver protrudes into the hernial sac. When it cannot be reduced, a more or less extended hepatectomy is necessary.

In the *polycystic liver*, resection is indicated when the disease only affects a limited portion of the liver or when complications develop, such as infection or hemorrhage.

Injuries. Damage to the liver produced by thoraco-abdominal injuries and especially by fire arm wounds are of vital importance. In 1954, R.S. Sparkman and M.J. Fogelman published 100 cases with a mortality rate of 10% and complications in 44% of the cases.

Immediately after the accident, the operative indication may be imposed by massive external and internal hemorrhage. The operation consists in evacuation of the blood clots, resection of the crushed part of the liver, hemostasis, hepatorrhaphy, drainage.

During the following days, secondary hemorrhage, biliary fistulas, more or less extensive necrosis and hepatic abscesses may develop. Any of these complications may necessitate hepatectomy. An interesting case is that published by Thomeret, Dubost et al. who performed a reoperation in a case of laceration of the liver because of prolonged hemobilia and secondary anemia. The arteriobiliary fistula found necessitated right planned hepatectomy, after which the patient recovered.

Inflammatory lesions. *Hepatic syphiloma*, exceptionally rare, sometimes takes on a pseudotumoral aspect. Whenever technically possible, it was extirpated being confused with a malignant tumor.

Tuberculosis of the liver must be limited to part of the liver to be treated surgically. The surgical forms of hepatic tuberculosis are single tuberculoma and the tuberculous cavern which follows. V. Pettinari extirpated a voluminous tuberculoma that had the aspect of a necrotic tumor. Rauber et al. (Nancy) extirpated an enormous cavern fistulized into the bile ducts.

Amebic or bacterial abscesses of the liver are treated by medical means and surgical drainage. When the abscess destroys a large area, hepatectomy may be necessary, as performed by R.W.Raven in one case. Abscesses with calcified walls that do not collapse after drainage should also be taken into consideration. In some cases, hepatectomy may give satisfactory results.

In the *infected, calcified or fistulized hydatid cyst* operations of the conservative type such as cystectomy, suture of the bile fistula are often difficult and followed by untoward complications. Hepatectomy may likewise be very difficult because of the anatomic alterations produced by the cyst and the operations should be based on the general indications mentioned. In other cases, hepatectomy may be a comparatively easy operation; for instance when the hydatid cyst has destroyed the left lobe almost entirely, there is a small sacrifice of glandular tissue and hemostasis is readily performed.

Alveolar echinococcosis. If technically possible, hepatectomy is obligatory, except when the hilus or a large part of the parenchyma has been invaded. Since this disease usually ends fatally when radical treatment is not applied, some surgeons carried out extensive resections in apparently inoperable cases. In a patient in whom alveolar echinococcosis had invaded this hilus, Chalnot and Groscidier successfully performed a right planned hepatectomy, resection of the confluence of the hepatic ducts and Y anastomosis of the left hepatic duct with a jejunal loop. In Romania, the first non-anatomic hepatectomy for alveolar echinococcosis was performed by us in 1955. The 27-year old patient fully recovered and was discharged on the 8th day after the operation. In France, the first resection of this kind was done in 1956 by J. Hepp (according to C. Couinaud).

Benign tumors. Angioma is a well-tolerated tumor but constantly threatens the patient with a spontaneous or traumatic intraperitoneal hemorrhage. Hepatectomy is indicated in hemangioma when the tumor is sufficiently well delimited and when it responds favorably to roentgentherapy. Levrat and Michaud of Lyon successfully extirpated a hemangioma of the right hepatic region, weighing 15 kg. H. B. Shumaker found in the literature 66 cases of hepatic hemangioma, to which he added a case of his own. In 56 cases the tumor was resected. Five of the 11 cases in which the tumor could not be resected died of spontaneous or intraoperative hemorrhage. In 1955, E. W. Raven added another 14 cases. A year earlier we performed a non-anatomic hepatectomy for hemangioma of the left lobe in a 40-year old patient who was discharged 10 days after the operation, fully recovered.

Hepatic adenoma and its variants: benign hepatoma, benign cholangioma and benign hepatocholangioma are tumors that must be extirpated since it appears to be on the borderline between benignancy and malignancy. The resection should include healthy tissue, and may sometimes imply a left hepatectomy.

Malignant tumors. Primary carcinoma of the liver is far less widespread in Europe than in Africa and Asia and is seldom discovered in time for surgical treatment. Hepatectomy can only be performed when there is a single tumor without invasion of the hilus or regional lymph nodes or distal metastases. The residual liver should present no traces of tumor tissue or signs of advanced cirrhosis. In most cases, diffuse macronodular or micronodular dissemination of the carcinoma is noted throughout the whole mass of the liver against a background of advanced cirrhosis. Extended resection, i.e. right or left hepatectomy, may ensure radical extirpation of the tumor. In certain favorable circumstances, a small carcinoma located on the anterior margin of the liver can be extirpated by limited anatomic or non-anatomic resection.

Primary sarcoma, *teratoma* and *malignant hemangioendothelioma* occur still more seldom than primary carcinoma and the same surgical treatment is applied.

W. S. Lorimer found 3 cases of teratoma in the literature, extirpated surgically, with one operative death; in 1915, he published a case of his own, in which right hepatectomy was performed. In 1951, P. F. Fox and L. E. Cella successfully resected a malignant hemangioendothelioma in a 10-month-old child. We, too, extirpated a malignant hemangioendothelioma from a child aged 4 and a half months.

Metastatic malignant tumors. One or several metastases may sometimes be found in a single hepatic region, the remaining portion being free of disease. As far back as 1902, H. Sérégé introduced the hypothesis that metastases of the intra-abdominal gastrointestinal tract are not randomly distributed within the liver; for instance tumors of the right colon produce metastases in the right hepatic region, and those of the left colon in the left part of the liver. However, recent investigations with radioisotopes appear to invalidate this hypothesis. In rare cases, when the tumor can be radically extirpated and there is a single secondary tumor, hepatectomy is indicated when technically possible. Hypernephroma is a kind of cancer that gives the highest proportion of single hepatic metastases. Since in secondary carcinoma the macroscopic aspect of the tumor does not exclude a possible microscopic dissemination in the residual liver, the success of hepatectomy is problematic. Notwithstanding, cases of survival for 15—17 years have been reported (O. Wangensteen, A. Brunschwig).

When a hepatic nodule is found in the course of an operation for malignant tumor and an extemporaneous examination cannot be performed, the nodule should be considered a metastatic tumor. However, when possible this examination should be performed as not all hepatic nodules are malignant and the patient would not have to undergo a useless operation.

Malignant tumors spreading directly to the liver from the neighboring organs. The hepatic tissue may be invaded by malignant tumors of the stomach, right flexure of the colon, esophagogastric junction and especially of the gallbladder, owing to its direct relationship with the liver. The principle of the treatment in these tumors is resection *en bloc* of the affected organ together with the adjacent hepatic tissue included in the neoplastic process. As invasion by contiguity has not such an extensive character as metastatic tumors proper, it is not necessary to sacrifice too much glandular tissue. A wedge-shaped resection is as a rule sufficient. In carcinoma of the gallbladder, G. T. Pack, Miller and Brasfield proposed extended right hepatectomy and cholecystectomy *en bloc*, plus lymph adenectomy of the hepatic pedicle. Until definite confirmation of the value of this method, we consider that it is excessively radical and does not comply with the balance between the operative hazard and the results expected. As only timid attempts at bilateral paramedian hepatectomy, which appears far more reasonable than extended right hepatectomy, have been made we consider cholecystectomy and wedge hepatectomy as the operations of election in cancer of the gallbladder.

Drainage hepatectomy. Resection of part of the liver, for anastomosis of one or more intrahepatic bile ducts to the stomach or intestine, is called a drainage hepatectomy. It is indicated in any mechanical obstruction of the extrahepatic ducts, of cicatricial or tumoral origin, when the biliodigestive transit cannot be reestablished because access to the hepatic hilus is blocked. In such circumstances, it is possible to expose one of the intrahepatic bile ducts and anastomose it to the jejunum. These anastomoses are seldom practiced at present. Drainage hepatectomy is chosen because it is more readily performed. For complete drainage, the confluence of the two hepatic ducts should be permeable; when it is blocked some authors propose drainage hepatectomy in both hepatic areas. In a case published by us, both hepatic ducts were obstructed; drainage hepatectomy of the left region was followed by a survival of 14 months, with a subclinical icterus due to biliary stasis in the right hepatic region.

At present three drainage hepatectomy procedures are used. Longmire's operation (intrahepatic cholangiojejunostomy) consists in resection of the left lobe or of part of this lobe (by lateral sagittal transection) and direct anastomosis of an ectatic branch of the left hepatic duct to the jejunum. Dogliotti's procedure is similar but the duct is anastomosed to the stomach. Our procedure (Făgărăşanu — hepatocholangiogastrostomy) consists in resection of segment III and anastomosis of the whole liver section to the stomach.

The indications for hepatectomy in cirrhosis. In view of the known regeneration capacity of the liver and starting from the idea that in cirrhosis a quantitative inbalance is produced between the parenchyma and the stroma, M. Mancuso, S. Messinetti and Napolitano (1957) reached the conclusion that hepatectomy might regenerate the cirrhotic liver and reestablish the balance between the epithelial and the connective tissue. In experimental cirrhosis induced in rats with carbon tetrachloride, F. C. Mann obtained unsatisfactory results after hepatectomy (1931). In 1958, A. H. Islami, G. T. Pack and H. J. Coleman noted that regeneration was more massive, but slower, the more severe the induced cirrhosis and the more extended the hepatectomy.

In man, M. Reifferscheid (1959) was not satisfied with the results obtained. According to L. Schalm, it is likely that Mann and Reifferscheid did not keep account of the factors underlined by Islami et al. Apart from Mancuso et al., partial hepatectomy for cirrhosis has also been performed by P. Valdoni et al., in 1957, and M. Lopez in 1959. Until 1962, the late results of these operations were not known.

HEPATIC HEMOSTASIS

Hemorrhage is the greatest risk of hepatectomy and a great number of hemostatic procedures have been developed, culminating in controlled hemostasis, characteristic of anatomic hepatectomy. Part of the older procedures are only of historical interest, but some are still useful after 70 years. Hepatic hemostasis may be divided into *temporary*, *definite* and *adjuvant*.

TEMPORARY HEMOSTASIS

Temporary hemostasis has a preventive character and attempts to avoid loss of blood until definite hemostasis can be performed.

Manual compression is the simplest procedure. Satisfactory results are obtained when manual compression of the liver beyond the edges of the wound is done by a skillful assistant (Fig. 191). The surgeon can then ligate the bleeding vessels directly or pass deep interlocking loop sutures through the liver mass.

Hepatic hemostatic clamps, still used today by some surgeons in non-anatomic hepatectomies are applied along the edges of the section surfaces (Fig. 192). Definite hemostasis is done after excision, under protection of these rubber-covered clamps which must be sufficiently elastic not to crush the friable liver tissue but resistant

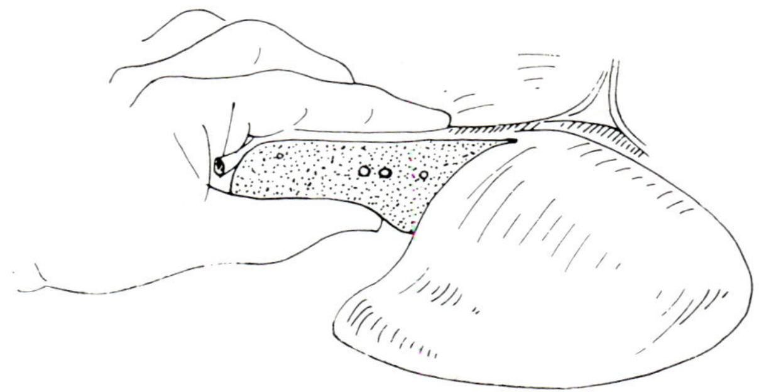

Fig. 191. — Manual compression for temporary hemostasis.

enough to exercise sufficient compression. Nakayama used a special hard clamp that crushed the liver tissue and compressed the vascular pedicles (Fig. 193 *a,b,c*). He applied this technique in 45 left lobectomies with good results, the operating time being very much shortened. The left hepatic vein and the two portal pedicles of the left lobe are ligated; a series of interlocking loop sutures close to the falciform ligament complete the hemostasis.

Congealing of the hepatic tissue. In 1955, A. Brunschwig and P. Serra published a procedure for temporary congealing of the hepatic section, by means of which a dry surface is obtained. The cautery had a fluid nitrogen reservoir; the vessels were ligated as they began to thaw and bleed. This procedure does not seem to have been used by other surgeons.

Temporary occlusion of the hepatic circulation. It is known that in the dog, experimental ligation of the vena porta is followed by death of the animal within an hour, due to accumulation of the blood in portal system and a steady fall in blood pressure. Since ligation of the portal vein produces disturbances comparable to those of an internal hemorrhage, irreversible central nervous lesions already develop 30 minutes after beginning the experiment. When the superior mesenteric artery is also clamped together with the branches of the celiac trunk or the aorta above the emergence of these arteries, clamping of the portal vein is tolerated within somewhat broader limits, restricted, however, by the onset of irreversible hepatic lesions. After interrupting portal circulation for 10 to 15 minutes, therefore below the safety threshold, recovery of the hepatic circulation necessitates more than 20 minutes. Clamping of the porta within this interval is lethal.

In man, attempts were made at clamping the afferent vessels at the beginnings of modern surgery. O. Wangensteen interrrupted the afferent circulation in 3 patients for 33, 24 and 12 minutes, i.e. the hepatic pedicle, superior mesenteric and gastroduodenal artery. After a 20-minute interval, the circulation was again interrupted

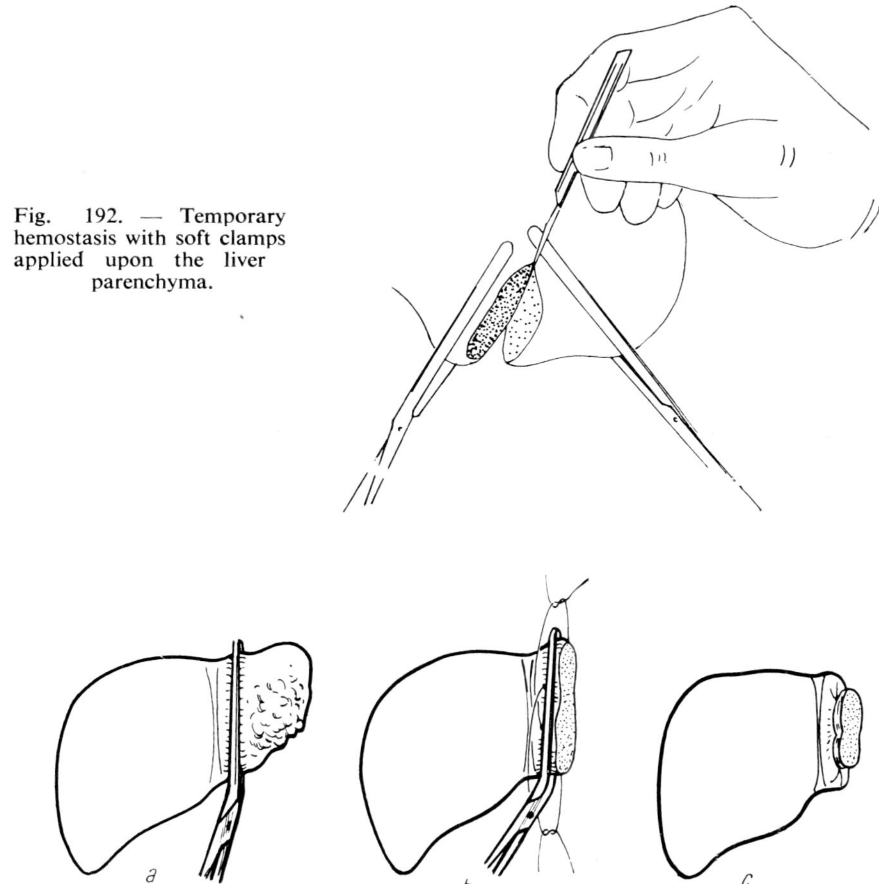

Fig. 192. — Temporary hemostasis with soft clamps applied upon the liver parenchyma.

Fig. 193 *a*, *b*, *c*. — Left non-anatomic lobectomy. Nakayama's procedure.

for 15 minutes, but one of the patients died from severe hepatic damage and the procedure is no longer used.

Temporary clamping of the portal pedicle together with the gastroduodenal and superior mesenteric artery is only indicated in emergencies, in severe hemorrhage in the course of hepatectomy and cannot be maintained for more than 10 minutes.

J. L. Lortat-Jacob who considered that the main danger in the course of right hepatectomy is hemorrhage from the inferior vena cava and hepatic vein, introduced into practice a procedure devised together with Vigneras: occlusion of the cava circulation with 2 loops passed around the cava above and below the confluence of the hepatic veins. Experimentally, it was demonstrated that the animals tolerated double clamping of the vena cava plus clamping of the afferent hepatic pedicle for 15 minutes. Beyond this interval, cardiac arrest occurs. The circulation and arterial pressure rapidly return to normal values, after removing the clamps. Triple clamping is also tolerated by man for 10—15 minutes until the accidentally damaged vena cava or the hepatic vein are ligated.

DEFINITE HEMOSTASIS

Interrupted ligature of Kuznetzov and Penski, who were the first to apply U-ligatures. By a series of ligatures close to the liver section plane, a hemostatic barrier is formed along the borderline between the residual liver and the part to be resected. A special round-tipped needle is threaded with long, double catgut which is passed through the thickness of the liver from the upper to the lower aspect, beyond the planned lines of incision. The suture end (*B*) is cut long enough to be able to tie it to the other end on the opposite part; the loop sutures are passed through the liver at about 2-cm distance. The loops are alternately cut on the upper and lower surfaces and tied. The liver is then sectioned at a sufficient distance from the suture barrier for the suture not to slip off, and only the large and medium bile ducts and vessels are ligated independently (Figs 194 and 195 *a, b,c*).

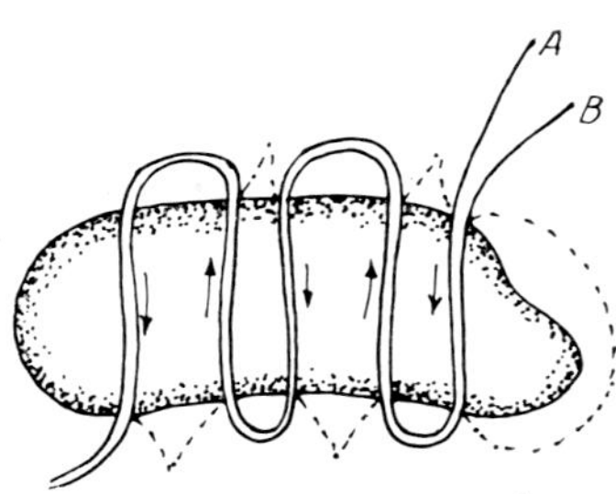

Fig. 194. — Hepatic hemostasis according to the Kuznetzov and Penski technique. The loops of suture *A* are cut on the upper surface of the liver and the ends are ligated. The same procedure is applied on the undersurface.

Chain ligature of M. Auvray. Two long sutures are passed through the liver from the upper to the lower aspect, at half the distance between the extremities of the planned section (*XY* and *AB*, Fig. 196). The two sutures are crossed, so as not to section the liver by divergent traction when they are tied. One end of *AB* is again passed through the liver at about 2-cm distance and the other end is threaded through the loop that is formed. This is repeated several times at 2-cm distance. The two ends are tied close together once the edge of the liver is reached. The same suture procedure is applied with the other suture (*XY*). The liver is then sectioned beyond the hemostatic barrier, leaving the biliovascular stumps sufficiently long for the sutures not to slip off.

Various ligations have been described which differ only in detail from the original techniques, the principle remaining the same. A simple technique is that of Wallich: a long, thick catgut is used for passing a series of deep loop sutures. The loops are then cut and the ends tied together. Wendel's technique is very similar (Figs 197, 198 and 199).

When small portions of the liver are excised, and there are no larger vessels, mass ligation can be used that do not section the liver tissue. The hemostatic effect of such ligation is greater the thicker the catgut and the denser the hepatic tissue. Thin catgut sections the liver tissue before obtaining satisfactory hemostasis.

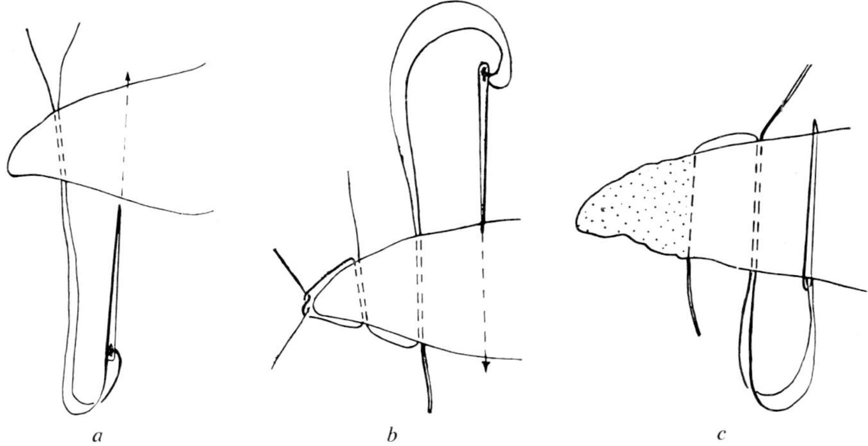

Fig. 195 *a*, *b*, *c*. — Hepatic hemostasis according to Kuznetzov and Penski. Sequence of the first four ligatures.

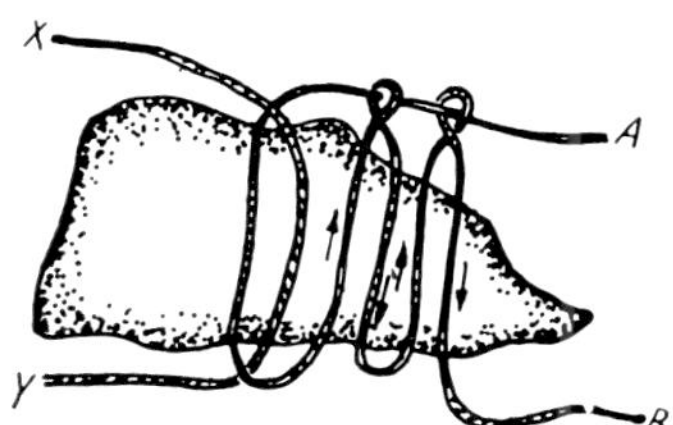

Fig. 196. — Hepatic hemostasis according to the Auvray procedure.

In non-anatomic hepatectomies, some authors substituted for the classical ligatures a kind of interrupted transfixing suture, drawn tight enough to compress the vessels without sectioning the liver tissue. J.R. Robinson and H.R. Butcher of St. Louis described such a technique in 1956. If the suture slips or weakens at one point, the whole suture relaxes. Hence, we consider this technique and other similar ones as contraindicated in hepatic resections.

Ligation of the vessels on the incised liver surface. Kuznetzov and Penski demonstrated that the hepatic vessels are not less resistant to traction than other vessels. The medium sized vessels on the incised hepatic surface can bear a weight of 600 gm. Due to their resistance and elasticity the clamped vessels can be drawn out about 1 cm to be ligated. These data were confirmed by Auvray in 1898. Individual vessels on the incised liver surface are closed by transfixing

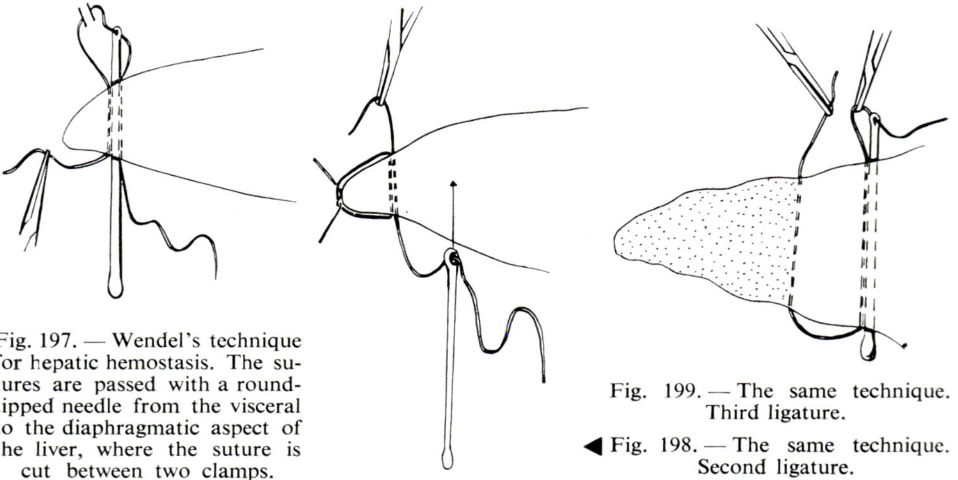

Fig. 197. — Wendel's technique for hepatic hemostasis. The sutures are passed with a round-tipped needle from the visceral to the diaphragmatic aspect of the liver, where the suture is cut between two clamps.

Fig. 199. — The same technique. Third ligature.

◀ Fig. 198. — The same technique. Second ligature.

sutures, including the surrounding hepatic tissue. These ligatures are still used today, especially to complete hemostasis by mass ligation when some vessels continue to bleed (Figs 200 and 201).

Transfixing ligatures on prostheses. Catgut sections the liver tissue when it is tied firmly holding together the larger vessels and bile ducts within the loop;

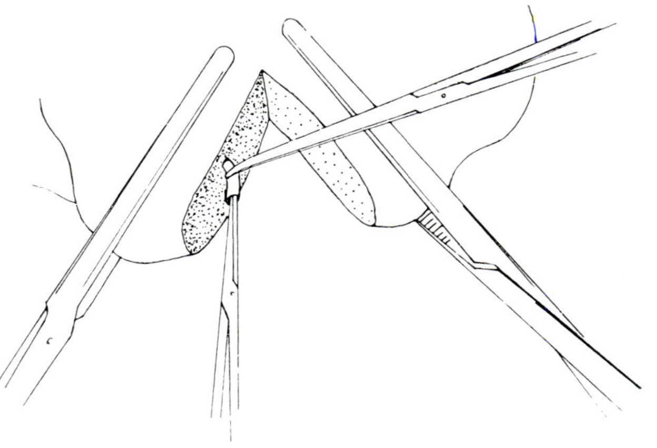

Fig. 200. — Ligation of the vessels on the incised hepatic surface. Clamping of a vessel for simple ligature.

however, massive bleeding may occur from the small vessels crossing the parenchyma. Therefore, several procedures were devised using prostheses of more or less resistant material, which were applied on the superior and inferior liver aspects, along the suture lines, below the loops, in order to prevent the suture from sectioning the liver tissue. The following have been used: chicken bones, whale bones, calf shoulderbone, cartilage, conserved flaps of urinary bladder and

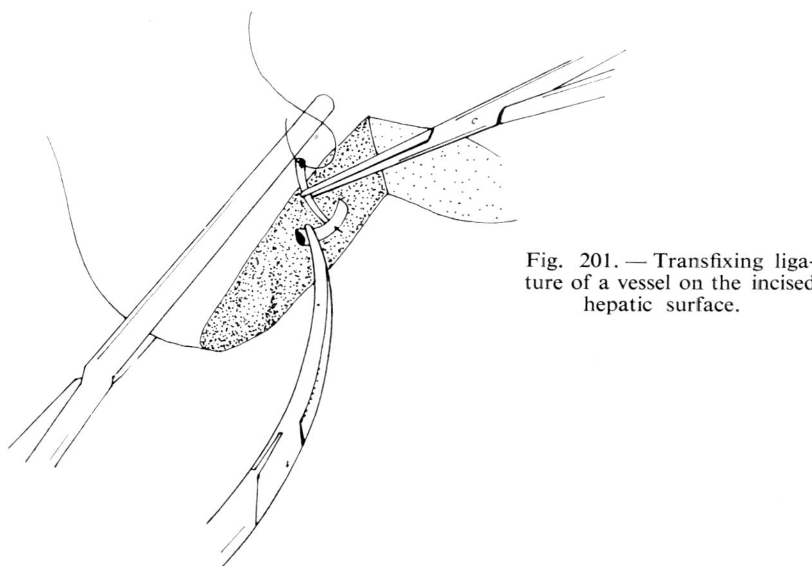

Fig. 201. — Transfixing ligature of a vessel on the incised hepatic surface.

intestine, pidgeon muscle, boiled tendons, wire, celluloid rods, magnesium bands, etc. At present, when the liver is extremely friable, catgut bundles or omentum fragments are successfully used.

Controlled hemostasis implies exposure and ligation of the main afferent and efferent vascular trunks supplying the region, lobe or segment to be resected. This type of hemostasis characterizes planned hepatectomy. Transfixing ligatures with U-sutures or ligature of the vessels on the incised surface are specific of non-anatomic resections but may also be used as complementary means in controlled hepatectomies. There are two routes of access to the vascular pedicles of the liver segments: the hilar and the fissural routes.

The *hilar route* offers direct access to the vascular pedicles that are visible on the lower aspect of the liver, belonging to the right and left region, left lobe and segment III. Meticulous dissection of the hilar plate is then necessary in order to expose the vascular pedicles. Before ligating and sectioning a pedicle, the surgeon should determine whether it actually supplies the condemned liver segment. The artery should never be ligated before clamping in order to see if the liver segment changes its color. The difficulties encountered in recognizing the distribution of the afferent pedicles may be partly overcome by intraoperative cholangiography and phlebography of the biliary and portal branches.

When the afferent vessels cannot be approached by intracapsular route, for various reasons, the extracapsular approach will be used. The lower aspect of the liver is visualized, approximately at the level of the afferent pedicle, at the site at which it is to be sectioned. The pedicle, sheathed in Glisson's capsule is detached from the liver tissue which covers it. Long blunt, curved needles passing between the pedicle and liver or even through the liver above the pedicle do not produce excessive bleeding. Temporary clamping of the partly isolated pedicle and changes in the color of the liver will show whether the level at which the pedicle is clamped was well chosen.

Fissural approach. In some cases, the intrahepatic vascular distribution is very difficult to unravel. There are numerous anatomical variants owing to reduplication of the branches or their transposition upon a neighboring pedicle. For instance, branches supplying the right liver may arise from the left hepatic artery and left branch of the vena porta. Ligation of these branches before the emergence of the other branches could also jeopardize the right hepatic region they are distributed to. Moreover, the topography of the vascular pedicles may be modified by certain pathologic processes to such an extent that they can no longer be compared to their normal aspect. In such cases fissural access is used, approaching the vascular pedicles indirectly, on their superior aspect, after exposing the fissure. This is done by ligating the hepatic vein. Before incising, a series of parallel interlocking deep sutures are placed and tied on both sides for preventive hemostasis and the liver is sectioned along the fissure; the upper aspect of the portal pedicle being reached, the liver tissue is detached from the pedicle. Ligation is done distal to the fissure plane.

Hepatectomy by manual crushing. Ton That Tung of Hanoi used a special hemostasis technique in the course of numerous left and right hepatectomies he performed, i.e. manual crushing (digitoclasis). The hepatic parenchyma is incised superficially along the main fissure, on the diaphragmatic and visceral aspects of the liver. The small, superficial vessels are isolated and ligated. The liver parenchyma is then crushed between the thumb and forefinger, starting with the anterior margin and advancing towards the hilus along the fissure plane. The large and medium sized vessels and ducts remain intact as they are more resistant than the liver tissue. In the hepatic hilus, the biliovascular pedicle is isolated along several centimeters to right or left according to whether a right or left hepatectomy will be performed. The vessels and bile ducts can then be ligated and sectioned under direct control.

J.P. Churet (Paris) checked this procedure experimentally and obtained satisfactory results especially when hemostasis was completed with locally applied hemostatics or suture points on the incised liver surface.

Adjuvant procedures. The thermal procedures used in the past have been abandoned as they produced deep bed sores with secondary hemorrhage and cholerrhage and could not arrest bleeding from the large or medium vessels (Paquelin's thermocauter, scalding vapors — Sneghirev and burning-hot air — Holländer).

Today, *electrocoagulation* may sometimes complete hemostasis that is insufficient following U-sutures, by controlling bleeding of the capillaries or arterioles and venules.

Tamponade with gauze is only indicated for temporary hemostasis of the capillary vessels. If the cut liver section continues to bleed, it is very likely that a large vessel is still open. It should be looked for and ligated directly or with the surrounding mass. When bleeding is massive, tamponade is illusory and only involves a high operative risk. Plugging with fibrin sponges gives better results owing to their specific hemostatic action; moreover, they are resorbable.

Omental grafts or pediculate parietal flaps (seromusculoaponeurotic) may be inserted to plug the liver defects; they are applied directly upon the incised hepatic surface or are used when the cut surface continues to bleed in spite of transfixing ligation. The parietal flaps used by C. Beck in 1902 are obsolete. In 1954, F. Lanzillo proposed to plug the liver with the diaphragm for instance in partial resection of the right hepatic area, where the two surfaces come in contact. C. Couinaud draws attention to the fact that coughing may cause the sutures fixing the two organs to loosen as they cut through the friable liver tissue.

Split skin grafts were recommended by F. Masters et al. (1954) who considered them, on the basis of experimental and clinical data, as excellent local hemostatics in hepatic surgery; applied upon the incised surface, they are able to control even severe bleeding. This method does not, however, seem to have been confirmed.

Hemostatics increase the efficiency of temporary or definite plugging. Among the numerous substances used, dry thrombin powder appears to be the most efficient.

CONTROL OF CHOLERRHAGY

Biliary peritonitis is a rare complication of hepatectomy. As a rule, there is a slight discharge of bile from the incised surface which is drained through a tube. However, in some cases an external biliary fistula develops when larger bile ducts are not well ligated. These fistulas may be favored by increased pressure in the bile ducts due to blocking of the extrahepatic bile ducts by a mechanical obstacle. When the extrahepatic bile ducts are not completely patent, hepatectomy should be followed by external drainage of the gallbladder or common bile duct.

PREVENTION OF AIR EMBOLISM

Attention was first drawn to the hazard of air embolism in the course of hepatectomy by Hochenegg and Israel and are recognized by most authors. In 1898, in the course of a hepatic resection for tumor, Hochenegg's patient had a massive venous hemorrhage. Autopsy revealed massive air embolism with a probable starting point in a hepatic vein. Theroretically, the amount of air aspirated in the inferior vena cava depends upon the caliber of the hepatic vein that has remained open, upon the time elapsed up to ligation of the vein and the negative pressure in the vena cava. A constant positive pressure excludes the possibility of air embolism. A negative pressure in inspiration and positive in expiration allows for successive hemorrhage and the aspiration of air in the hepatic veins. In the literature of the last few years we found no case of air embolism in the course of hepatectomy. However, the theoretical possibility of such a complication demands that certain precautions should be taken especially in right hepatectomy, where the imminent danger exists of opening the right hepatic vein or even the vena cava. Tightening of the ligature loops around the cava ensures good temporary hemostasis and favors definite hemostasis, also preventing the danger of air embolism. In other hepatectomies, correct measures of hemostasis on the cut hepatic surface may also be considered as measures for preventing air embolism.

PREOPERATIVE TREATMENT

Before operation an accurate balance must be drawn of the functional capacity of the liver, respiratory tract, circulation and excretory system. Any metabolic deficiencies, pathologic alterations of the figured elements of the blood, plasma components and coagulability disturbances must be detected. Correct treatment of the deficiencies raises the patient's resistance to an operation that is extremely severe in most cases. The operation may be contraindicated or put off when the patient does not respond to the treatment favorably (for instance decompensated heart failure).

ANESTHESIA AND RESUSCITATION

All the liver patients present a more or less accentuated degree of hepatic insufficiency, which is often latent, and that risks to become far more severe during and after hepatectomy. The anesthesiologist should bear in mind two particularly important factors:

1. The toxic action of the anesthetic on the liver cell;
2. Aggravation of the hepatocell damage due to hypoxia.

Of the premedication used, barbiturates and phenothiazines must be avoided or only used with the greatest caution. Their toxic action is protracted when the antitoxic capacity of the liver is reduced. In aged patients with advanced hepatic lesions these drugs may produce comatose phenomena. Hence, the premedication in surgery of the liver should be based upon weak sedatives, obtained from plants rather than synthetic, administered for a few days before the operation, to which pethidines are added on the day of the intervention.

Morphine and its derivatives are contraindicated because they produce spasms of Oddi's sphincter, modifying the peroperative cholangiographic results and favoring cholerrhagy of the sectioned hepatic surface.

Anesthesia with fluothane has low hepatotoxic effects provided a good oxygenation is obtained. Ether in large doses is toxic for the liver but may be administered in smaller amounts to patients with lesser hepatic lesions. Oxygen and 5% glucose perfusions must be administered, and the blood pressure constantly monitored. Anesthesia with volatile substances should always be administered by the endotracheal route and can be potentiated by fractional pethidine doses. Muscular relaxation is obtained with curarizing substances.

Blood loss is replaced by isogroup blood perfusions. The intensive care unit should be prepared to replace large quantities of blood, by rapid transfusion under pressure. In statistics on 53 hepatectomies performed in the Memorial Center for Cancer of New York, up to 1960, O. Schweitzer and W.S. Holland showed that 5 to 10 litres blood are lost in the course of right hepatectomy.

Drug-induced hypothermia and refrigeration have been used in hepatic surgery because of the advantage of a good hemostasis under controlled clamping of the hepatic pedicle. Most surgeons, however, consider the method risky. Li Pao-hua et al. experimented and applied in the clinic *intraperitoneal refrigeration*, with normal saline at a temperature of 0 to +4°C (32°—39.2°F), which permits prolonged clamping of the hepatic pedicles. Refrigeration is stopped when the body temperature falls below +30°C/86°F. Three patients were successfully operated by this method (2 hepatectomies and 1 lobectomy). In two of the cases the hepatic pedicle was clamped for 30 and 31 minutes, respectively. The body temperature was brought up to 33°C / 91.4°F with heated normal saline introduced into the peritoneal cavity. This method is considered superior to general refrigeration as lower temperatures are obtained at the level of the liver. The late results of such operations have not been reported.

ROUTES OF ACCESS

In surgery of the liver the surgical approach initially is explorative. The incision, limited at first, is only broadened after establishing the nature and extent of the lesions. The current incisions used can be sufficiently extended to permit a hepatectomy (Fig. 202 *a* through *k* and 203 *a* through *f*).

The left half of the liver is as a rule easily accessible exclusively by abdominal approach. The initial incision should be lengthened cranially and to the left. When the operation has started with a median supraumbilical laparotomy, it must be extended upward, resecting if necessary the xyphoid, or crosswise by a Grégoire left incision or Rio Branco left oblique incision. At the distal end of a medial incision Raven cut a cross T incision to the right and left of the median line. When the operation starts with a Sprengel incision it can be prolonged to the left for left lobectomy.

Right hepatectomy can only be practiced under good visibility when a broad thoracophrenolaparotomy is performed along the 8th intercostal space up to the posterior axillary line. The diaphragm is incised almost up to the inferior vena cava. When a right hepatectomy is envisaged, the operation should be started with an explorative abdominal incision running obliquely close to the

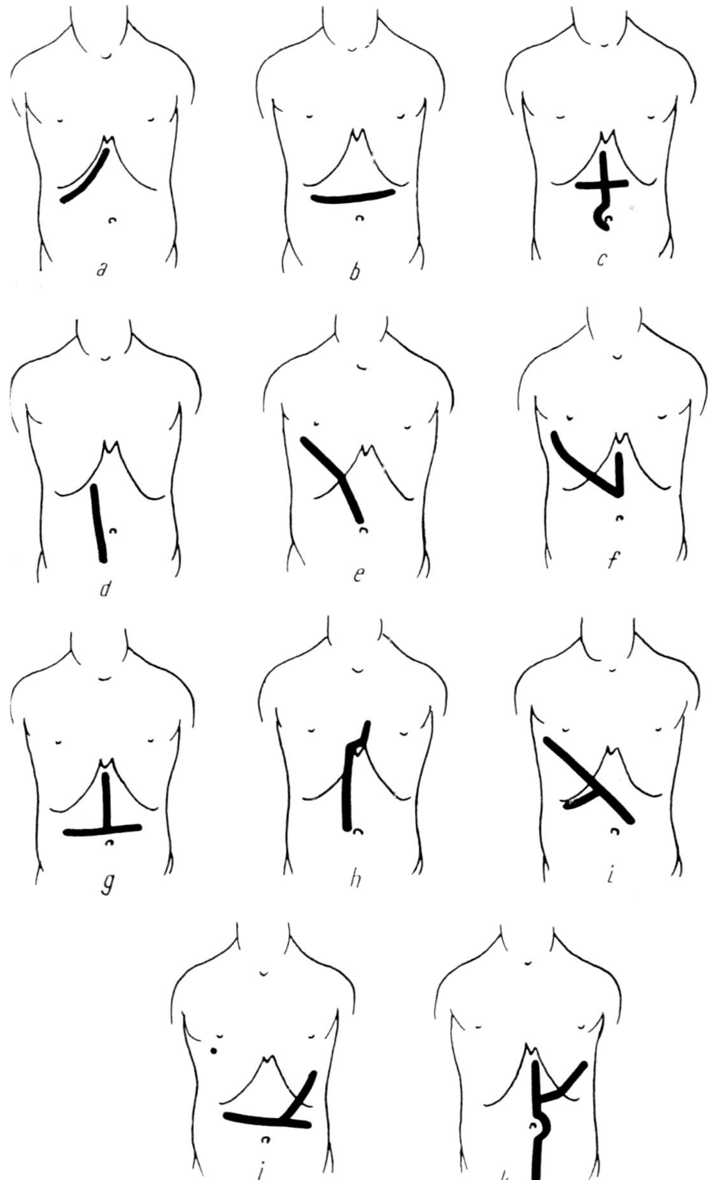

Fig. 202. — Different incisions for operations on the liver (according to M. Reifferscheid).

a) Classical subcostal incision; *b)* incision used by Sprengel, Bakes (1911), Tinker (1939), Warvi (1945), Sénèque (1950); *c)* A. Brunschwig (1955); *d)* J. K. Quattlebaum (1953), H. Gans (1955); *e)* Thoracophrenolaparotomy — M. Kirschner (1920), etc.; *f)* P. de Rio Branco (1912); *g)* R. W. Raven (1949); *h)* Tinker (1929), Quattlebaum (1953), etc.; *i)* H. Gans (1955); *j)* A. Brunschwig (1955); *k)* Rio Branco (1912).

umbilicus, towards the right costal margin, so that it can be prolonged up to the 8th intercostal space. Any other initial incision — subcostal, median or Sprengel — may be transformed into a thoracophrenolaparotomy.

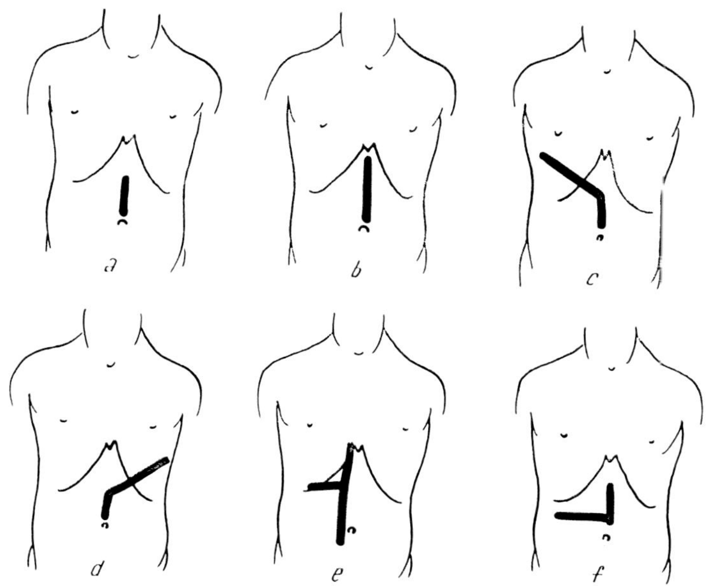

Fig. 203. — Prolongation of short median supraumbilical incision (after M. Reifferscheid).

a) short median supraumbilical explorative incision; *b)* incision extended towards the xyphoid process in order to have access to the left lobe of the liver; *c)* right thoracophrenolaparotomy for access to the right hepatic region; *d)* left thoracophrenolaparotomy for access to the left lobe; *e)* and *f)* other routes of access to the afferent pedicle.

HEPATECTOMY TECHNIQUES

RIGHT ANATOMIC HEPATECTOMY

After the abdominal incision the abdomen is explored, assessing the extent of the lesions, the technical and tactical possibilities, the immediate risk and late prognosis. When resection is possible the patient is turned to the left and the incision prolonged along the 8th intercostal space up to the posterior axillary line, sectioning the chondral border, then the diaphragm almost to the inferior vena cava. Visibility is increased after introducing the thoracic retractors and isolating the subhepatic viscera and right lung with moist surgical drapes.

Mobilization of the right hepatic region. The liver is rotated ventrally stretching the right triangular ligament which is then severed (Fig. 204). The two layers of the coronary ligament are then sectioned, one after the other after first separating them by introducing a finger or a tampon into the lax connective tissue between them. Particular attention should be paid not to injure the vena cava.

It is sometimes necessary to sever the round ligament as well in order to rotate the liver more easily.

Preventive hemostasis. As recommended by J.L. Lortat-Jacob, two suture loops should be passed round the vena cava in order to be ready in case of hemorrhage. The first loop is passed below the confluence of the hepatic veins. The vein is exposed below the posterior margin of the liver after sectioning the posterior parietal peritoneum. As the portion of the vena cava between the confluence of the hepatic veins and the pericardium is very short, the latter is opened over a distance of 3 cm and the second loop passed around the intrapericardiac portion

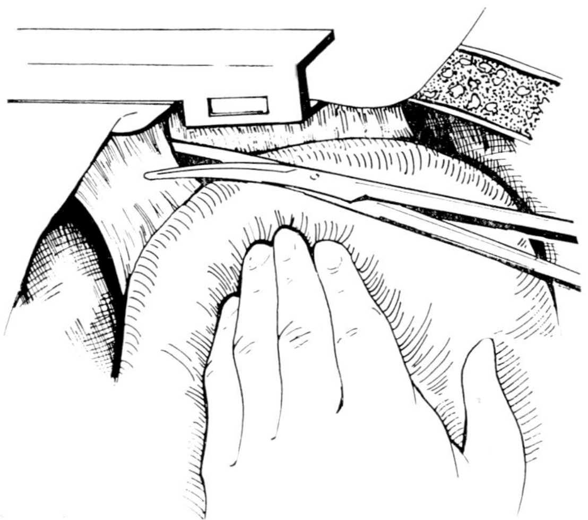

Fig. 204. — Right hepatectomy. Transection of the right triangular ligament.

of the inferior cava. A flexible clamp should be available so as to be able to clamp the afferent pedicle at any moment in case of severe hemorrhage.

The portal pedicle. In order to approach the pedicle of the right hepatic region it is necessary to detach the gallbladder from its hepatic bed, as for antegrade cholecystectomy. When local anatomic conditions are favorable to dissection of the vasculobiliary pedicle, the cystic duct and vessels are not severed. However, when the cystic vessels prevent exposure of the pedicle, the gallbladder must be removed. When the gallbladder is diseased there can be no question of leaving it *in situ.*

The portal pedicle is meticulously followed up toward the hilus, the hilar plate is then incised in order to expose the confluence of the hepatic ducts and bifurcation of the hepatic artery and vena porta and their right ramifications (Fig. 205). The right branch of the hepatic artery is clamped above the emergence of the cystic artery. Among the components of Glisson's capsule, the vein has the most sharp cut cleavage plane but is more readily damaged in the course of isolation. On the upper part of the vein, covered by the liver, dissection is sometimes difficult because there are many branches that can be injured. In

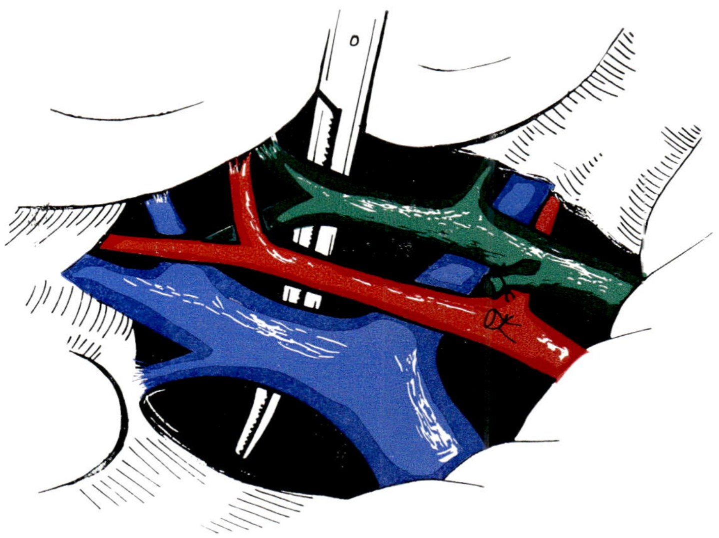

Fig. 205. — Meticulous dissection of the hilus and isolation of the three components of the pedicle, their bifurcation and left and right branches. The gallbladder is removed. Note the ligated stumps of the cystic duct and cystic artery. A forceps has been introduced below the right branches of the afferent pedicle components which can now be ligated and severed.

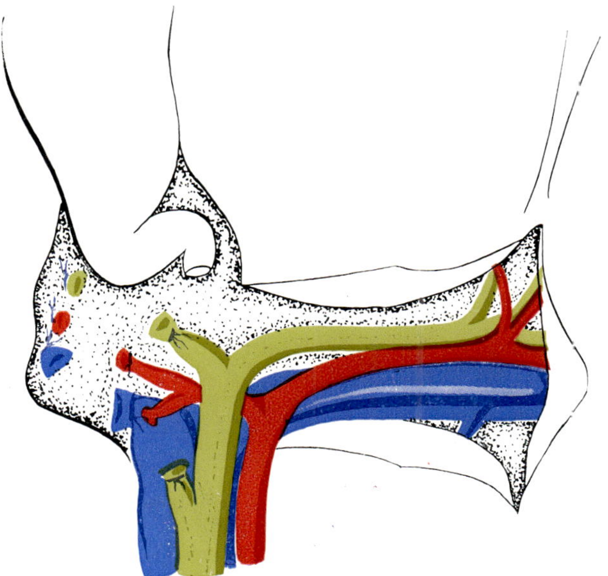

Fig. 206. — Right branches of the afferent pedicle after being sectioned (after Cl. Olivier).

order to establish whether the vein can be ligated and severed, the following precautions must be taken:

1. Clamping of the vein and artery is followed by a change in the color of the right hepatic region due to ischemia. If the dark, cyanotic area does not correspond to the right area, being more restricted or too extended then the artery and vein should be clamped more laterally or centrally, towards the bifurcation. Greater care should be taken the nearer one is to the original bifurcation of the trunks, dissecting the main branches meticulously so as not to make mistakes in choosing the site of the ligatures.

2. When there is any doubt as to the most favorable site of the ligature, a portal phlebography should be done, injecting the contrast medium into a vein on the lesser curvature of the stomach. The right branch of the portal vein, which is isolated but not yet clamped, is detected with the tip of a radioopaque probe. The radiographic image will show whether the vein can be ligated at this level. The artery and vein are severed between the ligatures. It is recommended to ligate the central end of the vessels with two nonabsorbable sutures.

3. In order to hasten hemostasis, or in the absence of corresponding technical means, the right pedicle can at first be ligated intra- or extracapsularly further away from the bifurcation. The only drawback of this procedure is the severe hemorrhage that may arise at the moment in which the liver is sectioned, from the ramifications of a longer portion of the artery and vein. Hemostasis is completed by direct ligation of the vessels upon the cut hepatic surface.

The right hepatic duct is severed between two ligatures. It is advisable to apply a double ligature with nonabsorbable suture to the central end in order to avoid a biliary fistula. Cholangiography may be necessary for establishing the level of the ligature, the same as phlebography for the right branch of the hepatic vena porta. When cholangiography cannot be carried out, the right hepatic duct should be severed in the last instance, after incision of the liver. Freed from the hepatic tissue to which it adheres, it should be sectioned laterally inasmuch as possible.

Ligation of the right hepatic vein. The liver is drawn to the left and downward in order to reveal the right hepatic vein which is short and thick (Fig. 207). Although with difficulty, a curved, blunt instrument can be passed around the vein, on the left side. This demands great skill and implies a fairly high risk, since the vena cava or one of the two hepatic veins may be damaged. Injury of the left hepatic vein is extremely dangerous and during its isolation the right hepatic vein should be constantly kept in view. After isolation the vein is severed between the ligatures. The central end is ligated with a double transfixing suture, as the caliber of the vein is large and the suture may slip.

The liver is then rotated to the left and upward in order to reveal the accessory hepatic veins that arise from the posterior aspect of the gland and join the right ventrolateral slope of the vena cava. Their variable number and size, their shortness and friability on traction of the liver demands particular attention in order to be ligated without loss of blood. Avulsion of one of these veins is equivalent to opening of the vena cava and should be treated as such. Hemorrhage is controlled by drawing close the loops around the cava.

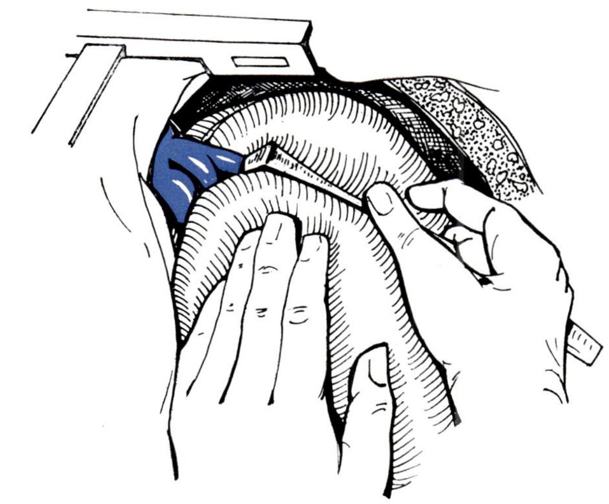

Fig. 207. — Approach to the right hepatic vein.

Resection of the liver. The liver is incised with the scalpel or cautery, along the main fissure, bearing in mind its inclination to the left and the reference points of this plane (Fig. 208). Lortat-Jacob considers that the incision should begin dorsally on the right side of the left hepatic vein, then continue ventrally along the right lateral aspect of the sagittal vein. During severance, the affluent ramifications of the sagittal vein, coming from the right paramedian lobe, are ligated (Fig. 209). The sagittal vein should not be denuded, leaving a cover of thin hepatic tissue, since the hazard of postoperative thrombophlebitis is greater after denudation.

The incision is gradually continued up to the superior aspect of the hilar region, which is disengaged laterally from the underlying liver tissue, then ligated and severed. The bleeding vessels and open bile capillaries on the sectioned surface are clamped and ligated. The transected surface may be covered by a free graft of parietal omentum or coronary ligament. The gallbladder, when not removed, is again attached to the liver. Any dynamic or mechanical obstacle in the common duct or Oddi's sphincter is removed. External biliary drainage is performed when necessary. Closed drainage of the abdominal cavity is followed by diaphragmatic suture and closure of the thoracoabdominal wall.

Several authors consider that the technique described by Lortat-Jacob endangers the lower vena cava although it is meant to lessen the danger. Apart from the difficulties encountered in passing the loops around the cava, below the liver and intrapericardially, there is also the danger of using the loops which may predispose to severe shock. Moreover, dissection of the right hepatic vein close to its junction with the vena cava is very difficult technically. According to Ton That Tung, whose experience includes 53 hepatectomies of all types, it is better

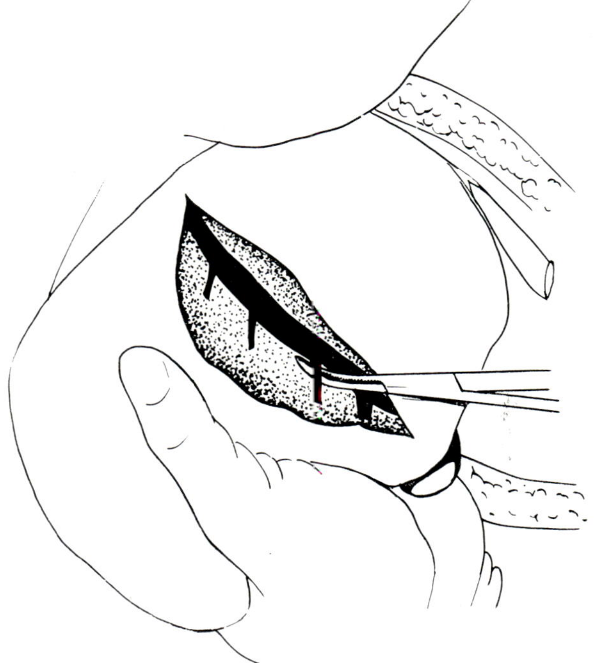

Fig. 208. — Transection of the liver on the diaphragmatic aspect, along the main fissure. The right branches of the sagittal vein are isolated and ligated.

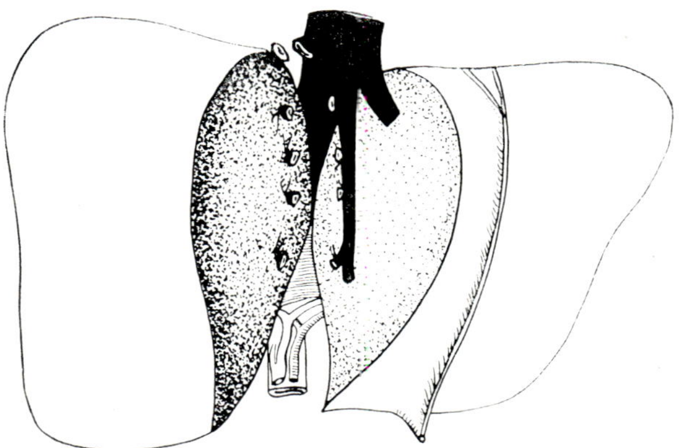

Fig. 209. — The right branches of the sagittal vein and right hepatic vein have been ligated and severed.

to ligate the right hepatic vein together with the surrounding hepatic tissue, at a distance from the vena cava, after ligating the pedicle of the afferent hepatic region and exposing the main fissure. Lortat-Jacob's procedure also includes resection of the caudate lobe. Dissection and ligation of the vena cava considerably increase the operative hazard. It is, therefore, preferable not to excise the caudate lobe. When it is affected by the pathologic process, hepatectomy is contra-indicated.

RIGHT HEPATECTOMY BY FISSURAL APPROACH

Hepatectomy by fissural approach is not an anatomic resection, but "secondary controlled" according to the expression of Lortat-Jacob. Actually, it represents an intermediate type between controlled and non-anatomic hepatectomies, especially as the fissure is generally opened under the protection of transfixing ligatures, characteristic of non-anatomic resections. Approach of the vascular pedicles in the hilus brings it close to the anatomic hepatectomies. The sequence of the procedure is the following:

The *right hepatic region*, is freed by severing the right triangular and the coronary ligament up to the inferior vena cava.

The *main fissure is opened* between two parallel rows of transfixing ligatures, placed to the right of the fissure so as not to damage the sagittal vein. Care must be taken that the ligatures through the liver substance should not injure the vein or compress it when tightened. The liver is then incised up to the superior surface of the hilar plaque.

Ligation of the pedicle of the right hepatic territory. The hilar plate is dissected laterally and to the right in order to free it from the underlying liver tissue. So as not to risk ligating the confluence of the portal components in the hilus, it is advisable to establish certain reference points by cholangiography. When this is not feasible, the hilar plate is detached as much as possible laterally, to the right, in order to be certain that the pedicle components within the dissected connective sheath strictly belong to the right liver. They are ligated all together, or each one separately and sectioned, after being dissected within Glisson's capsule in which they are enclosed.

Ligation of the right hepatic vein and eventually of the accessory hepatic veins belonging to the right hepatic region is carried out the same as in right hepatectomy by hilar approach.

EXTENDED RIGHT HEPATECTOMY

Extended right hepatectomy includes resection of the right hepatic region plus removal of the left paramedian segment or all the liver to the right of the left segmental fissure. The route of access, mobilization of the liver and the measures taken for preventing hemostasis succeed one another as in simple right hepatectomy. However, some of the operative moments present certain peculiarities.

Ligation of the portal components. This begins by broad exposure of the bifurcation of the main biliovascular triad, along the pedicle of both the right and left hepatic regions. The cystic duct and vessels are ligated and severed. The gallbladder is not excised separately, since it is removed together with the resected liver to which it adheres. The artery, vein and hepatic duct belonging to the right liver are ligated and divided separately. The bile duct and arterial branch of the paramedian segment of the left lobe, that join the left hepatic duct and left hepatic artery in the hilus, are then identified and ligated (Fig. 210). The portal branches of the quadrate lobe arise from the extremity of the venous trunk, from Rex' recessus umbilicalis, and are distributed to the lobe in a round-about way, running from left to right. Consequently, they are ligated on the incised surface after the liver is incised along the secondary fissure. When the bile duct and arterial branch of the quadrate lobe cannot be identified at their confluence with the main branches, they are ligated on the incised surface after opening the fissure.

Ligation of the hepatic veins. Not only the right hepatic vein but the sagittal vein should also be ligated (Fig. 211). Particular care should be taken as the risk of damaging the left hepatic vein into which it empties is fairly great. The liver is retracted downward and a sagittal incision is cut 2 cm from the vena cava. The incision is widened with blunt forceps in order to expose the left side of the sagittal vein. The liver is incised along the vein for a further 2—3 cm. The left part of the sagittal vein can now be freed, and the vein is severed between two ligatures.

Division of the liver is continued along the secondary fissure, 1 cm from the basis of the falciform ligament and left sagittal fissure, that remain to the left of the section. As the cleavage plane of the secondary fissure falls upon the left lobar pedicle, particular care should be taken not to divide it. This fatal mistake can be avoided by cutting the incision very obliquely in order to reach the undersurface of the liver to the right, up to the level where the right hepatic duct and vessels were sectioned. If, owing to the necessity of extirpating as much liver tissue as possible, the incision has been cut as close as possible to the left lobar pedicle and up to the superior aspect of the hilar plate that covers the left lobar pedicle, the hepatic tissue will be detached from the hilar plate, on the right, up to the right side of the bifurcation of the biliovascular triad, ligating the main trunks.

The other phases of the operation succeed one another as in the preceding operations, the only difference consisting in peritonealization of the incised hepatic surface with the falciform ligament separated from the diaphragm.

LEFT TOTAL HEPATECTOMY

Left hepatectomy implies resection of the left liver segment by an incision along the main fissure. There are two variations: total and subtotal left hepatectomy, with or without resection of the caudate lobe. As the former is far more difficult, it will only be performed if the pathologic process has affected the caudate lobe, or for prognostic reasons, for instance to extend the limits of oncologic

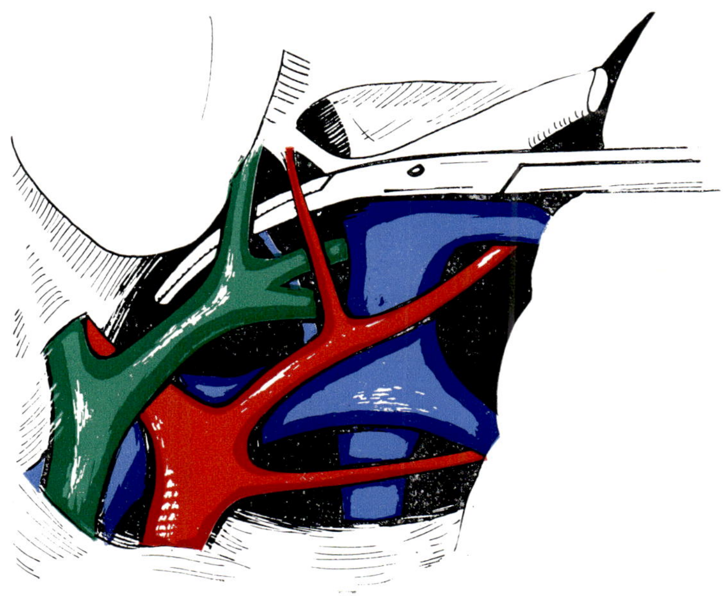

Fig. 210. — Extended right hepatectomy. The right branches of the afferent pedicle, as well as the branches supplying the left median lobe deriving from the main left branches of this pedicle,are ligated. For this purpose dissection is continued to the left, along the left branches of the bifurcation, up to the left sagittal fissure. The forceps passes below the arterial and biliary branches of the left paramedian lobe. After their ligation and transection the portal branch is isolated (after Reifferscheid).

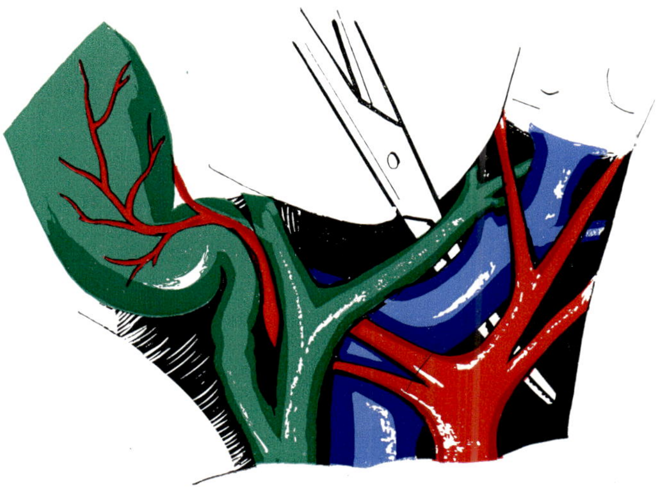

Fig. 211.—Left hepatectomy. The components of the left pedicle have been isolated. They will be ligated and severed separately.

safety on extirpating a malignant tumor in the immediate vicinity of the lobe. The caudate lobe belongs with certainty to the left liver when it protrudes into the *bursa omentalis*, to the left of the hepatic insertion of the lesser omentum. As a general rule, the caudate lobe should not be removed if possible.

The routes of access for left hepatectomy have been described in a previous chapter.

Mobilization of the liver. The left lobe is freed by severing the round ligament, then the falciform ligament along its diaphragmatic insertion. The surgeon

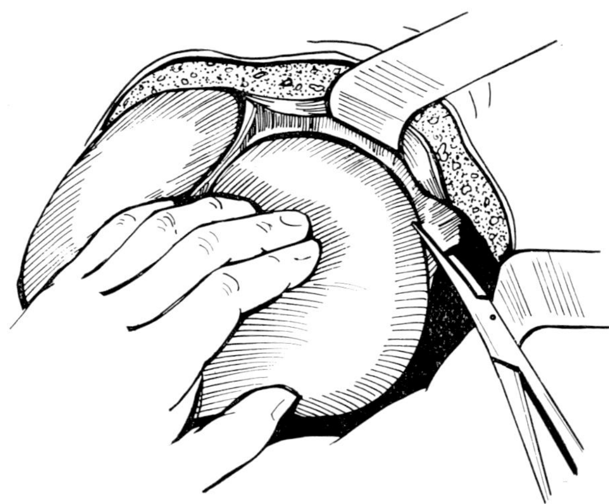

Fig. 212. — Mobilization of the left lobe of the liver. Transection of the left triangular ligament.

introduces his finger through the *pars flaccida* of the lesser omentum in order to pass a suture loop around the hepatic pedicle so as to prevent if necessary a severe hemorrhage. The *pars condensa omenti minoris* is incised towards the cardia. In this thicker portion of the omentum lies the left gastric artery that supplies part of the liver. It is divided between two ligatures. There are rare aberrant cases in which it distributes its ramifications to the whole liver (according to Couinaud, 1 case in 300). In this case, the artery must not be severed. The absence of arterial pulsations within the hepatic pedicle will draw attention to the possibility of exclusive coronary supply to the liver. The left lobe is drawn gently downward in order to extend the left triangular ligament which is then severed (Fig. 212), paying particular attention along the midline not to injure the left hepatic vein. As a measure of precaution, the folds of the ligament are detached and divided separately, as the left hepatic vein is thus more readily exposed to view.

Ligation of the afferent pedicle is performed in total left hepatectomy as close as possible to the bifurcation (Fig. 213). After dividing the peritoneum of the hepatoduodenal ligament close to the hilus, the hepatic artery lying posterior and to the left of the common bile duct is found. The artery is followed up to its bifurcation, then along the left branch, which is clamped 1 cm from the bifurcation in order to observe any changes in color. The pulsations of the right hepatic artery are also felt in order to be sure that it is patent. When it is certain that the artery belongs exclusively to the left hepatic segment, it is severed between the ligatures. Persistence of the initial color after clamping shows that supplementary arterial branches exist, as a rule a suprahilar anastomosis between the right and the left hepatic arteries which is ligated after opening the fissure.

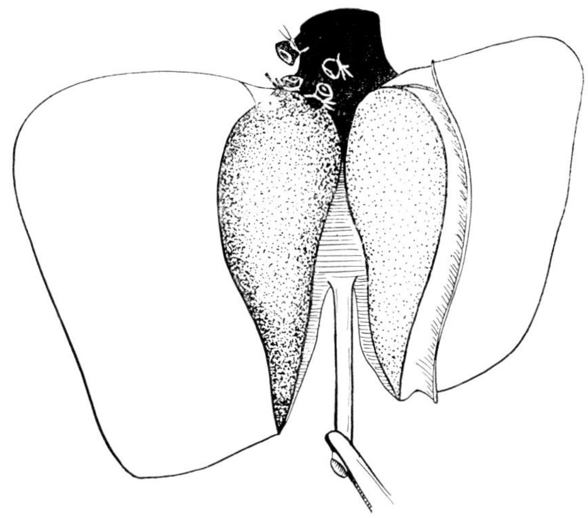

Fig. 213. — Extended right hepatectomy. The right hepatic vein and the sagittal vein have been ligated (after Cl. Olivier).

The left branch of the portal vein is exposed according to the procedure used for the artery, that is along the main trunk up to the bifurcation and then to the left. Clamping is likewise done close to the bifurcation. Portal phlebography may be very useful for checking correct application of the clamps. When the site has been well chosen, the vein is severed between two nonabsorbable suture ligatures, preferably with a double ligature on the central end. If clamping has been done too close to the bifurcation, dissection is continued. In general, the vein is readily detached from Glisson's capsule that covers it, but on the dorsocranial aspect several branches may emerge towards the caudate lobe and must be carefully divided in order to have sufficient space to ligate the vein.

The left hepatic duct can be isolated, ligated and divided concomitantly or later on. The choice of the site of ligation is greatly facilitated by cholangiography. A bile duct of the right segment may sometimes discharge into the left hepatic duct, as observed by us in one case. The presence of such a duct should be detected in order to ligate the left hepatic duct peripherally with respect to the aberrant branch.

Section of the liver. The gallbladder is detached from the liver, as for an antegrade cholecystectomy, leaving only the right lateral aspect adherent to the liver, the peritoneum not being incised at this site. The reference points of the main fissure are detected: the fundus of the cystic fossa and dorsally, the confluence of the left hepatic vein with the vena cava. The liver is incised along the main fissure in a ventrodorsal direction (Fig. 214). The incision should be made slightly to the left of the fissure so as not to injure the sagittal vein. The liver is

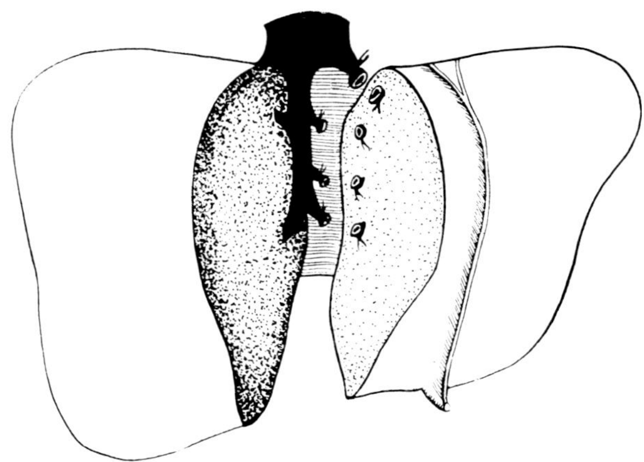

Fig. 214. — Left hepatectomy. The left branches of the sagittal vein and left hepatic vein have been ligated and severed.

drawn downwards, and the falciform ligament covering the angle between the liver and vena cava is transected. Between the liver and the vena cava there is a space filled with lax connective tissue, delimited laterally by the right and left hepatic veins. This gives a precise indication and facilitates incision of the liver in this dangerous area. Ventrodorsal transection almost up to the level of the hilus intercepts the main left branch of the sagittal vein, which should be ligated and divided. In order to continue the incision dorsally so as to mobilize the left hepatic lobe to a greater extent, the left hepatic duct and hilar plate are divided between ligatures, detaching the duct together with the hilar plate from the underlying liver tissue, as much as possible laterally and to the left. The two halves of the liver are drawn aside and incision of the main fissure is continued dorsally, ligating the left branches of the sagittal vein, which lies below the cut surface, covered by a thin layer or hepatic tissue.

Ligation of the hepatic veins. The left half of the liver is rotated upward, incising the peritoneum that descends from the caudate lobe upon the posterior abdominal wall. The accessory hepatic veins that supply the caudate lobe and discharge into the vena cava are severed. Finally the left hepatic vein is ligated and severed 1—2 cm before it joins the sagittal vein. When the vein is very short, it may be ligated together with a fragment of surrounding liver tissue.

The cut hepatic surface is controlled in order to ligate any open blood vessels or bile ducts and is then covered with omentum. Drainage with a rubber tube; suture of the abdominal wall.

LEFT HEPATECTOMY BY FISSURAL APPROACH

The technique of this variation resembles that of right hepatectomy by fissural approach. The liver is transected between two rows of interlocking deep sutures placed to the left of the main fissure so as not to damage the confluence of the two main branches of the sagittal vein at ist origin and the trunk of the vein itself. The portal pedicle and left hepatic vein are ligated separately after opening the fissure.

We have carried out left hepatectomy by fissural approach without previous transfixing ligatures, starting by ligation of the left hepatic vein, then dividing the liver along the left side of the sagittal vein and finally ligated Glisson's pedicle *en masse* or after previous dissection.

LEFT SUBTOTAL HEPATECTOMY

This is actually a left lobectomy, total left hepatectomy being very rarely performed. It is easier because the hepatic vessels and duct can be ligated laterally in a less dangerous area. Moreover, as the caudate lobe is not removed, it is no longer necessary to ligate the accessory hepatic veins.

The left branch of the vena porta is ligated and divided a little before the emergence of the left lateral vein and its ventral curve known under the name of *recessus umbilicalis*. The left hepatic duct and artery are likewise ligated more laterally than in total left hepatectomy. Left subtotal hepatectomy is a type of resection in which the whole vasculobiliary pedicle can be caught up in a Deschamps needle and ligated extracapsularly close to the left sagittal fissure. As the pedicle is ligated on the left border of the quadrate lobe and the hepatic incision following the fissural cleavage plane falls on the right border, the liver must be detached from the hilar plate that covers the vessels, from the lateral bifurcation leftwards up to the ligated and severed vessels. Several arterial branches and bile ducts belonging to the quadrate lobe must be ligated during this process. On the inferior aspect of the liver the incision skirts the left caudate lobe passing through the groove of the duct of Arantius.

The procedure is then the same as in left total hepatectomy.

PLANNED LEFT LOBECTOMY

Mobilization of the left lobe. The affected parts are examined in order to establish whether a left lobectomy is sufficient. The round ligament is severed, then the falciform ligament along its diaphragmatic attachment. The right and left folds of the posterior triangular expansion of the falciform ligament are incised almost up to the vena cava. The left triangular ligament is then incised along the midline so as to avoid injuring the left hepatic vein.

Ligation of the portal pedicles. The left lobe is supplied by two afferent pedicles, to which is added a segmentary bile branch. The ventral pedicle belongs to segment III of Couinaud's nomenclature, and the dorsal pedicle to segment II. The pedicle of segment III is formed of one or several veins that arise from the left horn of the umbilical recess, together with an arterial and a biliary branch that follow the same pathway. The pedicle of segment II is formed of the left lateral vein that arises from the bend of the left branch of the portal vein and courses ventrally under the name of *recessus umbilicalis;* to this is added an arterial and a biliary branch following the same course. All the vessels and bile ducts that form these pedicles run transversely to the left of the umbilical recess. Viewed from the

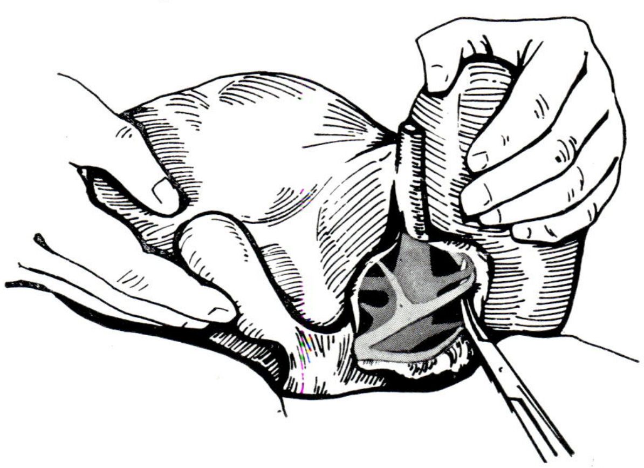

Fig. 215. — Left lobectomy. Isolation of the components of the portal pedicle of the left lobe.

underside of the liver, the most superficial component is the venous branch, then the artery and the bile duct. This is moreover, the general intrahepatic distribution of the vasculobiliary branches. In order to ligate the pedicles (Fig. 215) the hepatic end of the incised round ligament is pulled anteriorly and upward with the forceps and the visceral peritoneum is incised on the inferior aspect of the liver, to the left of the ligament. The round ligament must be detached with the greatest care not to injure the umbilical recess. It is easier to avoid the latter when Glisson's capsule is not opened. The ligament is now drawn anteriorly to the right and slightly upward, exposing the pedicle of segment III which is ligated together with the surrounding hepatic tissue on the left side of the left sagittal fissure. The same procedure is used for the pedicle of segment II which also lies in the left sagittal fissure 2—3 cm posterior to the pedicle of segment III. Each component should be ligated separately if possible.

Section of the liver. The secondary fissure is opened ventrodorsally, the incision passing 1 cm to the left of the insertion of the falciform ligament and inferiorly, to the left of the left sagittal fissure. The section must be done meticulously, with particular attention to the posterior border of the lobe so as not to open the left hepatic vein.

Ligation of the left hepatic vein. The incised lobe is retracted to the left in order to expose the left hepatic vein. When possible, it is separated from the hepatic tissue over a short portion, sufficient to divide it between suture ligatures; if it is too short it can be ligated by deep sutures, leaving the stump surrounded by a small portion of liver tissue (Fig. 216).

The bile ducts and vessels that still remain open on the cut surface are clamped and ligated. The raw area is covered by suturing the peritoneum of the falciform ligament to the inferior margin of the liver section (the falciform ligament is transected across its attachment to the diaphragm, its hepatic attachment remaining intact). Drainage with a rubber tube. Suture of the abdominal wall.

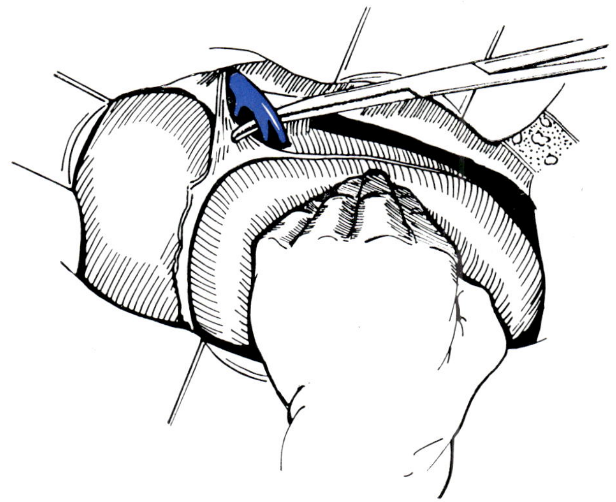

Fig. 216. — Left lobectomy. Dissection of the left hepatic vein.

If the undersurface of the liver is deformed by a pathologic process and the biliovascular pedicles are not accessible, they can be approached by the fissural route. The liver can be resected under control of manual hemostasis. When the incision reaches the upper part of the pedicles, these are detached from the liver laterally to the left, ligated with nonabsorbable sutures and severed. The posterior secondary fissure is then opened up to the left hepatic vein that is ligated and sectioned.

SEGMENTARY RESECTIONS

Controlled resection of the left lateral ventral segment or segment III according to Couinaud's nomenclature probably is the only possible controlled segmentectomy at present. Theoretically, it ought to be possible to excise by planned technique segments I, IV, V and VI. Actually, resection of the caudate lobe (segment I) is so difficult that its utility is far exceeded by the hazard of the operation. It is difficult to imagine a pathologic process strictly limited to the caudate lobe. The afferent pedicle of the left hepatic region is dissected in order to ligate the posterior branches of the left hepatic duct, left hepatic artery and left branch of the portal vein, as well as the numerous efferent hepatic veins that discharge into the inferior vena cava, without opening the main fissure. For these reasons excision of the caudate lobe has not been practiced in the clinic to date.

Couinaud asserts that resection of segment II is theoretically possible but he does not see its utility. In our opinion, resection of segment II is contraindicated by the principles of planned resections, the plane that separates segment II from segment III being crossed by the branches of the left hepatic vein which drain segment III.

Planned excision of segments IV, V and VI is theoretically possible but very difficult in practice. Planned resection can be successfully supplanted by non-anatomic hepatectomies, whose technique is less dangerous and more readily performed. Indeed, it is not only difficult but very risky to dissect the hepatic hilus and identify the segmentary branches. There is a constant risk of hemorrhage and injury to the main territorial branches.

The dorsal segments VII and VIII cannot be resected separately, either anatomically or non-anatomically. Any section passing through the portal fissures that separates them from the neighboring segments interrupts the efferent circulation of the ventral segements V and VI. However, bisegmentectomy VII and VIII or V and VI have been performed by some surgeons.

Controlled resection of segment III. This excision is comparatively readily performed and is used either in the presence of a limited pathologic process, or in order to expose the segmentary bile duct and anastomose it to the stomach or jejunum for retrograde biliodigestive drainage. The cleavage plane that separates segment III and IV forms part of the ventral half of the secondary fissure and lies in an oblique ventrocaudal direction. Hence a larger part of segment III is to be found on the diaphragmatic aspect of the liver, segment IV lying on the undersurface. The operation begins by a xyphoumbilical laparotomy. The round ligament is severed, then the falciform ligament along its attachment to the diaphragm. It is not necessary to section the falciform ligament up to the dangerous zone of the vena cava, as in left lobectomy.

Ligation of the afferent pedicle. The liver is exteriorized in the wound, by traction of the round ligament anteriorly and upward. The visceral peritoneum is incised to the left of the left sagittal fissure, along the round ligament, which is dissected up to the umbilical recess, without opening Glisson's capsule that envelops it. The round ligament is then retracted to the right for traction of the afferent pedicle of segment III formed of one or several portal branches that arise from the left horn of the umbilical recess, a segmentary arterial branch and bile duct, enveloped in Glisson's capsule. The pedicle can be ligated altogether extracapsularly passing the nonabsorbable suture around the pedicle with a Deschamps needle. The pedicle components can also be dissected intracapsularly and ligated separately. The most superficial on the undersurface of the liver are the venous branches, usually two, and deeper down is the segmentary artery and then the bile duct.

Section of the liver. Modification of the color that appears after ligation of the afferent pedicle is a valuable indication for delimitation of segment III and

IV. The liver is sectioned along the secondary fissure. On the lower aspect the section should not exceed posteriorly the pedicle of segment III by more than 2 cm since segment II might be injured. A frontal section is then cut obliquely forward and downward along the cleavage plane that separates segments III and II. The branches of the left hepatic vein draining segment III that appear on the cut hepatic surface, are ligated. The sagittal part of the sectioned surface is covered with the peritoneum of the falciform ligament, which is reflected downward and sutured to the lower border of the cut surface; the frontal portion is covered with the peritoneum of the omentum. Drainage with rubber tube. Suture of the abdominal wall.

NON-ANATOMIC HEPATECTOMIES

From the moment in which planned hepatectomies were defined theoretically and applied, the hepatectomy procedures used until then were considered non-anatomic. The erroneous opinion arose that in contrast to controlled resections, non-anatomic hepatectomies are only performed *sur demande* without keeping account of the intrahepatic distribution of the vascular and biliary branches. Along general lines, non-anatomic resections in the past complied with the knowledge of the times on the afferent and efferent circulation of the liver. The main danger zones were well known. The hepatic section could not lead to the intersection with the hilus or to the right or left branches of the bifurcation of the afferent pedicle. Section posterior to the hilus, where the large trunks of the hepatic veins might be intercepted, was likewise considered dangerous.

Today these areas are much better known, and the structural plan of the liver gives anatomic reference points that are readily detected. In addition, intraoperative cholangiography and portal phlebography have greatly modified our concept on non-anatomic hepatectomies (Fig. 217).

As a matter of fact, non-anatomic hepatectomy is just as well planned anatomically as a controlled hepatectomy, when the integrity of the liver circulation is complied with. The difference consists in a technical detail: separate isolation and ligation of the vascular pedicles of the portion to be resected, which is characteristic of anatomic resections, superior from this point of view, but only in certain circumstances but not in excision of the left lobe when many surgeons prefer the non-anatomic technique. The ventral half of the liver, anterior to the frontal cleavage plane that passes through the hilus, is much more readily accessible to non-anatomic resections. In benign lesions of the ventral segments, a controlled segmentectomy is seldom feasible, but it would be a tactical mistake to prefer a right or left hepatectomy, with useless sacrifice of liver tissue, to a non-anatomic resection.

With regard to the danger zones of hepatic excisions, their importance appears to have been exaggerated, not so much by surgeons with a vast clinical experience as by specialists in the anatomy of the liver. Actually the distribution of the intrahepatic vessels and bile ducts is extremely complex and exhibits so many anatomic variants and pathologic alterations that it is impossible to excise portions of the liver without injuring more or less the vessels of the neighboring regions. The true danger zone of non-anatomic hepatectomies is the whole of the hilus (in the transverse fissure on the undersurface of the liver). Deaths from hepatic coma have been attributed to necrosis of the liver when the danger zone has been exceeded without a serious anatomic checking. Bearing in mind the anatomic bases of hepatic vascularity, the following non-anatomic hepatectomies should be avoided:

1. Any wedge resection in the dorsal half of the liver.

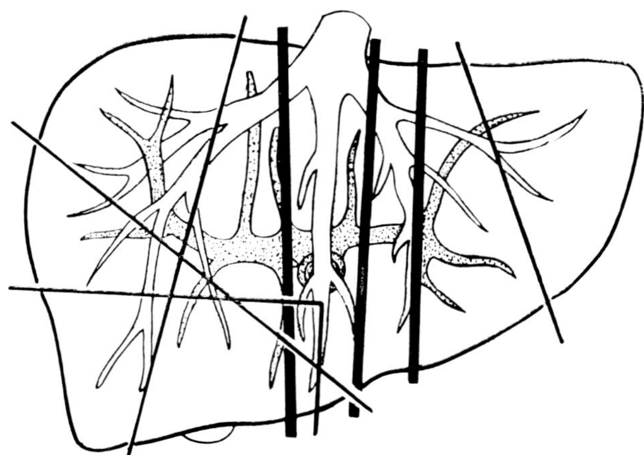

Fig. 217. — Schematic representation of the hepatic section planes. Full lines show the approximate lines of the main anatomic hepatectomies. The thin lines show some feasible non-anatomic resections (from K. Stucke after C. Popescu).

2. Wedge resections on the anterior half of the liver if they approach the hilus too much.

3. Wedge resection with the tip towards the umbilical recess (Fig. 218). The ventral extension of the left branch of the portal vein, together with the artery and biliary duct that accompany it, should be considered as a prolongation of the hepatic hilus and treated as such. Injury of the umbilical recess imposes resection of segments III and IV, which represent almost a quarter of the liver.

The following three categories of non-anatomic resections can be performed:

1. *Wedge resections* including the ventral aspect of the liver, and leaving intact the hilus and umbilical recess.

2. *Non-anatomic hepatectomies* of the undersurface of the liver, with a frontal and sagittal section plane. The frontal plane must leave the hilus intact. Peroperative cholangiography and portal phlebography will help to delimit this area more precisely. A large part of segments IV, V and VI together with the gallbladder can be excised *en bloc*. In this case the sagittal section should be carried out on the right side of the umbilical recess so as to severe only the right branches distributed to the quadrate lobe. Similarly, part of segment III and IV can be resected *en bloc*, the frontal section intercepting the umbilical recess; the sagittal section should be carried out on the left flank of the gallbladder. When necessary, the frontal section may be continued posteriorly in order to perform a wider marginal excision.

3. Non-anatomic hepatectomies with a *sagittal section* (hepatic "guillotine" resection). The prototype of this resection is total or subtotal left non-anatomic lobectomy. The liver is sectioned about 2 cm to the left of the falciform ligament, along a barrier of deep interlocking ligatures that include both the afferent and the efferent pedicles. Right non-anatomic hepatectomies can likewise be performed. A. Brunschwig used the non-anatomic technique in 7 of the 11 right hepatectomies performed until 1955.

The route of access in non-anatomic hepatectomies should be adapted to the site and volume of the part to be excised. In wedge-shaped anterior marginal

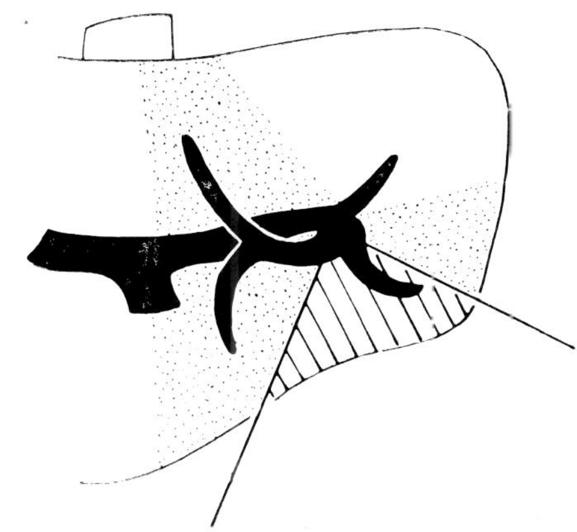

Fig. 218. — Ramification of the umbilical recess. Hatched area represents wedge resection of segment III. If due to a technical mistake the resection advances too much towards the recessus, the branches that supply the left lobe can be ligated distal to the resected part (dotted area) (after Reifferscheid).

resections, the Sprengel incision gives satisfactory access. When the resection includes large portions, as in left non-anatomic lobectomy or right non-anatomic hepatectomy, the incisions corresponding to the planned techniques can be prolonged: thoracophrenolaparotomy for right hepatectomy, Sprengel's incision continued to the left for left lobectomy, with or without a midline incision towards the xyphoid.

The section plane depends upon the nature of the lesion: it passes closer to the lesion when it is benign and distally when it is malignant, at the same time complying with the safety limits around the hilus. The scalpel or cautery is used under the protection of deep interlocking sutures previously passed along the section plane at about 1 cm distance. The way in which the catgut is tied depends upon the fragility of the liver tissue and the importance of the ligated vessels. When the hepatic tissue is friable and is criss-crossed by large vessels, the procedure of Kuznetzov and Penski or of Auvray is used, completing hemostasis by direct ligation of the vessels on the cut surface and by adjuvant hemostatics. When smaller portions are resected and the liver tissue has a normal or increased consistency separate ligatures with thick catgut can be used, as they do not cut through the tissue.

After wedge-shaped resections, the two sectioned surfaces are brought together and sutured with thick catgut. When the angle between the two sectioned surfaces is very broad and the surfaces cannot be brought in contact, they are covered with omentum. Simple, sagittal sections are likewise covered with omentum, or with the falciform ligament after left lobectomy, as in planned resections.

Drainage is necessary in extended resections which might predispose to postoperative hemorrhage or bile discharge, but is not applied in limited resections when good hemostasis has been obtained.

RESECTIONS OF THE LIVER IN CANCER OF THE GALLBLADDER

Cholecystohepatectomies *en bloc* are only indicated when the afferent hepatic pedicle is not invaded by the neoplastic process, therefore when the patient is anicteric. When the extrahepatic bile ducts are invaded, the operation — retrograde drainage of the bile into the gastrointestinal tract — is palliative. When the extrahepatic bile ducts are not invaded, the type of cholecystohepatic resection depends upon the extent of the liver lesions.

Cholecystectomy and wedge hepatectomy en bloc are indicated when the liver does not show signs of spread of the tumor process, or when the latter is limited. In the latter case the cystic duct is dissected and severed between two ligatures; the cystic vessels are then ligated and severed. By palpation or dissection of the hepatic hilus the point up to which the wedge resection can advance, without exceeding safety limits, is determined. Previous cholangiography may outline the topography of the hilus more precisely in order to avoid damaging the large vessels and their branches. Once the most advanced point of the resection is established, two thick catgut sutures are passed with a round tipped needle from the under to the upper surface of the liver. Two series of ligatures are then passed to the right and left of the gallbladder and as far as necessary from it, according to the procedure of Bălăcescu or A. Jianu. The gallbladder is resected *en bloc* with the underlying hepatic tissue between these ligatures. The two surfaces are approximated with several suture points or peritonealized with omentum.

Cholecystectomy and rectangular hepatectomy en bloc. When the neoplastic process extends very much to the right and left of the gallbladder, a broader hepatic resection is necessary, including the anterior segments, with the exception of segment III. After ligating and severing the cystic duct and cystic vessels, the anatomic formations of the hilus are exposed in order not to damage them, then a frontal barrier of sutures are passed from the right extremity of the liver up to 2 cm to the right of the left sagittal fissure. Here the line of the ligatures runs at right angle in a ventral direction. The gallbladder is excised together with the prehilar area of the quadrate lobe and segments V and VI. The sectioned surface is covered with omentum. Drainage.

Extended right hepatectomy performed by Pack, Miller and Brasfield has not proved useful in cancer of the gallbladder. The hazards are too great for a disease whose prospects are so little encouraging. It is more logical to perform a cholecystectomy with resection of the right and left paramedian segments. This is likewise risky and is still under study.

HEPATECTOMY IN GASTRIC CANCER EXTENDING TO THE LIVER

In many cases contiguous spread of a gastric cancer to the liver is not so extensive as to render impossible hepatogastric resection *en bloc*. As a rule the resection is contraindicated for other reasons: metastases, massive invasion of the lymph nodes, etc. Hepatogastric resection begins by dissecting the lesser and greater curvatures of the stomach, leaving intact, however, the continuity of the gastrohepatic tumor on the lesser curvature. The duodenum, then the stomach is incised as close as possible to the cardia. The stomach, being clamped at its extremity, still adheres to the liver. A barrier of deep sutures is passed in the liver beyond the macroscopic limits of the tumor, along a semicircular or semi-elliptic line. The liver is then resected together with the stomach. The gastro-intestinal continuity is reestablished.

DRAINAGE HEPATECTOMIES

Retrograde biliodigestive drainage is indicated in obstructive jaundice produced by congenital atrophy of the extrahepatic bile ducts, extensive stenosing sclerous cholangitis and neoplasm of the extrahepatic bile ducts when the pathologic process advances so much towards the hilus that any common biliodigestive anastomosis is impossible. Drainage hepatectomy has only a palliative role in cancer of the extrahepatic ducts. Although it is not an easy operation, it is more readily performed than the difficult dissection of the liver hilus in order to expose and anastomose one of the hepatic ducts to the intestine. The patency of the bile ducts at their confluence, one of the main conditions for a successful drainage hepatectomy, can be tested by intraoperative transhepatic cholangiography, when the hilus is inaccessible. The contrast substance is introduced by puncture of a bile duct in the left hepatic region. When the hepatic ducts are blocked at their confluence, a transhepatic cholangiography in the right hepatic region would expose it to a more or less accentuated inflammation of the bile tree due to the prolonged irritative action of the contrast substance that cannot be evacuated. Obstruction of the confluence of the hepatic ducts raises the question of biliary decompression of both regions, which is extremely difficult. As a rule only retrograde biliodigestive drainage of the left region is done, since the latter is more accessible. Drainage of both regions has been carried out by Longmire and by others in several cases. Bile stasis in the right hepatic region is partly compensated by the left region when the lesions are not too advanced. Cholangiography offers the advantage of visualization of the confluence of the hepatic ducts and of the bile ducts in the left lobe, which is of direct interest for drainage hepatectomy. The most accessible and dilated bile duct will be chosen.

The first attempts at transhepatic biliary drainage were made by Th. Kocher in 1882 and L. Langenbuch in 1886, who performed hepatostomies and hepatocholangiostomies, resecting a small portion of the left lobe and fixing it to the abdominal wall. This external drainage often failed because the cicatrix of the hepatoabdominal wound closed the external bile fistula. On the other hand, when the operation was successful and elimination of the bile satisfactory, the patient's condition improved but only for a short time, because the severe disturbances of constant bile losses appeared.

Drainage of the intrahepatic bile ducts into the gastrointestinal tract was practiced for the first time by Baudouin in 1897; he created a cavity in the left lobe of the liver which he anastomosed to the intestine *(hepatocholangioenterostomy)*. In 1909, at the Xth Congress of Russian surgeons and in a paper published in 1914, Alexandrov discussed the results obtained after seven such operations. Six of the patients died within a few days or months of the operation and one, operated by Garré, was still alive after 3 and a half years.

H. Kehr performed a hepatocholangioduodenostomy according to a similar procedure: after wedge resection of the anterior aspect of the left lobe he formed a cavity in the liver which he anastomosed to the duodenum. The icteric patient recovered his normal colouring but died 4 months after the operation. Kehr was probably the first to perform a *hepatogastrostomy* with retrograde drainage of the bile according to a procedure similar to that of hepatocholangioduodenostomy. He operated three patients successfully, one of whom followed up for more than 2 years. This type of operation was also used by Kocher and Chiari at that period.

In 1934, Gohrbandt of Berlin communicated a personal procedure of biliodigestive anastomosis. In 1932 he operated a colleague suffering from cancer of the extrahepatic bile ducts. On the liver surface he found a dilated bile duct, due to stasis. He anastomosed it to the stomach along a thin rubber tube. Later, in 1953 and 1957 Gohrbandt described a very difficult technique for *hepatogastrostomy*. In 1957, R. Jelinek of Vienna simplified this technique, applying only two suture layers between the liver and stomach.

In general, four different types of drainage hepatectomies are performed today:

1. Anastomosis of a dilated bile duct from the cut hepatic surface to the jejunum, i.e. intrahepatic cholangiojejunostomy (Longmire's procedure).
2. Dogliotti's operation, i.e. intrahepatic gastroductostomy, or anastomosis of a bile duct of segment II to the stomach after a non-anatomic resection of this segment.
3. Anastomosis of a hepatic sectioned surface, opening the duct of segment III to the stomach (Făgărăşanu procedure).
4. The idea of using the duct of segment III was taken up again by Soupault and Couinaud, who anastomosed this duct to a Roux-Y jejunal loop.

LONGMIRE'S PROCEDURE

A description of intrahepatic cholangiojejunostomy was first published by W.P. Longmire and M.C. Sandford in 1948. After an inverted V subcostal incision, the left lobe of the liver is freed from adhesions resulting from a possible previous operation and the left triangular ligament is sectioned. In the middle third of the left lobe, a ventrodorsal sagittal section is cut, controlling the hemorrhage by manual compression and U-ligatures. The transection is continued dorsally until a thick, dense chord is encountered in the hepatic parenchyma, marking the presence of a voluminous bile duct. The bile duct, dilated due to stasis, is dissected laterally, then severed leaving a 1 cm stump on the cut surface. Transection is then continued sagittaly in order to excise the lateral half of the lobe. If a more dilated bile duct is again encountered, it will be used for anastomosis and the stump of the first duct ligated. Hemostasis of the sectioned hepatic surface is done directly or by U-sutures. A Roux-Y jejunal loop is prepared, sufficiently long to bring it precolically up to the sectioned liver surface. The apex of the loop is ligated and invaginated, then the jejunum is anastomosed end-to-side to the bile duct, which is approximated laterally to the transectioned surface. The hepatic surface is covered with the jejunal loop whose peritoneal serosa is sutured to the liver, following the

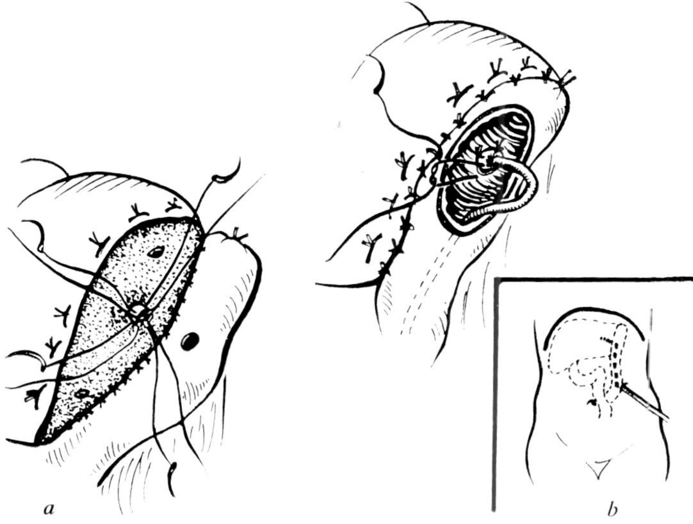

Fig. 219 *a* and *b*. — Longmire's intrahepatic cholangiojejunostomy. After excision of part of the left lobe, a large, dilated bile duct is isolated and anastomosed end-to-side to a Roux-Y jejunal loop. A drainage tube introduced through the jejunal anastomosis is exteriorized through the abdominal wall (after Flabeau).

contour of the raw section as close as possible. Drainage, suture to the abdominal wall.

After publication of Longmire's technique, it was modified by several surgeons: the sectioned hepatic surface was covered with resorbable fibrin sponge, or an end-to-end anastomosis was prefered (R.J. Baron and T. Yamashita, M.A. Andrade and R.M. Sibon). M. Reifferschied performed an end-to-side anastomosis of the bile duct to a double precolic jejunal loop. A side-to-side anastomosis of the Braun type, at the foot of the loop has likewise been recommended. Other surgeons have used the transmesocolic loop. A polyethylene T-tube is introduced, with one limb in the bile duct and the other in the jejunum. The vertical limb of the T is exteriorized through the jejunum and abdominal wall, like a Völker tube (Fig. 219 *a* and *b*).

DOGLIOTTI'S PROCEDURE

Intrahepatic ductogastrostomy was performed for the first time by A.M. Dogliotti in 1946 and published in 1949. The principle is the same as in Longmire's operation but another technique is used. After isolating the left lobe by transection of the triangular ligament, an assistant compresses the base of the lobe manually and the surgeon incises the liver with a scalpel along a sagittal plane, excising half or two thirds of the lobe. The larger vessels are clamped separately and ligated with silk sutures. Capillary hemorrhage is controlled by U-sutures. The dilated bile duct found in the center of the section is dissected

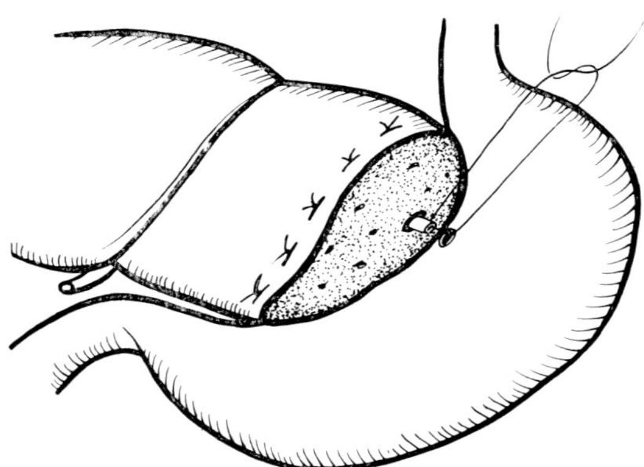

Fig. 220. — Dogliotti's intrahepatic ductogastrostomy. The first suture is placed for anastomosing the bile duct to the stomach. Hemostasis of the sectioned liver surface has been done with U-sutures and direct ligatures.

along 2 cm. End-to-side anastomosis with the stomach is performed where the anterior aspect of the stomach comes in contact with the bile duct, without being mobilized by traction (Fig. 220). The anastomosis is done with a double row of interrupted sutures, the superficial row including the gastric serosa and fibrous coat of the bile duct. The mucosa-to-mucosa approximation must be meticulously performed. Another row of sutures is passed between the stomach and liver along the contour of the transectioned surface, both for peritonealization and for a better protection of the anastomosis. Until 1954, Dogliotti applied this procedure in 6 patients suffering from fibrous stenosis of the common bile duct. There was no bile reflux, cholangitis or stenosis of the anastomosis.

HEPATOCHOLANGIOGASTROSTOMY (FĂGĂRĂŞANU PROCEDURE)

In 1955, at the XVIth Congress of the International Society of Surgeons held in Copenhagen we read a communication on the technique of hepatocholangiogastrostomy *(I. Făgărăşanu, L. Chitlaru, M. Cîrstea, "A propos de l'hépatectomie pour drainage: l'hépatocholangiogastrotomie dans les obstructions néoplasiques ou cicatricielles des voies biliaires; technique personnelle")* Our anatomic, pathologic and cholangiographic investigations showed that the largest, and also the most accessible intrahepatic bile ducts are not to be found towards the extremity of the lobe, but anteriorly, in the immediate vicinity of the round ligament. The left lobe has not a central bile collector duct but only one or two ducts for each segment. On resecting segment III, we generally discovered one or two ducts dilated by biliary stasis, located on the inferior aspect of the liver (Fig. 221).

For a hepatocholangiogastrostomy, segment III is excised according to the technique described. Total segmentectomy is not necessary and hence the section does not follow the cleavage plane between segment II and III very strictly. A wedge-shaped

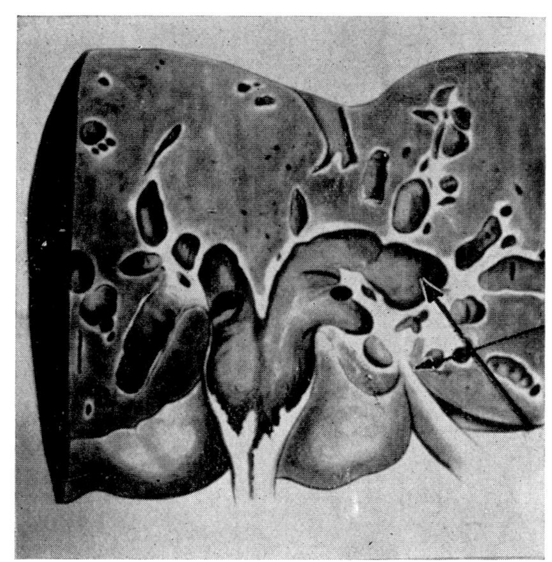

Fig. 221. — Section through the liver after prolonged obstruction of the bile ducts (laboratory specimen). Note dilated bile ducts.

or rectangular resection of segment III is sufficient, exceeding the segmentary biliovascular pedicle. Hemostasis is done by clamping and ligating the vessels separately on the cut hepatic surface, without U-sutures. A large amount of bile is discharged through the dilated bile duct or ducts. A polyethylene catheter is introduced in one of the bile ducts and cholangiography is performed in order to checkthe patency of the confluence of the hepatic ducts. The entire sectioned hepatic surface is anastomosed to the stomach, on the anterior aspect of the lesser curvature, close to the antrum, where the wall is incised lengthwise over a distance corresponding to the hepatic raw surface (Fig. 222). Anastomosis is done in a single layer, strengthened dorsally by the posterior parietal peritoneum, or the lesser omentum when it is not too friable. Anteriorly, the anastomosis is consolidated with the round and the falciform ligaments, previously transected (Fig. 223). Rubber drainage tube. Suture of the abdominal wall.

Technically, the operation is not difficult. Bleeding can be readily controlled. Particular attention should be paid to suture of the posterior aspect of the anastomosis. When the hepatic tissue is friable, two layers of interrupted sutures are necessary, tied sufficiently close, without however tearing the liver. The falciform and round ligaments, reflected along the anastomosis, likewise strengthen it.

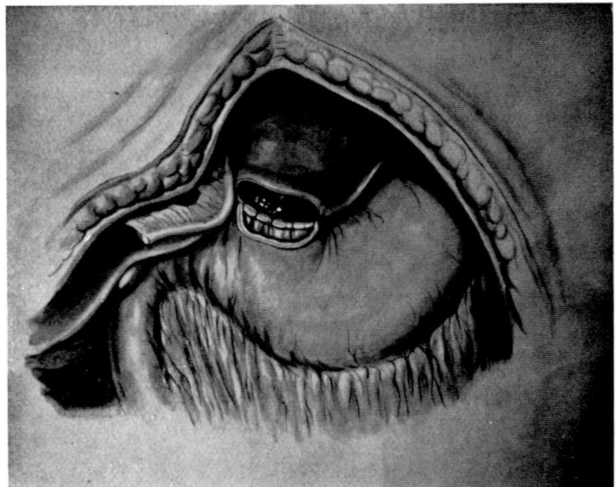

Fig. 222. — Hepatocholangiogastrostomy, Făgărăşanu procedure. After resection of segment III the raw liver surface is anastomosed to the stomach.

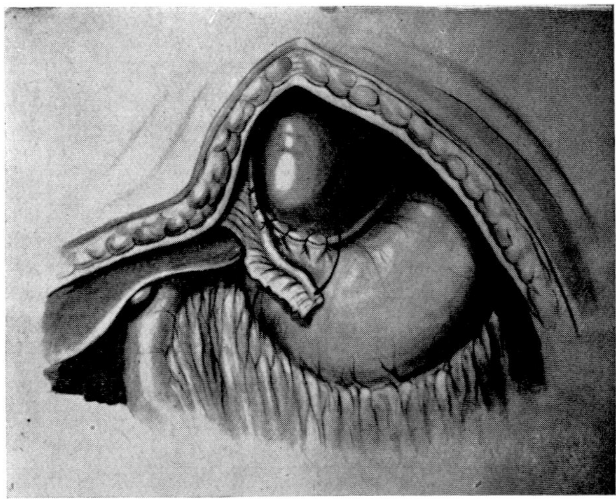

Fig. 223. — Hepatocholangiogastrostomy. The anterior aspect of the anastomosis is consolidated with the help of the round ligament.

INTRAOPERATIVE ACCIDENTS

Hemorrhage is the most feared accident in the course of hepatectomy. In the order of gravity, bleeding may occur from the incised hepatic surface, from the hilus, from the hepatic veins and from the vena cava. In spite of the measures taken (see the chapter on hemostasis) large amounts of blood may be lost and must be replaced by transfusions. Most operative deaths are caused by hemorrhage from the hepatic veins, which are very difficult to arrest because the veins lie so deep in the hepatic tissue.

Operative shock has multiple causes, common to all large operations. To these are added specific causes: clamping of the hepatic pedicle and vena cava; traction of the liver with partial or total arrest of the inferior cava circulation; sudden decompression of the vena cava by removal of tumor compressing it. In severe cases, shock may be followed by cardiac arrest.

Technical errors in applying the ligatures. In the course of right or left hepatectomies, the main bile ducts and vessels of the remaining hepatic region may be ligated by mistake, which is equivalent with a total hepatectomy. In left hepatectomy, the anatomy of the cleavage plane of the main fissure should always be borne in mind; on the undersurface of the liver it falls upon the bifurcation or a little to the right upon the pedicle of the right hepatic region. Therefore, transection continued along the fissure would be a fatal mistake.

In the course of wedge-shaped non-anatomic hepatectomies, the large biliary or vascular trunks, situated in the region of the hilus may be injured. When observed in the course of the operation it raises the question of resection of the portion of the liver supplied by the injured pedicle. The extent of the jeopardized area can be determined by dissection of the hilus, change in the color of the hepatic tissue and cholangiography. The surgeon must assume the responsibility of extending the operation to a hemihepatectomy in case of injury to the afferent pedicle of a whole hepatic territory.

Air embolism is a very rare accident. After the cases of Hochenegg and Israel we found no mention in the literature of such accidents.

POSTOPERATIVE CARE

After hepatectomy the patients must be looked after the same as following any severe intervention, bearing in mind the character of the operation and eventual injury of the residual liver. Apart from maintenance of the biologic constants within the limits of an acceptable equilibrium, it is necessary to keep account of the following factors, of particular importance in the postoperative care of hepatectomized patients:

The administration of antibiotics is obligatory after hepatic resections. However meticulously the technique is planned, there remain more or less devitalized portions of liver that risk necrosis and secondary infection. Antibiotics appear to have not only an antimicrobial action but also a neutralizing effect upon necrosing enzymes (Egers).

Morphine and its derivatives are strictly forbidden after hepatectomy since their spastic effect upon Oddi's sphincter produces hypertension in the biliary tree, increasing the risk of bile discharge and biliary fistula. Morphine can only be administered in case of external biliary drainage.

After hepatic resection, especially extended resection, the patients should be given as soon as possible a diet rich in proteins and carbohydrates and very poor in lipids in order to favor regeneration of the liver. The vitamin supply should not be neglected.

Some patients with a severe postoperative course were saved by the administration of cortisone (G.T. Pack and A.H. Islami). Cortisone is indicated in the patients threatened by hepatic coma.

POSTOPERATIVE COMPLICATIONS

Secondary hemorrhage and discharge of bile through the drainage tube: pseudocapillary hemorrhage and the discharge of bile from the small bile ducts are not excessive, last one or two days and stop spontaneously. Almost all patients lose small amounts of blood or bile through the drainage tube. However, when large amounts are discharged through the tube one must operate again in order to ligate the large vessels or bile ducts that were not ligated or off which the ligature slipped.

Shock. Except for the general causes of operative shock there appear to be certain specific causes in hepatic resections. According to Friedman et al. and Seneviratne, a greater or lesser degree of hypotension develops, probably due to vasoconstriction of the sinusoids and decrease of the blood flow through the liver, resulting in hypoxia and damage of the liver cell and shock that is often irreversible. Reifferscheid recommends a treatment with perfusions with glucose serum, hydrocortisone, sympathomimetics, vitamins B and C.

Jaundice. After extended hepatectomies, the intrahepatic branches of the portal vein, overcharged with the excessive blood supply that passes through the reduced liver, compress the neighboring bile branches producing temporary intrahepatic bile stasis. When the residual liver adapts itself to the new circulation conditions, the jaundice disappears.

Severe jaundice is caused by extensive hepatic necrosis, faulty ligation of the blood vessels and bile ducts of the remaining liver or thrombosis of the hepatic veins. The Budd-Chiari syndrome, produced by thrombosis of the hepatic veins may be avoided when in the course of a planned hepatectomy these veins are not injured or no denuded vein is left on the surface of the sectioned hepatic surface. In right and left hepatectomy, the sagittal vein must always remain covered by a thin layer of hepatic tissue.

Hepatic coma appears at the end of a severe jaundice, sometimes due to aggravation of the functional failure of the remaining hepatic tissue, that was already affected before the operation.

Progressive hepatorenal failure usually ends in death of the patient 10 to 14 days after the operation. Before the onset of uremic coma, the clinical picture is characterized by nausea, vomiting, subcutaneous and digestive hemorrhage. A treatment with levulose perfusions, injections with hydrocortisone, adrenocortical extracts, vitamin E, liver extracts, etc. has been recommended.

Thrombosis of the portal vein is characterized by abdominal distension, ascites and splenomegaly. According to Ton That Tung these signs appear too late to be able to start efficient treatment. This author does not hesitate to administer heparin as soon as the patient's temperature rises after the operation.

Septic complications. Zones of tissue necrosis may develop along the deep interlocking sutures, starting from the sectioned hepatic surface towards the hepatic parenchyma. When drainage is deficient and an infection develops not controlled by antibiotics, abscesses and prolonged suppuration of the hepatic recess may occur.

Biliary fistulas. The small intrahepatic bile ducts that remain open close spontaneously a few days after the operation. Discharge of the bile through the drainage tubes may sometimes be prolonged and the patient remains with an external bile fistula. These fistulas which close very difficultly and through which large amounts of bile are discharged, is generally caused by the slipping of a ligature off a large hepatic duct.

The increased pressure in the intra- and extrahepatic bile ducts, due to a mechanical or dynamic obstruction at the level of Oddi's sphincter, favors the development of biliary fistulas after hepatectomies. Hence, many surgeons consider it necessary to drain the common bile duct by a T-tube. We believe it necessary but not obligatory. The necessity of draining derives from the presence of an obstruction in the extrahepatic bile ducts, made evident by biliary manometry or cholangiography. The obstacle must be removed (sphincterotomy, choledochotomy according to the case).

RESULTS

The data published in the medical literature generally include small series of hepatectomies or isolated clinical cases. A. Brunschwig gathered about 1000 cases published up to 1955, in which resections for hydatid cyst were included. In the same year, A.V. Melnikov found in the Soviet literature 592 hepatectomies published during the preceding 15 years. According to K. Stucke, up to 1956 there were 1270 hepatic resections published, of which 198 planned hepatectomies (45 right and 153 left). J.L. Lortat-Jacob found only 43 controlled right hepatectomies, simple or extended, published up to the beginning of 1960. Lortat-Jacob appears to be more strict in his definition and probably excluded the operations which did not fully comply with the principles of anatomic resection.

The overall mortality rate according to Melnikov was 7% but is now higher because of the broader indications for resections of the liver. In controlled hepatectomies, the mortality is 10 to 20%, representing the maximum and minimum incidence of different statistics.

K. Stucke in statistics drawn up in 1956 shows that 94 patients suffering from primary carcinoma of the liver were operated; 13 survived for more than 3 years and 3 for 5 years; 136 hepatectomies were performed for metastatic cancer of the liver with a survival rate of over 5 years in 5.9% of the cases.

The late results of drainage hepatectomy are not well known. Up to 1956 there were 28 intrahepatic cholangiojejunostomies carried out, of which 9 by

Longmire. Dogliotti performed 6 intrahepatogastroductostomies up to 1954. In general, it is considered that intrahepatic biliodigestive anastomoses predispose to stenoses more than those of the extrahepatic bile ducts. However, they cannot be compared since intrahepatic anastomoses are only performed when the extrahepatic ones are not feasible. The few data available in the literature show that after drainage hepatectomies, the biliodigestive fistulas remain patent. R. Jelinek of Vienna performed two necropsies 19 and 50 days after hepatectomy according to the Gohrbandt procedure and found the bile ducts perfectly patent and able to drain the bile into the stomach.

At the XVIth Congress of the International Society of Surgery held in Copenhagen in 1955, the problem of hepatectomies was widely discussed on the basis of rich documentary material of particular statistical interest. Here are some of the results obtained by different authors:

A.V. Melnikov, in the U.S.S.R. performed 592 hepatic resections in the course of 15 years.

Superficial resections	336 (55%)
Wedge-shaped resection	165 (27.5%)
Left lobectomy	81
Massive resection of the right lobe	12
Resection of the quadrate lobe	3
Resection of Spiegel's lobe	5

These resections were indicated in the following cases:

Closed injuries	51
Open injuries	107
Hemangioma	32
Primary cancer of the liver	12
Metastatic cancer	22
Cancer of the gallbladder	7
Gastric ulcer penetrating into the liver and gastric cancer extending to the liver	188
Hydatid cyst of the liver	152
Other diseases	21

The mortality rate in this series was 13.7% (81 patients).

J.L. Lortat-Jacob collected from the literature only 13 right controlled hepatectomies up to 1955 of which 8 were for hydatid cyst and 4 for hepatic tumors. To this series, he added two cases of right non-anatomic hepatectomy, one of R. Soupault and the other a patient of J. Quénu, with a primary carcinoma, who was still alive 11 years and 5 months after the operation.

R.W. Raven reported on a statistics of 818 cases of primary carcinoma of the stomach, colon and rectum treated in the Marsden Hospital of London. Metastases were found in the liver in 176 cases (21.5%). Hepatectomy was considered feasible in 32 cases but was only performed in 4 cases.

V. Pettinari practiced 25 non-anatomic hepatic resections and a planned left lobectomy in 1940, considered to be one of the first operations of this kind. The patient was followed up 17 months after the operation, then was lost to view.

A. Brunschwig presented a personal series of 56 hepatectomies.

Benign tumors	5 cases
Primary malignant tumors	11 cases
Single metastases	14 cases
Multiple metastases	12 cases
Contiguity neoplastic invasion	14 cases

Brunschwig performed 33 wedge-shaped hepatectomies, 12 left lobectomies (1 death) and 11 right lobectomies according to the Lortat-Jacob procedure, but without thoracotomy.

The general mortality rate was 20% (11 cases): 6 of 23 patients (26%) died after lobectomies; 5 of 33 patients (15%) after wedge-shaped resections; 4 patients died in the course of right lobectomy.

R. Bourgeon performed 8 total or partial left hepatectomies and 10 right planned hepatectomies. All the patients suffered from hydatid cyst. Three patients died after right hepatectomy, one due to sudden decompression of the vena cava, after removal of the tumor (acute heart failure due to massive flow of the venous blood). Attention is drawn to the fact that this complication is not specific of hepatectomy and may also occur after the removal of a voluminous hydatid cyst by any method.

At the Memorial Center for Cancer of New York, O. Schweizer and W.S. Holland mention 53 different hepatectomies until 1960 with a mortality rate of 28% (15 deaths). The following were the causes of death:

hemorrhage	5 deaths
hepatorenal failure	5 deaths
peritonitis	2 deaths
ligation of both hepatic pedicles	2 deaths
heart failure	1 death

Our statistics. In the course of 14 years (1953—1966) we performed 48 hepatectomies in the Surgical Clinic of the Dr. Davila Hospital and the Elias Hospital. The first two cases were published in 1956: two left anatomic hepatectomies, one for hydatid cyst, the other for polycystic liver. These were the first operations of this kind published in Romania. In 1958 we published a series of 11 various hepatectomies, to which another 5 were added in 1960. Since then more than double the number of cases were operated. The longest survival after cholecystohepatectomy for neoplasm was of 7 years, and after drainage hepatectomy of one year and three months.

The following types of resection were performed:

Right controlled hepatectomy	4
Left controlled hepatectomy	7
Left controlled lobectomy	3
Resection of segment IV	2
Non-anatomic hepatectomy (4 simple resections; 11 cystoresections; 4 cholecystohepatectomies; 3 gastrohepatectomies)	22
Drainage hepatectomy (hepatocholangiogastrostomy)	10

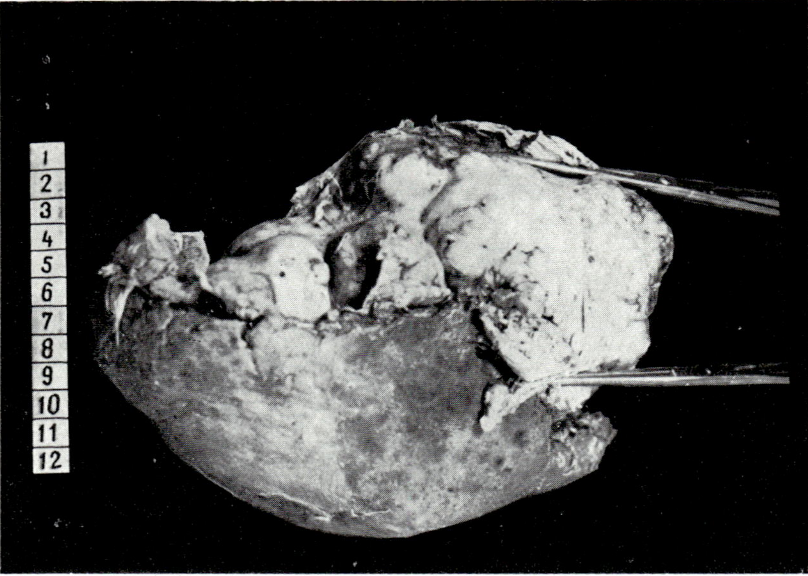

Fig. 224. — Operative specimen: right lobe of the liver with voluminous sarcoma. The patient *C.K.* survived two years and a month after right hepatectomy.

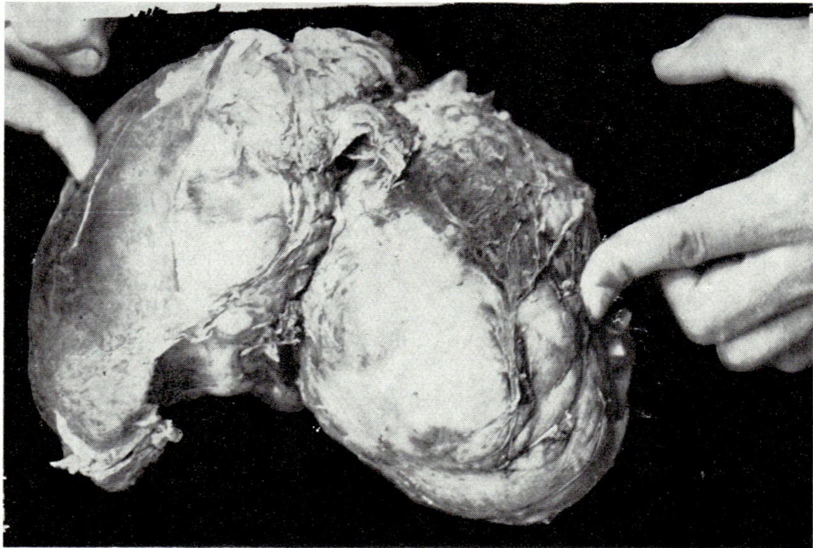

Fig. 225. — The same as in Fig. 224, viewed from another angle.

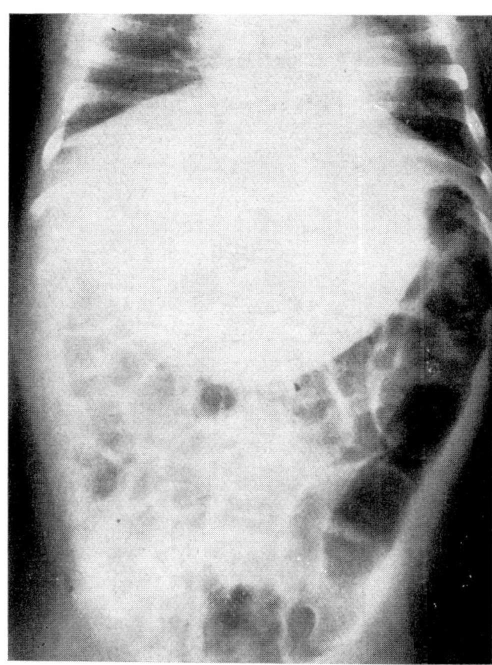

Fig. 226. — Preoperative X-ray of the child *B.I.* suffering from hemangiosarcoma of the left lobe of the liver.

Fig. 227. — Operative specimen after left hepatectomy (*B.I.*, hemangiosarcoma of the left hepatic lobe).

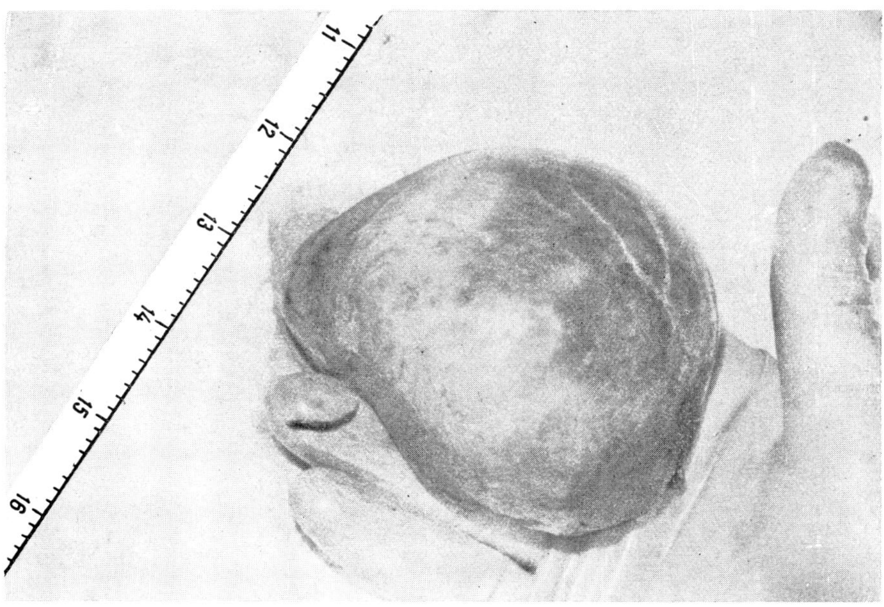

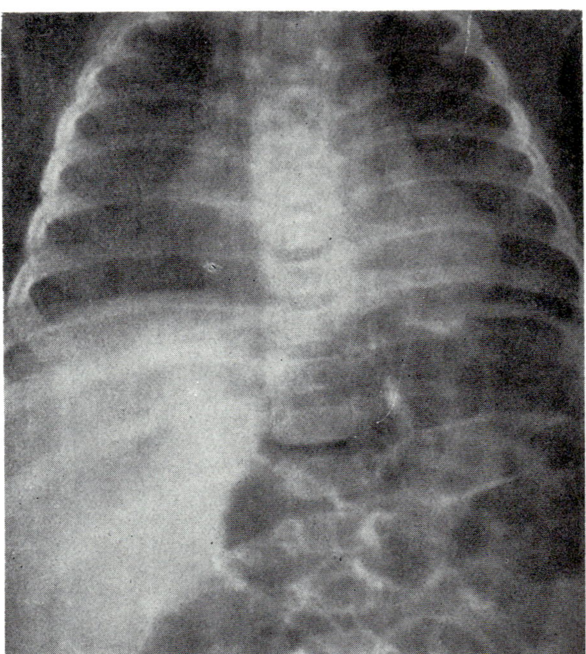

Fig. 228. — Postoperative X-ray of child *B.I.* Hepatic shadow much reduced in size, represents the remaining right hepatic region.

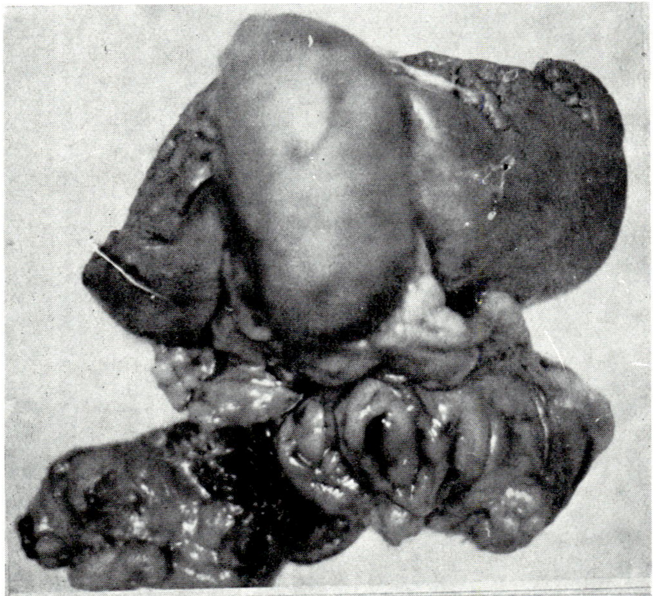

Fig. 229. — Operative specimen after wedge resection, cholecystectomy and transverse cholectomy, *en bloc* (patient *V.R.*).

These hepatectomies were performed for the following diseases:

Hydatid cyst	24 cases
Right controlled hepatectomy	3
Left controlled hepatectomy	3
Left non-anatomic hepatectomy	1
Left controlled lobectomy	3
Non-anatomic resection	13
Resection of segment IV	1
Alveolar echinococcosis	1 (simple non-anatomic resection)
Polycystic disease of the liver	1 (left planned hepatectomy)
Hemangioma	2 (resection of segment IV; simple non-anatomic resection)
Malignant hemangioma	1 (left planned hepatectomy)
Hepatic tumor (not identified)	1 (left planned hepatectomy)
Malignant tumor of the gallbladder	4 (cholecystohepatectomy)
Malignant tumor of the stomach extending to the liver	3 (gastrohepatectomy)
Cicatricial stenosis of the common bile duct	5 (drainage hepatectomy, hepatocholangiogastrotomy)
Primary or secondary malignant tumor of the extrahepatic bile ducts	5 (drainage hepatectomy, hepato cholangiogastrostomy).

In this series of patients there were 7 operative deaths (15% mortality rate). Two patients died in the operating theatre from hemorrhage of the hepatic veins in the course of planned hepatectomy (a right and a left one). One patient died from biliary peritonitis after right hepatectomy. Another three died postoperatively after gastrohepatectomy. Death of these patients was due to the major resection (total or subtotal gastrectomy) and to that of the liver. One of the 10 cases of drainage hepatectomy died from uremic coma. Analysis of these cases again shows that the major risk of extended excision of the liver is hemorrhage.

REFERENCES

1. ANDRADE M. A., SILVA R. M., Surgery, 1956, **40**, *5*, 913.
2. BĂLĂCESCU I., Rev. Chir., 1903, **10**, 433.
3. BIDULESCU ST., POPESCU I., MOCANU V., POPOVICI E., Chirurgia, 1962, **11**, 2.
4. BIER A., BRAUN H., KÜMMEL H., *Chirurgische Operationslehre*, vol. III, J. A. Barth, Leipzig, 1920, p. 543—550.
5. BOURGEON R. et al., Bull. Mém. Acad. Chir., 1953, **79**, *28*, 708.
6. BOURGEON R., PIETRI H., GUNTZ M., *Hépatectomies réglées pour kystes hydatiques*, in *16e Congr. Soc. Int. Chir.*, p. 1175—1178.
7. BRASFIELD D. R., Arch. Surg., 1962, **84**, *5*, 578.
8. BRUNSCHWIG A., *The surgery of hepatic neoplasms*, in *16e Congr. Soc. Int. Chir.*, p. 1122—1138.
9. BURGHELE TH., MOMICEANU D., IOACHIM H., Chirurgia, 1958, **7**, *3*, 415.
10. BURGHELE TH., PROCA E., Chirurgia, 1958, **7**, *6*, 909.
11. BURGHELE TH., PROCA E., MOMICEANU D., Mém. Acad. Chir., 1960, **86**, *1*, *2*, *3*, 65.
12. BURGHELE TH., PROCA E., Lyon chir., 1960, **56**, *2*, 258.
13. BURLUI D., RAȚIU O., NICULESCU I., Chirurgia, 1963, **12**, *1*, 29.
14. CHILD G. CH., *The hepatic circulation and portal hypertension*, W. B. Saunders, Philadelphia, 1954.

15. CHIPAIL GH., DIACONESCU M., WEXLER L., Chirurgia, 1953, **3**, *4*, 72.
16. * * * *Chirurgia*, vol. IV, Ed. medicală, Bucharest, 1958.
17. CIOBANU ST., Chirurgia, 1956, **5**, *2*, 163.
18. CIOBANU ST., Chirurgia, 1961, **10**, *2*, 301.
19. COUINAUD C., J. Chir., 1954, **70**, *12*, 933.
20. COUINAUD C., Presse méd., 1955, **62**, *21*, 417.
21. COUINAUD C., *Le foie. Études anatomiques et chirurgicales*, Masson, Paris, 1957.
22. COUINAUD C., Arch. Mal. App. digest., 1959, **48**, *11*, 1366.
23. DANICICO I., CIOBANU ST., PETRILĂ P., Chirurgia, 1959, **8**, *2*, 197.
24. DOGLIOTTI A. M., FOGLIATI E., Surgery, 1954, **36**, *1*, 69.
25. DROZDOV Z. S., KONTOROVICH I. A., Vestn. Khir., 1962, **85**, *6*, 83.
26. * * * *Encyclopédie Médico-Chirurgicale. Le foie*, ch. 7059.
27. FĂGĂRĂȘANU I., CHITLARU L., CÎRSTEA M., *A propos de l'hépatectomie pour drainage : l'hépatocholangiogastrostomie dans les obstructions néoplasiques ou cicatricielles de voies biliaires (technique personnelle)*, in *16e Congr. Soc. Int. Chir.*, Copenhagen, 1955, p. 1186.
28. FĂGĂRĂȘANU I., CHITLARU L., ROSENBERG A., POPESCU G., ALOMAN D., Chirurgia, 1956, **5**, *4*, 507.
29. FĂGĂRĂȘANU I., ALOMAN D., Chirurgia, 1957, **6**, *3*, 323.
30. FĂGĂRĂȘANU I., ALOMAN D., *Notre expérience concernant le cancer de la vésicule biliaire*, in *17e Congr. Soc. Int. Chir.*, Mexico, 1957.
31. FĂGĂRĂȘANU I., BURLUI D., Chirurgia, 1957, **6**, *4*, 483.
32. FĂGĂRĂȘANU I., ALOMAN D., Chirurgia, 1958, **7**, *1*, 15.
33. FĂGĂRĂȘANU I., POPESCU C., ALOMAN D., Probl. Terap., 1958, **9**, *1*, 9.
34. FĂGĂRĂȘANU I., ALOMAN D., Chirurgia, 1960, **9**, *4*, 495.
35. FOJANINI G., *Le epatectomie (parte fisiologica)*, in *Congr. Soc. Int. Chir.*, p. 1033—1043.
36. GALEEV M. A., Khirurghiya, 1961, *7*, 123.
37. GANS H., BAX H. R., *Partial resection of the liver in early carcinoma of the gall-bladder*, in *16e Congr. Soc. Int. Chir.*, p. 1147—1160.
38. GILORTEANU M., KÖVER GH., VELISARATU C., ZAHARIA M., Chirurgia, 1959, **8**, *3*, 419.
39. GOHRBANDT E., Arch. klin. Chir., 1953, **176**, 639.
40. GOHRBANDT E., Zblt. Chir., 1957, **82**, *16*, 641.
41. GOLDSMITH N. A., WOODBURNE R. T., Surg. Gynec. Obstet., 1957, **105**, *3*, 310.
42. GRIGORESCU I., MARINESCU L., IONESCU I., Chirurgia, 1957, **6**, *4*, 628.
43. HUARD P., MAYER-MAY J., *Les abcès du foie*, Masson, Paris, 1936.
44. ILIESCU G., POPA GH., *Hepatocolangiogastrostomia Făgărășanu*, Commun. Soc. Surgery, 17 Apr. 1963, Bucharest.
45. JELINEK R., Zblt. Chir., 1957, **82**, *16*, 645.
46. JIANU A., Rev. Chir., 1915, **3—4**, 163.
47. JUNÈS P., Rev. int. Hépatol., 1956, **6**, *1*, 129.
48. LI PAC-HUA, LI LI HSIEN, HSIEN TUNG., Chin. med. J., 1960, **80**, *3*.
49. LIPPMAN N. N., LONGMIRE W. P., Surg. Gynec. Obstet., 1954, **98**, *2*, 363.
50. LORTAT-JACOB J. L., ROBERT H.G., *Hépatectomies droites. Etudes cliniques*, in *16e Congr. Soc. Int. Chir.*, p. 1060.
51. MADDING F. G., PENISTON H. W., Surg., 1957, **104**, *5*, 417.
52. MALLET-GUY P. et al., Lyon Chir., 1953, **48**, *6*, 845.
53. MELNIKOV A. A., *O rezektsii pecheni*, in *16e Congr. Soc. Int. Chir.*, p. 1044.
54. MELNIKOV A. V., Anal. rom.-sov. (Chir.), 1956, **10**, *3 (11)*, 78.
55. MIRONOV P. S., Vestn. Khir., 1957, **79**, *6*, 129.
56. OTAKI A., READ A. E., STUBBS J., SCULTHORPE H., Brit. Med. J., 1960, *5194*, 256.
57. PACK G. T., ISLAMI A. H., Surgery, 1956, **40**, *3*, 611.
58. PANTALONI J., *Chirurgie du foie et des voies biliaires*. Inst. de Bibliogr., Paris, 1899.
59. PAOLUCCI R., *Le epatectomie*, in *16e Congr. Soc. Int. Chir.*, p. 1009.
60. PAPAHAGI E., CIOBANU ST., ȘTEFĂNESCU V., CONSTANTINOVICI AL., MUNTEANU S., Chirurgia, 1959, **8**, *2*, 281.
61. PATEL J., COUINAUD E., *Les bases anatomiques des hépatectomies réglées*, in *16e Congr. Soc. Int. Chir.*, p. 1015.
62. PETTINARI V., *La resezione epatica secondo la mia esperienza*, in *16e Congr. Soc. Int. Chir.*, p. 1169.

63. Popescu C., Suciu T., Chirurgia, 1953, **3**, *1*, 50.
64. Popescu C., Chirurgia, 1958, **7**, *2*, 263.
65. Popescu C., Chirurgia, 1958, **7**, *3*, 381.
66. Popescu C., Chirurgia, 1958, **7**, *5*, 733.
67. Raven R. W., *Hepatectomy*, in *16ᵉ Congr. Soc. Int. Chir.*, p. 1099.
68. Reifferscheid M., *Chirurgie der Leber*, G. Thieme, Stuttgart, 1957.
69. Robinson J. R., Butcher H. R., Surgery, 1966, **40**, *2*, 391.
70. Schalm L., Lyon Chir., 1962, **58**, *1*, 61.
71. Sénèque J., Roux M., Chatelin C. L., J. Internat. J. Chir., 1953, **13**, *1*, 59.
72. Stucke K., *Zur Anzeigestellung und Technik der Leberresektionen*, in *16ᵉ Congr. Soc. Int. Chir.*, p. 1160.
73. Stucke K., *Leberchirurgie*, Springer, Berlin, 1959.
74. Ton That Tung, *Chirurgie d'exérèse du foie*, Ed. Langues Etrangères, Hanoi, 1962.
75. Ţurai I., Gerota D., *Chirurgia căilor biliare extrahepatice*, Ed. Medicală, Bucharest, 1957.
76. Vasilescu V. et al., Fiziol. norm. patol., 1961, **7**, *1*, 27.

CHAPTER 11

TOTAL HEPATECTOMY. HEPATIC HOMOTRANSPLANTS

EXPERIMENTAL STUDIES

CLINICAL APPLICATIONS

PERSONAL INVESTIGATIONS

✦ Left liver or left lobe homotransplant in man (personal procedure)

The major controlled hepatectomies partly solve the problems raised by surgical pathology of the liver, but some diseases of the organ such as cirrhosis, primary cancer, congenital atresia of the bile ducts, generalized hemangiocavernoma, etc., can only be radically treated by total hepatectomy with immediate substitution of the diseased organ by a transplant taken from a donor (cadaver), after previous preparation.

In some cases hepatectomy might be useless, whereas grafting of a second healthy liver would, in principle, insure good clearance of the organism and supplement the deficient functions of the diseased liver, which under these conditions could remain *in situ*. In the former case the homograft would be *orthotopic*, in the latter *heterotopic*.

The experimental studies started in 1956 by Welch et al. raised extremely difficult problems not so much from the viewpoint of the technique as from that of the preservation and preparation of the graft. These investigations, taken up by different surgical centers (Starzl in Denver, Mikaeloff, Mallet-Guy in Lyon, Léger, Lortat-Jacob in Paris), led to encouraging conclusions, a survival of more than one year being obtained both in animals and humans.

The attempts in man came up against outstanding difficulties, the liver being a single organ, and a healthy live donor as in the case of the kidney being excluded. The immunologic barriers can be overcome with the kidneys by using a homotransplant from a twin, homozygote brother or sister, which gives very good results.

By analogy, as all the immunosuppressive methods used have not given satisfactory results, and until a safe method is found to avoid rejection of the graft, the only solution appears to be a transplant from a twin, i.e. the left lobe taken in the course of a controlled left lobectomy. This liver graft, experimented on the dog by Lortat-Jacob and Michoulier and on the human cadaver by us, in 1966, is feasible technically but actually hardly possible, since how many patients, suffering for instance from cirrhosis after chronic hepatitis have the luck of a twin who is willing to undergo a left lobectomy, involving greater hazard than a nephrectomy even in the hands of the most skilful surgeon?

The number of patients that would benefit by an orthotopic or heterotopic homograft is fairly high, and only an immunosuppressive medication or lymphocytic antiserum might make a homograft possible, without taking into account the question of consanguinity. Until an optimal solution is found, investigations have been centered upon the technical aspect of the procedure and especially upon certain problems of greater importance, such as:

1. The methods of collecting the homografts from the cadaver or perhaps even from the live subject in case of partial graft, which would meet both with technical difficulties and with moral objections.

2. The development of certain procedures for preserving the grafts which would permit transplantation of a liver that has not suffered, or only slightly, from arrest of the blood circulation, inevitable in the course of grafting.

Apart from rejection of the graft by the host organism, a problem that is common to all organ transplants, for the liver there exists an additional difficulty: that of the liver tissue which due to its extremely active metabolism resists anoxemia very poorly; the latter rapidly causes irreversible lesions both of the liver cells and of the intrahepatic circulation. Moreover, the suprahepatic veins in the dog have sphincters that react to anoxemia by spasms (Mason et al., 1959; Starzl et al., 1960; Kestens, 1964).

3. The development of a procedure that would avoid rejection of the graft, phenomenon that appears sooner or later, in the cases not treated by immunosuppressive means.

4. Finding of the most efficient means for improving the state of severe hepatic insufficiency of the receptor, which renders him incapable of standing such a difficult operation.

5. Finding of the most efficient means for preventing venous thrombosis, the cause of many failures due to embolism and infarction, or early fibrinolysis that may cause death by hemorrhage in the course of the operation.

EXPERIMENTAL STUDIES

History. The first experimental attempts followed by early success belong to C. S. Welch and E. O. Goodrich (1955—1956) who published the first technical results in the dog, after heterotypical transplantation of the liver.

Starting in 1959, F. D. Moore and T. E. Starzl published the first successful results obtained in animals, with orthotopic transplants the survival rate ranging between a few days to several months.

P. J. Kestens and W. V. Dermott (1961), Marchioro et al. (1963), P. J. Kestens (1964—1965) and M.D. Iacobescu et al. (1967) published important studies concerning perfusion of the isolated liver and its preservation in view of transplanting with or without selective hypothermia.

P. Hagihara and K. B. Absolon, Mehrez et al. (1964—1965) reported on their experimental and clinical investigations with heterotopic liver homografts.

During the same period, the extremely interesting works of Mikaeloff (Lyon), L. Léger et al., Lortat-Jacob et al. (Paris), Mallet-Guy and Michoulier (Lyon), Gilbertini et al. (Modena), etc., supplied new technical solutions, with a survival of several months in the cases treated with immunosuppressives.

The technique of liver homotransplants in animals. The animal most often experimented upon is the dog. Of late, some investigators have used the pig whose liver is more resistant to anoxia than that of the dog and more adequate for clearance perfusion.

Transplant of the liver from one animal to another is done as follows:

1. Total hepatectomy in the recipient and transplant of a whole liver from a donor of the same species (orthotopic homotransplant).

2. Grafting of a second whole liver from the donor animal, the liver of the recipient remaining *in situ*.

3. Heterotopic transplant of part of the donor liver (as a rule two lobes), the recipient liver remaining *in situ.*

Orthotopic transplants are extremely difficult because they must be preceded by total hepatectomy, an operation which usually demands a thoracophrenolaparotomy.

This hepatectomy involves excising the whole retrohepatic segment, the graft being likewise taken with a segment of the retrohepatic cava as the anastomoses are more readily carried out on these vascular segments than on the suprahepatic veins.

On the other hand, as clamping of the portal vein is very difficult to bear by the experimental animal, especially the dog, a temporary portacaval anastomosis must be performed prior to the operation in order to shunt the portal blood towards the inferior vena cava (or a portajugular shunt both in animals and man), and suppressed at the end of the operation.

Starzl et al. used in their experiments both portacaval anastomosis and extracorporeal femurojugular shunt.

Orthotopic homograft in the dog. Various procedures for grafting the liver to the recipient dog have been described (Moore, Starzl, L. Léger, etc.).

These procedures resemble one another along general lines.

A description will be given of Moore's technique. The operation should be performed by two teams, one for the donor, the other for the recipient.

General anesthesia (pentothal) with intubation is necessary in all the cases.

Operating table 1 : Donor dog :

Thoracophrenolaparotomy in the 7th right intercostal space. Isolation of the posterior vena cava above the liver, freeing it from its diaphragmatic orifice, then posteriorly and below the liver. Transection and ligation of the common bile duct; freeing of the hepatic artery and part of the aorta at its emergence from the diaphragm.

Dissection and severing of the portal vein as low down as possible. Through the hepatic end of this vein Ringer-Locke serum, cooled to 4°C/39.2°F is immediately perfused. The temperature of the liver is thus brought down to between 12°C/53.6°F and 18°C/64.4°F (Fig. 230).

Mikaeloff and McDermott as well as Léger used in their later experiments extracorporeal perfusion of the liver *in situ* with heparinized blood, oxygenated and cooled with the help of a pump similar to that used in cardiac surgery. The blood is taken either from the donor dog or from some larger dogs with the same blood group (Fig. 231).

According to the technique of Starzl et al., the donor is bled completely, introducing a polythene tube in one of the primary iliac arteries, ligating and severing the other terminal and collateral arteries. The vena cava is then sectioned below and above the liver, as close as possible to the pericardium. The aorta is then sectioned along 10—12 cm, in continuation with the hepatic artery, ligating the other tributaries of the celiac trunk, thus performing total hepatectomy.

Operating table 2. Recipient dog: thoracophrenolaparotomy in 7th right intercostal space. Isolation of the posterior vena cava above, at the back of and

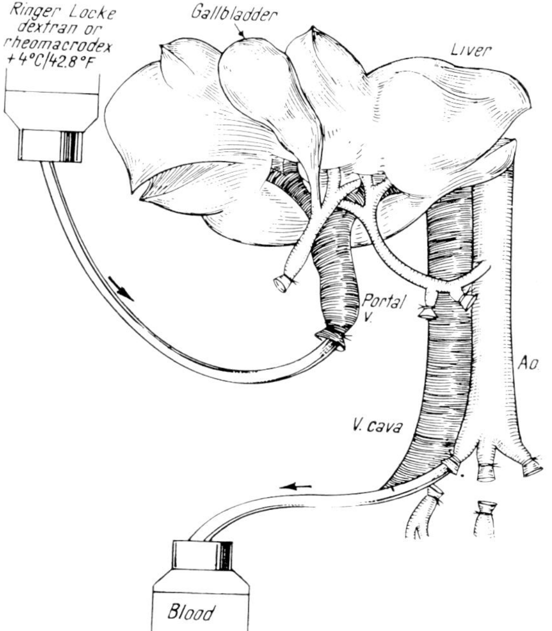

Fig. 230. — Perfusion *in situ* of the liver before removal (after T. E. Starzl, modified).

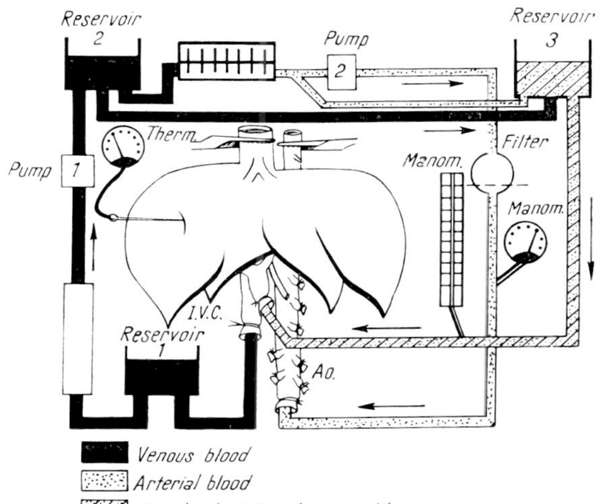

Fig. 231. — Perfusion of the liver with an oxygen pump (after Kestens and McDermott, T. E. Starzl, P. Mikaeloff).

below the liver. Dissection of the hepatic pedicle, with ligation and transection of the common bile duct.

The hepatic artery and trunk of the portal vein are freed. Temporary portacaval anastomosis (Starzl, Mehrez, Mikaeloff) is performed or, after section of the portal vein, a portajugular bridge (Léger) that will permit temporary shunt of the splanchnic blood. Before sectioning the posterior vena cava a second

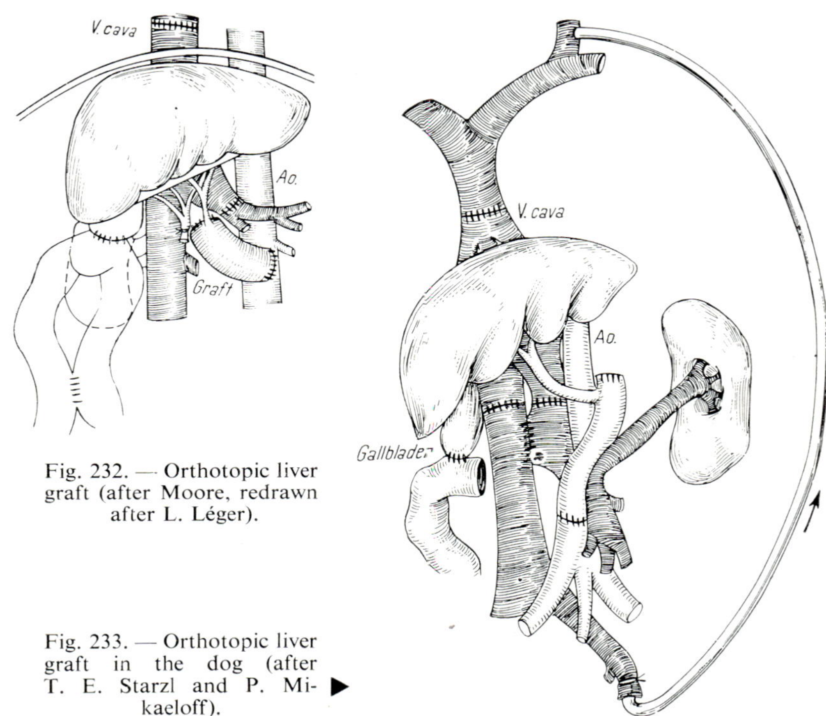

Fig. 232. — Orthotopic liver graft (after Moore, redrawn after L. Léger).

Fig. 233. — Orthotopic liver graft in the dog (after T. E. Starzl and P. Mikaeloff). ▶

extracorporeal cavacaval bridge, joining the femoral to the right jugular vein, is carried out. Finally, total hepatectomy is completed by sectioning the vena cava above and below the lower, and the portal vein above, the temporary portacaval shunt, which is suppressed closing the two openings separately.

Graft. Cavacaval anastomosis above and below the liver, then portaportal, with an anterior and a posterior silk suture (0000).

End-to-side anastomosis of the aorta segment of the graft to the aorta of the recipient, below the renal arteries (Figs 232 and 233).

The bile is drained by cholecystoduodenostomy or cholecystojejunostomy, with a Braun anastomosis at the foot of the loop. Suture of the diaphragm. Closure of the thoracoabdominal wall, with pleural drainage.

E.W. Fonkalsrud, G.H. Stevens, W.L. Joseph, D. Rangel, Y. Yakeishi and W.P. Longmire Jr. used a double internal vascular shunt in order to avoid prolonged venous clamping while arranging the homograft (Fig. 234) and heparinization of the recipient.

Heterotopic transplants. *Technique.* In these transplantations the difficulty arises at the moment in which the whole mass of the liver must be introduced into the abdomen of the recipient.

This may be avoided by using very small dogs (6—10 kg) as donors and very big dogs (20—30 kg) as recipients. Several surgeons (Lortat-Jacob et al., Michoulier et al.) avoided this drawback by grafting only two liver lobes.

For heterotopic graft of the whole liver several techniques have been proposed (Mehrez, Starzl, Léger).

Removal of the graft. Along general lines, the same procedure as for the orthotopic homograft is used. The donor liver is perfused *in situ* with a Ringer-Locke solution at +4°C/39.2°F or with a macromolecular solution. Léger prefers a Rhéomacrodex solution (with a molecular weight of 40,000). Similarly, dextran or another solution with large molecules, to which procaine or heparin are added.

Grafting procedure. Mehrez puts the supplementary liver with its convex aspect into the pelvis with the hilus facing the diaphragm. The portal vein of the graft is anastomosed end-to-end to the splenic vein of the recipient, after splenectomy. For the portal blood to perfuse the graft, it is necessary to ligate the portal vein of the recipient incompletely; the portal blood is thus obliged to change its direction, perfusing the graft.

In man, in the patient suffering from cirrhosis with portal hypertension, this condition is met with by the cirrhosis itself. The suprahepatic vena cava is anastomosed end-to-end to the left iliac vein. The aortic graft removed from the continuation with the hepatic artery is sutured end-to-end to the left primary iliac artery. The gallbladder can be anastomosed to an intestinal loop or drawn up to the wall after its intubation with a Pezzer tube (Léger) in order to be able to follow the secretion of the bile (Fig. 235).

Starzl et al. prefer to raise the hepatic graft with part of the retrohepatic vena cava which is sutured above and below the liver to the vena cava of the recipient. In this case the portal vein is anastomosed end-to-side to the mesenteric vein.

Starzl also used another method, that of anastomosing the portal vein to the distal extremity of the sectioned vena cava, and the suprahepatic vena cava to the proximal end of the vena cava. L. Léger removes the graft with a very short segment of the suprahepatic vena cava which he anastomoses end-to-side to the vena cava of the recipient, below the renal veins; the portal vein is anastomosed end-to-end to the distal extremity of the right primary iliac vein. The hepatic artery with its aortic continuation is anastomosed end-to-end to the left external iliac artery (Fig. 236). The operation is terminated by bringing the gallbladder in contact with the wall by means of a Pezzer tube. Aspiration drainage from the abdominal cavity.

Partial liver homotransplants. Apart from total liver grafts in ortho- or heterotopic position, certain very interesting experiments were centered upon the possibility of grafting only part of the liver, for instance two lobes in the

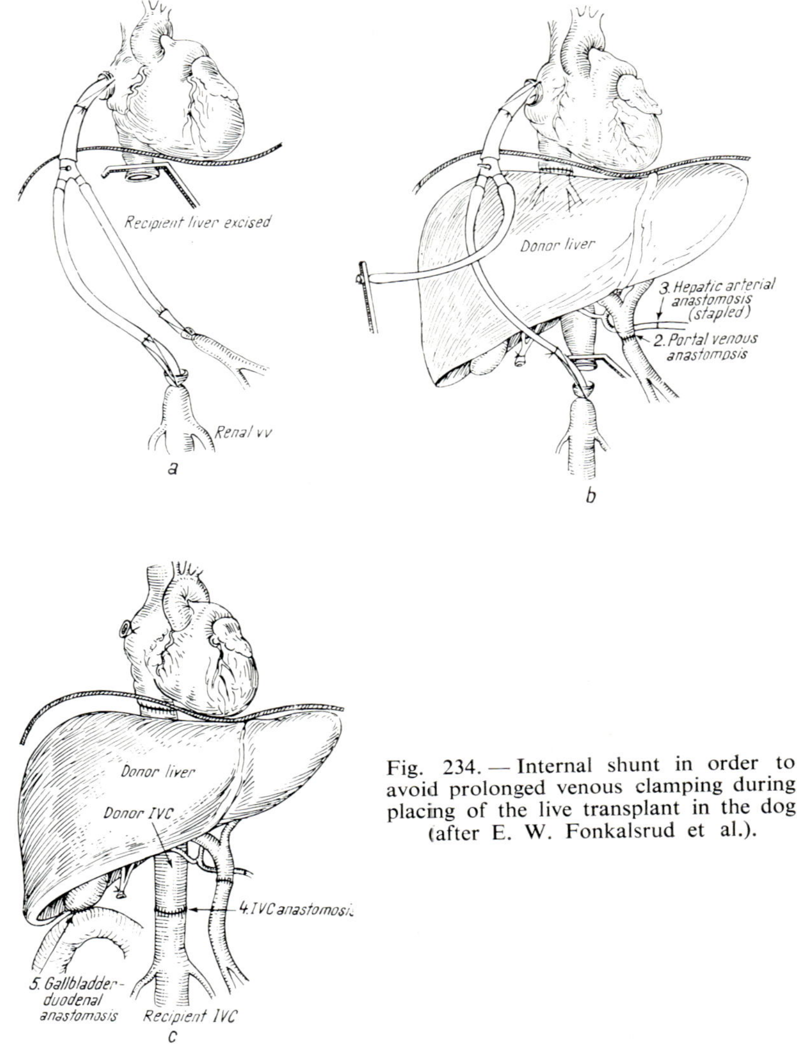

Fig. 234. — Internal shunt in order to avoid prolonged venous clamping during placing of the live transplant in the dog (after E. W. Fonkalsrud et al.).

dog (J.L. Lortat-Jacob, P. Mallet-Guy, J. Michoulier) or the left lobe in man (I. Făgărăşanu).

Removal of the whole liver is a difficult problem and will probably remain so in the future. The removal of the liver from a cadaver even when performed under optimal conditions, is restricted by certain legal, ethical and moral codes. The maximum preservation time, by extracorporeal circulation, does not exceed a few hours.

The ideal solution would be fresh grafts from a healthy, live man, the quality of the graft being better and more readily obtainable from a donor related to the patient.

As left hepatectomy is today a current operation with a very low mortality rate and as one fourth of the normal liver is sufficient to insure its function, grafting of the left lobe would be sufficient to save the patient's life, for instance in severe, reversible liver insufficiency, cirrhosis with hypertension or digestive hemorrhage due to esophageal varices.

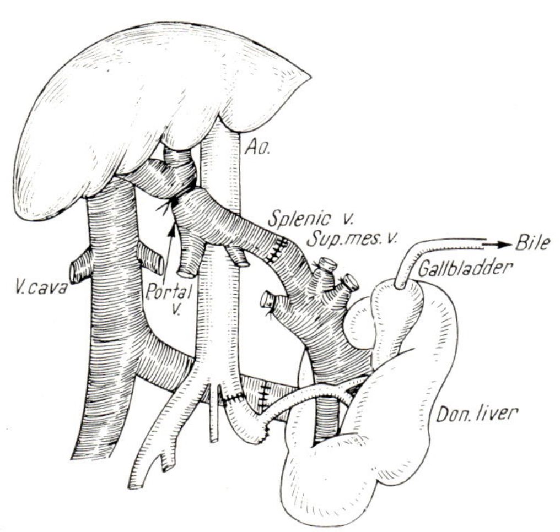

Fig. 235. — Total heterotopic liver graft in the dog (after Mehrez).

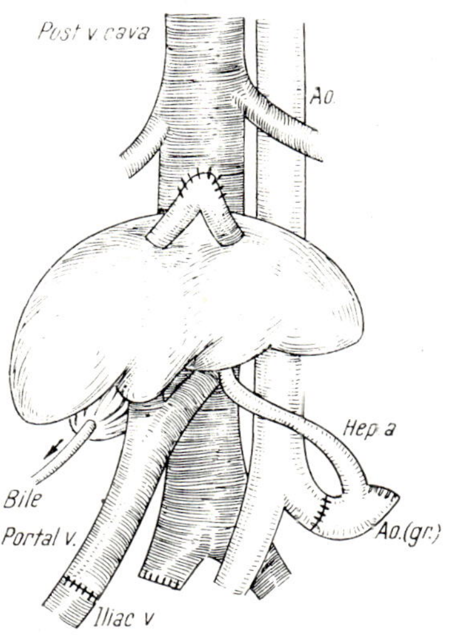

Fig. 236. — Total heterotopic liver homotransplant in the dog (as performed by L. Léger et al.).

The experimental investigations of Lortat-Jacob et al. revealed the difficulties of these partial transplants in the dog, and first of all the impossibility of reimplanting the hepatic artery; for this, arterialization of the portal blood or even portal vein would be necessary. The authors tried five different variants without finding a satisfactory solution. Notwithstanding, by anastomosis of the iliac vein to the portal branch of the transplanted liver segment, after previous femurofemural shunt, the suprahepatic vein being anastomosed to the inferior vena cava, a satisfactory bile flow was obtained.

In all the 5 variants, the common bile duct was not anastomosed to a segment of the gastrointestinal tract but catheterized, the bile being collected exteriorly. One of these variants is not applicable in humans in the authors' opinion.

Mallet-Guy, J. Michoulier et al. (Lyon) developed a partial grafting technique (1966), anastomosing the portal vein of the transplant formed of two lobes to the distal end of the splenic vein, sectioned close to the confluence with the portal vein. The spleen is left *in situ*, the hepatic artery supplying this organ sufficiently, and therefore obtaining a good portal venous return, supplying the graft with portal blood. The inferior vena cava is anastomosed end-to-side to the vena cava of the recipient. The hepatic artery, which is raised together with a ring of aorta is anastomosed by the aorta segment to the anterior aspect of the recipient's aorta; the common bile duct is anastomosed to an intestinal loop (Fig. 237).

This differs from Mehrez' procedure, in which the portal vein of a total liver graft is anastomosed to the proximal end of the splenic vein after splenec-

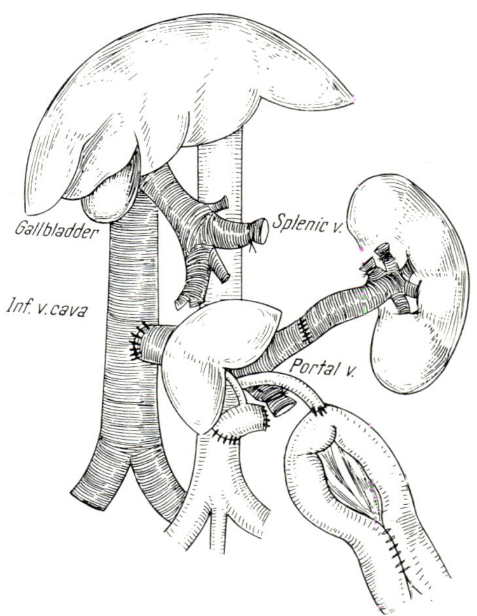

Fig. 237.—Heterotopic liver homotransplant (only 2 lobes) (after Michoulier et al.).

tomy, thus offering the graft ideal hemodynamic conditions since at normal pressures it receives the total amount of blood that normally reaches the portal vein through the splenic vein, as checked by angiography.

This procedure does not endanger the patient's life if the graft is rejected because the hemodynamic conditions of the liver left *in situ* are not jeopardized.

Welch and L. Léger showed that in this, as in other procedures, the intestinal blood does not pass through the graft; it appears that blood of intestinal origin is absolutely necessary for survival of the graft as it probably contains an as yet unknown factor upon which the success of the graft depends.

The investigations of Mikaeloff, Michoulier and Bernard have shown that the portal vein of the liver transplant should be in all cases anastomosed to a venous trunk with portal circulation (splenic vein, large mesenteric vein) and not to an arterial trunk or a branch of the inferior vena cava.

However, phenomena of rejection of the graft appeared sooner or later in the course of their experiments (between the 6th and 24th day). Three dogs survived and were sacrificed in perfect health on day 32, 90 and 150 after the operation. In all three cases complete resorption of the graft had taken place, a sclerous, retractile nodule with several nonabsorbable sutures alone remaining.

The angiographies performed showed perfect circulation through the liver left *in situ* and the systemic veins.

P.M. Daloze et al., working with T.E. Starzl (Denver), and using an auxiliary liver homograft according to an inversed Welch procedure (Fig. 238) demon-

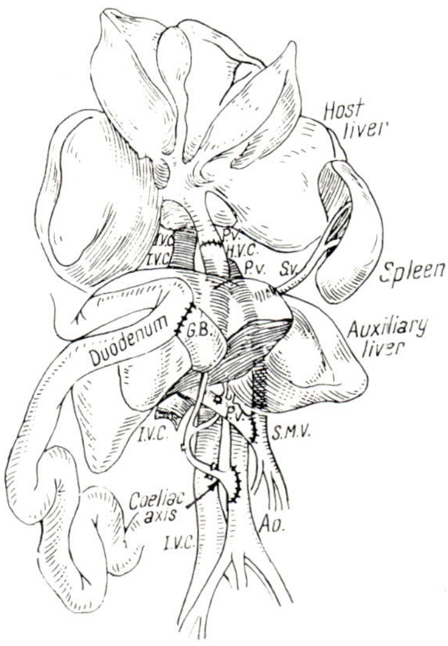

Fig. 238. — Procedure for suppressing the passage of portal blood through the host liver to the benefit of the grafted liver (Daloze, Huguet, Porter, Starzl).

strated that rapid atrophy of the liver cannot be prevented by implantation of the transplant upon the host portal vein, which shows that a competition exists between the grafted and the host liver.

Orthotopic liver transplant in the pig. Lately, in experimental liver transplants other animals besides the dog have been used, especially the pig and the rat. The pig whose liver has been successfully used in extracorporeal clearance transfusions has proved to be an adequate experimental animal, probably due to the close anatomic and physiologic resemblance with man.

Certain difficulties arose because of the large size of this animal and a dwarf breed was produced weighing approximately the same as man (50—100 kg). Thanks to this, R.Y. Calne et al. (Cambridge) were able to develop a technique of orthotopic liver transplant in the pig that gave excellent results: in a series of 24 transplantations 22 animals survived, some still being alive 4 months later (British Journal of Surgery, 1968, **55,** 203—206).

Calne et al. used the following technique:

A. *Donor animal.* General anesthesia with halothane, with tracheal intubation. The donor animal is immersed in ice water in order to obtain a temperature of 33° to 34°C (91.4°—93.2°F). Median laparotomy. The portal vein is dissected and isolated, then the hepatic artery; after ligation of the left gastric and splenic artery, the celiac trunk together with its origin in the aorta is freed. The common bile duct is ligated and severed immediately above the duodenum. The inferior vena cava is isolated above the liver where it crosses the diaphragm.

Perfusion of the liver *in situ* with a Ringer-Hartmann solution at +4°C/39.2°F after intubation of the aorta for bleeding the animal and of the portal trunk for washing the liver. During this interval, total hepatectomy is rapidly terminated, sectioning the portal vein, vena cava above and below the liver and the aorta wall around the origin of the celiac trunk.

B. *Recipient animal.* It is anesthetized and prepared concomitantly, exposing the two jugular veins which will serve for the systemic caval and portal shunts. A perfusion catheter is introduced in the left subclavicular vein.

Broad xyphopubic laparotomy and incision of the peritoneum retrohepatically, to the right of the inferior vena cava, which is freed from the diaphragm up to its discharge into the right supraarcuate vein. The aorta is dissected and freed up to the origin of the celiac trunk. The hepatic artery proper is then ligated, taking care not to injure the gastroduodenal artery. Juxta duodenal ligation of the common bile duct; bilateral vagotomy and gastroduodenostomy, in view of the predilection of pigs for postoperative gastroduodenal ulcer.

Heparin treatment of the recipient is followed by cava and portajugular shunts. Hepatectomy is then rapidly carried out.

The washed liver from the donor is then transplanted by anastomosing first of all the suprahepatic cava, then performing a portaportal anastomosis, suppressing in the last instance the portajugular shunt, after which the circulation is released in the liver by removing the clamp from the portal vein and the suprahepatic vena cava. The celiac trunk is then anastomosed to the aorta, the subhepatic cava is anastomosed and then the cavajugular shunt is suppressed.

The operation is terminated by establishing the continuity of the bile ducts by a cholecystoduodenostomy, or still better by an end-to-end choledochocholedochostomy.

For the control of shock and acidosis, the transplant is perfused with 1 liter 5% dextrose, 1 liter of homologous blood and 150 ml 5% sodium bicarbonate.

CLINICAL APPLICATIONS

Until April 1969, 55 attempts were made at orthotopic homotransplants and 21 heterotransplants in man.

The results may be considered encouraging since Starzl in his last series reported 5 survivals of over a year and 7 of over 6 months at the date of his report.

Bearing in mind that not only cancer patients might benefit by liver grafts but also newborn children with congenital atresia of the bile ducts, patients with cancer of the bile ducts, cirrhosis of the liver, diffuse hemangioma, alveolar echonococcosis, etc., this would imply after a brief calculation of the mortality rate from these diseases at least 4000 liver grafts in the U.S.A., one thousand in Great Britain, 800—900 in France and several thousands in the rest of the world. These figures are eloquent and fully explain the interest shown in finding a means of avoiding rejection of the liver transplant, especially if account is kept of the fact that most of the failures are due to fibrinolysis or rejection of the graft, an immunologic phenomenon that it has not yet been possible to avoid completely, or to the consequences of the immunosuppressive treatment which lowers the defense potential of the organism against infection. Hence, it is normal that clinical and experimental investigations should be centered upon finding safe immunosuppressive means that will not harm the recipient.

PERSONAL INVESTIGATIONS

Starting from the idea that the future of liver grafts in man does not stand in total transplants but in partial ones from living donors, we carried out experiments on cadavers on the various possibilities of grafting to man a liver transplant obtained by left anatomic hemihepatectomy or by left anatomic lobectomy, with intact left suprahepatic vein, left branch of the portal vein, left hepatic artery and left hepatic bile duct. The experience gained in over 40 anatomic and non-anatomic hepatectomies performed until now shows that left hepatectomy and especially left lobectomy can be carried out without undue risk.

After various attempts we found that the best means of grafting a hepatic homotransplant to man is that illustrated in Figs 239 and 240.

LEFT LIVER OR LEFT LOBE HOMOTRANSPLANT IN MAN (PERSONAL PROCEDURE)

1. After splenectomy, leaving intact the splenic artery and vein, the left renal vein is exposed up to discharge of the central capsular vein into the renal vein.

2. A second surgical team concomitantly performs a left anatomic hepatectomy or lobectomy (Figs 241, 242 and 243).

3. The graft is perfused *in situ* after transection of the left portal vein in which a polythene catheter is introduced, attached to a perfuser containing dextran, Rhéomacrodex or Ringer-Locke solution cooled to +4°C/39.2°F. In this sterile solution procaine and heparin can be added (Fig. 230). Perfusion can also be carried out extracorporeally.

4. The graft is mounted as follows: the left suprahepatic vein is anastomosed to the left renal vein close to the discharge of the left central capsular vein by an anterior and a posterior side-to-end suture (Fig. 244).

The portal vein of the graft is anastomosed end-to-end to the splenic vein, and the hepatic artery to the splenic artery (Fig. 245).

The left hepatic duct is anastomosed to a Roux-Y loop or a jejunal loop by the Braun procedure (Fig. 246).

Fig. 239. — Heterotopic homograft of left human liver (anatomic experiment). The left liver collected from a donor or from a cadaver is grafted after splenectomy. Anastomosis of Glisson's pedicle to the splenic vessels, of the suprahepatic vein to the left renal vein (end-to-side), of the left hepatic duct to a jejunal loop (Făgărăşanu).

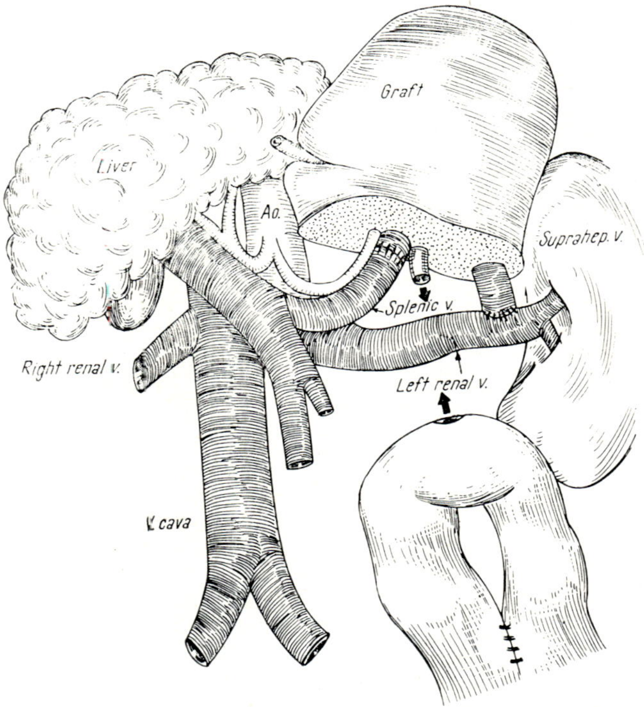

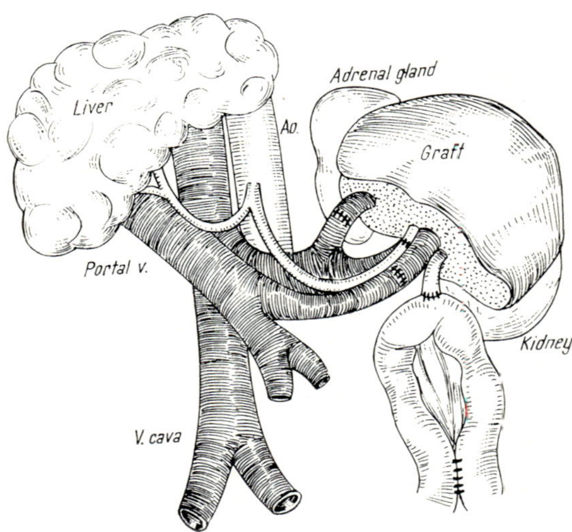

Fig. 240. — Left liver lobe homograft in man, mounted heterotopically on the splenic vessels and accessory renal vein. In this case the left renal vein is duplicated. The left hepatic duct is anastomosed to an intestinal loop (Făgărăşanu).

In this way a good venous return is obtained through the left suprahepatic vein and left renal vein, and good arterial vascularization through the splenic artery. The portal circulation is ensured by counter flow from the splenic vein, the portal blood trying to find an outlet, especially as most cases are operated for cirrhosis of the liver and portal hypertension. This return takes place through the left portarenal anastomosis which at the same time perfuses the grafted liver.

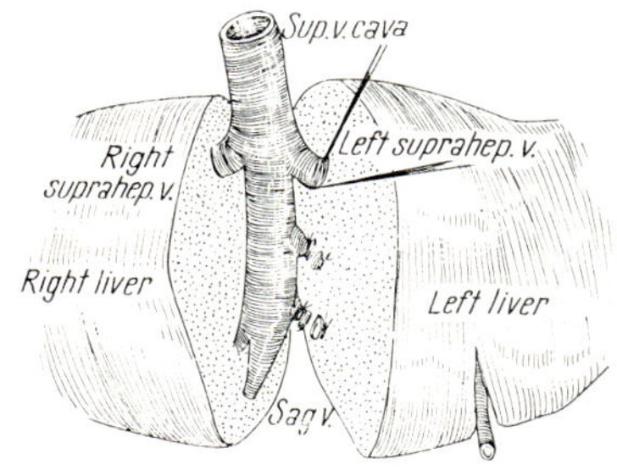

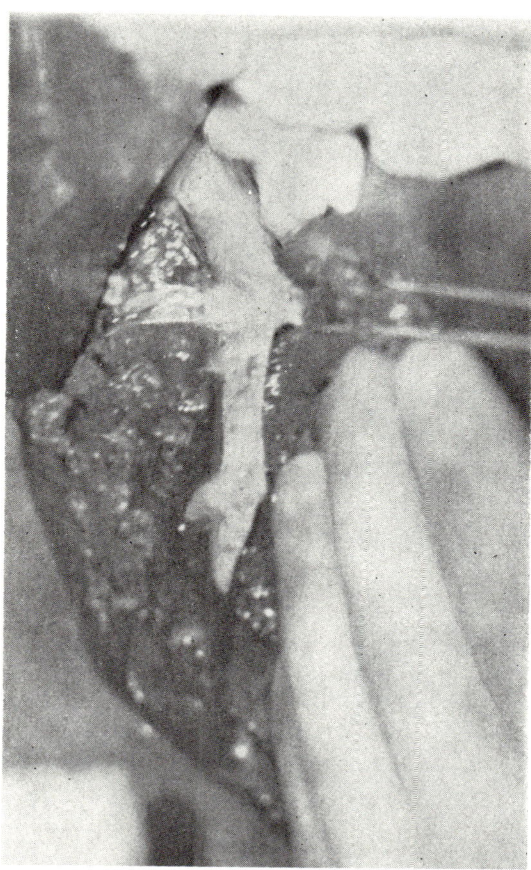

Fig. 241. — Left hepatectomy. Opening of the sagittal fissure in order to obtain a left liver transplant in man. Note the right and left suprahepatic veins, sagittal vein and inferior vena cava. A stay suture reveals the site where the left suprahepatic vein will be severed (anatomic experiment).

In hypertension, the portal blood does not contain splenic blood, but that of the portal system which looks for a vicarious pathway towards the systemic veins. As shown by L. Léger, one of the conditions of success of liver homografts is their obligatory perfusion with portal blood and not with the blood of the systemic veins, as done by other surgeons. The portal blood and especially the blood coming from the intestines contains an as yet unknown factor that appears to be indispensable to the success of liver transplants.

The grafting proposed by us presents no hazard for the recipient. The postoperative care consists in daily perfusions with 1 to 1½ liters glucose serum, antibiotics of the teramycin type, penicillin and streptomycin in sufficient doses and an immunosuppressive treatment starting on the day of the operation and consisting in parenteral injections with Imuran (5 mg/kg in the first days), Azaserin

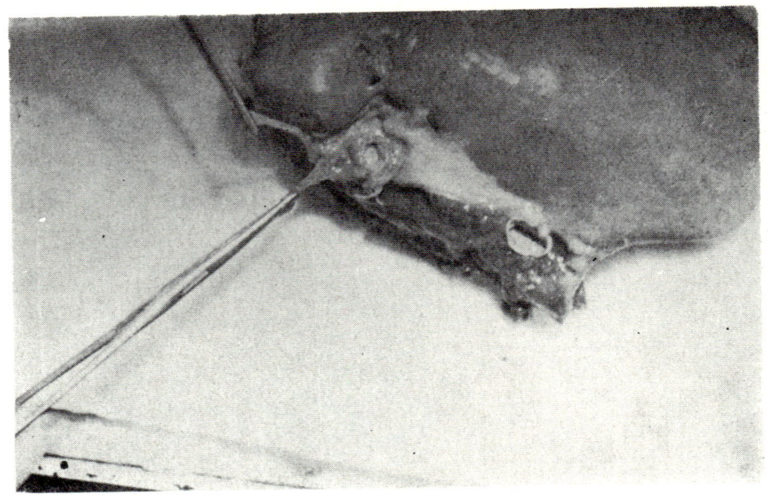

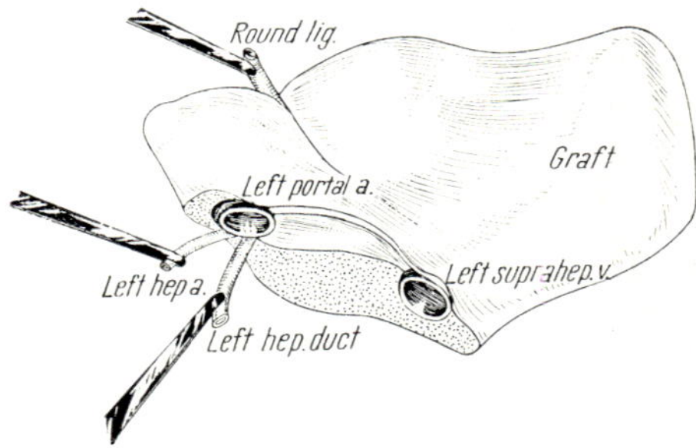

Fig. 242. — Left human liver homotransplant. The two clamps are placed on the left hepatic artery and left hepatic duct. Between them is the left portal vein. To the right, the suprahepatic vein (anatomic experiment).

(1 mg/kg during the following 2—3 weeks) and local irradiation of the graft at peak moments of rejection; these will ensure viability of the graft.

In case of rejection and resorption of the graft, the anastomoses created and the collateral circulation that develops between the portal and the inferior cava systems will improve the patients condition by lowering the portal pressure.

The key problem that still remains to be solved is that of finding willing donors and of perfecting postoperative care, especially immunosuppressive therapy and the control of infection.

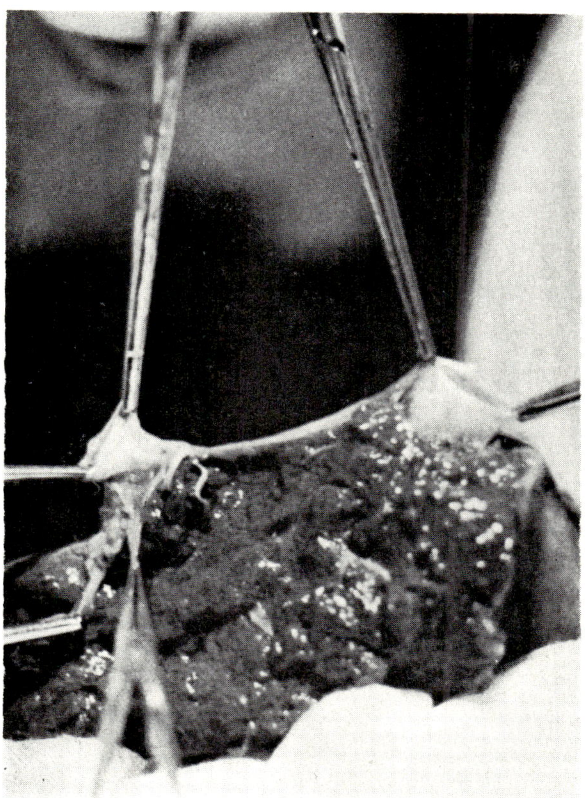

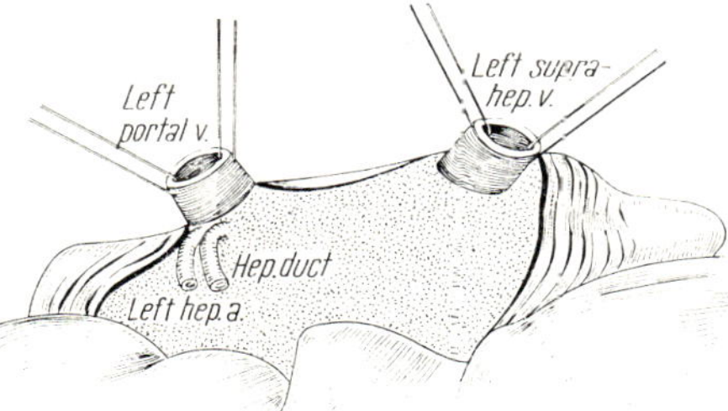

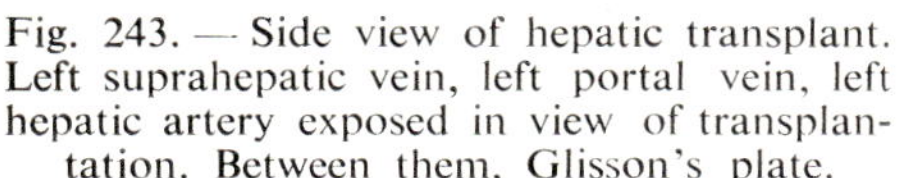

Fig. 243. — Side view of hepatic transplant. Left suprahepatic vein, left portal vein, left hepatic artery exposed in view of transplantation. Between them, Glisson's plate.

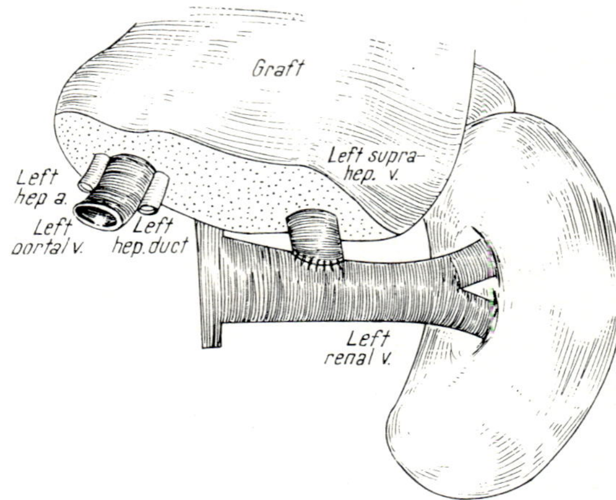

Fig. 244. — The left suprahepatic vein is anastomosed side-to-end to the left renal vein (Făgărăşanu, anatomic experiment).

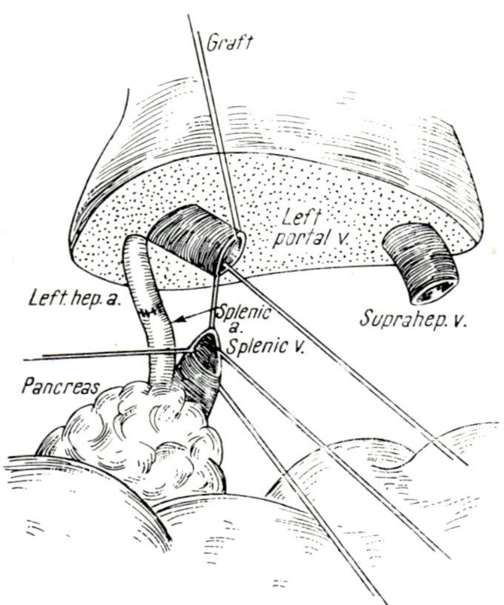

Fig. 245. — End-to-end anastomosis of the splenic artery to the left hepatic artery. Now, end-to-end anastomosis of the splenic vein to the left portal vein follows.

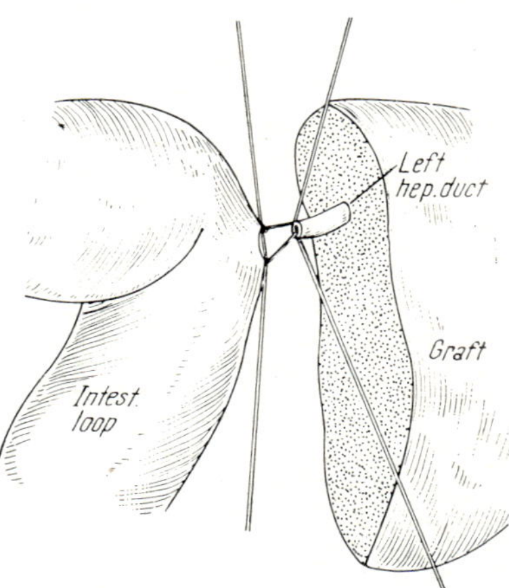

Fig. 246. — Left hepatic duct is anastomosed to a jejunal loop, Braun anastomosis to the foot of the loop (Făgărăşanu).

REFERENCES

1. Absolon K. B., Hagihara P. H., Griffon W. D., Lillehei R. C., Rev. int. Hépatol., 1965, **15**, *8*, 1481.
2. Dermileau et al., Mém. Acad. Chir., 5 Febr. 1964.
3. Făgărășanu I., *Procedure for heterotopic homograft of left lobe or left liver in human (Experimental studies)*, in *Internat. Meeting on liver regeneration, Montecatini Terme, 29—30 Oct. 1966*.
4. Gibertini G., Lodi R., Zambarda E., Montanari C., Ferrari P., Bondioli A., Rev. int. Hépatol., 1965, **15**, *8*, 1516.
5. Goodrich E. O., Welch H. F., Nelson J. A., Beecher T. A., Welche C. S., Surgery, 1956, **39**, 244.
6. Hagihara P., Absolon K. B., Surg. Gynec. Obstet., 1965, **119**, 1297.
7. Iacobescu M.D., Rădulescu I.M., Nazarian P.A., Alexandru S.S., Rev. int. Hépatol., 1967, **17**, *2*, 99.
8. Kestens P. J., Mc Dermott W. V., Surgery, 1961, **50**, 196.
9. Kestens P. J., *La perfusion du foie isolé. Son application à l'étude de quelques problèmes de biologie*, Arscia, Bruxelles, 1964.
10. Kestens P. J., Acta chir. belg., 1965, **64**, 326.
11. Kestens P. J., Haxhe J. J., Alexandre G. P. J., Hassoun A., Lambotte L., Rev. int. Hépatol., 1965, **15**, *8*, 1382.
12. Léger L., Marcenac N., Tubiana M., Patel J. Cl., Neveux J. Y., Chapuis J., Lenriot J. P., Leroy G., Frenoy P., Mém. Acad. Chir., 1965, **91**, *4—5*, 148.
13. Léger L., Marcean N., Mathé G., Patel J. Cl., Neveux J. Y., Chapuis J., Lenriot J. P., Tubiana M., Leroy G., Lemaigre G., Frenoy P., Mém. Acad. Chir., 1965, **91**, 289.
14. Léger L., Chapuis J., Neveux J. V., Lenriot J. P., Patel J. Cl., Langrand L., Woell G., Frenoy P., Mém. Acad. Chir. Paris, 1966, **92**, *10—19*, 497.
15. Lortat-Jacob J. L., Maillard J. N., Giuli R., Benhamon J. P., Leandri J., Rev. int. Hépatol., 1965, **15**, *8*, 1491.
16. Mallet-Guy P., Michoulier J., Bernard L., Imbert J. C., Lyon chir., 1966, **62**, *4*, 481.
17. Marcenac N., Léger L., Patel J. Cl., Neveux J. Y., Chapuis Y., Lenriot J. P., Tubiana M., Leroy G., Lemaigre G., Frenoy P., Presse méd., 1964, **72**, 811.
18. Marchioro T. L., Hintley R. T., Waddell W. R., Starzl T. L., Surgery, 1963, **54**, 900.
19. Mehrez I. P., Nabsteh B. C., Kekis B. P., Apostolu K., Gottlieb L. S., Deterling R. A., Ann. Surg., 1964, **159**, 414.
20. Mikaeloff Ph., Dureau G., Rassat J. P., Chabert M., Dumont L., Belleville J., Tronchon J., Malluret J., Descotes J. (rapp. Werthelmer), Mém. Acad. Chir., 1965, **91**, *8—9*, 286.
21. Mikaeloff Ph., Kestens P. J., Dureau G., Rassat J. P., Haxhe J. E., Alexandre C. P. J., Dubernard M., Cuilleret J., Hassoun A., Maldague P., Morian M., Rev. int. Hépatol., 1965, **15**, *8*, 1401.
22. Michoulier J., Bernard L., Imbert J. C., Foroy J., Leroy J., Mém. Acad. Chir., 1966, **92**, *20—21*, 548.
23. Moore F. D., Smith L. L., Burnap T. K., Dallenbach F. D., Dammin G. J., Gruber V. P., Schiemayer W. C., Steenburg R. W., Ball M. R., Belko J. S., Transplant. Bull., 1959, **6**, 103.

24. Moore F. D., W. Leeler H. B., Demissanos H. V., Smith L. L., Balankura O., Abel K., Greenberg J. B., Dammin G. J., 1960, **152**, 374.

25. Moore F. D., Birth A. G., Dagher F., Veith F., Krisher J. A., Order S. E., Shucart W. A., Dammin G. J., Couch N. P., Ann. N. Y. Acad. Sci., 1964, **120**, 729.

26. Moore F. D., Smith L. L., Burnap T. K., Dallenbach F. D., Dammin G. J., Gruber U. F., Shoemaker W. L., Steenburg R. W., Bali M. R., Belko J. S., Transplant. Bull., 1958, **6**, *1*, 103.

27. Starzl T. E., Kaupp H. A., Brock O. R., Lazarus R. E., Johnson R. U., Surg. Gynec. Obstet., 1960, **111**, 733.

28. Starzl T. E., Marchioro T. L., von Kaulia K. V., Hermann G., Brittain R. S., Waddel W. R., Surg. Gynec. Obstet., 1963, **117**, *6*, 659.

29. Starzl T. E., Marchioro T. L., Lowlands D. T., Kirkpatrik C. H., Welson W. E. C., Rifkind D., Waddel W. R., Ann. Surg., 1964, **160**, *3*, 411.

30. Starzl T. E., Marchioro T. L., Porter K. A., Rev. int. Hépatol., 1965, **15**, *8*, 1447.

31. Welch C. S., Transplant. Bull., 1955, **3**, *2*, 54.

PRINTED IN ROMANIA